SHEEP & GOAT
Medicine

SHEEP & GOAT
Medicine

Edited by

D.G. Pugh, DVM, MS
Diplomate, American College of Theriogenologists
Diplomate, American College of Veterinary Nutrition
Professor
Food Animal Section
College of Veterinary Medicine
Auburn University, Alabama

With 150 *illustrations*

SAUNDERS
An Imprint of Elsevier

SAUNDERS
An Imprint of Elsevier

The Curtis Center
Independence Square West
Philadelphia, Pennsylvania 19106

NOTICE

Pharmacology is an ever-changing field. Standard safety precautions must be followed, but as new research and clinical experience broaden our knowledge, changes in treatment and drug therapy may become necessary or appropriate. Readers are advised to check the most current product information provided by the manufacturer of each drug to be administered to verify the recommended dose, the method and duration of administration, and contraindications. It is the responsibility of the licensed prescriber, relying on experience and knowledge of the patient, to determine dosages and the best treatment for each individual patient. Neither the publisher nor the editor assumes any liability for any injury and/or damage to persons or property arising from this publication.

Library of Congress Cataloging in Publication Data

Sheep and goat medicine / [edited by] D.G. Pugh.—1st ed.

p. ; cm.

Includes bibliographical references and index.

ISBN-13: 978-0-7216-9052-0   ISBN-10: 0-7216-9052-1

1. Sheep—diseases. 2. Goats—diseases.   I. Pugh, D.G. (David G.)
[DNLM: 1. Sheep diseases—therapy. 2. Goat diseases—therapy. 3. Veterinary medicine. SF 968 S5405 2002]

 SF968 .S54 2002

 636.3′089—dc21   2001034176

Editor-In Chief: John A. Schrefer
Editorial Manager: Linda L. Duncan
Senior Developmental Editor: Teri Merchant
Project Manager: Linda McKinley
Senior Production Editor: Jennifer Furey
Designer: Julia Ramirez

SHEEP AND GOAT MEDICINE

FIRST EDITION

Permissions may be sought directly from Elsevier's Health Sciences Rights Department in Philadelphia, PA, USA: phone: (+1) 215 239 3804, fax: (+1) 215 239 3805, e-mail: healthpermissions@elsevier.com. You may also complete your request on-line via the Elsevier homepage (http://www.elsevier.com), by selecting 'Customer Support' and then 'Obtaining Permissions'.

ISBN-13: 978-0-7216-9052-0
ISBN-10: 0-7216-9052-1

Printed in the United States of America

Last digit is the print number: 9 8 7 6

Contributors

David E. Anderson, DVM, MS
Diplomate ACVS
Associate Professor, Food Animal Medicine and Surgery
Department of Veterinary Clinical Sciences
College of Veterinary Medicine
The Ohio State University
Columbus, Ohio

A.N. Baird, DVM, MS
Diplomate ACVS
Associate Professor, Veterinary Clinical Sciences
Purdue University
West Lafayette, Indiana

Ellen B. Belknap, DVM, MS
Diplomate ACVIM
Associate Clinical Professor, Department of Clinical
    Sciences
College of Veterinary Medicine
Auburn University, Alabama

Christopher Cebra, VMD, MA, MS
Diplomate ACVIM
Department of Large Animal Clinical Sciences
College of Veterinary Medicine
Oregon State University
Corvallis, Oregon

Margaret Cebra, VMD, MS
Diplomate ACVIM
Philomoth, Oregon

Undine Christmann, DMV
Large Animal Internal Medicine
Department of Clinical Sciences
College of Veterinary Medicine
Auburn University, Alabama

Carmen M.H. Colitz, DVM, PhD
Diplomate ACVO
Assistant Professor of Ophthalmology
School of Veterinary Medicine
Louisiana State University
Baton Rouge, Louisiana

Barbara C. Diffay, DVM
Special Assistant to the Dean
College of Veterinary Medicine, Nursing, and Allied
    Health
Tuskegee University
Tuskegee, Alabama

Virginia R. Fajt, DVM, PhD
Collaborator, Veterinary Antimicrobial Decision Support
    System
Animal Medicine
College of Veterinary Medicine
Iowa State University
Ames, Iowa

Alan M. Heath, DVM, MS
Diplomate ACT
Assistant Professor, Department of Clinical Sciences
College of Veterinary Medicine
Auburn University, Alabama

Bruce L. Hull, DVM, MS
Diplomate ACVS
Professor and Head, Food Animal Medicine and Surgery
College of Veterinary Medicine
The Ohio State University
Columbus, Ohio

Hui-Chu Lin, DVM, MS
Diplomate ACVA
Associate Professor, Department of Clinical Sciences
College of Veterinary Medicine
Auburn University, Alabama

Michael Q. Lowder, DVM, MS
Diplomate ABVP
Associate Professor, Department of Large Animal
    Medicine
College of Veterinary Medicine
University of Georgia
Athens, Georgia

Margo R. Machen, DVM, PhD
Associate Professor, Department of Clinical Sciences
College of Veterinary Medicine, Nursing, and Allied
    Health
Tuskegee University
Tuskegee, Alabama

David McKenzie, DVM, MS
Assistant Professor, Department of Clinical Sciences
School of Veterinary Medicine
Tuskegee University
Tuskegee, Alabama

Seyedmehdi Mobini, DVM, MS
Diplomate ACT
Professor of Veterinary Science
Research and Extension Veterinarian
Georgia Small Ruminant Research and Extension Center
Agricultural Research Station
College of Agriculture, Home Economics, and Allied
    Programs
Fort Valley State University
Fort Valley, Georgia

Christine B. Navarre, DVM, MS
Diplomate ACVIM
Associate Professor, Food Animal Section
Department of Clinical Science
College of Veterinary Medicine
Auburn University, Alabama

Darrell L. Rankins, Jr., PhD
Associate Professor, Department of Animal and Dairy
    Sciences
College of Agriculture
Auburn University, Alabama

Laura K. Reilly, VMD
Diplomate ACVIM
Adjunct Assistant Professor of Medicine,
New Bolton Center
University of Pennsylvania
Kennett Square, Pennsylvania

D. Michael Rings, DVM, MS
Diplomate ACVIM
Professor, Food Animal Medicine and Surgery
Department of Veterinary Clinical Sciences
College of Veterinary Medicine
The Ohio State University
Columbus, Ohio

Debra C. Ruffin, DVM, MS
Diplomate ACVIM
Department of Clinical Sciences
College of Veterinary Medicine
Auburn University, Alabama

Bryan M. Waldridge, DVM, MS
Diplomate ABVP
Department of Clinical Sciences, Equine Section
College of Veterinary Medicine
Auburn University, Alabama

Lisa Helen Williamson, DVM, MS
Diplomate ACVIM
Associate Professor, Department of Large Animal
    Medicine
College of Veterinary Medicine
University of Georgia
Athens, Georgia

Cindy Wolf, DVM, MS
Small Ruminant Clinical Specialist
Department of Clinical and Population Sciences
College of Veterinary Medicine
University of Minnesota
St. Paul, Minnesota

To Jack and Terry, who raised my sister, brother, and me to do the best we could in order to glorify the Lord.

To Jayne, my soul mate, best friend, and love of my life.

To Rebekah, Natalie, and Dylan, who are truly gifts from God. They give me a wonderful desire to work hard.

Preface

The desire to work with and learn about goats and sheep can be traced to my life well before veterinary school. The first animals I ever purchased with my own money were two cross-bred Nubian goats, and the first animal I traded work for was a Hampshire ewe. Over the years my family and I have been involved before and after veterinary graduation as sheep breeders, in sheep 4-H and FFA showing, as meat goat breeders, and as pet goat and sheep owners. As a veterinarian both in private and academic practice, my primary interest has been in small ruminants. Over the years several good books on either goat or sheep medicine have been published. Chapters in discipline-oriented texts deal with disease, surgery, or reproduction of sheep and/or goats. However, I have always thought it difficult to find information dealing with the *whole* of sheep and goat medicine, surgery, reproduction, and nutrition in a single text. This is where the roots of this book began—as an attempt to fill that void. As a faculty member and small ruminant clinician at Auburn University, the phone calls I receive from other university clinicians, practicing veterinarians, and producers are based on an inability to easily locate applicable information. The goal of this book is to provide a text on sheep and goat medicine, nutrition, surgery, and theriogenology in an easily usable form.

When W.B. Saunders first contacted me, I was apprehensive about committing to such a major undertaking. I knew I would be unable to write this book alone. I contacted people I knew would be able to bring a wide range of experience and ability to their writing. I am proud that several former veterinary or graduate students who rode in ambulatory trucks with me (Drs. Cindy Wolf, Ellen B. Belknap, Alan M. Heath, Bryan M. Waldridge, Virginia R. Fajt, and Michael Q. Lowder) and who have gone on after graduation to excel in large animal medicine and practice and become experts in a wide range of disciplines are included as authors. I also asked colleagues at Auburn University (Drs. Christine B. Navarre, Alan M. Heath, Debra C. Ruffin, Ellen B. Belknap, Hui-Chu Lin, and Bryan M. Waldridge) to help me in this endeavor. I included clinicians with a sheep focus (Drs. Wolf and Heath), those who focus on goats (Drs. Diffay, Waldridge, and Mobini), and academicians who treat them both (Drs. Ring, Machen, Anderson, Hull, Belknap, Navarre, Christopher and Margaret Cebra, Reilly, Baird, and Williamson). I also included professionals with specific specialty areas (Drs. Lin [anesthesia], Colitz [ophthalmology], and Rankins [nutrition]). Also included were those who had practical experience in production, not only as veterinarians, but also as producers of sheep (Drs. Wolf, Navarre, and Rankins) and goats (Drs. Mobini, Diffay, Waldridge, Navarre, and Rankins).

In addition, I tried to ensure that the writers represented different areas of North America so as to bring both geographic and production perspectives to the contents of this text (Northeast—Dr. Reilly; Northwest—Drs. Cebra and Cebra; Midwest—Drs. Anderson, Baird, Hull, Rings, and Wolf; and Southeast—Drs. Navarre, Belknap, Diffay, Mobini, Heath, Rankins, Ruffin, Lin, and Williamson).

Although the book is entitled *Sheep and Goat Medicine,* it covers surgical and diagnostic procedures, basic nutrition, diet formulations, theriogenology, ophthalmology, and anesthesiology. The book is designed so the private practitioner, academic clinician, graduate student, veterinary student, animal scientist, and some producers can easily access applicable information. To enhance the reader's ability to use this book as a reference, I tried to incorporate as many pictures, charts, and tables as space would allow.

The book includes 17 chapters and 3 appendices. The first chapter (on handling and examination of sheep and goats) and the last chapter (on flock health) are the only two chapters in which sheep and goats are discussed completely separately. Because of specific concerns in restraint and examination as part of a health care program, I felt it was better to discuss the two species separately in these two chapters. Dr. Cindy Wolf, an excellent clinician, academician, and sheep producer, wrote much of the sheep sections of those two chapters. My good friend and colleague, Dr. Seyedmehdi Mobini, wrote the bulk of the goat sections of the last chapter, and Drs. Barbara C. Diffay and David McKenzie wrote most of the physical examination and handling information on goats for the first chapter. Dr. Diffay has spearheaded goat 4-H projects in Alabama and is the veterinary advisor to the Alabama Meat Goat Association. Dr. McKenzie is a very fine clinician at Tuskegee University.

In portions of Chapter 2 (Feeding and Nutrition) and Chapter 6 (Theriogenology of Sheep and Goats), sheep and goats are discussed separately, but only in situations where the topic material does not apply to both. Throughout the remaining chapters and appendices, sheep and goats are discussed together.

Three appendices are included in the book to provide quick reference information for the reader. Appendix I provides drug dosage information, Appendix II helps the reader administer fluid therapy, and Appendix III lists normal clinical diagnostic values.

Chapter 2 includes information on ways to formulate and implement a total parenteral nutrition program, three methods for balancing a ration using a hand-held calculator, and ways to balance the mineral component of the diet.

Drs. Christopher and Margaret Cebra took on the arduous task of writing the catch-all chapter (Chapter 14—Diseases of the Hematologic, Immunologic, and Lymphatic Systems [Multisystem Diseases]). It covers some of the same diseases discussed elsewhere, albeit from a systemic viewpoint. The two chapters by Drs. Cebra and Cebra and the chapters by Drs. Waldridge and Colitz (Diseases of the Ophthalmologic System) and Dr. Belknap (Diseases of the Respiratory System) were written solely by those authors. I served as editor and layout designer only. All these folks did an outstanding job.

The rest of the book chapters have my "fingerprints" all over them. I was fearful that the book might too closely reflect my personal ideas and experiences as a sheep and goat producer and veterinarian. However, I truly believe that the co-authors have balanced out the text with their collective expertise. In the final months of preparation the original author of Chapter 11 (Diseases of the Neurologic System) had to step down due to other commitments. With less than 2 months before the book was due to the publisher, Dr. Margo R. Machen took on the task of coordinating and writing much of the chapter. I cannot thank her enough for the outstanding job she did putting this chapter together with little notice.

I wish to thank all of the contributing authors who put up with my constant hounding to complete their portions of the book; none complained and all worked very hard! I want to give special thanks to Drs. Navarre, Heath, Ruffin, and Belknap (as well as Dr. Bob Carson, theriogenologist extraordinaire), who were my constant sounding boards throughout the book's writing and editing. In addition, Dr. Gatz Riddell helped in the review of Chapter 13 (Diseases of the Mammary Gland) and Dr. Chris Johnson helped review Chapter 9 (Diseases of the Musculoskeletal System). All of these colleagues gave me valuable insight and criticism that greatly improved the final version of the book.

Special thanks go to those who helped me with organizing, typing, and laying out the book: Debbie Burelle at Auburn University's College of Veterinary Medicine and my dear wife, Jayne Pugh. These ladies deserve the best "thank you" I can offer because they worked tirelessly on this endeavor. The staff at the Learning Resource Center at Auburn University helped with pictures and drawings.

Last but by no means least important, I want to thank my teachers in veterinary and graduate school that have had a profound influence on my life and career. They include Drs. Dilmus Blackmon, John McCormack, and the late Tom McDaniel, all of whom taught me in veterinary school at the University of Georgia, as well as Dr. Ronnie Elmore, who directed me as a resident at Texas A & M University. Also, I want to thank Dr. LaRue Johnson, from whom I learn something new every time we talk. These gentlemen are my mentors in veterinary medicine and over time and space have greatly influenced the writing and editing of this book more than they will ever know.

D.G. Pugh

Contents

Chapter 1

Handling and Examination of Sheep and Goats

BARBARA C. DIFFAY, DAVID McKENZIE, CINDY WOLF, AND D.G. PUGH

PHYSICAL EXAMINATION OF SHEEP

The clinician should note the *signalment* of the sheep at the start of the examination. Signalment is a significant part of the examination process because certain differential diagnoses are more common in sheep of a particular age, breed, pregnancy status or stage, or sex. Although this statement may seem obvious, it bears repeating—consideration of the signalment often provides the practitioner with information useful in prioritizing the list of differential diagnoses.

Specific body systems may require further clinical scrutiny after the initial examination. This is especially important if the system in question was difficult to assess during the first examination. For example, a 5-month-old, crossbred wether that weighs 110 pounds and is on ad lib feed (95% concentrate) in a feedlot presents with the complaint of being off feed. Obstruction of the urethra caused by urolithiasis is a high-ranking differential diagnosis, but the diagnosis may be missed if no urination or straining is noted on the initial physical examination. Reexamination as clinical signs worsen may yield the correct diagnosis at a later time.

The art of taking a useful history improves with experience. The clinician should avoid asking leading questions. Questions need to be thorough enough to address all important points, but not so lengthy that they inhibit the development of a good relationship with the client. When taking an animal's history, the clinician needs to consider the client's knowledge base. Clients with more experience provide better observations. The clinician should remember to ask for details regarding the previous treatment history and responses to that treatment.

The following elements are particularly important parts of the animal's history:

Purchase and source(s)
Transportation history
Stays off the premises (e.g., shows and fairs, breeding)
Feeding and watering history, including consistency
Water source
Management (grazing or confined)
Procedural history (vaccinations, castration, docking, drenching)
Stage of pregnancy or lactation

Handling Before and During Examination

A good understanding of normal sheep behavior is useful when working with this species. Taking advantage of their desire to escape is a fundamental part of successful handling. Sheep will readily follow one another; will move away from things that frighten them; will move better around slight corners or curves; will move away from buildings; prefer to move uphill; prefer lighted areas and resist dark barns, alleys, and chutes; and will respond to well-trained herding dogs. Handling areas should be well lighted and free of objects that may project shadows into the animals' visual path and should have solid sides. For ease in catching an individual animal, the clinician should first move the group into a small yard or enclosure. The wool or hair should not be grabbed. A crook or lariat is an acceptable catching device. Regardless of the method of capture, excitement and stress should be avoided. A sheep can be handled by various handling points—for example, under the mandible, tail, and flank (Figure 1-1). After it has been caught, a sheep can be "set up" on its rump for examination, shearing, and foot trimming (Figure 1-2). Dairy sheep and hand-reared, bottle-fed lambs are more used to human contact than most other sheep and as a rule are more curious about and less wary of people.

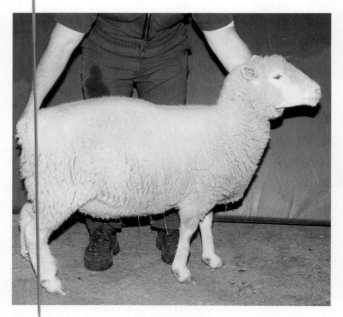

Figure 1-1 The handler is on the left side of the sheep with his left hand under the jaw and his right hand holding the tail. It would be acceptable for him to be kneeling with one knee (usually the right) on the ground and the right hand holding the right rump.

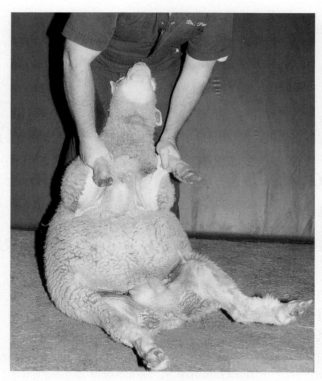

Figure 1-2 There are many variations to sitting a sheep on its rump. The left arm should be placed around the animal's neck at the level of the shoulder. The right hand reaches under the sheep, grasping the right hindfoot and setting it on its rump.

Mismothering of lambs and ewes can readily occur if they are disturbed, particularly during the first few weeks of life. Handling of lambs and ewes should occur with a minimum of stress, and it may be prudent to house the pair together during treatment to maintain a strong bond.

"Over the Fence" Examinations

The flocking instinct in sheep is very strong. Therefore any individual animal that separates itself from the flock should be suspect. Sheep are relatively undemonstrative animals; a sick animal may show few signs apart from isolation and possibly drooping ears and a decreased flight response (Table 1-1). Any animal that lags behind (even for a short distance) when the group is moved rapidly should be examined. Abnormal respiratory signs may be detected by moving animals rapidly for short periods. In sheep with respiratory disease, both respiratory rate and effort increase as the animals are moved— even at a fast walk. Sheep should be observed for evidence of diarrhea or soiling of the breech area while on pasture. Normal fecal pellets are free of blood and mucus. Because sheep are either fed as a group or graze pasture, their natural feeding behavior should be observed. Reluctance to feed may result from disease, parasitism, or dental disease, but inability to feed because of lack of bunk space and bullying is not uncommon. Sheep usually chew their cud more rapidly than cattle. Compared with goats, sheep are not as particular about the cleanliness of feeders and waterers. Signs of wool or hair abnormalities should be noted. Loss of wool may indicate recent stress from fever, external parasitism, insufficient dietary fiber, or some neurologic diseases. The animals should be observed for any signs of lameness. Feet and joint abnormalities are common in sheep flocks. Common nervous signs in sheep include circling, head pressing, and apparent blindness.

A diagnosis of pathology in an individual may alert the clinician to a condition affecting other animals in the flock subclinically. In cases in which no clinical diagnosis can readily be made, the clinician should try to persuade the owner to allow a full necropsy. This is of paramount importance if a large number of animals are at risk.

A visual judgment of the body condition of sheep cannot be made if they are carrying a heavy fleece. Therefore the clinician should palpate the dorsal spinous and transverse spinous processes of the first lumbar vertebra as well as the loin musculature of several animals in the flock to estimate body condition. Open ewes and ewes in early pregnancy are often purposely kept in light condition. Nevertheless, emaciated sheep may be heavily para-

TABLE 1-1

SOME BEHAVIOR PATTERNS OF SHEEP AND GOATS

	Behavior Pattern	
ACTIVITY	SHEEP	GOATS
Food preference	Grass and succulent herbage	Browse (weeds, leaves, and twigs)
Food variety	Accept monotonous diet	Need variety
Habitat selection	Lowlands or hilly grasslands	Climb on rocks and elevations
Antagonistic behavior	Butt head on	Sideways hooking motion
Fighting	Butt	Rear on hind legs
Sexual behavior	Less herding	Herding of females
Newborn young behavior	Remain by mother ("lying in")	Freezing some distance from mothers ("lying out")
Alarm signal	Snort and stamp one forefoot	Frequent high pitch ("sneeze")
Alarm	Form a compact bunch	Form a thin line
Hornless condition	Fertile	Sterile (usually) in males
Tail	Hangs down	Stands up (erect)
Beard	Absent	Present in buck and in some females
Wattles	Absent	May be present
Hears a low-flying plane	Frightened and likely to run herd	Often stand and watch
Stress (elevated blood cortisol)	Results from isolation or subjection to an unfamiliar environment	More of a problem with young kids and doelings

sitized or suffering from various diseases such as paratuberculosis, caseous lymphadenitis, and ovine progressive pneumonia (OPP).

A very strong maternal relationship develops in sheep. Most ewes vigorously reject any attempt by other lambs to suckle, although some (even before lambing) will "steal" lambs. In North America confined ewes are routinely "jugged" for as long as 48 hours to ensure maternal bonding. A "jug" is a 4- or 5-square-foot pen in which just-lambed ewes are placed to allow the bonding process to occur. Nearly all lambs suckle within 2 hours of birth. Lambs suckle very frequently—at least 60 to 70 times a day.

The clinician should walk or drive through the grazing land to examine animals under undisturbed conditions. Sheep do not graze or defecate randomly but select campgrounds (generally under trees and near water) to rest and ruminate. In very hot weather sheep tend to graze more often in the early morning and evening.

External Examination

Examination for body condition score. Body condition scoring of sheep is an important management tool. The scoring scheme depends on assessing fat and muscle over and around the first lumbar vertebra. The traditional system uses a six-point system, with a 0 representing emaciation and a 5 representing extreme obesity. Target body condition scores are crucial to flock productivity. Ewes should have a body condition score of 2.5 to 3.5 at breeding to achieve an optimal ovulation and lambing rate. Ewes that are overly fat at breeding tend to be open at pregnancy checking.

To assess the body condition score of a sheep, the clinician must evaluate four areas of the lumbar region:

1. The prominence of the dorsal spinous process
2. The prominence of and degree of fat covering on the transverse spinous process
3. The amount of muscle and fat under the transverse spinous process—this is assessed based on the ease with which the examiner's fingers pass beneath the transverse processes
4. The fullness of the loin eye muscle (longissimus dorsi) and degree of fat covering between the transverse and dorsal spinous process

Sheep must be confined to a pen or chute to allow adequate palpation for body condition scoring (see Figure 2-1).

Examination of Body Systems

While examining the animal, the clinician may observe a number of problems. The following paragraphs list and discuss some common abnormalities and their associated etiologies.

Wool and hair. Animals with excess wool should be examined for wool blindness. Wool-blind sheep or those with wool hanging over their eyes have difficulty competing for feed in unconfined settings. Snow can freeze on the surface of their wool, making the wool-blindness more pronounced. Shearing the wool from around the faces of ewes in the late fall helps ensure better body condition after a harsh winter.

Wool loss. If the clinician observes wool loss, he or she must then discern whether it is a generalized or local phenomenon. Chewing of the wool generally implies a shortage of roughage, particularly if many of the flock are engaged in this activity. A "break" in the wool indicates a weakness in the wool fiber at the actively growing site. This occurs secondary to systemic disease or some marked nutritional stress.

Skin disease. The clinician should look for evidence of irritation from ectoparasites (e.g., lice, keds, mange mites, fly strike), parting the wool for close inspection of the skin. Specific sites are usually rubbed and scratched by sheep with clinical scrapie. In endemic areas, the clinicians also should examine for evidence of screw-worms. Myiasis (fly strike) most commonly affects the perineal area, poll, breech, and preputial area.

Wool changes. If matted wool with exudation is noted by the clinician, a diagnosis of mycotic dermatitis is likely. If the wool is matted without exudation, the sheep probably have more than 1 year of wool growth or have been chronically sick or underfed. With the onset of warm weather and sweating, wool can become even more matted. When numerous sheep are found to have a loss of crimp and their wool takes on a steely appearance, a nutrient (copper) deficiency should be suspected. Fleece rot results from prolonged wetness accompanied by bacterial multiplication. Grass seed infestation may occur in range- and browse-grazing sheep. Hairiness and/or abnormal wool pigmentation such as brown fibers over the nape of the neck in wool sheep may indicate border disease infection.

Hair and Skin in Hair Sheep Breeds

Normal shedding—Hair sheep (Barbados, Gulf Coast Native) shed their winter coat in spring.
Pruritus—Mange, allergy, and scrapie are three common causes of pruritus.
Hair loss—Ringworm, mange, and poor nutrition can all result in loss of hair over the entire body or in small, circumscribed areas.
Skin nodules—Abscesses, pustules, and demodectic mange cause most skin nodules.
Dandruff—Dandruff and skin flecks are generally nonspecific signs of illness or poor nutrition.

Crustiness—Crustiness, especially under the dew claws, is a common result of chorioptic mange.
Sunburn—Animals with white, thin skin can become sunburned, especially on their udders.

Photosensitization causes head shaking, restlessness, itching, swelling, peeling of white or unprotected portions of the skin, and sloughing of the tips of the ears. The ears of older sheep may show damage from torn-out ear tags or predators. Frostbite often affects the extremities, including the ears, limbs, and tail. Skin damage from freezing appears as swelling followed by the loss of the tips of ears, tails, and even distal portions of the limbs.

Examination of the Head

Head injuries from fighting are not uncommon in rams, and these injuries are prone to secondary infections and myiasis. Injuries caused by fighting are most frequently seen during the breeding season, before the rams are put with the ewes, and when new rams are first added to a ram group. Rams do not appear to be able to recognize one another immediately after shearing. Separating rams for 24 hours after shearing may help prevent fight-associated injuries. Horn growth can impinge on or grow into the skull or eye; horns should therefore be trimmed when necessary.

The clinician should always look for any signs of dyssymmetry during examination. Nervous dysfunction such as a lip droop, an eyelid droop, or a tongue deviation often results from trauma or listeriosis. Any facial swelling should be evaluated for abscesses secondary to puncture wounds, abscessed lymph nodes *(Corynebacterium pseudotuberculosis)*, trauma, hematomas, or seromas.

The eyes should be examined for watery discharge and conjunctival inflammation. These conditions may be apparent from a distance as blepharospasm and wet cheeks. The presence of keratoconjunctivitis suggests a contagious condition, especially if the pathology is bilateral and numerous animals in the group are affected. The animal should be examined for signs of anemia (nematode infections), jaundice (copper toxicity), and congestion (fever, septicemia, toxemia). Certain breeds (e.g., Hampshire) normally have black pigment in some of the mucous membranes, requiring the clinician to use other mucous membranes for examination (sclera, inside the mouth, inside the vulva, inside the prepuce). Entropion, or inverted lower eyelid, is a common heritable defect seen in young lambs. It is often present at birth but not detected until the affected lamb is 1 or more days old. Animals with entropion are usually brought to the clinician's attention because of corneal inflammation. The clinician should examine the sheep's lips and gums for vesicles and scabs. The presence of vesicles is suggestive of contagious ecthyma (sore mouth). Similar lesions also may be found on the muzzle, around the eyes, near the coronary band, on the prepuce, around recently docked tails, and at the base of the udder and teats.

Teeth.   If any incisors are missing, as is common in aged ewes, the descriptive term is *broken mouth.* This pathology can result in poor body condition in grazing animals, although lost incisors are less of a problem in sheep being fed harvested feedstuffs. Mottling and pitting of enamel may indicate fluorosis. Grinding of the teeth may indicate abdominal pain or nervous disease. The bottom incisors should meet the upper pad of the mandible. If the molar teeth are missing, overgrown, or not apposed, the clinician may note poor body condition, draining or fistulous tracks from the mandible, or bony enlargement over the affected tooth (Figure 1-3).

Teeth wear varies greatly with diet and soil types. Older sheep develop periodontal disease and are prone to tooth loss. Molar or cheek teeth are most important to the welfare of the sheep; they can be examined by careful palpation of the cheeks or by using a mouth speculum and a light source. However, molar examination may be difficult because sheep are unable to open their mouths very wide and usually resist this type of examination. Replacement breeding stock (ewe and ram lambs) should be evaluated for overshot or undershot jaws. Mild cases will not affect the ability to grow and maintain body condition, but these animals should not be used for breeding. Excessive salivation (ptyalism) may indicate local irritation caused by glossitis from a foreign body or trauma; the gingival lesions of contagious ecthyma also may produce excessive salivation. An inability to swallow because of a neurologic disorder (e.g., tetanus, rabies) is another cause of ptyalism. Nasal bot migration may result in sneezing and serous nasal discharge. A cyanotic tongue is strongly suggestive of bluetongue especially if it occurs in regions of the country where the disease is prevalent.

Body Systems

Digestive system.   The clinician should palpate the pharynx for injuries, particularly those that may result from improper use of drenching equipment. Bloat often occurs in sheep, especially those with diets high in legumes (alfalfa). Anesthetized sheep should be evaluated throughout anesthesia for the development of bloat, which may impinge on their ability to breathe. Usually, if a handful of skin can be grabbed in the left paralumbar fossa, the sheep is not bloated sufficiently to affect respiration. If the skin cannot be grabbed, the bloat should promptly be relieved to prevent respiratory arrest. Normal rumen contractions for sheep occur at the rate of one or two per minute. Percussion of the abdomen is rarely as useful in sheep as in cattle because sheep do not usually develop the gas-filled viscus (displaced abomasum) that is commonly noted in dairy cattle.

The clinician should carefully palpate the abdomens of young lambs for pain and swelling, particularly in the umbilical area (omphalophlebitis). The perineal area should be examined for evidence of active diarrhea. The nature of the diarrhea can be helpful in generating a list of differential diagnoses. The presence of blood may suggest coccidiosis in lambs older than 4 weeks of age. A foul odor suggests salmonellosis in sheep of any age. Diarrhea caused by cryptosporidiosis is often grayish-yellow, may contain blood, and usually occurs in 2- to 4-week-old lambs. Rectal prolapse is not uncommon in fattening lambs, especially those whose tails were docked excessively short. Normal rectal temperature in sheep is 101.8 to 103.5 degrees Fahrenheit (° F), but it may transiently exceed 104° F during periods of excitement (Table 1-2).

Respiratory system.   A clear, bilateral, watery nasal discharge is relatively common in sheep; it generally occurs during times when sheep are housed in poorly ventilated buildings. This serous nasal discharge is most frequently seen in areas where the temperature fluctuates considerably during the day. Discharge from just one nostril is less common but can occur with *Oestrus ovis* (nasal bot) infections, tumors, or foreign bodies. Sheep with nasal bot infections sneeze and have an intermittent, clear serous nasal discharge. Bilateral purulent nasal discharge may indicate upper or lower respiratory tract infection. Bilateral bloody nasal discharge is seen with some infectious conditions (e.g., anthrax) or after the ingestion of root crops that have undergone freezing and thawing before consumption. Sheep that have pneumonia cough intermittently, have an elevated respiratory rate (above 20 breaths per minute), and may show increased respiratory effort. Pneumonia is more common in young and very old animals. The normal respiratory rate for a healthy unexcited sheep is 12 to 20 breaths per minute (see Table 1-2).

Cardiovascular system.   Damp wool can make auscultation difficult. Therefore the clinician should attempt the heart examination in a quiet area with the use of a good quality stethoscope. The normal heart rate for a healthy unexcited sheep is 70 to 80 beats per minute. The pulse can best be evaluated by palpating the femoral artery on the medial aspect of the rear leg (see Table 1-2).

Urinary system.   Urine samples can usually be obtained from ewes by briefly occluding their nostrils. The urethral process of a male can be examined after the ram lamb reaches puberty and the preputial adhesions have detached. Placing the ram in a sitting position and manually reflecting the prepuce caudally allows exteriorization of the penis. A gauze placed around the penile shaft makes grasping and examination easier. Uroliths can occasionally be palpated and/or seen in the urethral process.

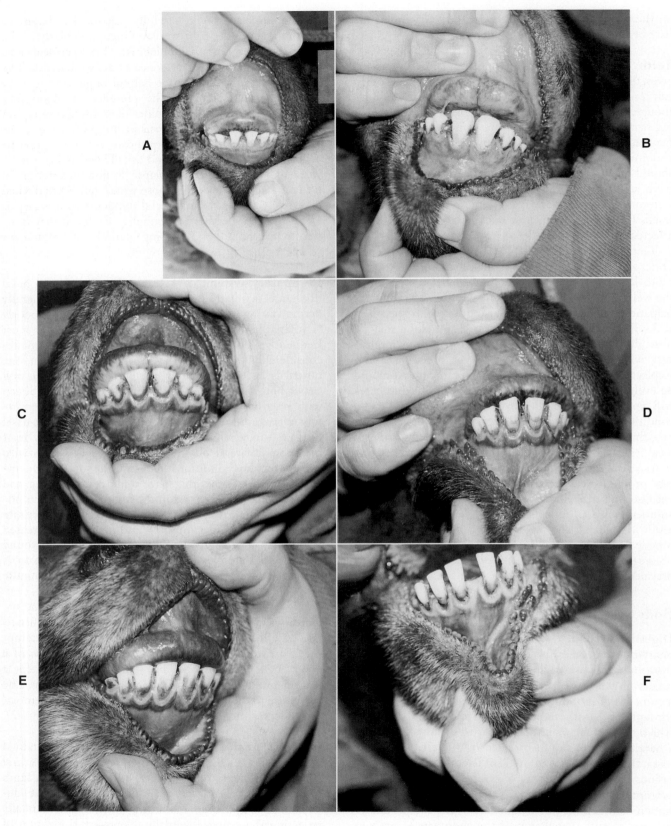

Figure 1-3 The dentition of sheep. **A,** Dentition at 6 months to 1 year. **B,** Dentition at 1 to 1.5 years. **C,** Dentition of a 2-year-old. **D,** Dentition of a 3-year-old. **E,** Dentition of a 4-year-old. **F,** Dentition of an aged or a broken-mouthed ewe.

TABLE 1-2

SOME PHYSIOLOGIC PARAMETERS OF SHEEP AND GOATS

PARAMETER	SHEEP	GOATS
Rectal temperatures (vary according to ambient temperatures and fleece or hair coat)	102° F (with a range of 101.5° to 104° F)	102° to 104° F
Ruminations	2 per minute	1 to 2 per minute
Pulse	70 to 80 beats per minute	70 to 90 beats per minute
Respiration	12 to 20 breaths per minute	15 to 30 breaths per minute
Puberty	5 to 12 months	4 to 12 months
Estrus	36 hours	12 to 24 hours
Estrus cycle	16 to 17 days	18 to 23 days
Gestation	147 days	150 days
Average birth weight	Breed dependent	Breed dependent
Single	8 to 13 pounds	
Twins	7 to 10 pounds	
Fleece weight	7 to 15 pounds	

Passing a catheter in male sheep is difficult because of the presence of the urethral diverticulum where the urethra crosses the caudal border of the pelvic floor. Dribbling of urine, abdominal straining, or urethral pulsing noted on digital palpation of the rectum all indicate urethral obstruction. As urolithiasis progresses, abdominal distension develops. Enlarged urinary bladders can be visualized by ultrasonographic examination, and urine may be drained by cystocentesis. If the urethra remains obstructed, the urethra and bladder will usually rupture. Scabs or ulceration on the prepuce may indicate ulcerative posthitis. This condition is most commonly found in wethers being fed high concentrations of protein.

Genital system. The scrotum should be examined by palpating its contents and noting its external appearance. The skin and wool or hair covering should be intact and uniform. A ram's scrotum can have chorioptic mange infestations, localized injuries, frostbite, and hernias. Close examination helps detect these abnormalities. The testes and epididymes must be palpated carefully for abnormalities of shape (epididymitis), size (orchitis, hypoplasia), freedom of movement in the scrotum (adhesions, spermatocele or varicocele, abscesses), and turgidity (poor testicular tone is usually associated with suboptimal sperm production). The phrase that "big is beautiful, mobility meaningful, resilience respectable, softness suspicious" is helpful to remember when evaluating rams for breeding soundness. Rams selected for breeding should always have symmetric scrotal contents and meet the breed and age criteria for scrotal circumference measurements (see Chapter 6). The urethral process is normally visible at the end of the penis. This structure may be absent in some

rams—presumably because of a previous subclinical episode of urolithiasis or trauma. The urethral process may slough secondary to urolithiasis. Vaginal prolapse is seen in ewes in the last 2 weeks of pregnancy. If the prolapse is not replaced within approximately 12 hours, it may enlarge to contain the bladder, the cervix may be traumatized, and the mucus plug may be disrupted. All ewes with a vaginal prolapse should be carefully monitored for anorexia, depression, and ascending uterine infection. Such infections are usually fatal for the fetus and can result in toxemia and death of the ewe. Uterine discharge or lochia is normally seen after lambing for up to 3 weeks. Normal lochia should be reddish-brown in color and nonodorous. Any other discharge from the vagina warrants further evaluation and may indicate an abortion. Ewes that have recently aborted should be considered infectious to other animals and should be examined and quarantined.

Sheep are seasonal breeders. In the Midwest, breeding season begins in late summer and continues throughout the fall, with lambing in late winter and spring. The breeding season and lambing period in other locales is based on season and demand for sales and markets.

Mammary glands. If a lamb is starving or a ewe resists suckling by her own lamb, the clinician should carefully examine the udder for bilateral symmetry and abnormalities of color, pliability, temperature, turgidity, and volume of milk produced. Both teats should be evaluated for patency and milk flow. A physiologic prepartal udder edema occurs in some sheep. A diffusely hard or firm udder in the first few days after lambing may indicate OPP. Affected glands secrete scant quantities of normal-appearing milk. No signs of inflammation are present in most cases of OPP, and both glands are equally affected. The udder should be carefully palpated for evidence of acute or chronic bacterial mastitis lesions. Mastitis generally affects only one gland. Abscesses commonly form as a result of chronic mastitis. A California Mastitis Test (CMT) is useful for diagnosing the condition. The first sign of acute bacterial mastitis may be an abduction of the rear leg in order to minimize contact with the inflamed gland. This is often perceived as lameness. Contagious ecythma, udder impetigo, and bites or abrasions from suckling can cause external lesions at the base of the udder or on the teats. Lamb-induced injuries often occur on the medial aspect of the teat, and generally at the base of the udder.

Locomotor system. The stance and gait should be carefully observed. Sheep should be forced to walk away from the examiner. Observation from the side greatly aids in diagnosis. Lameness is best determined with the animal at a walk rather than a run. Difficulty in walking or lameness in young lambs can result from septic arthritis or white muscle disease, among other causes. Arthritis can be a problem in older rams and has a variety of causes. Carpal swellings are commonly seen in older animals; however, some thickening of the skin over the carpi (hygromas) can occur naturally when sheep are housed on hard surfaces. Enlargement of the epiphyseal areas is seen in lambs with rickets and those that have developed calluses from healing rib fractures.

Sheep with footrot commonly graze on their knees. Feet should be examined, pared, and smelled during the routine examination. Virulent footrot produces a characteristic foul odor. Initially the examiner observes an interdigital dermatitis, followed by necrosis and underrunning of horn. The footrot lesions start at the abaxial part of the heel and move proximally toward the toe. The entire sole may be underrun and sloughed if the virulent strain of *Dichelobacter nodosus* is present or if affected sheep do not receive timely treatment. In most cases of footrot, more than one foot is affected; the condition more commonly affects the front feet. Secondary myiasis is a common finding during fly season in some parts of North America.

Acute pain and swelling often accompany foot abscesses. Over time, suppuration occurs, often on the lateral aspect of the coronary band of the affected claw. Foot abscesses usually affect only one foot. Abscess of the foot is a sporadic condition, whereas footrot occurs in outbreaks.

Nervous system. To begin an evaluation of the nervous system, the clinician should observe the sheep carefully from a distance. Behavioral abnormalities may be associated with either primary nervous system disease or a metabolic condition. For example, ewes with pregnancy toxemia exhibit ataxia and blindness. Sheep observed in sternal recumbency with the head deviated toward the flank may be hypocalcemic, severely anemic, or profoundly dehydrated and acidotic (secondary to rumen acidosis), or may suffer from meningitis. When sheep circle to one side, the practitioner must consider listeriosis, brain abscesses, and parasitic lesions. Sheep with grass tetany (hypomagnesemia) generally stagger. Hypomagnesemic animals are often grazing rich, fast-growing forage. Ataxia in lambs may be caused by copper deficiency, spinal abscesses resulting from an ascending tail docking infection, nematode larval migration *(Paralephastrongyles tenuis)*, or trauma.

Tetanus is common on some farms. Affected sheep initially demonstrate a localized stiffness such as a semierect tail, erect ears, and prolapsed third eyelids. As the disease progresses, the animal's entire body becomes stiff and goes into tetanic spasms secondary to external stimulation. Affected animals also develop opisthotonos. Sheep usually have the paralytic form of rabies rather than the furious form. Pseudorabies also occurs in animals in direct contact with infected swine. Sheep that are clinically affected with scrapie may have an abnormal gait. Scrapie-infected sheep may bunny hop, be hypermetric on the rear legs, or have proprioceptive deficits of the forelimbs. They are generally weak. They also may be emaciated yet interested in eating, have wool rubbed off of their hindquarters and flanks, and may even have areas of skin excoriation. Ewes in late pregnancy that have clinical scrapie are often misdiagnosed as having pregnancy toxemia, and vice versa.

Lymphatic system. The superficial lymph nodes of sheep are hidden beneath their wool and fiber. The clinician should palpate them to assess for size and consistency. Lymph nodes that are infected with *Corynebacterium pseudotuberculosis* enlarge and rupture. They drain a thick yellowish-green, nonodorous purulent fluid. External lymph nodes that should be palpated during a routine examination include the mandibular, parotid, retropharyngeal, prescapular, prefemoral, supramammary, and popliteal lymph nodes. The internal lymph nodes can only be evaluated by ultrasound and radiographic examination or necropsy examination.

Examination of the Environment

The clinician should evaluate the environment for its fitness for the particular group of sheep. Questions to consider include: Does the environment contain an appropriate diet and water source? Does it provide suitable shelter? Do the sheep have enough space to meet their needs? The practitioner must be familiar with the needs of the particular production group to answer these questions correctly. Objective data such as a forage analysis may be required to address the group's needs.

Examination of the Ration

Many producers describe the diet of their sheep in terms of buckets of grain and bales of hay fed per day. Practitioners should work to help clients discuss the sheep diets as follows:

- Production group being fed such diet
- Number of sheep in that group
- Average body condition score and body weight
- Pounds of grain fed per day
- Feed analysis of that grain
- Pounds of hay (or other roughage source such as haylage or silage) given and consumed each day
- Forage analysis of the hay
- Availability, form, and analysis of trace mineral salt

The water source and its cleanliness and delivery system also are important features of the diet. The amount of roughage fed compared with the amount consumed is not the same because of wastage, which varies depending on the quality and feed delivery system. Placing feed on the ground or in some styles of round bale feeders generally results in more wastage than feeding in sheep-proof bunks and collapsing bale feeders.

Necropsy Findings

Wherever possible, the practitioner should perform necropsy on recently dead sheep. The gross necropsy findings of a thin adult sheep with no well-described signs is frequently sufficient to make a diagnosis regarding the cause of weight loss. If no gross lesions are evident, major tissues (fresh and fixed) should be submitted to a diagnostic laboratory for further investigation. The practitioner can improve the chance for a diagnosis by providing a thorough case history and requesting specific tests where indicated.

*F*URTHER READING

Hindson JC, Winter AC: *Outline of clinical diagnosis in sheep*, Cambridge, MA, 1996, Blackwell Science.

Martin WB, Aitken ID: *Diseases in sheep*, ed 3, Malden, MA, 1999, Blackwell Scientific.

Boden E: *Sheep and goat practice*, London, 1991, Bailliere Tindall Publishing.

Leahy J, Barrow P: *Restraint of animals*, Ithaca, NY, 1953, Cornell Campus Store.

RESTRAINT AND HANDLING OF GOATS

Safety and Health Considerations

According to the United States Department of Agriculture, agriculture ranks as one of the three most hazardous industries in the United States along with mining and construction. The safety and welfare of animals and personnel must be considered when planning working facilities. Poorly designed and maintained facilities contribute to inefficiency and can lead to livestock and human injuries and loss of time and money. When performing veterinary procedures, the clinician must recognize the potential for zoonoses. An assessment of the herd's health status through histories and physical examinations guards clinicians, technicians, and farm personnel and families against zoonotic infections.

Stress and trauma to the livestock are to be avoided. Producers who are able to have frequent, nonthreatening interactions with their goats will reduce the herd's apprehension of being handled.

Physical Restraint

When planning procedures that require physical restraint of goats, practitioners should consider the layout and surroundings of the working facility, the physical condition and temperament of the animals, and human and animal safety. One person can easily restrain and carry out certain procedures on goats that have been frequently handled in a quiet, nonaggressive manner. However, for efficiency and safety, when goats have had only occasional human contact, animal restraint and procedures should be performed with an assistant. If a goat has been mishandled, it will be wary of future attempts to confine and constrain it. Patience and an easygoing manner of treatment hold rewards for the clinician.

Restraint for Physical Examination

To catch and lead a goat, it is acceptable to use the horns, beard, collar, or halter (Figure 1-4). The techniques of

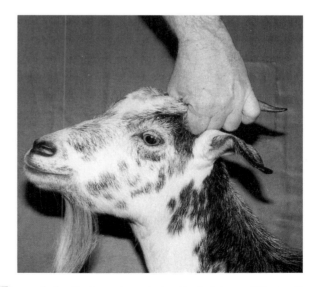

Figure 1-4   Goats can be restrained by their horns, if the handler grasps near the skin and keeps the rear of the animal under control. If the handler does not control the animal's rear and the goat flips around, it may injure its neck. Grasping the horn near the tip may result in breaking the horn and possibly fracturing the skull.

looping an arm around the goat's neck or grabbing its gastrocnemius tendon can be used to catch and hold a goat (Figure 1-5). A goat being held by a hind limb may possibly dislocate a hip joint in an attempt to jerk itself free. Goats find restraint by their ears painful and owners consider it abusive.

The use of an assistant or restraining devices facilitates physical examinations, vaccinations, blood collections, artificial insemination, hoof trimming, and other procedures. Equipment such as stanchions, tilt tables, squeeze chutes, cages, and raceways can be used. Some procedures can be completed while an assistant steadies the goat against a wall or fence by firmly holding a leg against the goat's flank or thorax behind its elbow. A handler can gently flip, place, and then hold a goat in lateral recumbency by placing a knee on the goat's neck. Another useful strategy is to have the handler straddle the goat, then back it into a corner and firmly press his or her knees against the goat's shoulders or neck. Kids weighing up to 30 pounds that are used to being handled can be placed with their legs folded under them on the lap of an assistant while the clinician examines the head of the kid.

Restraint of the Head

While straddling the goat's withers or neck, the clinician can control the animal's head by gripping its cheeks, beard, or horns. One method for head restraint is to place one hand on each cheek and wrap the fingers under the mandible, being careful to avoid pressure on the trachea. Alternatively, the clinician can hold the beard with one hand and wrap the other arm around the goat's neck. A third method involves gripping the horns. The ability to control a horned goat's head depends on the temperament of the goat as well as the skill and strength of the handler.

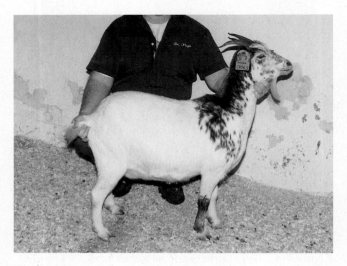

Figure 1-5 In this case the handler uses his left hand to hold the jaw–throat latch area and his right hand to hold the tail. If the goat tries to free itself, the handler can move the left hand onto the jaw and pull the animal closer to help control it.

After the head is stabilized, the goat's ears, eyes, nose, and mouth can be inspected. For an oral examination, the use of a speculum is recommended to ensure a clear view of the oral cavity and prevent the goat from biting instruments or the clinician's fingers.

Restraint for Administration of Medications

The administration of oral and injectable medications and the collection of blood samples are best accomplished by positioning the goat as described previously for physical examination and head restraint.

Oral drugs. When drenching, dispensing boluses, or passing an orogastric tube, the clinician should hold the goat's head in a straight, natural position with the mandible parallel to the ground. The dose syringe is inserted well into the cheek pouch via the commissure of the lips. The goat must be given time to swallow as the fluid is slowly dispensed. Tilting the head upward can lead to aspiration pneumonia. To safely and properly place a bolus, the clinician moves the balling gun over the base of the tongue, but not into the pharynx. After administering the tablet, the clinician maintains the position of the head and holds the goat's mouth closed until the goat swallows. This prevents the animal from spitting out the medication. Using a speculum, the clinician can pass a 1.2- to 1.5-cm diameter stomach tube through the mouth of an adult goat. An 8 French red rubber urethral catheter with an attached 60-cc catheter-tip syringe can be used as an orogastric tube to feed or provide oral medications to very young and weak kids.

Injectable drugs. The veterinarian should ask the owner the purpose for which he raises the goats (e.g., leather, meat, breeding, exhibition, pet). Reactions to vaccines and antibiotics can cause lesions in commercially valuable skin and muscle and cosmetic flaws in hobby, pet, and show goats. Meat producers prefer that injections be placed in the neck, a meat cut of low value. Breeders prefer the axilla, where a nodular mass of scar tissue is not visible and cannot be readily mistaken for caseous lymphadenitis.

INTRAMUSCULAR INJECTIONS: Intramuscular injections are commonly given in the area of the neck enclosed by the cervical vertebrae ventrally, nuchal ligament dorsally, and shoulder caudally. Other muscles used for injections include the longissimus in the lumbar region as well as the gluteals, semitendinosus, semimembranous, and triceps (Figure 1-6). The clinician must pay special attention to the location of the sciatic nerve in the thighs because irritating drugs can cause permanent damage. Additionally, the small muscle masses in young goats limit the volume of the injectable substance.

SUBCUTANEOUS INJECTIONS: Subcutaneous injections can be given in the axilla or on the chest wall (Figure 1-7). The triangular area of the neck described previously also is used. However, shot reactions near the prescapular lymph node may be erroneously diagnosed as caseous lymphadenitis.

ADDITIONAL INJECTION ROUTES: The jugular vein is often used to administer intravenous drugs and collect blood samples. It is advisable to use a 4-cm, 20-gauge needle for venipuncture. Intradermal injections call for 1.8-cm, 25-gauge tuberculin needles. Intraperitoneal injections, primarily used in neonates, are given with 1-inch, 18- or 20-gauge needles inserted no deeper than 1.8 cm. While the kid is held hanging by its front legs, the clinician inserts the needle perpendicular to the skin about 1 cm to the left of the navel.

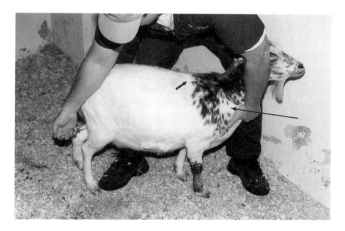

Figure 1-6   An injection is being made into the semimembranosus/semitendinosus area. Injections in this area can result in lameness from local muscle irritation or nerve damage. However, this is a good intramuscular injection site in animals not being raised for meat if a large volume of medication is required. Other preferred sites, particularly for small dose volumes, are indicated by the *arrows.*

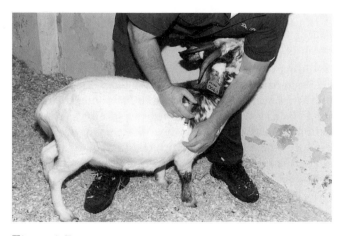

Figure 1-7   Administering a subcutaneous injection in the chest region of a goat.

Before giving intramammary infusions, the clinician should clean and swab the teat with alcohol. Single-use teat cannulae are used for each teat and inserted just deep enough to gain entry into the teat cistern. In does with small teat orifices, sterile tomcat catheters can be used to infuse medications.

Restraint for Hoof Trimming

With the goat standing, the clinician flexes the pastern and raises the foot and limb until the sole faces upward. The clinician can then work facing the head or tail of the goat while positioned at the animal's side (Figure 1-8). An assistant can hold the goat, place the goat in a stanchion, or halter tie the goat while the clinician trims the hooves. In caring for fractious animals, sitting them on their rump (as is done with sheep) may be useful.

Facilities

An important goal of well-planned working facilities is to gather, restrain, and handle animals with minimal stress and prevent injuries to animals and personnel.

Fencing.   Fencing is used to confine stock, separate animals into management subgroups, exclude predators, and protect ornamental and commercial crops from consumption by goats. The selection of appropriate fencing material is dictated by purpose, size, and cost. When planning permanent enclosures, owners may want to consult fence contractors and suppliers of commercial handling equipment, as well as other goat keepers who may have proven ideas for consideration. Smooth-wire, high-tensile, multiple-strand electric fencing deters goats and predators alike and is easily maintained. However, if

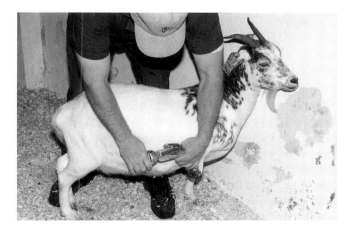

Figure 1-8   Goats can be restrained in a variety of ways for hoof trimming. In this case the handler is restraining the goat by pressing his left and right legs and knees into the goat's side while pressing the left arm and elbow into the goat's shoulders and neck. The left hand is holding the foot and the right hand is doing the trimming.

the power source fails, goats may find freedom by stepping through the wire strands.

Goats can damage field fencing by standing on their hindlimbs and leaning their front feet against the fence. A single strand of electric wire placed near the top and bottom of a woven wire fence discourages goats from leaning on the fence and may prevent predators from crawling underneath. Horned goats, particularly those with backward-pointing horns, are likely to get caught when withdrawing their heads from the 6-inch wide by 5-inch high spaces in the fencing. This renders the goat indefensible against being butted by herd mates or attacked by predators. A possible fatal outcome is strangulation of the entrapped goat. Similarly, a goat can catch its foot in the open spaces of a chain-link fence and fracture a leg in its struggle to free itself.

Although welded-wire panels can withstand the pressure of goats, they can entrap horned goats if the panel openings are the standard size of 8 inches wide by 6 inches high. Furthermore, kids weighing less than 15 pounds can step through these spaces to escape confinement. Welded-wire panels with openings smaller than 8 inches wide by 4 inches high can eliminate these concerns.

Housing. Housing facilities provide shelter for livestock; storage for feed, equipment, and supplies; and a work area for routine animal care procedures. Shelter that provides warmth, shade, and protection from wind, precipitation, and predators establishes an environment of comfort and calmness in the herd. Unlike cattle, goats will interrupt their grazing to seek cover from rain. The shelter should promote the productivity and well-being of goats.

Heating and cooling, ventilation, flooring, and water supply should be considered under the guidance of a person knowledgeable and experienced in farm building construction. Additionally, space should be planned for loafing areas, feed and water troughs, kidding stalls, and shelter for disabled goats and animal groupings specific to the facility (e.g., young does and bucks, recently shorn goats, research study groups). Feed and equipment storage areas must be designed to eliminate the potential for consumption of excessive amounts of grain and ingestion of stored chemicals.

Floor space alone does not determine adequate living space for animals. Enclosure shape, floor type, ceiling height, the location and dimensions of feeders and waterers, and other physical and social elements affect the usefulness of the space. Mature does require an average of 16 square feet of stall space, excluding troughs. A buck may need as much as 30 square feet, whereas a kid needs approximately 10 square feet. Shelters in outside pens or pastures should allow 5.5 square feet per goat. Fence heights vary between 4 to 5 feet for does and 5 to 6 feet for bucks in rut.

A clean, dry, draft-free, well-bedded stall or pen is ideal for kidding and bonding of the dam with her off-spring. Housing for does at parturition enables the goat keeper to manage difficulties experienced by the doe or her kids in a timely manner. Limiting the doe to a stall gives her a quiet, undisturbed environment for bonding, a crucial event that calls for a minimum of 5 minutes.

In large herds, it may be impractical to provide individual stalls for preparturient does. In such cases, does may be group-penned 2 to 4 weeks before parturition, giving the owner ample opportunity to monitor for potential problems. Neonates are highly susceptible to hypothermia in cold or wet weather; therefore owners should take precautions against their does delivering in the field.

Feed and water. Good feed and water hygienics should be practiced to promote healthy goats and reduce wastage of feed. In contrast to tales of tin can–eating goats, goats will decline wet or moldy feed and dirty water. Feedstuffs should be provided in well-designed troughs that minimize contamination with feces, urine, and dirt deposited by hooves.

A 15-inch-long feed trough space can accommodate one adult goat. Kids, when penned or pastured with mature goats, should have free access to a creep feeder, effectively eliminating competition with adult animals. Bunk space in the creep area should be 10 inches per kid. Despite ample trough space and the use of creep feeders, goats low in the herd hierarchy may not be allowed access to feed. To alleviate the effect of dominance, multiple feeders may be used, or distressed goats can be isolated and fed individually. Alternatively, goats simultaneously restrained and fed in individual stanchions or keyhole mangers will be unable to dominate or be dominated by herd mates.

The volume of water consumed by livestock is influenced by the water content of feed sources, environmental temperature, and water quality. To encourage consumption, the keeper should offer clean water ad lib. Typical water troughs or self-waterers can be used. In cold climates the use of water heaters improves intake. Adequate drainage should be provided under watering devices.

Avoiding drug residues in meat and milk. Veterinarians and goat producers working as a team can ensure that only wholesome meat and milk products enter the human food chain. Extra-label drug use and chemical contamination of feed and pasture give rise to drug residues in products for human consumption. Veterinarians should advise their clients on the ethical and legal limitations of not following all labeled guidelines for drugs used in food-producing animals.

Particular effort should be made to educate livestock producers who administer pharmaceuticals without an established veterinary-client-patient relationship (VCPR). Conscientious record keeping is essential in residue avoidance. Records should include animal identification numbers; drug names; dates, amounts, and routes of administration; withdrawal times; and contact information for the person who administers treatment. Awareness of potential risk factors for disease and conscientious management practices on the part of the keeper lead to reduced disease incidence and the subsequent need for drug use. In these ways an individual owner can ensure that his or her goats are wholesome and safe to enter the human food chain.

Biosecurity

Sick or injured animals.   Goat keepers should provide an area separate from the herd where disabled animals can be housed while receiving veterinary and nursing care. The potential is great for disease transmission to herd mates that may later occupy a previously contaminated stall or pen. Consequently, the area reserved for disabled animals must be easily cleaned and disinfected after discharge of recovered animals.

Introducing new animals to the herd.   A pre-purchase health examination by a veterinarian is an important aspect of disease prevention and the establishment of a new VCPR. Taking precautions to reduce the risk of introducing disease in a stable herd is a sound business decision that contributes to increased profitability through reduced veterinary expenses, time, and effort.

A pre-purchase evaluation includes a health assessment of the herd of origin. Based on the history, physical examinations, and knowledge of diseases occurring on nearby livestock farms, the veterinarian may perform diagnostic tests to assess the health and reproductive soundness of animals offered for sale.

Veterinarians should advise owners to restrict a recently purchased goat to clean housing that minimizes physical and aerosol contact with the owner's existing herd. An isolation period of 4 weeks allows the animal to become acclimated to its environment with minimal stress. In addition, the owner is better able to observe the goat for incubating disease conditions, nutritional requirements, and behavior patterns.

*F*URTHER READING

The American Sheep Industry Association, USDA Extension Service: *Producing high quality consumer products from sheep,* Englewood, CO, 1995, Colorado State University.

Bell HM: *Rangeland management for livestock production,* ed 2, Norman, OK, 1978, University of Oklahoma Press.

Bowen JS: Bringing quality assurance concepts to goat producers, *Large Animal Practice,* p 24, July/August 1997.

Diffay BC: *Avoiding introduction of contagious diseases on your goat farm,* fact sheet no. 2, Tuskegee, AL, 1996, Tuskegee University Press.

Federation of Animal Science Societies: *Guide for the care and use of agricultural animals in agricultural research and teaching,* Savoy, IL, 1999, Federation of Animal Science Societies.

Forte VA, Jr, Devine JA, Cymerman A: Research stanchion and transporter for small ruminants, *Lab Anim Sci* 38:478, 1988.

Gubernick DJ: Maternal "imprinting" or maternal "labeling" in goats, *Appl Anim Behav* 28:124, 1980.

Houpt KA: *Domestic animal behavior for veterinarians and animal scientists,* ed 3, 1998, Ames, IA, Iowa State University Press.

Lager K: Apparatus and technique for conditioning goats to repeated blood collection, *Lab Anim Sci* 27(3):38, 1998.

Leahy JR, Barrow P: *Restraint of animals,* ed 2, Ithaca, NY, 1953, Cornell Campus Store.

National Research Council (Grossblatt N, editor): *Guide for the care and use of laboratory animals,* Washington, DC, 1996, National Academy Press.

O'Brien PH: Feral goat home range. Influence of social class and environmental variables, *Appl Anim Behav* 12:373, 1984.

Smith MC, Sherman DM: *Goat medicine,* Malvern, PA, 1994, Lea & Febiger.

Sonsthagen TF: *Restraint of domestic animals,* Goleta, CA, 1991, American Veterinary Publications.

Stricklin WR, Gonyou HW: Housing design based on behavior and computer simulations. In Stricklin WR, Gonyou HW, editors: *Animal behavior and the design of livestock and poultry systems,* Ithaca, NY, 1995, Northeast Regional Agricultural Engineering Service.

PHYSICAL EXAMINATION OF GOATS

Clinical diagnosis begins with history taking and the performance of a systematic physical examination.

History information obtained from the client falls into two main categories. The first is the presenting complaint, which includes the duration, onset (acute, chronic, seasonal), and associated signs of disease. The second is management factors, which include pasture and soil type, diet and diet changes, sources of water, housing (hygiene, shelter from weather, ventilation, humidity, temperature), previous diseases, treatments, vaccinations and tests in individual animals or in the herd, recent transportation and introductions to the herd, and separation of different age groups.

Physical examination enables the identification and localization of a problem to a particular organ system or systems. Problem identification is the most crucial component of successful diagnosis and treatment. To form an overall impression of the goat's general condition, the veterinarian should observe it from a distance. Parameters to be assessed include posture, gait, body condition and conformation, alertness, breathing pattern, and interaction with the herd (sick animals often isolate themselves). The animal should then be restrained for the hands-on examination, which begins at the head and ends at the tail.

Head and Neck

Skin and musculoskeletal systems.   The clinician should note the general symmetry of the lips, nostrils, muzzle, cheeks, eyes, and ears. Next, wearing gloves if suspicious of a zoonotic disease, the clinician examines the lips and muzzle for raised lesions such as vesicles, pustules, crusted lesions (e.g., contagious ecthyma), papules, or nodules (e.g., papillomas). Diseased animals often have a dry, rough, and dull hair coat. Matted hairs may be a sign of dermatophilosis. Scratching the base of the ears and shaking the head may indicate ear mites, as may the presence of debris deep within the ear canal. Circumscribed areas of hair loss without pruritus also may indicate dermatophilosis. Areas of hair loss and excoriations may be a sign of pruritus. Parting the hairs allows closer examination of the skin. External parasites and areas of erythema, hyperpigmentation, and raised lesions should be identified and examined.

The hydration status should be assessed by pinching the skin of the upper eyelid and noting the presence or absence of tenting (the upper eyelid should retract rapidly on pinching). Color and vascular engorgement of the sclera and conjunctiva also are to be evaluated. Reddened conjunctiva with an ocular discharge suggests keratoconjunctivitis, corneal ulceration, foreign body, or entropion. The clinician should examine the ears for raised lesions and skin color. Erythema of the ear tips in light-skinned breeds suggests photodermatitis. Hornless goats should be examined to determine whether they are naturally horned (horn buds and whorls of hair over the horn buds) or polled (no horn buds and central whorl of hair). The naturally polled phenotype may be associated with the intersex genotype. Wattles may be found in either sex, occurring on the neck and sometimes the face and ears. Benign cysts may occasionally be found at the base of the wattles and should not be confused with abscessed lymph nodes.

The male goat commonly urinates on his head and forequarters when sexually aroused. Clinicians should wear gloves and protective clothing when handling them.

Digestive and gastrointestinal systems.   Incisors can be used to determine the age of goats. Deciduous incisors erupt as follows:

I_1 at birth to 1 week
I_2 at 1 to 2 weeks
I_3 at 2 to 3 weeks
I_4 at 3 to 4 weeks

Permanent incisors erupt as follows:

I_1 at 1 to 1.5 years
I_2 at 1.5 to 2 years
I_3 at 2.5 to 3 years
I_4 at 3.5 to 4 years

Foul breath suggests dental disease (alveolar periostitis or root abscess). Dropping feed from the mouth or constant drooling of saliva may indicate uneven tooth wear, stomatitis, or neurologic disease. Regurgitation may result from pharyngeal or esophageal obstruction. Milk regurgitation in a kid suggests a cleft palate. Pallor of the conjunctiva and mucous membranes suggests anemia caused by gastrointestinal parasitism. Congestion may indicate fever or toxemia. Icterus may be a sign of liver disease, as may repeated yawning (which also is suggestive of pregnancy toxemia or hepatic lipidosis).

Prognathism or brachygnathism should be readily apparent. A soft fluctuant mass in the maxillary region may be a salivary mucocele or retained cud (the differentiation is made by oral examination). Submandibular edema suggests hypoproteinemia (such as that caused by gastrointestinal parasitism). A firm mass behind the laryngeal area may be an enlarged thyroid gland secondary to iodine deficiency.

The clinician should carefully palpate the jugular furrows. The esophagus may be palpable in the left jugular furrow if it is distended by a bolus of food or a foreign body.

Respiratory system.   Symmetry of airflow from the nostrils can be assessed with the back of the hand or a feather. Uneven airflow may be caused by a nasal passage blocked by a foreign body or nasal adenocarcinoma (rare). The character of any nasal discharge should be noted (i.e., consistency, volume, unilateral or bilateral, continuous or intermittent). Food and water containers should be examined for nasal exudate. The appearance of "scalded" skin or hair loss below the nostrils suggests an intermittent discharge. A serous discharge may be a sign of nasal inflammation or early viral infection. A mucoid discharge may result from early pneumonia, lungworm infestation, *Oestrus ovis* larval infection (occasionally seen in goats), trauma, or abscess formation. A mucopurulent nasal discharge may be seen in advanced pneumonia with bacterial superinfection. A hemorrhagic discharge usually indicates more severe nasal trauma.

The clinician should auscultate the trachea for wheezing (collapsed trachea, obstructive lesion) and crackling sounds (tracheitis). A cough can be elicited by palpating the larynx and squeezing the trachea. A normal animal coughs once or twice, whereas a diseased animal may cough repeatedly after tracheal compression. Upper airway disease (e.g., early pneumonia, foreign body, compressive lesion) is usually characterized by the acute onset of a loud, harsh, dry, nonproductive cough. Affected goats do not swallow after coughing. Lower airway disease is usually characterized by a chronic, soft, productive cough. The goat swallows after coughing and coughs only occasionally. Examples of lower airway disease include chronic pneumonia, lung abscess, and lungworm infection. Coughing up blood suggests aspiration pneumonia or pharyngeal abscess.

A foul, rotten breath suggests pharyngitis, laryngitis, or fungal pneumonia. A dull sound produced on percussion of the sinus area indicates fluid accumulation caused by an inflammatory disease (e.g., tooth root abscess [maxillary sinuses], infected dehorning site, ascending respiratory infection [frontal sinuses]).

Cardiovascular and hemolymphatic systems. Enlarged submandibular, retropharyngeal, parotid, and prescapular lymph nodes may indicate regional inflammation or abscessation (caseous lymphadenitis). The ears should be warm to the touch. Cold ears may result from decreased peripheral blood flow (toxemia or hypocalcemia).

The clinician should observe and palpate the jugular furrows. In normal animals a jugular pulse may be noted extending about one third of the distance from the thoracic inlet toward the mandible. A distended jugular vein with a pulse extending all the way up the neck may indicate congestive heart failure and/or tricuspid valve insufficiency.

Neurologic systems. Signs of neurologic disease include asymmetric pupil size and face, nostril, ear, and eye positions. Additional signs include depression or hyperexcitability, head pressing, facial tremors, and retention of feed in the buccal pouches (see Chapter 11).

Thorax and Forelimbs

Skin and musculoskeletal systems. Examination of the skin over the thorax and forelimbs is the same as that for the head and neck. Careful observation for abnormal conformation is crucial for long-term production and survival of animals in range-grazing programs. Goats should be observed for gait abnormalities; a goat walking on its carpi may have footrot or caprine arthritis-encephalitis (CAE) virus infection. Excessive growth or wear on the lateral and medial surfaces of each claw should be noted. The clinician should check the coronary band for inflammation or separation from the foot and assess odors and discharges from the interdigital space. The joints should be palpated for swelling or pain and moved through a full range of motion. Swollen carpi may be caused by a carpal hygroma (no pain on manipulation) or CAE (painful when manipulated).

Respiratory system. The clinician can note the respiratory rate without disturbing the goat by observing the movements of the costal arch or nostrils at a distance. The average respiratory rate for an adult goat is 15 to 30 breaths per minute; kids have a respiratory rate of 20 to 40 breaths per minute (see Table 1-2). An increased respiratory rate may be a sign of excitement, high environmental temperature or humidity, pain, fever, respiratory or cardiovascular disease, or respiratory compensation for metabolic acidosis. A decreased respiratory rate may result from respiratory compensation for metabolic alkalosis. The clinician should carefully note signs of dyspnea or respiratory distress, including tachypnea, extended head and neck, open-mouth breathing, flaring nostrils, abducted elbows, and anal pumping.

The cranial border of the lung field is deep to the triceps, the dorsal border extends from the point of the shoulder to the last rib, and the caudoventral border arches from the point of the elbow to the last rib. The clinician can place a stethoscope well forward under the triceps to auscultate the cranial lung fields. Because of the goat's relatively thin chest wall, normal breath and bronchial sounds are readily detectable and may sound harsh (louder on inspiration than expiration). Bronchial sounds are usually loudest over the craniodorsal lung field at the level of the tracheal bifurcation. Increased breath sounds suggest the conditions listed previously as causing tachypnea. Decreased breath sounds may be appreciated with pneumothorax.

Abnormal lung sounds include crackles (air moving through inflammatory fluid in the airways) and wheezes (air moving through inflamed, narrowed airways). Respiratory conditions causing abnormal lung sounds include pulmonary edema and pneumonia. Because significant lung disease can be present without causing an audible abnormality, other signs of respiratory disease (e.g., signs of dyspnea along with fever, cough, and nasal discharge) must be assessed. The clinician should be aware of the interrelationship of the respiratory and cardiovascular systems; detection of disease in one system warrants careful examination of the other.

Cardiovascular and hemolymphatic systems. Auscultation of the heart is performed by slowly moving the stethoscope over the valves and locating the point of maximal intensity. On the left side of the thorax, the clinician can auscultate the pulmonic valve (low third intercostal space, below the elbow), the aortic valve (high fourth intercostal space, above the elbow), and the left atrioventricular (A-V) or mitral or bicuspid valve (low fifth intercostal space, at the level of the elbow). On the right side of the thorax the clinician auscultates the right A-V or tricuspid valve (high fourth intercostal space, above the elbow). Rate, rhythm, character, and intensity of the heart sounds should be assessed. Tachycardia (the normal heart rate ranges between 70 to 90 beats per minute in an adult goat and 90 to 150 beats per minute in a kid) may occur as a normal condition in young, ruminating, lactating, late-pregnant, or excited goats. Abnormal conditions causing tachycardia include anemia, congestive heart failure, pain, and inflammation. Bradycardia may result from a conduction block (A-V node block). A sinus arrhythmia is often detectable during late inspiration, and is normal. Abnormal arrhythmias may be noted (e.g., in atrial fibrillation).

Neurologic system. Signs of neurologic disease include incoordination and ataxia, proprioceptive deficits such as knuckling, stumbling, adduction, abduction, circumduction, abnormal postural placement, and flaccid limbs following repeated joint flexion.

Abdomen

Skin and musculoskeletal systems. A goat's body condition score can be estimated by palpating the lumbar vertebrae, rib cage, and sternum (see Chapter 2). Goats tend to deposit most of their body fat internally, around the abdominal viscera, so that an animal in normal health may appear thin on lumbar palpation. Examination of the abdominal skin is essentially the same as that described for the head and neck.

Digestive and gastrointestinal systems. Standing behind the goat, the clinician should observe the contours of the abdomen, looking at the left and right sides and upper and lower quadrants. These areas should be auscultated with alternating percussion and ballottement.

Distention of the left upper quadrant, with a gaseous "ping" on percussion, suggests ruminal tympany or bloat. A severely bloated rumen may distend the left upper, left lower, and right lower quadrants. Distention of the lower left quadrant with a firm feel on ballottement may indicate rumen impaction. Rumen contractions are counted by auscultating the left upper quadrant while gently placing a hand on the area to hear and feel the contractions. Normally one or two primary contractions occur each minute, associated with mixing of the ingesta. In addition, one secondary contraction occurs per minute, associated with eructation. Indigestion, metabolic or mineral imbalances, or generalized pain may decrease the rate of contraction.

Distention of the right upper quadrant, with a fluid wave on ballottement or a gaseous sound on percussion and auscultation, suggests distention of the cecum or spiral colon. Distention of the lower right quadrant with a firm feel on ballottement may result from a severely impacted abomasum or an advanced pregnancy.

Ventral abdominal distention of the lower left and right quadrants suggests chronic indigestion or ascites secondary to hypoproteinemia resulting from gastrointestinal parasitism or severe liver disease. A grossly enlarged liver (such as that seen in severe congestive heart failure) may be palpable on the right side of the abdomen behind the costal arch. Generalized abdominal distention, with no audible gastrointestinal motility, may be a sign of gastrointestinal ileus.

Respiratory system. Pronounced abdominal movements may be observed in an animal with dyspnea.

Cardiovascular and hemolymphatic systems. Bilateral ventral abdominal distention may indicate ascites resulting from congestive heart failure.

Urogenital and reproductive systems. Bilateral ventral abdominal distention also may indicate uroperitoneum caused by a ruptured bladder (common in castrated males). In urethral obstruction the clinician may note a solid-feeling distended bladder on deep palpation of the caudal abdomen. The left kidney also may be noted on deep palpation of the mid-dorsal abdomen and assessed for size, shape, and consistency. In young goats the umbilicus should be examined for signs of inflammation from an umbilical infection or dripping urine from a patent urachus.

Pelvis and Hindlimbs

Skin and musculoskeletal systems. The ventrum, teats, and genitalia should be examined for papules (papillomas), pustules, and ulcerations (contagious ecthyma). The skin and musculoskeletal examination of the pelvic limbs is similar to that performed for the forelimbs.

Digestive and gastrointestinal systems. The normal rectal temperature of a goat ranges between 38° and 40° C (see Table 1-2). Hyperthermia may result from elevated environmental temperature and humidity, stress and excitement, or inflammatory disease. Hypothermia may occur in malnourished or older animals. The perineum and the back of the hindlegs should be examined for fecal soiling. In young kids the presence or absence (atresia ani) of the anus should be noted.

Cardiovascular and hemolymphatic systems. The clinician should palpate the prefemoral and supramammary (female) or scrotal (male) lymph nodes and note any enlargement (caseous lymphadenitis). The rate and character of the pulse can be assessed by gentle palpation of the femoral artery in the inguinal region. An irregular pulse is occasionally noted in cases of atrial fibrillation or myocarditis. A strong pulse may occur in young, excited, lactating, ruminating, or late-pregnant animals, or in animals with anemia or inflammation. Recumbent animals or animals with hypovolemia, hypocalcemia, or left ventricular failure often have weak pulses.

Urogenital and reproductive systems. The clinician observes the scrotum for lesions, assesses the testicles for firmness and heat, and examines the prepuce and penis. Ulceration or occlusion of the preputial orifice suggests ulcerative posthitis (which occurs most commonly in goats on a high-protein diet). The preputial hairs should be examined for the presence of crystals or blood and for unusual dryness (in urethral calculi or obstructive urolithiasis). Anal pumping and perineal urethral pulsations (with the goat unable to urinate or dribbling urine) also may indicate obstructive urolithiasis. Edema in the prepuce and ventral abdomen, with tissue sloughing, may be a sign of a ruptured urethra.

The penis of the male goat is difficult to examine directly without sedation. However, the clinician may be able to exteriorize the penis by placing the goat on his

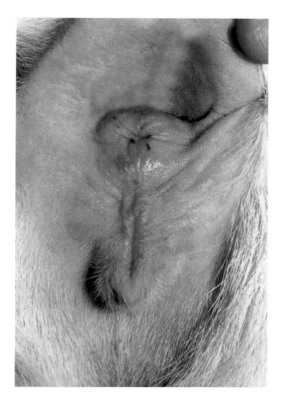

Figure 1-9   The vulva of a pluripara dairy doe. A subtle dermatitis is visible on the dorsal vulvar lips, but it is of no consequence in this case. No discharge, erythema, or enlargement of the clitoris is evident. After the area has been carefully washed and dried, a sterile vaginal speculum can be introduced to visualize the cervix.

The vulva and udder of the female should be examined for color and size (Figure 1-9). Swelling and hyperemia may indicate estrus or impending parturition. Crystals on the vulva hairs below the urethral orifice suggest a urinary tract infection. The clinician should note the color, consistency, and volume of any discharge from the vulva. A moderate, serous to cloudy discharge is common in late estrus. A reddish-brown, odorless discharge seen 1 to 3 weeks after parturition is probably lochia, the normal breakdown product of the cotyledonary attachments. The finding of large protruding vulva lips or clitoris or a short anogenital distance is suggestive of an intersex.

The udder should be palpated for symmetry, size, shape, and texture. A cold, dark udder suggests gangrenous mastitis. If the animal is lactating, the clinician should examine the teats for patency by expressing a small amount of milk, and note the color and consistency of the milk. Discolored, thick, or clumpy milk can indicate mastitis.

Neurologic system.   Findings suggestive of neurologic disease include posterior paresis with a distended bladder on deep palpation, as well as loss of anal and tail tone.

FURTHER READING

Gay CC: Clinical examination of sheep and goats. In Radostits OM, Mayhew IGJ, Houston DM, editors: *Veterinary clinical examination and diagnosis,* Philadelphia, 2000, WB Saunders.

Kelly WR: Clinical examination and making a diagnosis. In Radostits OM et al, editors: *Veterinary medicine,* ed 9, Philadelphia, 2000, WB Saunders.

Kelly WR: *Veterinary clinical diagnosis,* ed 3, London, 1984, Bailliere Tindall.

Smith BP: *Large animal internal medicine,* ed 2, St Louis, 1996, Mosby.

Wilson JH: The art of physical diagnosis, *Vet Clin North Am: Food Animal Pract* 8(2):169, 1992.

side and pulling back on the prepuce while pushing forward on the sigmoid flexure at the level of the perineum, then gently grasping the penis to keep it extended. The surface of the penis should be examined first. The clinician can then examine the urethral process for calculi or other lesions.

Chapter 2

Feeding and Nutrition

DARRELL L. RANKINS, JR., DEBRA C. RUFFIN, AND D.G. PUGH

Sheep and goats are small ruminants with a worldwide range. They are found under varying production schemes—from backyard pets to expansive range land grazing operations. The common goal of goat or sheep production units is conversion of forage to usable animal products (e.g., meat, milk, fiber). With regard to their grazing preferences, ruminants are categorized as browse selectors, grass and roughage grazers, or intermediate types.[1] Sheep are predominantly grass and roughage grazers, whereas goats are generally classified as intermediate types. Sheep tend to graze selectively and prefer higher-quality portions of the plant. As sheep age, they may be unable to consume adequate forage in range conditions because of dental disease. Goats have small mouths and prehensile lips and are active foragers that will readily consume flowers, fruits, and leaves. Goats can use browse that has woody stems or thorns. Similar to sheep, goats tend to select highly digestible portions of grasses. They will graze, but prefer to eat at head height, which is a natural protection mechanism against some nematode parasites. When given a choice, goats tend to select grass over legumes and browse over grass. They prefer to graze along fence lines and rough or rocky pasture areas. Goats flourish in areas featuring browse or numerous plant species to graze. However, they usually perform poorly compared with sheep or cattle on flat, improved, monoculture pastures. If given a choice, many meat goats (e.g., Boer, Spanish) prefer a diet of 80% to 85% browse and 15% to 20% grasses. Both sheep and goats use their mobile lips and tongue to consume their diets selectively. Goats have been mistakenly labeled as animals that will eat anything and subsist on feedstuffs of inadequate nutrient content. To the contrary, goats are extremely particular about their diet and refuse to consume feeds that have been soiled. The goat's inquisitive feeding habits result in their use of most species of forage present in the environment. The nutritional content of the diet selected by goats is greater than the average of the vegetation present on a pasture. These attributes have led to the use of goats for brush management in many regions of the world, whereas sheep are maintained in mostly pasture settings. Use of goats for weed and brush control predispose this specie to the ingestion of toxic plants. Some of the browse consumed by goats contains high concentrations of essential oils, lignin, or tannins, all of which depress digestion or are poorly digestible. Whenever browse is the predominant forage consumed, mineral uptake may be better than that expected from grasses grown on the same land. Many species of browse tend to have deeper roots, resulting in rich mineral content, possibly to the point of toxicity. Therefore goats maintained for brush control should be closely monitored for changes in body weight, body condition score, and hair coat; the clinician should note any signs of toxicosis. Sheep also are excellent converters of browse and brush to meat, fiber, and milk, but they are raised mostly as grazing animals.

WATER

Although it is often taken for granted, water is an extremely important nutrient. It is the major constituent of an animal's body. If an animal were deprived of all nutrients it would succumb to water deprivation first. Although sheep and goats may lose most of their body fat and 40% to 50% of their total body protein and survive, a water loss of only 10% can prove fatal. Both sheep and goats are particular about the quality of their water sources. In general, a clean, fresh source of water should be available at all times. Each ewe or doe should have at least 1 foot of water trough space; a paved surface 8 to 10 feet around the water source helps prevent unsanitary conditions conducive to many diseases, including footrot. Daily water intake can be affected by several factors.

Pregnancy and lactation increase water requirements and consumption—water intake is increased by the third month of gestation and is doubled by the last month. In addition, water intake is greater for females carrying twins than for those carrying only a single.[2] Likewise, lactating ewes or does consume twice as much water as nonlactating females: 7 to 15 liters compared with 3.5 to 7 liters per day, respectively. Animals grazing lush spring pastures where the forage water content may exceed 80% consume markedly less water than those consuming dry hay, which may be only 10% to 12% water. Obviously, lactating dairy animals require even greater quantities of water. When high-protein diets are being fed or when mineral consumption increases, water consumption also increases. Sheep may increase their water intake by twelve-fold during summer compared with intake during the winter months.[2] Water quality also can affect daily water consumption. For maintenance, individual goats and sheep usually consume 3.5 to 15 liters of water per day.[3]

Water varies in quality according to the amount and type of contaminant. The most common dissolved substances in water are calcium, magnesium, sodium chloride, sulfate, and bicarbonate.[3] If the salts of these minerals are present in high enough concentrations, depressed performance, illness, and occasionally death can result. In addition to causing various problems in animals, dissolved salts are additive in their suppression of production and health. As salt concentrations increase, water consumption is usually depressed, with young animals generally being more affected than adults. Over time, animals tend to adapt to water with high concentrations of dissolved salts. However, quick or abrupt changes from water with relatively low concentrations to water with high concentrations of dissolved substances are poorly tolerated.[3] Table 2-1 provides general guidelines for total dissolved solids in drinking water.[4-6] High sulfate concentrations in the 3500 to 5000 parts per million (ppm) range may result in suppressed copper absorption from the intestine. Nitrates, and less commonly, nitrites, are occasionally encountered in toxic concentrations from ground water (Table 2-2). Most safe, drinkable water has a pH of 7 to 8. As the alkalinity of water increases, its suitability for consumption decreases. Table 2-3 provides standards for various other water contaminants.

Although water contaminated with coliform bacteria has been associated with disease in humans, only rarely is coliform contamination of drinking water implicated as a causal agent of disease in sheep and goats. Only very young animals are generally affected.

Maloiy and Taylor[7] observed that goats are quite efficient at water conservation. Goats tend to adapt to high ambient temperatures better than other domestic ruminants and require less water evaporation to control body temperature. In addition, they possess the ability to reduce urine and fecal water losses during times of water deprivation.

In summary, sheep and goats should have access to a continuous supply of fresh, clean water in order to ensure that productivity is not compromised.

TABLE 2-1

GENERAL RECOMMENDATIONS FOR TOTAL DISSOLVED SOLIDS IN DRINKING WATER

TOTAL DISSOLVED SOLIDS (PPM)	COMMENTS
Less than 3500	Safe
3500-5000	May take animals time to adapt to this concentration; if sulfates are the predominant type of solid, some diarrhea may occur
5000-10,000	Safe for nonpregnant, nonlactating adults; may cause depressed water intake or production in young animals
More than 10,000	Unsafe

From Bauder J: When is water good enough for livestock? *Montana State Extension Bulletin,* 2000; Guyer PQ: *Livestock water quality,* University of Nebraska Extension Service Bulletin G79-46A; Meyer KB: *Water quality in animals,* 1999, Purdue University Extension Bulletin WQ9.

TABLE 2-2

POTENTIALLY DANGEROUS CONCENTRATIONS OF NITRATE NITROGEN IN DRINKING WATER*

NITRATE NITROGEN (PPM)	COMMENTS
Less than 100	Safe
100 to 300	Potentially unsafe when animals are consuming high-nitrate feedstuffs (e.g., during a drought)
More than 300	Not safe

*High sulfate concentrations in the 3500 to 5000 ppm range may result in copper absorption abnormalities.

From Bauder J: When is water good enough for livestock? *Montana State Extension Bulletin,* 2000; Guyer PQ: *Livestock water quality,* University of Nebraska Extension Service Bulletin G79-46A; Meyer KB: *Water quality in animals,* 1999, Purdue University Extension Bulletin WQ9.

TABLE 2-3

RECOMMENDED STANDARDS FOR UPPER LIMITS OF POTENTIALLY TOXIC CONTAMINANTS THAT MAY OCCUR IN WATER

CONTAMINANT	UPPER LIMIT OF CONTAMINATION (PPM)
Aluminum	5
Arsenic	0.2
Cadmium	0.01-0.05
Chromium	0.05-1
Cobalt	1
Copper	0.5
Fluoride	2-3
Iron	1-3
Lead	0.05-1
Mercury	0.01
Selenium	0.05
Vanadium	0.1
Zinc	25
Carbonate and bicarbonate	2000

From Bauder J: When is water good enough for livestock? *Montana State Extension Bulletin,* 2000; Guyer PQ: *Livestock water quality,* University of Nebraska Extension Service Bulletin G79-46A; Meyer KB: *Water quality in animals,* 1999, Purdue University Extension Bulletin WQ9.

ENERGY

Energy is probably the first limiting nutrient of most practical conditions where sheep and goats are maintained throughout the world. Energy requirements vary greatly depending on level and stage of production, level of activity, and intended animal use. Except in situations where rapid growth rates are desired or milk production is to be maximized, the energy requirement can usually be met with medium- to high-quality forage. However, under maximal production pressures, some sort of supplementation may be required. Energy-deficient diets can result in poor growth rates, lower body condition scores, decreased fiber production, decreased fiber diameter, decreased immune function, and increased susceptibility to parasitic diseases and other pathologies. Angora goats and many wool breeds of sheep are prone to various fiber production changes, whereas cashmere goats may be less susceptible.

The majority of the energy that is used by sheep and goats comes from the breakdown of structural carbohydrates from roughage. Therefore roughage should comprise the bulk of their diet. Energy can be expressed in terms of the net energy system (calories) or in terms of total digestible nutrients (TDN) as a percentage of the feed. The two expressions are interchangeable by use of various prediction equations; this chapter uses TDN as the measure. Currently, most feed and forage testing laboratories estimate TDN using the Van Soest fiber analysis. A representative sample is analyzed for neutral and acid detergent fiber contents, and then TDN is predicted based on one or both of these values. This system works effectively for most forages but is less reliable for feeds that are high in starch (e.g., corn). In general, warm-season, perennial grass hays are about 50% to 54% TDN, whereas many of the cereal grains are usually 80% to 90% TDN. Most forages in the green, vegetative state are about 62% to 70% TDN on a dry matter basis. Stemmy, dry, poor-quality hay is less than 50% TDN. By comparing these typical values with the requirements of various classes of sheep and goats, keepers can ascertain when supplemental energy sources are needed for forage-based rations. For example, a 150-pound ewe requires a diet containing 55% TDN for maintenance, 59% for late gestation, and 65% for the first 6 weeks of lactation. Therefore the dry, non-pregnant ewe could use low-quality forage, but the pregnant or lactating ewe needs a diet of lush, vegetative forage. If a good to excellent forage is unavailable, some type of energy supplement is required for the late pregnant or lactating ewe. Similarly, a 110-pound doe requires a diet containing 56% TDN for maintenance.[2,8]

A variety of choices are available for energy supplementation. The most common choice is cereal grains, corn being the most common of these. Corn is dense in energy, and most of that energy is in the form of starch. When appreciable levels of starch are supplemented to ruminants consuming forage-based diets, the general response is a decrease in forage intake and digestibility. However, the sheep or goat receiving corn supplementation still has a higher energy status because of the energy from the corn. Several other feedstuffs are available for use as energy supplements for ruminants consuming forage-based diets (e.g., oats, barley, rye). Two other non-traditional energy supplements are soybean hulls and wheat middlings. Soybean hulls are the outermost layer of the soybean and are comprised of abundant quantities of digestible fiber. Unlike corn, soybean hulls do not suppress fiber digestion but may increase hay digestibility. Even though soybean hulls have a TDN value 62% less than corn, they produce similar results when used as an energy supplement for ruminants consuming forages. Wheat middlings, a by-product of wheat milling, elicit similar responses. Often these by-product type feeds are much more economical than corn.[2,8]

Another source of energy supplementation is fat. In general, total fat content should not exceed 8% of the diet, or 4% to 5% as supplemental fat. In the southern

United States, where cotton production is prevalent, whole cottonseed (which contains approximately 24% fat) is used as an energy supplement for both sheep and goats. Sheep or goats should be supplemented with no more than 20% of their daily intake as whole cottonseed, assuming that the remainder of the diet contains no fat.

PROTEIN

As a general rule, a minimum of 7% dietary crude protein is needed for normal rumen bacterial growth and function for sheep and goats. If dietary protein drops below 7%, forage intake and digestibility are depressed. Protein deficiency is associated with decreased fiber production, slowed growth, decreased immune function, anemia, depressed feed use, edema, and death. All of the protein reaching the small intestine is in the form of bacterial or protozoal protein or dietary protein that escaped ruminal digestion. The quality (amino acid content) of the bacterial protein is, surprisingly, quite good. Therefore the quantity of dietary protein provided to adult ruminants is much more important than the quality. The opposite is true of the pre-ruminant lamb or kid. If lambs or kids are fed a milk replacer, it should be composed of milk by-products in order to have an adequate amino acid composition for maximal growth.

Crude protein content varies widely among the various feedstuffs. Warm-season, perennial grass hay samples can range from less than 6% to more than 12% crude protein, whereas legumes in the vegetative state may occasionally be more than 28% crude protein. The protein content of plants declines with maturity. Similar to energy needs, crude protein requirements vary with the animal's stage of production. For maintenance, a 150-pound ewe requires a diet including 8% to 9% protein, and a 110-pound doe needs a diet with 7% to 8% protein. During lactation both the ewe and doe require in excess of 13.5% protein, depending on the number of offspring suckling or, in the case of dairy goats and sheep, level of milk production. Supplementation of protein may be necessary for the heavy producing animals. Whenever grass hay is fed, protein deficiency should be a concern, particularly for growing or lactating animals. The most consistent sign of protein deficiency in lactating animals is poor weight gain or slow growth in their lambs or kids, particularly for twins or triplets.[2,8]

Typical protein supplements include the oilseed meals (cottonseed meal, soybean meal), commercially blended supplements containing both natural protein and non-protein nitrogen (range cubes or pellets, molasses-based products), and various by-products (whole cottonseed, corn gluten feed). Protein should be fed to meet, but not greatly exceed, requirements. Excess protein usually results in increased feed costs and higher incidences of diseases (heat stress, pizzle rot, urolithiasis).

Non-protein nitrogen (NPN) is an inexpensive way to increase the protein concentration of rations for sheep or goats. NPN is any source of nitrogen in the non-protein form, but the most commonly used type is urea. Whenever NPN is used, the diet should have sufficient amounts of highly fermentable energy components. Feeding grain with NPN can result in a decrease in rumen pH. This depresses the ability of the ruminal urease enzyme to ferment urea, resulting in a slower release or breakdown to ammonia and carbon dioxide (CO_2). Slowing this metabolic pathway allows more efficient protein synthesis by the rumen microbes. On the other hand, diets of poor quality roughage result in a higher rumen pH and enhanced urease activity. This results in a quicker release of ammonia, a poorer "marriage" of chains of carbon atoms and nitrogen for microbial protein synthesis, and a potential increase in the incidence of urea/ammonia toxicity. Whenever NPN is added to the diet, feeds containing a urease enzyme should be limited or avoided. Such urease-containing feeds include raw soybeans and wild mustard. Signs of urea-ammonia toxicity include dull or depressed demeanor, muscle tremors, frequent urination and defecation, excessive salivation, increased respiration, ataxia, tetanic spasms, and death. Treatment includes the infusion of a 5% acetic acid solution (vinegar and water) into the rumen through a stomach tube. In severe cases, rumenotomy and fluid therapy may be required.

The following rules of thumb are useful when feeding urea as a protein source:

1. Never use urea for more than one third of the protein in the diet or 3% of the grain portion of the diet.
2. Ensure that a highly fermentable source of carbohydrates (e.g., corn, milo) is fed along with NPN.
3. Avoid the sudden introduction of urea into the diet (allow at least 8 to 10 days for its introduction).
4. Ensure proper mixing of feedstuffs whenever urea is used.
5. If 1 pound of urea and 6 pounds of ground corn are cheaper than 7 pounds of cottonseed meal (CSM) or soybean meal (SBM), then the former diet may be efficiently fed. However, if 7 pounds of either CSM or SBM is less expensive, the urea should be avoided.
6. If the crude protein of the diet is greater than 14% of the dietary TDN, NPN is of little value. For example, if TDN is 45%, which is typical of many dry hays during winter, NPN is of limited or no value if the crude protein of the diet is greater than 6.3% ($45 \times 0.14 = 6.3$).

Because of varying dietary intakes and their relationship to body condition scoring, NPN is best used in sheep or goats with body condition scores greater than 2.5; they should be avoided in animals with a body condition score of less than 2. If NPN is offered to animals, it should be fed daily; less is used for protein synthesis if the supplement is fed less frequently. In an Australian study[9] the inclusion of NPN in poorly digestible forage diets for lambs resulted in increased weight gain and wool production and decreased signs of parasitic nematode infestation.

MINERALS

Clinicians generally consider seven macrominerals and eight microminerals when assessing mineral nutrition for sheep and goats (Table 2-4). The designations *macro* and *micro* do not reflect the minerals' relative importance, but rather the amount of each that is required as a portion of the diet. Macromineral needs are usually expressed as percentages of the diet, whereas micromineral needs are generally expressed as ppm or mg/kg. The seven commonly assessed macrominerals are calcium, phosphorus, sodium, chlorine, magnesium, potassium, and sulfur. The eight microminerals are copper, molybdenum, cobalt, iron, iodine, zinc, manganese, and selenium. Trace mineral deficiency is less common than energy, protein, or macromineral deficiency. They occur slowly over time and rarely cause the dramatic effects on productivity and body condition seen in protein deficiency.[2,8] In some cases of mineral deficiency a liver biopsy is the diagnostic

TABLE 2-4

MINERAL REQUIREMENTS OF SHEEP AND GOATS

MINERAL	SHEEP	GOATS
Sodium, %	0.09-0.18	0.09-0.2
Calcium, %	0.20-0.82	0.20-0.90
Phosphorus, %	0.16-0.38	0.14-0.40
Magnesium, %	0.12-0.18	0.12-0.18
Potassium, %	0.50-0.80	0.50-0.80
Sulfur, %	0.14-0.26	0.16-0.32
Iodine, ppm	0.10-0.80	0.60
Iron, ppm	30-50	more than 30
Copper, ppm	7-11	10
Molybdenum, ppm	0.10-0.5	0.10
Cobalt, ppm	0.10-0.20	0.10
Manganese, ppm	20-40	20-60
Zinc, ppm	20-33	45-50
Selenium, ppm	0.10-0.20	0.10-0.3

From *Nutrient requirements of sheep,* Washington, DC, 1985, National Academy Press; Bratzlaff K, Henlein G, Huston J: Common nutritional problems feeding the sick goat. In Naylor JM, Ralston SL, editors: *Large animal clinical nutrition,* St Louis, 1991, Mosby.

tool of choice. The technique for liver biopsy is covered in Chapter 4.

Calcium and **phosphorus** are interrelated and are therefore discussed together. Nearly all of the calcium in the body and most of the phosphorus is found in the skeletal tissues. Diets deficient in calcium and phosphorus may delay growth and development in young lambs and kids and predispose them to metabolic bone disease (e.g., rickets, osteochondrosis) (see Chapter 9). Likewise, calcium and phosphorus deficiencies in lactating ewes and does can dramatically reduce milk production. Serum phosphorus concentrations are not highly regulated but are still maintained between 4 and 7 mg/dl for sheep and between 4 and 9.5 mg/dl for goats. Phosphorus deficiency is the most commonly encountered mineral deficiency in range or winter pastured animals. Most forage tends to be high in calcium and relatively low in phosphorus; this is especially true in legumes. Beet pulp and legumes (such as clover and alfalfa) are good to excellent sources of calcium. For lactating dairy goats and sheep, supplemental calcium and phosphorus are necessary to meet high demands for milk production. Range goats may need less supplemental phosphorus than sheep because of their preference for browse and plants that tend to accumulate phosphorus. Phosphorus serum concentrations of less than 4 mg/dl may indicate phosphorus deficiency.[2] Phosphorus deficiency results in slow growth, listlessness, an "unkempt" appearance, depressed fertility, and depraved appetite or pica.[2]

Sheep and goats fed high grain or concentrate diets typically need supplemental calcium and little to no additional phosphorus. Grains are relatively low in calcium but contain moderate to high concentrations of phosphorus. Although serum calcium is tightly held in a narrow range, serum concentrations consistently below 9 mg/dl are suggestive of chronic calcium deficiency.[2] Chronic parasitism can decrease the body stores of both calcium and phosphorus.[2] Common calcium supplements include oyster shells and limestone. Defluorinated rock phosphate is an excellent source of phosphorus. Dicalcium phosphate or steamed bone meal (where available) are good sources for both. The calcium-to-phosphorus ratio should be maintained between 1:1 and 2:1.[2,8]

Sodium and **chlorine** are integral components of many bodily functions. Salt (sodium chloride [NaCl]) is the carrier for most ad lib mineral supplements. If salt is not offered ad lib, it should be incorporated into a complete ration at a level of 0.5% of the diet. Sodium is predominately an extracellular ion and is important for normal water metabolism, intracellular and extracellular function, and acid-base balance. Conversely, chloride is an intracellular ion, functions in normal osmotic balance, and is a component of gastric secretions. Sheep or goats that are deficient in salt intake routinely chew wood, lick the soil, or consume other unlikely plants or debris. The

NaCl content of feeds may be increased to 5%, particularly for feeding males, to help increase water intake and reduce the incidence of urolithiasis.

Salt is commonly used as a carrier to ensure trace mineral intake because sheep and goats have a natural drive for NaCl. If the clinician, nutritionist, or rancher elects to use a salt-containing mineral mixture to ensure mineral intake, he or she should be aware that individual consumption may vary drastically. Furthermore, improperly prepared salt mixtures or blocks, feed supplements, liquid feeds, or certain types of food or water contamination can drastically alter mineral consumption. Salt also is useful as an intake limiter for energy-protein supplements. A 10% to 15% NaCl mixture of two parts ground corn and one part soybean meal is approximately 20% crude protein. The added salt usually limits intake to 0.45 kg of this mixture per adult goat per day. Whenever using salt-limited feeding, the keeper should take care to introduce the feedstuffs slowly over 2 to 3 weeks and provide access to adequate quantities of fresh clean water. Only white salt should be used as in intake limiter. If trace mineral salt or ionized salt is used, mineral (e.g., copper, iodine) toxicity is likely, particularly in sheep.

Magnesium is important for normal functioning of the nervous system and is required for many enzymatic reactions. Skeletal magnesium can be used by the animal during times of deficiency, but the skeletal magnesium reserve is much smaller than the calcium reserve. Most fast-growing, heavily fertilized cereal grains or grass pastures are deficient in magnesium. Magnesium absorption is depressed by high concentrations of plant potassium and/or rumen ammonia. Legume and legume-grass mixed pastures are good sources of magnesium. A magnesium deficiency can lead to a condition known as *grass tetany* in either sheep or goats. Magnesium toxicity is very rare.

Potassium is required for normal acid-base balance and is an integral component of many enzymatic pathways; it functions as an intracellular ion. The requirement is between 0.5% and 0.8% of the diet depending on the stage of production. Most grains contain less than 0.4% potassium, whereas fresh green forages generally contain more than 1%. However, dormant forages may have much lower potassium concentrations. Potassium deficiencies or toxicities are rare for sheep and goats. However, deficiencies may occur in highly stressed animals being fed diets composed mostly of grain. Therefore, under stressful situations (such as weaning), supplemental potassium may be indicated for animals fed predominantly on grain.[2,8]

Sulfur is a component of many bodily proteins. It is found in high concentrations in wool and mohair because of the large amounts of sulfur-containing amino acids (cystine, cysteine, and methionine) in keratin. Sulfur deficiency can reduce mohair production in Angora goats.[10] The general recommendation is to maintain a 10:1 nitrogen-to-sulfur ratio in sheep and goat diets.[2,8] This has been recently substantiated by Qi et al,[11] who reported ideal ratios of 10.4:1 for maximal gains and 9.5:1 for maximal intake in growing goats. However, a ratio as low as 7.2:1 has been suggested for optimal mohair production.[12] If the forage is low in sulfur content or large quantities of urea are used in the diet, weight gain and fiber production can be increased by providing supplemental sulfur. In sheep and goats, sulfur deficiency may result in anorexia, reduced weight gain, decreased milk production, decreased wool growth, excessive tearing, excessive salivation, and, eventually, death. Browsing animals such as goats may ingest enough tannins to decrease sulfur availability. Sulfur deficiency also depresses digestion, decreases microbial protein synthesis, decreases use of NPN, and lowers the rumen microbial population. Whenever NPN is fed to fiber-producing animals, sulfur supplementation is indicated. With the possible exception of oats and barley, the sulfur content of most cereal grains is usually low to deficient, although corn-soybean diets usually meet requirements for the ruminal synthesis of sulfur-containing amino acids.

Sulfur toxicity is occasionally seen where calcium sulfate is used as a feed intake limiter. It also occurs when ammonium sulfate is fed as a source of NPN or as a urinary acidifier. If sulfur is supplemented in the form of sulfate, toxicity may occur, particularly if the sulfur content is greater than 0.4% of the diet.[2] Sulfate can be reduced to sulfide in the rumen or lower bowel. Sulfide in large enough concentrations can result in polioencephalomalacia that is only partially responsive to thiamine.

Copper deficiencies can be primary (as a result of low intake) or secondary (caused by high concentrations of molybdenum, sulfur and iron, or other substances in feedstuffs). In the rumen, copper, molybdenum, and sulfur form thiomolybdates, which reduce copper availability. Copper's ability to function as part of the enzymes needed for specific biochemical reactions is depressed. This impairment in metabolism results in clinical signs of deficiency. Other factors that alter copper absorption include high concentrations of dietary cadmium, iron, selenium, zinc, and vitamin C in the animal, as well as alkaline soils. Roughage grown on "improved pastures" (fertilized, limed) is more likely to be deficient. Liming reduces copper uptake by plants, and many fertilizers contain molybdenum. Good quality lush grass forages have less available copper than most hays, and legumes have more available copper than most grasses. Liver copper reserves last up to 6 months in sheep.[2,8]

Signs of copper deficiency include microcytic anemia, depressed milk production, lighter or faded hair color, poor quality fleeces, heart failure, infertility, increased susceptibility to disease, slowed growth, enlarged joints, lameness, gastric ulcers, and diarrhea. These signs appear to be more severe with primary copper deficiencies than with a lowered copper-molybdenum ratio. Sheep with copper deficiencies have inferior wool, which is usually characterized as "stringy" or "steely." Such wool lacks both tensile strength and crimp. Growing lambs and kids are more susceptible to copper deficiency, followed by lactating females.

Several breed differences have been observed with regard to copper metabolism. For example, some Finnish-Landrace sheep may have lower serum copper concentrations than Merinos, which in turn have lower serum copper levels than British breeds at similar levels of intake.[13] Milk is usually deficient in copper, and molybdenum is concentrated. Lambs suspected of having the swayback condition usually have a liver copper concentration of less than 80 ppm dry weight.

Anecdotal reports indicate that goats offered only sheep mineral (with low to absent added copper and added molybdenum) may succumb to copper deficiency. This deficiency may be magnified in pygmy goats and young, growing animals. Merino sheep and dwarf goat breeds require 1 to 2 ppm more copper than other breeds. Copper is absorbed more efficiently by young animals than adults.[2,8]

Very young lambs or kids can present with **enzootic ataxia**. Affected animals are born from copper-deficient ewes or does. The swayback condition of lambs or kids is usually seen at birth but may be diagnosed in animals up to 3 months of age. Neonates may experience a progressive ascending paralysis. Signs of this ataxia include muscular incoordination (especially in the hindlegs), lack of nursing, and death. Most neonates die within 3 to 4 days of the first symptoms. Affected older animals may survive or die, depending on severity. Rear limb ataxia, muscle atrophy, and weakness are seen in lambs or kids from 2 weeks to 3 months of age. A definitive diagnosis is made with necropsy. Histopathologic examination of the spinal cord reveals myelin degeneration and cavitations of cerebral white matter. Liver copper concentrations are invariably depressed. Prevention and treatment require copper supplementation (oral supplements, copper needles, a trace mineral mixture, or injectable copper) and attaining a good dietary copper-to-molybdenum ratio.

If copper deficiency is suspected, the copper, molybdenum, sulfur, and iron concentrations of the diet should be determined. To confirm copper deficiency, the nutritionist or clinician should measure body tissue concentration. Serum copper is commonly used to determine body copper status, but much of the copper is bound in the clot, making plasma a more reliable indicator of body copper status. Unfortunately, from a body assessment standpoint, blood copper concentrations may be falsely increased by stress or disease. If serum copper is overtly low and animals were not stressed during sampling, copper deficiency is likely. If serum copper concentrations are used for assessment, and copper concentrations fall within normal ranges, additional copper supplementation is of little or no value. An exception is if serum copper is normal but dietary molybdenum is high or if the copper-to-molybdenum ratio is less than 4:1. In this case the assayed copper may not be available for use in body metabolism. The dietary copper–to-molybdenum ratio should be maintained between 5:1 and 10:1. Liver is the best tissue to determine body copper status, but it has limitations and is a poor indicator of short-term copper balance. If liver copper is marginal, but plasma or serum copper is in the normal range, the animal may have a favorable response to copper supplementation. In such a case, dietary copper is probably deficient, and the liver stores of copper are being depleted. If the clinician suspects a herd problem, he or she should sample not only a cross-section of ages and production status, but also as many animals who are showing clinical signs as possible.

Forage samples should be taken for copper and trace mineral analysis. Core samples of hay should be properly collected. Feed samples should be placed in plastic bags, not brown paper boxes or bags. Dietary copper should range between 4 and 15 ppm. In areas where copper deficiency is a problem in goats, a mineral mixture with 0.5% copper sulfate should be offered free choice. However, this level of copper may be toxic for sheep.[2,8] In extremely deficient areas, copper needles can be administered orally or copper can be injected parenterally.

Copper toxicity is a much larger problem in sheep than goats. The magnitude of difference between copper deficiency and copper toxicity is quite small. Copper toxicity can occur in sheep as a result of simple mixing errors during the formulation of mineral premixes or by feeding mineral mixes formulated for species other than sheep. Sources of toxic concentrations of copper include premixes, trace mineral supplements made for species other than sheep, copper sulfate–containing foot baths, high copper-containing feedstuffs (horse, hog, or chicken feeds), and some nontraditional feedstuffs (broiler litter). Signs of copper toxicity include increased respiration, depression, weakness, hemoglobinuria, icterus, and acute death. Gross pathology of affected animals includes signs of a massive hemolytic crisis and dark, hemoglobin-filled kidneys. Treatment includes the use of D-penicillamine (50 mg/kg once a day) and ammonium tetrathiomolybdate (3.4 mg/kg every other day)(see Chapters 4 and 10). Goats are closer to cattle than sheep in susceptibility to copper toxicity.

Cobalt is used by rumen bacteria in the formation of vitamin B_{12}. It is deficient in some highly organic and/or poorly drained soils. Cobalt deficiency in sheep or goats is characterized as a classic B_{12} deficiency, with symptoms including lack of appetite, emaciation, anemia, and "wasting disease." Cobalt deficiency is associated with white liver disease, although phosphorus and copper deficiencies and chronic parasitism also play roles in pathogenesis. Animals with this condition have excessive ophthalmic discharge and become extremely pale. Necropsy reveals a fatty liver (see Chapter 4). To determine whether a cobalt deficiency exists, the clinician must evaluate the complete diet. Serum or urinary methylmalonic acid is increased, and serum vitamin B_{12} and liver cobalt concentrations are depressed in cobalt deficiency. However, diagnosis may be difficult because of the normally low tissue concentration of cobalt. A diet with a cobalt concentration of 0.1 ppm is adequate in most instances, but dietary levels below 0.06 ppm should be considered deficient. If a frank deficiency exists, a cobalt-supplemented trace mineral mixture should be fed ad lib. Cobalt toxicity is of minimal concern for sheep and goats under practical conditions in North America.[2,8]

Iron deficiency in sheep and goats is quite rare under grazing conditions. Lambs or kids raised in total confinement and deprived of access to pasture and earth-floored stalls or paddocks may become deficient. Iron deficiency is exacerbated when young animals are fed a milk replacer deficient in iron. Newborn kids and lambs are born with minimal iron stores. Iron is an important component of hemoglobin, and a deficiency can result in microcytic-hypochromic anemia. Iron deficiency is a rare problem in adults, except in cases of excessive parasitism. In kids and lambs with diagnosed iron deficiency, iron dextran (150 mg intramuscularly) at 2- to 3-week intervals may prove a valuable therapy.[10] Parenteral iron dextran may be toxic, and clinicians should exercise caution when using it.[10] If selenium deficiency also exists, the use of iron dextran can result in painful muscle reactions. The iron requirement is generally 30 to 40 ppm of the diet.

Iodine deficiency is more common in certain geographic regions of North America, particularly the northern tier states of the United States. Iodine availability is depressed by methylthiouracil, nitrates, perchlorates, soybean meal, and thiocyanates. Minerals that interfere with iodine absorption include rubidium, arsenic, fluorine, calcium, and potassium. Iodine appears to be most available for use by the body during winter months and during lactation. The form or "state" in which iodine exists in the feed alters availability—iodates are absorbed more readily than iodides. Signs of iodine deficiency include goiter, poor growth, depressed milk yield, pregnancy toxemia, and reproductive abnormalities (e.g., abortion; stillbirth; retained placentas; irregular estrus; infertility; depressed libido; birth of small, weak, and either hairless or short, fuzzy-haired newborns). Lambs or kids born to iodine-deficient dams may have enlarged thyroid glands. Affected kids can be treated with 3 to 6 drops of iodine (Lugol's solution) daily for 7 days. Commonly the enlarged thyroid in the kid is a congenital problem unassociated with dietary iodine (see Chapter 7). After a thorough examination of the diet, if iodine deficiency is still suspected, the clinician can use serum or plasma thyroxine to assess the body status; these markers are lowered in deficient states. Iodine is readily absorbed, so most sources will work well in salt-mineral mixtures or feed supplements. Iodine levels of 0.8 ppm for lactating animals and 0.2 ppm for nonlactating ewes or does are usually sufficient. Applying iodine (tincture or Lugol's, 1 to 2 ml) to the skin of a pregnant female once each week is a labor-intensive but rewarding method of preventing iodine deficiency–induced hypothyroidism. Occasionally hyperiodinism is associated with the feeding of kelp or related plants in mineral mixtures. This is a clinical problem in the occasional pet or dairy goat. Simply removing the iodine source may be all that is required for treatment of toxicity.[2,8]

Zinc is associated with deficiency-related disease or dysfunction in sheep and goats. Zinc availability is improved by the presence of vitamin C, lactose, and citrate in the diet. Oxalates, phytates, and large dietary concentrations of calcium, cadmium, iron, molybdenum, and orthophosphate all depress zinc availability. Zinc concentrations are usually higher in legumes than in grasses, but legumes invariably contain large concentrations of calcium, which can depress zinc availability. Zinc tends to be less available from cereal grain. Signs of zinc deficiency include dermatitis and parakeratosis, depressed milk production, impaired appetite, poor feed utilization, slowed growth, increased susceptibility to footrot, less hair on legs and head, swollen joints, poor growth, deceased reproductive performance, reduced testicular development, impaired vitamin A metabolism, and increased vitamin E requirements. Male goats appear more sensitive to marginal zinc intake.

When zinc deficiency is suspected, the clinician should carefully sample all constituents of the diet. Serum or plasma should be properly collected into tubes specifically designed for trace mineral analysis (royal blue top or trace mineral tubes). Hemolysis alters the accuracy of serum and plasma samples, because red blood cells have high zinc concentrations. Liver samples yield the most reproducible measurements of the zinc status of the animal. Both polystyrene containers and brown paper bags may be contaminated with zinc and should not be used for sample collection. Diets containing 20 to 50 ppm of zinc are usually sufficient except for animals that consume a high percentage of legumes in their diets. In these cases a chelated form of zinc is indicated. Trace mineral-salt mixes with 0.5% to 2% zinc usually prevent deficiency. The difference between required and toxic amounts is quite large, and therefore zinc toxicity is rare under most conditions.[2,8]

The absorption of **selenium** from the small intestine is enhanced by adequate dietary levels of vitamins E and A and histidine. Large dietary quantities of arsenic, calcium, vitamin C, copper, nitrates, sulfates, and unsaturated fats inhibit selenium absorption. Legumes are usually better sources of selenium than are grasses, which, in turn, are superior to cereal grains (see also Chapter 9).

The signs of selenium deficiency include nutritional muscular dystrophy, particularly of the skeletal and cardiac muscles of fast-growing young lambs or kids, and retained placentas. Signs associated with insufficient selenium include poor growth, weak or premature lambs or kids, depressed immune function, mastitis, and metritis. Most often, selenium deficiency is observed in lambs between birth and 8 weeks of age. Serum selenium concentrations are difficult to interpret because they may reflect the dietary intake in the past 2 to 4 weeks. Whole blood selenium is reflective of dietary selenium intake over the past 100-plus days. Liver concentration is the measurement of choice for diagnosing selenium deficiency. However, the authors of this chapter prefer to use whole blood selenium to determine selenium adequacy. Diets containing 0.1 to 0.3 ppm of selenium are usually adequate. The upper limit (0.3 ppm) should be fed during the final trimester of pregnancy. Mineral-salt mixes should contain between 24 and 90 ppm selenium in deficient regions. Of course, dietary limits may be restricted to different levels in different countries and states of the United States. In cases of frank deficiency, injectable vitamin E and selenium preparations may be given. Selenium toxicity may occur, but deficiency is the more prevalent problem. Toxicity is characterized by wool break, anorexia, depression, incoordination, and death[2,8] (see Chapter 9).

VITAMINS

Because the rumen normally synthesizes B vitamins in healthy sheep and goats, the only vitamins needed in the diets of nonstressed animals are the fat-soluble vitamins: A, D, E, and K. If an animal has altered rumen function, is parasitized, is on a low-fiber diet, or is being given long-term antibiotic therapy, supplemental B vitamins may be of value.

Vitamin A is involved in numerous bodily functions. It is essential for growth, proper skeletal development, normal reproduction, vision, and epithelial tissue integrity. Signs of vitamin A deficiency include weight loss, depressed immune function, night blindness, decreased fertility, and hair loss. Vitamin A can be stored in the liver for 4 to 6 months or longer. Green, vegetative forage meets the daily vitamin A requirement of all classes of sheep and goats, which is 45 to 50 IU per kg of body weight per day for nonlactating animals.[2] During late gestation and lactation the requirement increases to 85 IU per kg of body weight per day. Plants do not contain preformed vitamin A, but instead have vitamin A's carotenoid precursors.[2,8] Hay that is brown and dry and has been stored for long periods is probably deficient. Vitamin-mineral supplements that also contain oxidizing agents (e.g., copper, iron) are subject to oxidative destruction during storage. Although the label may suggest that vitamin A is present, its activity may be minimal.

Vitamin D requirements are generally met if the animals are exposed to sunlight. In confinement feeding operations or during sustained overcast or cloudy conditions, vitamin D should be supplemented. Vitamin D deficiency can occur in heavily wooled lambs raised with limited access to sunlight or sun-cured forages. Winter months tend to be the most common time for marginal blood vitamin D concentrations. Vitamin D, along with calcium and phosphorus, is important for normal bone integrity. Deficiencies can result in rickets (see Chapter 9). Plants, both fresh and in the form of hay (particularly sun-cured hay), contain abundant quantities of ergocalciferol (vitamins D_2 and D_3). The vitamin D requirement for sheep is 5 to 6 IU per kg of body weight per day, except for early weaned lambs, which have a requirement of 6 to 7 IU per kg of body weight per day.[2] For conversions, 1 IU of vitamin D equals 0.025 μg of crystalline D_3.[2,8]

Vitamin E is a biologic antioxidant that plays a major role in cell membrane integrity. It is closely associated with selenium in its mode of action, and a deficiency of either can lead to white muscle disease, depressed immune function, and depressed fertility in sheep and goats. Lambs from vitamin E–deficient ewes may experience stiffness, paralysis, and pneumonia. If a higher than expected incidence of infection and disease is noted in lambs or kids, the keeper or clinician should investigate the herd's vitamin E intake. In selenium-deficient areas, young lambs should generally be given extra vitamin E and selenium by injection. Vitamin E is poorly stored in the body, so daily intake is crucial. Although vitamin E is found in most good-quality forages, if females are consuming poor-quality hay (particularly in selenium-deficient areas), supplementation is required. Feeds rich in vitamin E include alfalfa meal, cottonseed meal, and brewer's grain. Some feedstuffs (e.g., corn, high sulfur-containing feeds, onions) decrease vitamin E availability. The current National Research Council (NRC) recommendations for vitamin E requirements of sheep are 20 IU per kg of feed in dry matter for lambs weighing less than 20 kg. Lambs heavier than 20 kg and ewes require 15 IU per kg of feed in dry matter.[2]

If a ruminant animal is healthy, the keeper does not need to supplement **vitamin K.** Vitamin K is important for normal blood clotting and vision. In healthy animals it is produced in sufficient quantities in the rumen and lower gut.

MINERAL FEEDING

A salt block or loose salt is just that—a block or loose mixture of NaCl. Trace mineral salt in block or loose form is composed of NaCl (usually 98% to 99%) with added trace microminerals. The adequacy or content of certain minerals in the block or loose salt mixture is generally not specified. The nutritionist or clinician should carefully evaluate the type of salt-mineral supplement that is being offered to sheep or goats.

Most adult ewes consume around 0.3 to 0.8 kg of a mineral mix per month, or about 10 to 28 g daily. Sheep and goats maintained in dry lots usually consume more than this, whereas those that graze or browse on range consume less. Although commonly used, salt blocks are inappropriate for both sheep and goats, and their use can lead to inadequate mineral intake and the occasional broken tooth. A commonly used mixture of 40% dicalcium phosphate and 60% trace mineral salt offered ad lib generally provides an effective yet inexpensive salt-mineral supplement. If vitamin E supplementation is required, 1 kg (2¼ lb) of a vitamin E supplement containing 44,100 IU per kg can be combined with 22.7 kg (50 lb) of trace mineral salt. If animals consume 10 to 17 g of the mixture daily, requirements for vitamin E should be met. If the keeper is concerned that sheep or goats are not consuming enough of the mineral, he or she can monitor intake by weighing the mineral being offered weekly. If animals are not consuming enough of the supplement, the addition of corn, molasses, or soybean meal may enhance uptake. If too much of the mixture is being consumed, the addition of white salt will curtail intake.

FEED ADDITIVES

To date, very few feed additives have been approved in the United States by the Food and Drug Administration for use in sheep and goats (see Appendix I). Two antibiotics, chlortetracycline and oxytetracycline, have been approved as feed additives for sheep in the United States. Dietary antibiotics may improve average daily gain, increase feed conversion, and reduce the losses associated with certain diseases (e.g., pneumonia, enterotoxemia) of lambs and kids when incorporated into creep feeds or finishing diets. Responses are variable and depend on management and the degree of stress the lambs are experiencing. Chlortetracycline and tetracycline are labeled in the United States for increased feed efficiency and improved body weight gain (20 to 60 g per ton of feed), for the prevention of *Campylobacter fetus* abortion in breeding ewes (80 mg per animal per day), and for the treatment of bacterial pneumonia caused by *Pasteurella multocida* and enteritis caused by *Escherichia coli* (22 mg per kg of body weight per day). Both of these antibiotics have been successfully used in similar dosages in goats (off label) to treat the conditions listed for sheep. These antibiotics may be milled into complete diets or top-dressed onto feeds to treat footrot or conjunctivitis in situations where individual animal treatment is difficult. Individual animal intake may vary, with resultant alterations in response to therapy. Whenever feed-based antibiotics are used, anorexic animals will have insufficient intake for proper therapy.

Two ionophores, lasalocid and monensin, are approved in the United States as feed additives for control of coccidiosis in sheep and goats, respectively. Both are approved only for confinement feeding, and neither are approved for use in animals whose milk is to be used for human consumption in the United States. If the ionophores are fed to ewes or does 30 days before they give birth, they can reduce the shedding of infective oocysts and may reduce pasture contamination and resultant coccidiosis infection in young lambs or kids. Both have value in improving weight gain and feed efficiency in adults and young growing animals. Ionophores also enhance proprionic acid fermentation in the rumen, thus increasing the pool of glucose precursors and aiding in the prevention of pregnancy toxemia in late-term ewes and does. These drugs have the added benefit of decreasing the incidence of free-gas bloat in animals on high grain–low forage diets (show lambs, feedlot lambs).

Decoquinate is another anticoccidial feed additive that is licensed for use in sheep and goats in the United States. However, it is not approved for use in animals producing milk for human consumption. Decoquinate acts early in the life cycle of coccidia, before they can cause gastrointestinal damage, therefore preventing some of the more serious consequences of infection. Decoquinate is very safe and can be added to feed, mineral mixtures, and milk or milk replacers. Lambs or kids at risk of developing coccidiosis because of stress or environmental contamination and ewes or does in late gestation are likely candidates for the use of this feed additive. To maximize their effectiveness, decoquinate-containing feeds should be fed continually for a minimum of 28 days.

The dewormer morantel is approved as a feed additive for goats to control gastrointestinal nematodes. Feed additive anthelmintics are valuable for use in animals that are difficult to handle individually because of demeanor or lack of facilities. However if anthelmintics are fed continuously and consistent therapeutic intake is not met, anthelmintic resistance will occur.

The anionic salts ammonium chloride and ammonium sulfate are both urinary acidifying agents, that help prevent certain types of urolithiasis when added to the diets of rams, bucks, and wethers. Urolithiasis may occur in males (who have smaller urethral diameters than females) consuming high-grain diets. This is particularly true in pet goats, breeding bucks or rams, and feedlot lambs. However, these anionic salts tend to be unpalatable, and because of their effective dosage rate (200 mg per kg per day), their use may result in depressed feed intake.

The term *yeast culture* refers to yeast and the medium on which it is grown. It can be dried, preserved, and used as a feed additive. Although the mode of action has not yet been determined, it appears that the feeding of some yeast cultures may stimulate dry matter intake and fiber digestion, especially in mildly stressed animals. These yeast cultures may stimulate the growth of ruminal bacteria, which utilize lactic acid. The quality of these products should be examined closely before their use. Yeast culture may be useful in easing animals onto grain-rich diets and minimizing rumen upset during the diet transition phase.

Buffers are salts that resist pH changes, whereas neutralizing agents neutralize acid and therefore increase pH. Some feed-grade buffers include sodium bicarbonate, sodium sesquicarbonate, sodium bentonite, and calcium carbonate. Magnesium oxide, sodium carbonate, and sodium hydroxide are neutralizing agents. Buffers and neutralizing agents can be added to high-grain diets (e.g., diets fed to feedlot lambs, show lambs, and dairy animals) to help ease the rapid changes in ruminal pH associated with the ingestion of excessive concentrates. Sodium bicarbonate is probably the most widely used of these chemicals. The response to feeding buffers appears to be variable except when they are used in dairy animals receiving high-grain diets. Buffers are of less value when forage-based diets are fed. In dairy goats and sheep, buffering agents improve milk production, minimize milk fat depression, decrease the incidence of lactic acidosis-rumenitis complex, and improve overall health. These buffers may be fed ad lib to dairy goats, included in a total mixed diet at around 1%, or top-dressed onto the feed.[10]

FIBER

Fiber is an important component of the diet of a ruminant animal. Without adequate fiber in the diet, normal rumination does not occur. In sheep, feeding a concentrate-based diet with limited amounts of fiber results in "wool pulling" as the animals seek a roughage source. To promote a healthy rumen, the dietary fiber content should generally be greater than 50%.

Fiber also is required in the diet to maintain acceptable levels of milk fat. The particle size of the fiber is important. It is generally suggested that a minimum particle size of 1 to 2.5 cm be fed to stimulate normal rumination, although the effect of smaller particles is not well documented in sheep and goats. Pelleted roughage does not meet the requirement for fiber size. Animals being fed pelleted forage or lush pasture should be offered hay.[14]

PELLETED FEEDS

The process of pelleting compacts feeds by forcing them through a die. Pelleting of feeds decreases waste, allows for easier storage and mechanization, and decreases labor. However, it usually increases the total feeding cost. Compacting the feed ingredients reduces or eliminates fines and dust particles and therefore increases palatability. The pelleting process reduces separation and feed sorting, preventing the intake of only certain parts of the total feed. Because pelleting usually entails grinding, particle size is usually reduced, somewhat improving digestibility. However, feeding pellets can result in decreased milk fat in dairy animals, urolithiasis in males, and an increased incidence of ulcers and choke. Pelleting also may reduce or destroy much of the vitamins A, E, and K in the feed. Therefore, when pelleting feeds, manufacturers should fortify these nutrients in the pellet.

FEED ANALYSIS

Both sheep and goats can derive nutritional value from numerous feeds. A listing of a wide array of feeds and their nutritional content can be found in Table 2-5. For simplicity, energy values are reported as TDN. Many feeds have limitations on their use because of such factors as fat content, palatability, moisture content, antinutritional factors, and other attributes beyond the scope of this chapter.

To analyze the nutrient content of a given feedstuff, the clinician must obtain a representative sample. For hay samples, random sampling of approximately 10% of the bales is adequate. For large round bales a core sample into the round side of the bale to a depth of approximately 78 cm is ideal. Most sampling devices provide an approximate 2.5-cm diameter core from the bale. All of the core samples should be combined into one container and thoroughly mixed. From this combined mix, the clinician should properly package a subsample of approximately 0.22 kg and send it to a laboratory for analysis. Samples of silage and other high-moisture feeds should be frozen before shipment to the testing laboratory. To analyze bulk feeds that are stored in bins or other storage facilities, the clinician should take several random grab samples as the feed is being augered or unloaded. Forage can be evaluated by appearance, albeit with much less accuracy than with some sort of analysis. Green, leafy forage that is free of mold or weeds is usually more nutritious.

After a representative sample arrives at the laboratory, it is analyzed for a variety of nutritive components. First, the sample is assayed for moisture content. Most feeds contain approximately 10% to 15% moisture, possibly less in arid environments. The dry matter of a feed is therefore important, and for comparison the nutrient content of the feed is reported as a percent of its dry matter. If the moisture content exceeds 15%, mold contamination is a problem. In addition, total ash content also may be determined and individual minerals measured. Total ash content may be of value for various by-product feeds in which dust or soil contamination may be a problem.

The fiber content also should be determined. Most laboratories use the Van Soest procedure, which is based on the use of detergents. The first step is to boil the sample in a neutral detergent solution and separate the cell contents from the fiber. The undissolved fraction is referred to as the *neutral detergent fiber (NDF)*. This NDF fraction is then boiled in an acid detergent solution, dissolving the hemicellulose and leaving behind the remaining fraction, the *acid detergent fiber (ADF)*. This fraction is dissolved in 72% sulfuric acid, which solubilizes the cellulose. The remaining lignin and silica are separated by

TABLE 2-5

NUTRIENT COMPOSITION OF VARIOUS FEEDSTUFFS FOR SHEEP AND GOATS*

FEEDSTUFF	DRY MATTER %	TOTAL DIETARY NUTRITION %	CRUDE PROTEIN %	CALCIUM %	PHOSPHORUS %
ALFALFA					
Fresh	26.0	59.8	20.3	1.88	0.27
Hay, sun-cured, early bloom	90.5	56.5	19.2	1.39	0.21
Hay, sun-cured, mature	91.2	55.0	14.5	1.17	0.21
Meal, dehydrated	91.8	60.4	19.1	1.5	0.24
BAHIA GRASS					
Fresh	28.7	54.7	12.5	0.45	0.31
Hay, sun-cured	90.0	50.9	9.4	0.45	0.22
BAKERY					
Waste, dehydrated	91.2	89.1	11.1	0.15	0.24
BARLEY					
Grain	88.6	82.7	13.0	0.06	0.38
BEET, SUGAR					
Pulp, dehydrated	91.0	74.4	9.8	0.68	0.1
BERMUDA GRASS, COMMON					
Fresh	28.9	56.1	12.7	0.48	0.28
Hay, sun-cured	91.2	48.1	9.7	0.47	0.18
BERMUDA GRASS, COASTAL					
Fresh	30.3	58.8	12.8	0.5	0.26
Hay, sun-cured	91.6	54.4	12.2	0.42	0.21
CANOLA (RAPE)					
Seeds, meal mechanically extracted	92.0	78.6	38.4	0.72	1.13
CITRUS					
Pomace (citrus pulp)	91.1	81.3	6.7	1.88	0.13
CLOVER, CRIMSON					
Fresh	17.5	64.0	17.1	1.37	0.28
Hay, sun-cured	87.8	61.2	16.7	1.35	0.22
CLOVER, LADINO					
Fresh	17.7	70.2	24.8	1.39	0.38
Hay, sun-cured	89.1	63.5	22.4	1.35	0.31
CORN (MAIZE)					
Cobs, ground	89.8	48.5	3.1	0.12	0.04
Gluten, meal	91.3	86.8	47.5	0.16	0.50

*Values are shown as a dry matter basis.

TABLE 2-5

NUTRIENT COMPOSITION OF VARIOUS FEEDSTUFFS FOR SHEEP AND GOATS—cont'd

FEEDSTUFF	DRY MATTER %	TOTAL DIETARY NUTRITION %	CRUDE PROTEIN %	CALCIUM %	PHOSPHORUS %
CORN (MAIZE)—cont'd					
Gluten, with bran (gluten feed)	89.9	82.8	25.4	0.35	0.84
Grits byproduct (hominy feed)	90.2	87.9	10.3	0.05	0.57
Grain, grade 2	87.3	88.1	10.0	0.02	0.33
Silage, well-eared	34.1	70.1	8.2	0.26	0.21
COTTON					
Hulls	90.4	45.1	4.2	0.14	0.08
Seeds, meal mechanically extracted	92.6	79.5	44.3	0.2	1.17
Seeds, whole	92.2	90.3	23.5	0.15	0.73
FESCUE, TALL					
Fresh	24.0	62.5	10.8	0.51	0.46
Hay, sun-cured, early bloom	92.0	54.2	10.3	0.3	0.27
FISH, MENHADEN					
Meal, mechanically extracted	91.7	77.2	66.6	5.70	3.28
GRASS					
Hay, sun-cured, full bloom	89.3	54.9	9.5	0.57	0.24
JOHNSON GRASS					
Hay, sun-cured	90.5	55.7	7.7	0.89	0.31
MOLASSES					
Sugar cane	74.3	82.2	5.8	0.99	0.11
OATS					
Grain	89.2	77.4	13.2	0.09	0.38
Hay, sun-cured	90.7	60.3	9.6	0.32	0.26
ORCHARD GRASS					
Hay, sun-cured	89.6	57.9	11.8	0.41	0.28
PEANUT					
Hay, sun-cured	90.7	51.1	11.5	1.12	0.14
Hulls	91.0	21.9	8.7	0.27	0.07
RICE					
Bran	91.0	73.8	14.1	0.08	1.66
Hulls	91.9	12.5	3.0	0.12	0.08
RYE					
Grain	87.5	82.6	13.7	0.08	0.39

Continued

TABLE 2-5

NUTRIENT COMPOSITION OF VARIOUS FEEDSTUFFS FOR SHEEP AND GOATS*—cont'd

FEEDSTUFF	DRY MATTER %	TOTAL DIETARY NUTRITION %	CRUDE PROTEIN %	CALCIUM %	PHOSPHORUS %
RYEGRASS					
Fresh	22.6	70.1	17.6	0.66	0.4
Hay, sun-cured, early bloom	89.9	58.0	14.4	0.56	0.35
SORGHUM (MILO)					
Grain	89.4	85.4	11.3	0.03	0.3
Silage	28.8	57.3	6.6	0.35	0.21
SOYBEAN					
Seed coats, hulls	90.3	76.7	11.2	0.53	0.19
Seeds, meal mechanically extracted	90.0	85.4	48.1	0.26	0.62
Seeds, meal extracted in solution	89.9	83.6	49.9	0.26	0.64
TRITICALE					
Grain	89.2	77.5	13.2	0.05	0.3
WHEAT					
Fresh, early vegetative	22.2	78.3	22.1	0.4	0.4
Grain	89.0	87.3	15.1	0.05	0.38
WHEY					
Dehydrated	93.3	79.7	14.1	0.91	0.82

*Values are shown as a dry matter basis.

ashing the sample. The NDF is an estimate of the amount of hemicellulose, cellulose, and lignin the sample contains, whereas the ADF estimates only the amount of cellulose and lignin. As the NDF content of a feedstuff rises, the bulkiness of the feed also increases—that is, NDF is negatively correlated with dry matter intake. As the ADF content of a feed rises, its digestibility is decreased. Pelleting or grinding usually results in a greater dry matter intake, even for feedstuffs with relatively high NDF contents. Based on the determined levels of the various fiber fractions, prediction equations are used to compute TDN content and various other values for energy content (e.g., metabolizable energy, net energy).

The last major nutrient that is measured is crude protein. The sample is analyzed for nitrogen content, and then crude protein is calculated as percent nitrogen multiplied by 6.25. The crude protein value cannot indicate if any or how much of the protein has been damaged by heat. Heat damage often results in decreased digestibility. This method of protein analysis does not differentiate between NPN and natural protein. If the protein is reported as digestible protein, this is formulated from the crude protein content. Unfortunately, digestible protein is of limited practical value in developing rations. Additionally, samples may sometimes be analyzed for fat. Table 2-6 illustrates sample hay analyses.

Different testing laboratories use different equations to predict energy values. One common equation is as follows:

$$TDN\ (\%) = 88.9 - (0.79 \times ADF\ [\%])$$

The equation balances using either the ADF (39%) or the TDN (58.09%) values from the analysis provided in Table 2-6. This is a simple equation, but the various net energy prediction equations use cubic and quadratic terms that are much more complex. The NDF fraction can be used to estimate the animals' voluntary dry matter intake:

$$\text{Dry matter intake (\% of body weight)} = 120 \div NDF\ (\%)$$

Again, using the information from Table 2-6, the equation is solved as follows:

$$\text{Dry matter intake} = 120 \div 62\% = 1.94\%\ \text{of body weight}$$

TABLE 2-6

A SAMPLE ANALYSIS FOR FESCUE HAY

CONSTITUENT	DETERMINED DRY-MATTER BASIS
Moisture	12.75%
Dry matter	87.25%
Crude protein	12.31%
Fiber	
NDF	62.00%
ADF	39.00%
Total digestible nutrients*	58.09%
Net energy—lactation*	1.31 mcal/kg
Net energy—maintenance*	1.25 mcal/kg
Net energy—grain*	0.58 mcal/kg

*Calculated from prediction equations.

In other words, animals consuming the hay in Table 2-6 would consume about 1.9% of their body weight in dry matter.

Another calculated figure that may be reported on a forage analysis is relative feed value (RFV). This is calculated as follows:

$$\text{RFV} = \text{digestible dry matter (\%)} \times \text{dry matter intake (\%)} \div 1.29$$

where digestible dry matter (%) = 88.9 − (0.779 × ADF[%]). Therefore, for this example the equation is completed as follows:

$$\text{RFV} = (58.52 \times 1.94) \div 1.29 = 88$$

RFVs can exceed 100 and often do for good-quality alfalfa. However, they do not take into account the crude protein content of the forage, which must be evaluated separately. The poorer the quality of a forage, the longer it requires for digestion. Poor-quality forage remains in the rumen for a longer period, thereby limiting feed intake. Keepers purchasing feeds would do well to make decisions based on RFV. However, during diet formulation, TDN and protein concentrations are used most often as guidelines.

BALANCING A RATION

Substitution Method

The substitution method for balancing a ration works best when only two or three feedstuffs are to be used on a farm or ranch. (The authors of this chapter use pounds, not kilograms, in demonstrating this method of ration calculation.) As an example, the following paragraphs il-

lustrate the method for calculating a diet for a group of ewes with an average body weight of 150 pounds. These animals also are in the last trimester of pregnancy, with a high expected twinning rate (Table 2-7, *A* and *B*). Some grass hay is available and has been analyzed; it contains 51% TDN and 8.8% crude protein. Both corn and soybean meal can be purchased as needed. The ewes' daily requirements can be determined from this information. Table 2-7 illustrates that a 154-pound ewe with a 180% to 225% expected lambing rate consumes 4.2 lb of dry matter per day and requires 2.8 lb of TDN and 0.47 lb of protein. If x = lb of hay, then 4.2 − x = lb of corn. TDN can then be determined as follows:

$$0.51(x) + 0.881(4.2 - x) = 2.8$$

where *0.51* and *0.881* are the proportion of TDN in the hay and corn, respectively. As noted in the table, *2.8* is the daily TDN requirement in pounds. Solving for x indicates that feeding 2.4 lb of hay and 1.8 lb of corn per day (dry matter basis) provides the ewes' energy needs.

The next step is to determine the protein adequacy. The provided hay contributes 0.21 lb of protein (2.4 × 0.088); the corn contributes 0.18 lb of protein (1.8 × 0.1). Total daily intake of protein is therefore 0.39 lb (0.21 + 0.18). However, because the protein requirement was determined to be 0.47 lb, the diet is still deficient by 0.08 lb (0.47 − 0.39). A protein source such as soybean meal can be used to supplement the grain (corn). The net gain in protein for this substitution is 0.34 lb for every pound of soybean meal substituted for corn (0.44 − 0.1). Dividing the deficiency (0.08 lb) by the net gain in protein gained by substituting soybean meal for corn (0.34 lb) indicates that the ration can be balanced by adding 0.23 lb of soybean meal and subtracting 0.23 lb of corn. The final daily ration is therefore 1.57 lb of corn, 0.23 lb of soybean meal, and 2.4 lb of hay.

To convert this to an as-fed basis, and for simplicity's sake in this example, the keeper should assume that all feeds are 90% dry matter. Therefore the amount of each feedstuff should be divided by 0.9, resulting in 1.7 lb of corn, 0.25 lb of soybean meal, and 2.7 lb of hay.

From a practical standpoint, the authors of this chapter would probably offer the ewes free-choice hay and supplement them with 2 lb of a corn-soybean meal mixture that contains 87.5% corn and 12.5% soybean meal. This ration is fed until lambing commences, at which time the diet is reformulated to meet the demands of lactation.

Fixed Ingredients

The next example illustrates a method of balancing a ration using a fixed set of ingredients. In this example, three different grain sources are used: corn, oats, and wheat. The diet is balanced for 30-lb kids growing at a

Text continued on p. 38

TABLE 2-7, A

DAILY NUTRIENT REQUIREMENTS OF SHEEP (NUTRIENTS PER DAY)

Body Weight		Weight Change Per Day		Dry Matter			Total Dietary Nutrition		Digestible Energy	Metabolizable Energy	Crude Protein		Calcium	Phosphorus
KG	LB	G	LB	KG	LB	% BODY WEIGHT	KG	LB	MCAL	MCAL	G	LB	G	G
EWES														
Maintenance														
50	110	10	0.02	1.0	2.2	2.0	0.55	1.2	2.4	2.0	90	0.21	2.0	1.8
60	132	10	0.02	1.1	2.4	1.8	0.61	1.3	2.7	2.2	104	0.23	2.3	2.1
70	154	10	0.02	1.2	2.6	1.7	0.66	1.5	2.9	2.4	113	0.25	2.5	2.4
80	176	10	0.02	1.3	2.9	1.6	0.72	1.6	3.2	2.6	122	0.27	2.7	2.8
90	198	10	0.02	1.4	3.1	1.5	0.78	1.7	3.4	2.8	131	0.29	2.9	3.1
Flushing—2 weeks prebreeding and first 3 weeks of breeding														
50	110	100	0.22	1.6	3.5	3.2	0.94	2.1	4.1	3.4	150	0.33	5.3	2.6
60	132	100	0.22	1.7	3.7	2.8	1.00	2.2	4.4	3.6	157	0.34	5.5	2.9
70	154	100	0.22	1.8	4.0	2.6	1.06	2.3	4.7	3.8	164	0.36	5.7	3.2
80	176	100	0.22	1.9	4.2	2.4	1.12	2.5	4.9	4.0	171	0.38	5.9	3.6
90	198	100	0.22	2.0	4.4	2.2	1.18	2.6	5.1	4.2	177	0.39	6.1	3.9
Nonlactating—first 15 weeks of gestation														
50	110	30	0.07	1.2	2.6	2.4	0.67	1.5	3.0	2.4	112	0.25	2.9	2.1
60	132	30	0.07	1.3	2.9	2.2	0.72	1.6	3.2	2.6	121	0.27	3.2	2.5
70	154	30	0.07	1.4	3.1	2.0	0.77	1.7	3.4	2.8	130	0.29	3.5	2.9
80	176	30	0.07	1.5	3.3	1.9	0.82	1.8	3.6	3.0	139	0.31	3.8	3.3
90	198	30	0.07	1.6	3.5	1.8	0.87	1.9	3.8	3.2	148	0.33	4.1	3.6
Last 4 weeks of gestation (130% to 150% lambing rate expected) or last 4 to 6 weeks' lactation suckling singles														
50	110	180(45)*	0.40(0.10)	1.6	3.5	3.2	0.94	2.1	4.1	3.4	175	0.38	5.9	4.8
60	132	180(45)	0.40(0.10)	1.7	3.7	2.8	1.00	2.2	4.4	3.6	184	0.40	6.0	5.2
70	154	180(45)	0.40(0.10)	1.8	4.0	2.6	1.06	2.3	4.7	3.8	193	0.42	6.2	5.6
80	176	180(45)	0.40(0.10)	1.9	4.2	2.4	1.12	2.4	4.9	4.0	202	0.44	6.3	6.1
90	198	180(45)	0.40(0.10)	2.0	4.4	2.2	1.18	2.5	5.1	4.2	212	0.47	6.4	6.5

Last 4 weeks of gestation (180% to 225% lambing rate expected)

50	110	225	0.50	1.7	3.7	3.4	1.10	2.4	4.8	4.0	196	0.43	6.2	3.4
60	132	225	0.50	1.8	4.0	3.0	1.17	2.6	5.1	4.2	205	0.45	6.9	4.0
70	154	225	0.50	1.9	4.2	2.7	1.24	2.8	5.4	4.4	214	0.47	7.6	4.5
80	176	225	0.50	2.0	4.4	2.5	1.30	2.9	5.7	4.7	223	0.49	8.3	5.1
90	198	225	0.50	2.1	4.6	2.3	1.37	3.0	6.0	5.0	232	0.51	8.9	5.7

First 6 to 8 weeks of lactation suckling singles or last 4 to 6 weeks of lactation suckling twins

50	110	−25(90)	−0.06(0.2)	2.1	4.6	4.2	1.36	3.0	6.0	4.9	304	0.67	8.9	6.1
60	132	−25(90)	−0.06(0.2)	2.3	5.1	3.8	1.50	3.3	6.6	5.4	319	0.70	9.1	6.6
70	154	−25(90)	−0.06(0.2)	2.5	5.5	3.6	1.63	3.6	7.2	5.9	334	0.73	9.3	7.0
80	176	−25(90)	−0.06(0.2)	2.6	5.7	3.2	1.69	3.7	7.4	6.1	344	0.76	9.5	7.4
90	198	−25(90)	−0.06(0.2)	2.7	5.9	3.0	1.75	3.8	7.6	6.3	353	0.78	9.6	7.8

First 6 to 8 weeks of lactation suckling twins

50	110	−60	−0.13	2.4	5.3	4.8	1.56	3.4	6.9	5.6	389	0.86	10.5	7.3
60	132	−60	−0.13	2.6	5.7	4.3	1.69	3.7	7.4	6.1	405	0.89	10.7	7.7
70	154	−60	−0.13	2.8	6.2	4.0	1.82	4.0	8.0	6.6	420	0.92	11.0	8.1
80	176	−60	−0.13	3.0	6.6	3.8	1.95	4.3	8.6	7.0	435	0.96	11.2	8.6
90	198	−60	−0.13	3.2	7.0	3.6	2.08	4.6	9.2	7.5	450	0.99	11.4	9.0

EWE LAMBS

Nonlactating—first 15 weeks of gestation

40	88	160	0.35	1.4	3.1	3.5	0.83	1.8	3.6	3.0	156	0.34	5.5	3.0
50	110	135	0.30	1.5	3.3	3.0	0.88	1.9	3.9	3.2	159	0.35	5.2	3.1
60	132	135	0.30	1.6	3.5	2.7	0.94	2.0	4.1	3.4	161	0.35	5.5	3.4
70	154	125	0.28	1.7	3.7	2.4	1.00	2.2	4.4	3.6	164	0.36	5.5	3.7

*Values in parentheses are for ewes suckling lambs in the last 4 to 6 weeks of lactation.

TABLE 2-7, B

DAILY NUTRIENT REQUIREMENTS OF SHEEP (NUTRIENTS PER DAY)*

Body Weight		Weight Change Per Day		Dry Matter			Total Dietary Nutrition		Digestible Energy	Metabolizable Energy	Crude Protein		Calcium	Phosphorus
KG	LB	G	LB	KG	LB	% BODY WEIGHT	KG	LB	MCAL	MCAL	G	LB	G	G
Last 4 weeks of gestation (100% to 120% lambing rate expected)														
40	88	180	0.40	1.5	3.3	3.8	0.94	2.1	4.1	3.4	187	0.41	6.4	3.1
50	110	160	0.35	1.6	3.5	3.2	1.00	2.2	4.4	3.6	189	0.42	6.3	3.4
60	132	160	0.35	1.7	3.7	2.8	1.07	2.4	4.7	3.9	192	0.42	6.6	3.8
70	154	150	0.33	1.8	4.0	2.6	1.14	2.5	5.0	4.1	194	0.43	6.8	4.2
Last 4 weeks of gestation (130% to 175% lambing rate expected)														
40	88	225	0.50	1.5	3.3	3.8	0.99	2.2	4.4	3.6	202	0.44	7.4	3.5
50	110	225	0.50	1.6	3.5	3.2	1.06	2.3	4.7	3.8	204	0.45	7.8	3.9
60	132	225	0.50	1.7	3.7	2.8	1.12	2.5	4.9	4.0	207	0.46	8.1	4.3
70	154	215	0.47	1.8	4.0	2.6	1.14	2.5	5.0	4.1	210	0.46	8.2	4.7
First 6 to 8 weeks of lactation suckling singles (wean by 8 weeks)														
40	88	−50	−0.11	1.7	3.7	4.2	1.12	2.5	4.9	4.0	257	0.56	6.0	4.3
50	110	−50	−0.11	2.1	4.6	4.2	1.39	3.1	6.1	5.0	282	0.62	6.5	4.7
60	132	−50	−0.11	2.3	5.1	3.8	1.52	3.4	6.7	5.5	295	0.65	6.8	5.1
70	154	−50	−0.11	2.5	5.5	3.6	1.65	3.6	7.3	6.0	301	0.68	7.1	5.6
First 6 to 8 weeks of lactation suckling twins (wean by 8 weeks)														
40	88	−100	−0.22	2.1	4.6	5.2	1.45	3.2	6.4	5.2	306	0.67	8.4	5.6
50	110	−100	−0.22	2.3	5.1	4.6	1.59	3.5	7.0	5.7	321	0.71	8.7	6.0
60	132	−100	−0.22	2.5	5.5	4.2	1.72	3.8	7.6	6.2	336	0.74	9.0	6.4
70	154	−100	−0.22	2.7	6.0	3.9	1.85	4.1	8.1	6.6	351	0.77	9.3	6.9
REPLACEMENT EWE LAMBS														
30	66	227	0.50	1.2	2.6	4.0	0.78	1.7	3.4	2.8	185	0.41	6.4	2.6
40	88	182	0.40	1.4	3.1	3.5	0.91	2.0	4.0	3.3	176	0.39	5.9	2.6
50	110	120	0.26	1.5	3.3	3.0	0.88	1.9	3.9	3.2	136	0.30	4.8	2.4
60	132	100	0.22	1.5	3.3	2.5	0.88	1.9	3.9	3.2	134	0.30	4.5	2.5
70	154	100	0.22	1.5	3.3	2.1	0.88	1.9	3.9	3.2	132	0.29	4.6	2.8

REPLACEMENT RAM LAMBS

40	88	0.73	1.8	4.0	4.5	1.1	2.5	5.0	4.1	243	0.54	7.8	3.7
60	132	0.70	2.4	5.3	4.0	1.5	3.4	6.7	5.5	263	0.58	8.4	4.2
80	176	0.64	2.8	6.2	3.5	1.8	3.9	7.8	6.4	268	0.59	8.5	4.6
100	220	0.55	3.0	6.6	3.0	1.9	4.2	8.4	6.9	264	0.58	8.2	4.8

LAMBS FINISHING—4 TO 7 MONTHS

30	66	0.65	1.3	2.9	4.3	0.94	2.1	4.1	3.4	191	0.42	6.6	3.2
40	88	0.60	1.6	3.5	4.0	1.22	2.7	5.4	4.4	185	0.41	6.6	3.3
50	110	0.45	1.6	3.5	3.2	1.23	2.7	5.4	4.4	160	0.35	5.6	3.0

EARLY WEANED LAMBS—MODERATE GROWTH POTENTIAL

10	22	0.44	0.5	1.1	5.0	0.40	0.9	1.8	1.4	127	0.38	4.0	1.9
20	44	0.55	1.0	2.2	5.0	0.80	1.8	3.5	2.9	167	0.37	5.4	2.5
30	66	0.66	1.3	2.9	4.3	1.00	2.2	4.4	3.6	191	0.42	6.7	3.2
40	88	0.76	1.5	3.3	3.8	1.16	2.6	5.1	4.2	202	0.44	7.7	3.9
50	110	0.66	1.5	3.3	3.0	1.16	2.6	5.1	4.2	181	0.40	7.0	3.8

EARLY WEANED LAMBS—RAPID GROWTH POTENTIAL

10	22	0.55	0.6	1.3	6.0	0.48	1.1	2.1	1.7	157	0.35	4.9	2.2
20	44	0.66	1.2	2.6	6.0	0.92	2.0	4.0	3.3	205	0.45	6.5	2.9
30	66	0.72	1.4	3.1	4.7	1.10	2.4	4.8	4.0	216	0.48	7.2	3.4
40	88	0.88	1.5	3.3	3.8	1.14	2.5	5.0	4.1	234	0.51	8.6	4.3
50	110	0.94	1.7	3.7	3.4	1.29	2.8	5.7	4.7	240	0.53	9.4	4.8
60	132	0.77	1.7	3.7	2.8	1.29	2.8	5.7	4.7	240	0.53	8.2	4.5

*These values represent different weight losses and sizes than in Table 2-7, A.

rate of 0.20 lb per day. In addition, cottonseed hulls are available as a roughage source and cottonseed meal as a source of protein. The wheat was purchased at a bargain price, but potential problems exist with feeding large amounts of it. Therefore wheat is limited to 15% of the diet. In this example the owners have requested that equal quantities of corn and oats be used in the diet formulation. Table 2-8 describes the daily requirements for these goats as follows: dry matter intake of 0.9 lb, protein intake of 0.119 lb, and TDN of 0.59 lb. First, the nutrients being provided by the fixed level of wheat should be taken into account:

$$\text{Daily intake} = 0.90 \text{ lb} \times 15\% = 0.135 \text{ lb of wheat per day}$$
$$\text{TDN from wheat} = 0.135 \text{ lb} \times 0.873 = 0.12 \text{ lb of TDN}$$
$$\text{Protein} = 0.135 \text{ lb} \times 0.151 = 0.020 \text{ lb of protein}$$

Subtracting these amounts from the requirement yields the following results:

$$\text{Dry matter} = 0.90 - 0.135 = 0.765$$
$$\text{TDN} = 0.59 - 0.12 = 0.47 \text{ lb}$$
$$\text{Crude protein} = 0.119 - 0.020 = 0.099 \text{ lb}$$

An equation similar to the previous example, in which x = pounds of cottonseed hulls and $0.765 - x = 1{:}1$ mixture of corn and oats is now used to solve for TDN:

$$0.451(x) + 0.8275(0.765 - x) = 0.47$$

where 0.451 is the TDN content of the cottonseed hulls and 0.8275 is the TDN content of a mixture of equal parts of corn (0.881) and oats (0.774) [0.881 + 0.774] ÷ 2 = 0.8275.

Solving for x reveals that balancing the ration requires 0.52 lb of cottonseed hulls and 0.24 lb of the corn/oats mix, which equates to 0.12 lb (0.24 lb divided by 2) of each.

So far, the ration consists of 0.52 lb of cottonseed hulls, 0.135 lb of wheat, 0.12 lb of corn, and 0.12 lb of oats. The hulls provide 0.022 lb of protein (0.52 lb × 0.042), the corn provides 0.012 lb of protein (0.12 lb × 0.10), and the oats provide 0.016 lb of protein (0.12 × 0.132). Total protein in the ration thus far is 0.05 lb (0.022 + 0.012 + 0.016). The requirement is 0.099 lb, leaving a deficit of 0.049 lb.

Cottonseed meal can be substituted for some of the grain. An equal mix contains 11.6%, so the net gain of the

TABLE 2-8

DAILY NUTRIENT REQUIREMENTS FOR GOATS

CLASS OF GOAT	BODY WEIGHT (LB)	DRY MATTER INTAKE* (LB)	TOTAL DIETARY NUTRITION (LB)	CRUDE PROTEIN (LB)
Dry doe, early pregnant	50	1.25	0.64	0.091
	70	1.75	0.83	0.117
	90	2.25	1.00	0.141
	110	2.75	1.17	0.164
	130	3.25	1.32	0.186
Doe, late pregnancy	50	1.25	1.12	0.159
	70	1.75	1.45	0.205
	90	2.25	1.75	0.248
	110	2.75	2.04	0.288
	130	3.25	2.31	0.327
Doe, lactating	Add 0.35 pound of total dietary nutrition and 0.072 pound of protein per pound of 4% milk produced			
Kid, growing at 0.2 lb/day	30	0.9	0.59	0.119
	40	1.2	0.70	0.134
	50	1.5	0.79	0.148
Kid growing at 0.3 lb/day	30	0.9	0.66	0.147
	40	1.2	0.77	0.162
	50	1.5	0.86	0.176
Kid growing at 0.4 lb/day	30	0.9	0.74	0.176
	40	1.2	0.85	0.191
	50	1.5	0.94	0.205

*Daily dry matter intake for does is estimated at 2.5% of body weight but can be as high as 2.75% of body weight. For growing kids, intake is estimated at 3% of body weight but can be as high as 4.5% depending on diet and types of kids being fed.

substitution is 32.7% (44.3% − 11.6%). Therefore to balance the ration the keeper should add 0.15 lb (0.47 lb divided by 0.327) of cottonseed meal and take out 0.075 lb of corn and 0.075 lb of oats from the diet.

The final daily ration is as follows:

	LB DRY MATTER	LB AS FED*	% AS FED
Cottonseed hulls	0.52	0.58	58.0
Wheat	0.135	0.15	
Corn	0.045	0.05	5.0
Oats	0.045	0.05	5.0
Cottonseed meal	0.15	0.15	17.0

*To determine this column, the keeper should determine the percentage of dry matter and divide it into the amount of dry matter being fed (e.g., cottonseed hulls 0.52 lb dry matter at 90% dry matter, or 0.52 divided by 0.9 = 0.58 lb of feed). In this example, all the feeds are 90% dry matter.

Pearson Square

The Pearson square is a simple technique that is quite useful for blending two ingredients on the basis of one nutrient. In the following example, corn and soybean meal are blended to attain a concentrate mixture of 16% crude protein. The square is formed by placing the percentage of the nutrient that is desired in the center and then placing the percentage of the nutrient present in the two feeds at the left corners:

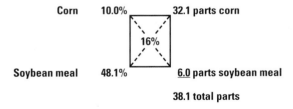

The square is solved by subtracting diagonally across the square without regard to the sign of the differences (in other words, *no* negative numbers) and recording the difference at the right corners. Using the individual and total parts, the percentage of each ingredient can be calculated:

32.1/38.1 = 84.25% corn

6/38.1 = 15.75% soybean meal

Therefore a mixture composed of 84.25% corn and 15.75% soybean meal mixture yields a feed with a crude protein content of 16%. This quick method can be used for any class of nutrient.

Calculating for Phosphorus and Calcium Supplementation

The next example illustrates the way to calculate requirements for phosphorus and calcium supplementation. The 84.25% corn and 15.75% soybean meal mixture from the previous example is used. Values for the calcium and phosphorus content of these two feedstuffs are provided in Table 2-5:

	CALCIUM	PHOSPHORUS
Corn grain, grade 2	0.02%	0.33%
Soybean meal, mechanically extracted	0.26%	0.62%

All values are provided on a dry matter basis. Calcium supplementation is to be made with limestone, and phosphorus supplementation is to be made with dicalcium phosphate. The corn/soybean meal mixture comprises 97% of the diet. This allows for the addition of a calcium and phosphorus source (dicalcium phosphate) and a calcium source (limestone) for needed trace minerals, as well as a urine acidifier (if needed). Corn is therefore 81.7% of the diet (84.25% × 0.97), whereas soybean meal comprises 15.3% of the diet (15.75% × 0.97). Assuming a requirement of 0.5% for phosphorus and knowing the percentage of phosphorus in dicalcium phosphate (18.5%) allows the calculation of the amount of phosphorus supplementation (as dicalcium phosphate) by multiplying each feed ingredient by the percentage of phosphorus in that feed and adding the results:

$$0.5\% = (81.75\% \times 0.0033) + (15.3\% \times 0.0062) + (x \times 0.185\%)$$

where *0.5%* is the daily phosphorus requirement, *81.75%* is the percentage of corn in the diet, *0.0033* is the percentage of phosphorus found in corn, *15.3%* is the percentage of soybean meal in the diet, *0.0062* is the percentage of phosphorus found in soybean meal, *x* is the amount of dicalcium phosphate required for supplementation, and *0.185%* is the percentage of phosphorus in dicalcium phosphate. The equation is solved as follows:

$$0.5\% = 0.27\% + 0.095\% + (x \times 0.185\%)$$
$$0.5\% = 0.365\% + (x \times 0.185\%)$$
$$(0.5\% - 0.365\%) \div 0.185\% = x$$
$$x = 0.73\%$$

Therefore dicalcium phosphate must comprise 0.73% of the diet to satisfy the phosphorus requirement.

It is now possible to solve for the required calcium supplementation in the form of limestone, assuming a daily requirement of 0.6% and knowing both the amount of dicalcium phosphate in the diet (0.73%) and the percentage of calcium in limestone (38%):

$$0.6\% = (81.75\% \times 0.0002) + (15.3\% \times 0.0026)$$
$$+ (0.73\% \times 0.22\%) + (x \times 0.38\%)$$

where *0.6%* is the daily calcium requirement, *81.75%* is the percentage of corn in the diet, *0.0002* is the percentage of calcium found in corn, *15.3%* is the percentage of soybean meal in the diet, *0.0026* is the percentage of calcium found in soybean meal, *0.73%* is the percentage of dicalcium phosphate in the diet, *0.22%* is the percentage of calcium in dicalcium phosphate, *x* is the amount of limestone required for supplementation, and *0.38%* is the percentage of calcium in limestone. The equation is solved as follows:

$$0.6\% = 0.016\% + 0.04\% + 0.16\% + (x \times 0.38\%)$$
$$0.6\% = 0.216\% + (x \times 0.38\%)$$
$$(0.6\% - 0.216\%) \div 0.38\% = x$$
$$x = 1\%$$

Therefore limestone must comprise 1% of the diet to satisfy the calcium requirement.

The ration calculated in the previous examples would therefore be composed of the following:

Corn	81.7%
Soybean meal	15.3%
Dicalcium phosphate	0.73%
Limestone	1%
Total ration	98.73%

This is on an as-fed basis. Given that a standard 0.5% (0.5 lb) of sodium chloride and 0.05% (0.05 lb) of trace minerals are usually added, the resultant mixture is 99.28% complete on a dry matter basis.

References

1. Hofmann RR: Anatomy of the gastrointestinal tract. In Church DC, editor: *The ruminant animal digestive physiology and nutrition,* Englewood Cliffs, NJ, 1988, Prentice-Hall.
2. *Nutrient requirements of sheep,* Washington, DC, 1985, National Academy Press.
3. *Water requirements for livestock,* 2000, Alberta Agriculture Food and Rural Development Extension Bulletin.
4. Bauder J: When is water good enough for livestock? *Montana State Extension Bulletin,* 2000.
5. Guyer PQ: *Livestock water quality,* University of Nebraska Extension Service Bulletin G79-46A.
6. Meyer KB: *Water quality in animals,* 1999, Purdue University Extension Bulletin WQ9.
7. Maloiy GMO, Taylor CR: Water requirements of African goats and haired sheep, *J Agric Sci* 77:203, 1971.
8. *Nutrient requirements of goats: angora, dairy and meat goats in temperate and tropical countries,* Washington, DC, 1981, National Academy Press.
9. Knox MR, Steel JW: The effects of urea supplementation on production and parasitological responses of sheep infected with *Haemonchus contortus* and *Trichostrongylus colubriformis, Vet Parisit* 3:123, 1999.
10. Bratzlaff K, Henlein G, Huston J: Common nutritional problems feeding the sick goat. In Naylor JM, Ralston SL, editors: *Large animal clinical nutrition,* St Louis, 1991, Mosby.
11. Qi K, Lu CD, Owens FN: Sulfate supplementation of growing goats: effects on performance, acid-base balance, and nutrient digestibilities, *J Anim Sci* 71:1579, 1993.
12. Qi K et al: Sulfate supplementation of Angora goats: metabolic and mohair responses, *J Anim Sci* 70:2828, 1992.
13. Hayter S, Wiener G: Variation in the concentration of copper in the blood plasma of Finnish-Landrace and Merino sheep and their crosses with reference to reproductive performance and age, *Anim Prod* 16:261, 1973.
14. Holland C, Kezar W: *Pioneer forage manual. A nutritional guide,* Des Moines, IA, 1995, Pioneer Hi-Bred International.

Further Reading

Naylor JM, Ralston SL: *Large animal clinical nutrition,* St Louis, 1991, Mosby.

Ensminger ME, Oldfield JE, Heineman WW: *Feeds & nutrition,* ed 2, Clovis, CA, 1990, Ensminger Publishing.

BODY CONDITION SCORING

Theoretically, the exact amount of nutrients required for each stage of production should be provided; however, this is usually not practical under field conditions. Therefore the animal is subject to seasonal periods of undernutrition and overnutrition. A useful system to help assess the overall nutritional status of the flock is to assign a body condition score to the animals. The body condition score system most commonly used for sheep and goats has a range of 1 to 5, with 1 being extremely thin and 5 being extremely obese. Body condition scoring is accomplished by palpating a relaxed ewe or doe for the degree of fat covering on the spinous processes and transverse processes in the lumbar region (Figure 2-1).[1] Because more than 85% to 90% of all healthy ewes receive a score of 2, 3, or 4, half-scores are often assigned for greater accuracy. For example, if the animal scores higher than a 3, but not quite a 4, it should be classified with a condition score of 3.5. Ideally, the majority of the flock should have a condition score of 2.5 to 3 at breeding and parturition.

If the flock was scored 45 days before parturition, and the average was less than 2.5 to 3, the keeper should increase the flock's energy intake so that the animals reach an average of 2.5 to 3 by the time of parturition. Animals in thin body condition at parturition give birth to weaker babies and generally produce less milk during early lactation. An ideal body condition score is especially important in accelerated breeding systems in which the females are rebred within 60 to 90 days after parturition. Likewise, if the average condition score 30 days before breeding is less than 3, the keeper should consider flushing the females. Moreover, condition scoring all the females allows the keeper to move the thin females (those with a score less than 2) into one feeding group while leaving the others (those with a score higher than 3) in another feeding group. In this way the thin females can receive additional supplementation without the others becoming overconditioned. A universally accepted condition scoring system is not available for goats. The authors follow the system in Table 2-9 and use many of the same principles described for sheep.[2] Figure 2-2 shows a crude

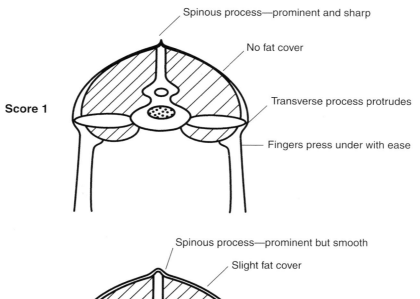

Score 1

Spinous process—prominent and sharp

No fat cover

Transverse process protrudes

Fingers press under with ease

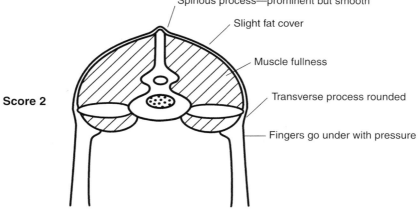

Score 2

Spinous process—prominent but smooth

Slight fat cover

Muscle fullness

Transverse process rounded

Fingers go under with pressure

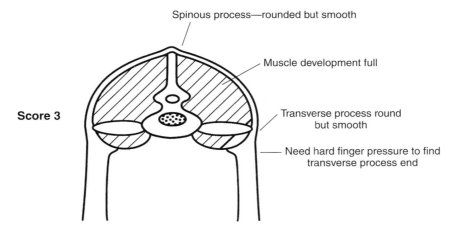

Score 3

Spinous process—rounded but smooth

Muscle development full

Transverse process round but smooth

Need hard finger pressure to find transverse process end

Figure 2-1   Body condition scores for sheep. These drawings show a cross-section through the lumbar region and depict the fat covering (or lack thereof). *Score 1,* The spinous and transverse processes are sharp and no fat is detectable on the loin area. These animals are emaciated. *Score 2,* Animals are still thin with prominent spinous and slightly rounded transverse processes. The examiner's fingers can be passed under the edge of the transverse processes. *Score 3,* Animals have smooth, slightly rounded spinous and transverse processes. Slight pressure is required to palpate the transverse process.

Continued

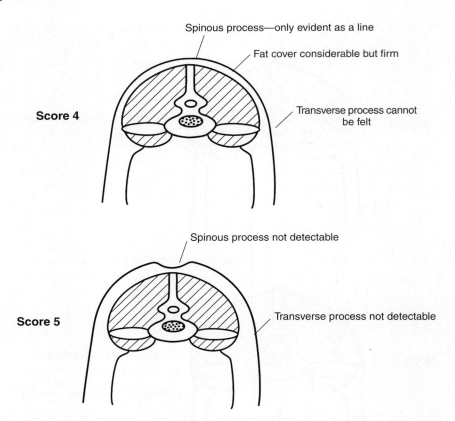

Spinous process—only evident as a line

Fat cover considerable but firm

Score 4

Transverse process cannot be felt

Spinous process not detectable

Score 5

Transverse process not detectable

Figure 2-1, cont'd *Score 4,* These animals are fat. The spinous processes are barely palpable. *Score 5,* These animals are obese, with a midline concavity running over the spinous process. Because these scores are broad, many owners or managers round up to half-scores (e.g., 2.5) if the animal has more fat covering then one score but not quite as much as the next whole-number score up.

TABLE 2-9

THE BODY CONDITION SCORING SYSTEM FOR GOATS

SCORE	APPEARANCE
0	No subcutaneous tissue seen.
1	Dorsal aspect of vertebral column forms a continuous ridge, hollow flank, ribs easily seen. Sternal fat easily moved laterally. Chondrosternal joints easily palpable. No muscle or fat between ribs or bones. Transverse processes of lumbar vertebrae easily visualized, and articular processes easily palpable.
2	Sternal fat moveable, but 1 to 2 cm thick. Tissue visible between skin and chondrosternal joints. Some tissue around transverse processes of lumbar spine, but it is more difficult to palpate than in Score 1. Need slight pressure to palpate articular processes.
3	Dorsal aspect of vertebral column is less prominent. Sternal fat is thick and barely moveable. Chondrosternal joints are difficult to palpate. Lumbar vertebrae have thick tissue covering. Articular processes of transverse processes not palpable.
4	Sternal fat, costochondral fat, and rib fat continuous. Transverse process difficult to palpate. Spinous processes not palpable.
5	Sternal fat and rib fat bulges between pressed fingers. Spinous and transverse processes not palpable.

From Santucci PM et al: Body condition scoring of goats in extensive conditions. In Morand-Fehr P, editor: *Goat nutrition,* Wageningen, Netherlands, 1991, Pudoc.

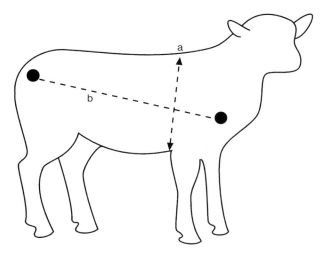

Figure 2-2   The clinician can estimate the weight of a sheep or goat by measuring the circumference or heart girth just behind the shoulder and elbow *(a)* and the body length from shoulder to rump or tuber ilium *(b)* in inches. ***Heart girth*** $\times$ ***heart girth*** $\times$ ***body length*** $\div$ ***300*** $=$ ***weight in lb***. The wool of unshorn animals should always be compressed during this estimation. One of the authors (Dr. Pugh) uses this formula on sheep and goats of varying size with acceptable results. (Adapted from Ensminger ME, Oldfield JE, Heinmann WW: *Feeds and nutrition,* ed 2, Clovis, CA, 1990, Ensminger Publishing.)

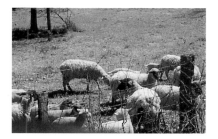

Figure 2-3   These mixed breed sheep are grazing a fescue pasture. They have free range to the pasture and, in this case, no pasture rotation is being used.

method of estimating the body weight of sheep and goats.

FEEDING PROGRAMS

In North America, most farm flocks of sheep and goats are maintained on pasture- or range-based systems. Worldwide, about 80% of all nutrients for sheep and goats are derived from forage.[3] Both species are adept at converting forage into high-quality products for human consumption and use. Whenever sheep (and possibly goats) graze large pastures or range, their maintenance energy requirements may be more than 60% higher than those of animals raised in dry lots.[5] The more walking required or the larger the range, the more work the animal must perform to consume enough forage to support maintenance, growth, lactation, and fiber production.

PASTURES

Producing and providing good-quality forage ultimately reduces feeding costs, increases overall health, and usually results in a more profitable farming operation. In a typical fall breeding/spring lambing operation, supplemental grain feeding can be kept to a minimum if a good forage management program is followed. A variety of perennial grasses (e.g., fescue, orchard) can be used by sheep and goats. Strategic incorporation of legumes (e.g., clover) and some annual grasses (e.g., rye grass) can provide excellent nutrition for the flock. The addition of 30% legumes to a grass pasture improves the nitrogen content of the soil and increases pasture productivity. Legumes improve the nutritional value of a pasture, but may predispose to calcite calculi or bloat. Still, the benefits far outweigh the problems if the legumes are used judiciously.

Where possible, a pasture grazing system should include warm-season perennial grasses for use by the ewes after weaning. During early gestation, these same grasses can be used as mature forage. Approximately 60 days before parturition and through the first 90 days of lactation the females can graze on cool-season, annual grasses. In some environments the warm-season grasses then begin their seasonal production. With this system, very little supplemental feeding is required. As long as quantity of the various forages is not limited, grain supplementation is usually not required. However, under most practical settings, weather limits forage quantity for 60 days or longer each year. A good-quality, pasture-based forage feeding system often requires minimal energy and protein supplements for non-lactating, non-growing animals.

For proper forage management, adequate amounts of grazeable land and several pastures are needed for a rotational grazing program (Figure 2-3). Forage must have some periods of rest from grazing to maintain optimal productivity. Therefore pasture rotation is essential. The pasture layout does not need to be elaborate or comprised of many small paddocks. However, pastures do need to be divided for proper maximization of forage production. Approximately 6 to 10 separate paddocks or pastures are desirable, and further subdivisions can be added as needed (Figure 2-4). The divisions should be based on the productivity of the soil and natural breaks in the topography. They will not necessarily be of equal size. The forage should be grazed in a way that optimal leaf material is produced. Depending on the time of year and amount of moisture, the length of time grazing an area and rest between each rotation vary. For example, the keeper might have his or her flock graze each of 10 paddocks for an average of 3 days at a time; at the end of the rotation the first paddock has had 30 days of rest and

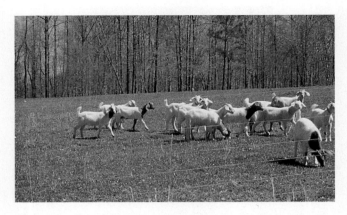

Figure 2-4 These Boer and Boer-crossed goats are in a pasture rotation program in which they are moved every 5 days.

should have good forage regrowth. This type of grazing management may not necessarily increase animal gains, but it may increase the land's carrying capacity as well as the overall quality of the pastures. Pasture rotation systems that increase grass production do not necessarily aid in parasite control. Between four and six ewes (and their lambs) and five to eight does (and their kids) can be maintained on the same amount of land that will support one cow and her calf. However, in woodland or brushy areas the same land that will nutritionally support one cow and her calf will provide enough forage for about 10 goats and their kids.

A complete mineral supplement should be offered at all times. An adequate mineral supplement for animals grazing grass pasture contains 15% to 30% salt, 6% to 12% calcium, 6% to 12% phosphorus, and 1% to 4% magnesium (except in early spring when magnesium should be 8% to 14% of the minerals). Trace minerals suitable for the area and soil type also should be offered.

RANGE

Many of the world's sheep and goats graze on range lands. The common goal among all range land enterprises is to use as much standing forage as possible with little use of harvested forage or other supplements. Supplemental feeding should only be practiced when nutrient demands far exceed the nutrient supply of the forage. Some deficiencies are acceptable because of the female's ability to regain body condition during the period from weaning until breeding. The amount and type of supplementation needed are variable across range conditions. The two most important factors in supplementation decisions are stage of animal production (lactation) and weather conditions (moisture or snow cover). A good range mineral mixture includes equal parts of dicalcium phosphate and trace mineral salt. The trace mineral salt component should be designed for the local forage and

soil types. In general, phosphorus should be supplemented under most range land conditions. Regardless of its composition the salt-mineral supplement should be made available free choice as the only source of salt.

Additional supplements containing protein or energy may be used as needed. Body condition scoring can help in making the decision to supplement energy. If the level of desirable performance can be attained by using a supplemental grain less than or equal to 0.5% of body weight, feeding grain can be economical. However, if greater quantities of grain are needed, negative effects of the grain on forage use will occur (depressed digestibility of forage). Several grain by-products are acceptable supplements for ruminants consuming a forage-based diet. For example, soybean hulls and wheat middlings can provide economical supplies of energy without negative effects on forage use. Protein supplements in the form of soybean meal or cottonseed meal are often used and may actually enhance the digestibility of moderate- or poor-quality forage.

Whenever hand feeding is difficult, salt-limited rations may be useful for range-fed sheep or goats used for brush control. Depending on requirements, supplemental energy (e.g., corn, oats) or protein (e.g., cottonseed meal, soybean meal) should be ground and mixed with salt in a 3:1 to a 6:1 salt-to-grain ratio, depending on intake. If intake is too great, more salt should be added. If intake is too low, salt should be removed. In all cases only white salt (NaCl) should be used. The use of salt-limited feeds decreases trace mineral intake. If trace mineral deficiencies exist locally, and salt-limited feeds are to be used, the keeper should add a suitable trace mineral salt to the feed at a level where trace mineral consumption does not exceed 0.02% of the animal's weight. Salt-limited supplemental feeding should be introduced slowly over 2 to 3 weeks, and the animals should be monitored daily, particularly in times of stress (predator attacks, weather changes).

CONFINEMENT FEEDING

Confinement feeding of sheep or goats in various small vegetation-free enclosures or dry lots is used in certain locales for all or part of the year. In climates with colder winters and areas that lack winter grazing, some producers move sheep (and occasionally goats) to a sheltered dry lot or barn for protection. Such situations usually require more start-up money (for construction of a barn to house animals, feeding floor or lot, and water system) than range or pasture operations. Confinement management also may increase the incidence of some contagious diseases, external parasites (particularly during winter), feeding costs, bedding costs, and the need to handle and dispose of manure. Still, the advantages can more than outweigh the disadvantages in operations where a cheap source of feed and labor is available.

TABLE 2-10

EXAMPLE RATIONS FOR DRY LOT FEEDING FOR NON-DAIRY ANIMALS (LB/DAY)

Ingredient*	150-Pound Ewe						70-Pound Doe					
	MAINTENANCE		GESTATION		LACTATION		MAINTENANCE		GESTATION		LACTATION	
	A†	B†	A	B	A	B	A	B	A	B	A	B
Alfalfa hay	2.9		4.25		5.5		2.0		2.8		2.6	
Grass hay		2.9		3.6		4.8		1.67		2.3		2.2
Corn			0.25	0.75	1.0	1.0		0.33		0.5	0.4	0.4
Soybean meal				0.15		0.75						0.4

*See Table 2-5 for average nutrient contents for each ingredient.
†A and B are different sample diets for each stage of production.

When properly performed, confinement or dry lot feeding can all but eliminate two of the most serious problems with sheep and goat production: internal parasites and predators. However, during confinement feeding, some access to outdoor dry lots is needed to improve hoof and udder health and decrease the need for supplemental vitamin D. Because no grazing is allowed and feedstuffs (hay, silage, grains) are fed in bunks or other types of feeders, production losses resulting from parasites can be curtailed. Also, less energy is required for maintenance (walking to a feed bunk versus grazing). Animals require 2 to 4 hours to consume the same amount of dry matter from hay that they do in 16 to 22 hours of grazing pasture. Heavy-wooled breeds of sheep in full fleece require 1.5 times more space in a confined area than those that have been shorn. Adult sheep and goats require 0.6 and 0.3 m of linear bunk space per animal, respectively.

With confinement systems, ewes and does are more easily separated by age (ewe lambs, adult ewes) and production (lactating, dry or early lactation, late lactation). The ability to feed groups separately can improve the use and efficiency of available feedstuffs and help decrease the incidence of some production diseases (e.g., pregnancy toxemia, hypocalcemia). A dry lot program can be used not only during winter; but also when pasture becomes scarce or when feeding young lambs or kids for rapid gains.

In dry lot feeding, sheep or goats may be fed hay, silage, haylage, or green chop, just as would be used for cattle. The dietary habits of sheep and goats vary and affect intake. However, dietary preference appears to limit the use of certain feedstuffs more greatly in goats. The smell, taste, and variety of feeds also affects intake. Silage can be fed to sheep and goats, but both may take time to adapt to its smell and consistency. Silage that has been poorly packed, exposed to air, or has not attained a low enough pH (less than 5.5) may mold or be contaminated with *Listeria monocytogenes*. Such silage should be avoided, as should bundle-fed, uneaten, frozen, moldy, or spoiled silage. Where possible, the use of square bales of hay results in less wastage than large round bales, but they usually cost more and require more labor to use.

Feed bunk design should minimize animal contamination. Adults and kids (lambs) should be prevented from crawling into feed containers and soiling the feed.

Dry lot feeding is also of value when implementing a parasite control program. If oral anthelmintics of the benzimidazole class are to be used in a deworming program, forcing the animals to fast or feeding dry hay for 12 to 24 hours before deworming and then providing dry lot feeding for as long as 72 hours improves the results. This technique also allows for parasite egg–laden feces to be "cleaned" or "passed" from the bowel before placing animals on a safe pasture. Therefore animals may be moved to pasture after deworming in a relatively parasite-free state, reducing pasture contamination. Examples of confinement or dry lot rations are shown in Table 2-10.

FEEDING THE ADULT MALE

Males should enter the breeding season in good body condition without excessive fat. Rams and bucks should be maintained at a prebreeding body condition score of 3 to 4 because they may lose more than 10% of their body weight in 1½ months of a breeding season. Condition scores should be assessed as part of a breeding soundness evaluation about 2 months before breeding. It is usually beneficial to feed a concentrated energy-protein supplement to the males beginning approximately 4 to 6 weeks before the breeding season. Depending on the body condition and size of the males, 0.5 to 1 kg (1 to 2 lb) of concentrate usually suffices. A good-quality supplement for grass-based forage is 80% corn and 20% soybean meal. After the breeding season some concentrate may need to be fed to help the males regain an adequate body condition. For the remainder of the year, adult males can be fed at a maintenance level. If grass forage is fed, animals should have free access to a mixture of 50% dicalcium phosphate and 50% trace mineral salt. If legumes are a significant portion of the diet, a mixture of 50% trace mineral salt, 25% dicalcium phosphate, and 25% defluorinated rock phosphate can be offered. In both instances, these mineral-salt mixtures should be the only source of salt offered to encourage adequate intake. The trace mineral component should be designed for the local soil types. For sheep, low-copper mineral mixtures are optimal, but goats can safely consume trace mineral mixtures made for cattle. Because of the possibility of urolithiasis in males, the keeper should take steps to prevent stone formation by adding ammonium chloride or other urine acidifiers to the mineral mixture (see Chapter 10).

FEEDING THE FEMALE

Breeding females have different nutrient requirements as the stage of production changes. Although requirements are much lower for maintenance than they are for lactation, meeting these requirements is important for efficient production. Body condition scoring all females every 2 to 3 weeks is an important and cost-effective management tool. Mineral feeding as described for the adult male is applicable for the female.

Maintenance

During maintenance the objective is to maintain the female's weight and health and replenish any losses experienced during lactation. Most pasture or range settings provide adequate levels of nutrient intake to maintain dry, non-pregnant sheep and goats for this entire period. If extremes in environmental conditions occur (e.g., drought, snowfall), some supplemental feeding is required.

Breeding

At the time of breeding, the practice of flushing the females has been used with some success. The basic premise is that increased nutrition, specifically energy, just before and during the early breeding season increases the ovulation rate and therefore the lambing or kidding rate. The female's age and body condition and the time of year all affect the response to flushing. Mature females in marginal body condition usually respond best to flushing. Moreover, the practice appears to be more beneficial when trying to breed the group early or late as opposed to during the peak of breeding season. Overconditioned females either do not respond or appear to respond only marginally to flushing. Flushing can be accomplished by the provision of lush pastures or by supplementation with about 0.14 kg (0.33 lb) to 0.45 kg (1 lb) of a 10% to 12% crude protein grain per head per day. It is best to begin approximately 2 weeks before the males are introduced

and continue for an additional 2 to 3 weeks into the breeding season.

The effects of flushing include increased body condition, increased ovulation rate, and increased number of lambs born. Adequate body condition is necessary for acceptable conception rates. Outside certain biologic limits a flushing effect cannot be observed. For example, an extremely thin (condition score 1) female would probably not have an increased ovulation rate because she is too thin to have normal reproductive cycles. However, within normal ranges (condition score 2.5 to 3) the ovulation rate appears to respond to a short-duration increase in energy, and, to a lesser extent, to increased protein intake (see Figure 2-1). Flushing does not always increase lambing or kidding rates; however, it does increase the number of females cycling early in the breeding season, resulting in a greater proportion of the offspring being born early in the lambing or kidding season. Females at or just under a body condition score of 2.5 to 3 are optimal for most breeding flocks.

Early to Middle Gestation

After the female has conceived, early gestation is the time of partial fetal and placental development. Nutrition is important for adequate development, but requirements are not greatly increased over those of maintenance. If the diet is lacking in energy, protein, and certain minerals, poor placental development may occur, resulting in poor fetal growth. A reduction in lamb survival rates at birth can result from inadequate feeding during early gestation. Likewise, adequate nutrition is required for proper attachment of the embryo to the uterus. Mid-term stress abortions can occur in Angora goats as a result of energy deficiency. This is more common in range conditions, particularly after a weather change, predator attack, or decreased feed intake. The incidence can be minimized by not breeding the female until she has attained 60% to 70% of her projected mature weight, and by maintaining a steady nutritional state during pregnancy[4] (see Chapters 6 and 7). During early gestation ewes and does can be maintained on winter range or pasture or moderate-quality hay. As seasonal decreases in feed availability or weather-associated increases in feed requirements occur, some supplemental grain may be required. Females should be fed to maintain a body condition score of 2.5 to 3 during early gestation. The scores should be assessed every 2 to 3 weeks, and any flock condition score change acted on immediately.

Late Gestation

The nutrition of the female during the last 6 weeks of gestation is extremely important. Approximately 70% of fetal growth occurs during this period. Undernutrition can result in poor colostrum production, low birth–

weight lambs and kids, lower energy reserves in the newborn animals, and increased death loss, especially during cold and inclement weather. Birth weight is an important factor affecting newborn survival. It can be influenced by breed, number born, age of dam, and the dam's preparturient diet. Extremely low birth weights (lambs weighing less than 2 kg) can result in an increased incidence of death during the first 24 hours. Conversely, overfeeding of energy can result in obesity and contribute to dystocia. Proper nutrition is crucial. In general, more problems result from underfeeding than from overfeeding during late gestation.

The process of converting dietary energy into fetal growth is quite inefficient. Because 70% to 80% of fetal growth occurs during the final 6 weeks of gestation, the dam's energy requirements increase substantially. In many instances the only way to provide the extra nutrition is to increase the amount of concentrate being offered. This sharp increase in energy requirements is compounded if the dam has multiple fetuses. A large uterus filled with several fetuses physically limits rumen capacity. This can result in a situation whereby the mature female cannot consume enough forage to meet her needs. Under these conditions the keeper may wish to feed between ⅓ to 1 lb of grain per day, depending on the size of the dam.

During late gestation, feeding regimens should be designed to minimize the energy being supplied by body fat reserves. This is especially crucial for late-gestating ewes. Excessive catabolism of body fat can result in pregnancy toxemia. The dam is at greater risk for this condition if some environmental or disease stressor is occurring concurrently. Pregnancy toxemia is characterized by a buildup of ketones in the blood as a result of accelerated fat catabolism. Affected ewes appear listless and have a distinct acetone smell. Maintaining the flock at a body condition score of 2.5 to 3 and promoting adequate energy intake during late gestation help prevent pregnancy toxemia. During late gestation, ewes with a single fetus may consume as much as 3.5% to 4% of their body weight in dry matter in grain or excellent-quality forages. Intake may reach 5% in some does. If poor-quality forage is fed, these pregnant females may only be able to consume 2% to 3% of their body weight in dry matter. Treatment can be successful, but as is the case with all nutritional problems, prevention is the best strategy. Ewes should be fed approximately 1 kg (2.2 lb) of a cereal grain (e.g., corn, oats) during the final month of gestation to prevent pregnancy toxemia. Goats also can develop pregnancy toxemia but appear to be more resistant (see Chapter 4). Dairy goats that are grazing or being fed good-quality grass hay can be fed 0.5 to 1 kg (1 to 2 lb) of a 16% crude protein grain per 100 lb of body weight daily the final 1½ months of gestation. The amount of grain may need to be adjusted depending on body condition.

In addition to encouraging healthy lambs and preventing pregnancy toxemia, adequate nutrition during this time frame promotes significant mammary development during the last 30 days of pregnancy. Stillbirths, pregnancy toxemia, and poor milk production are all indicators of feeding an energy-deficient diet in late gestation. Adequate nutrition should be provided to support milk and colostrum production.

Feed or mineral supplements that contain added ionophore, antibiotics, or decoquinate may help control or prevent coccidiosis, abortion, and pregnancy toxemia (see the section on Feed Additives in this chapter, as well as Chapters 4 and 6 and Appendix I).

Lactation

In both sheep and goats, milk production peaks within 2 to 3 weeks after parturition, then declines rather rapidly to a low by 8 to 10 weeks after parturition. In dairy animals this drop in milk production is less profound. A dam nursing a single kid or lamb produces less milk than a female nursing twins or triplets. This is because one lamb or kid is unable to consume the amount being produced, allowing a reduction of total mammary output. A dam nursing twins produces approximately 30% more milk than one nursing a single. Likewise, a lactating dairy goat being milked two to three times per day for maximal milk production also produces greater amounts. A dairy goat usually weighs 10% of a dairy cow's weight, but may require 12% to 14% of the nutrients. Lactating does may be capable of consuming 4% to 5% or more (up to 10% to 11% in some females) of their body weight in dry matter, making feed intake the most important limiting factor affecting milk production.

Milk production during the first 4 weeks of lactation is important for good lamb and kid growth. If milk production is lacking, the lamb or kid can compensate by increasing solid feed consumption. However, because feed is less digestible than milk, suckling animals cannot consume enough feed to make up for a milk deficiency and may therefore exhibit suppressed growth rates during early lactation.

Underfeeding energy during late gestation or early lactation results in greater than expected death losses in lambs, particularly twin lambs. Depressed milk production results in lambs that are "scruffy," poorly kept, thin, and weak. Necropsies of affected lambs show nondescript signs—the gastrointestinal tract is filled with straw, and the lambs have little or no abdominal fat. Lambs older than 1 month are less likely to starve as they begin to eat on their own.

During peak lactation it is nearly impossible for a ewe or doe to consume enough feed to meet their nutrient demands. During this time, good to excellent dairy animals use body fat to make up for this deficit and therefore experience a downward shift (often by more than 1 point) in body condition score. This is why an adequate body condition before parturition is paramount. To make efficient use of her body fat a ewe or doe must have adequate levels of protein in the diet. For example, the NRC[5] recommends a protein concentration of 13.4% for ewes nursing a single versus 15% for those nursing twins. Likewise, for does producing milk containing 3.5% fat, the NRC[6] recommends an additional 68 g of protein per day for each additional kg of milk being produced. Many producers feed dairy goats 0.23 to 0.4 kg (0.5 to 1 lb) of a 16% to 18% crude protein grain per 0.5 kg of milk produced up to 1.8 kg (4 lb); they then feed 0.5 to 1 kg (1 to 2 lb) of grain for each additional 1.8 kg (4 lb) of produced milk. Whenever diets containing large quantities of cereal grain are fed, some form of rumen buffer should be included in the diet or offered free choice.

Because feed intake can limit production in heavy producing dairy animals, increasing the diet's energy density in early lactation may be required. The addition of fat to the diet is an excellent way to increase the energy density of the diet. As a general rule, supplemental fats should not exceed 4% to 5% of the diet. Oil seed (whole cottonseed), where locally available, is an excellent way to add energy to the diet. About 2% to 3% of the added fat can effectively come from oil seeds. If more fat is needed, 2% to 3% more fat can be added in the form of specialty fats, including calcium or magnesium salts or fatty acids. These specialty fats are expensive, but for the most part bypass the rumen. The fatty acids and calcium or magnesium salts are broken apart for digestion in the small intestine.

Obviously, the concentrate portion of the grain can be adjusted based on body condition scores. These recommendations show the importance of adequate protein concentrations for maximal milk production. Whole cottonseed can be included in the diets of lactating animals as an excellent energy (greater than 90% TDN) and protein (21% to 23% crude protein) source. Whole cottonseed should account for no more than 20% of the diet. The requirements of most lactating ewes can be met by feeding 3.2 to 3.6 kg (7 to 8 lb) of a 12% to 14% crude protein, 55% to 60% TDN diet. If hay is fed, a grass-legume or legume only hay helps supply protein demands. If silage is fed, it usually takes 1.36 kg (3 lb) to supply the equivalent amount of energy in 0.68 kg (1.5 lb) of good-quality hay.

With the exception of dairy goats or ewes, milk production decreases quickly; by 8 to 10 weeks postpartum it has become an insignificant nutrition source for the suckling lambs or kids. During this time the dam's requirements can be met by grazing moderate- to good-quality pasture or range. If animals are grouped and fed by production, first-lactation dams with one kid or lamb should be fed with mature females with twins. Also, if these first-lactation dams have twins, they should be fed with mature dams with triplets.

Some dairy goats are susceptible to "off-flavor" milk production. Cabbage, onions, wild garlic, and some species of weeds or browse can all negatively affect milk flavor. If certain feed sources cannot be avoided, feeding these off-flavor producers just after milking may reduce some of their ill effects. Still, avoiding the offending feedstuffs is the best method of prevention. Other non-feed influences on milk flavor are disease (metritis, mastitis), filthy living conditions, and gastrointestinal upset.

NUTRITIONAL DISORDERS

The most common nutrition-related diseases seen in late gestation in goats and sheep are pregnancy toxemia (see Chapter 4), hypocalcemia, and hypomagnesemia.

Hypocalcemia

Hypocalcemia can be a problem in dairy goats and to some extent in ewes, meat and fiber goats, and pet animals. It usually occurs shortly before or after parturition and is a result of low concentrations of serum calcium. Some cases also are complicated by hypophosphatemia and hypermagnesemia or hypomagnesemia. Ewes appear most susceptible in late gestation and early lactation, particularly when experiencing some sort of stress (e.g., hauling, predator attack, no feed). Sheep may succumb to hypocalcemia 6 weeks before to 10 weeks after parturition. The greatest demand for calcium for the non-dairy animal occurs 3 to 4 weeks before parturition in females with more than one fetus, as a result of the calcification of fetal bones. Goats may have hypocalcemia before parturition; however, in high-producing dairy goats the disease generally occurs after the dam gives birth. Whenever an abrupt demand for calcium occurs, the body requires 1 or more days to accrue the enzyme systems capable of mobilizing bone stores of calcium. High intake of calcium, phosphorus, or some cations (potassium, sodium) decreases the production of parathyroid hormones. During decreased parathyroid function, less 1,25 dihydroxycholecalciferol is produced. This results in lowered absorption and mobilization of calcium from the intestines and bones. Low dietary calcium or increased amounts of dietary anions enhances the production and release of parathyroid hormones.

Clinical signs. Early in the course of the disease animals have a stiff gait, tremors, and tetany. Affected animals may be ataxic or constipated and have decreased rumen motility. As the disease progresses, an increased heart and respiratory rate, regurgitation of rumen content, bloat, and depression to the point of opisthotonos can occur. Corneal and pupillary light reflexes appear normal at first, but become depressed before disappearing entirely. The rectal temperature usually remains in the normal range, but may be slightly low.

Diagnosis. Diagnosis is usually based on a history and signalment conducive to hypocalcemia, as well as response to therapy. Serum calcium concentrations less than 4 to 5 ml/dl in sheep and goats are fairly diagnostic of this disease.

Treatment.   In clinical cases, immediate treatment is needed, usually in the form of intravenous (IV) administration of calcium borogluconate (50 to 100 ml of a 23% solution). Subcutaneous delivery of these calcium solutions or the oral administration of a calcium gel designed for cattle, but based on sheep or goat body weight, helps prevent relapse. If the subcutaneous route is chosen to supply a "reservoir" of calcium for affected animals, solutions containing dextrose or numerous electrolytes should be avoided if possible, because some result in abscesses. During treatment, the clinician should monitor the animals' hearts and slow or stop therapy if arrhythmias occur. If the treatment is successful, the animals should stand and urinate within 20 minutes. If left untreated, affected animals usually die.

Prevention.   To prevent or minimize hypocalcemia, particularly in dairy goats, the diet should be low in calcium and have a low cation-to-anion ratio. The dietary modifications used for the prevention of milk fever in cattle may be of value in dairy sheep and goats. Therefore reducing or eliminating diets rich in cations (alfalfa) or calcium and phosphorus in the late dry period may aid in prevention. Many legumes are rich sources of potassium and calcium and can therefore contribute to hypocalcemia. Immediately after parturition the calcium levels in the diet should be increased. This strategy improves calcium reabsorption for bones and absorption from the intestine. Hauling or other forms of stress should be minimized in sheep during the final 8 weeks of gestation. Even with this strategy some incidence of hypocalcemia may be experienced.

Hypomagnesemia

Hypomagnesemia (grass tetany) can be a problem in sheep and, to a lesser extent, goats grazing on lush, rapidly growing forage. It usually occurs during the early spring on pastures that are well fertilized with nitrogen and potassium. A combination of elevated nitrogen and potassium levels in the forage leads to a reduced absorption of magnesium from the gastrointestinal tract of the animal. The primary problem in hypomagnesemia is reduced absorption by the animal rather than low plant concentrations. Cattle, sheep, and goats that graze lush cereal grains (e.g., wheat, rye), particularly in early lactation or late gestation, are predisposed to this condition. Any type of stress (e.g., weather changes, transportation, predator attack) can increase blood concentrations of free fatty acids, and excess blood from fatty acid concentrations depresses blood magnesium. Other forms of hypomagnesemia occur during winter when animals are fed poor-quality grass hay (with low magnesium content) and in lambs or kids fed only low-magnesium milk replacers. Kids or lambs with access to grain or legume-grass hay are more resistant to hypomagnesemia. Ewes with poor dentition and those that lose excessive weight during winter are prone to the condition.

Clinical signs.   Hypomagnesemia generally occurs in ewes 2 to 4 weeks after lambing. It is more common in females with twins. Affected animals are excitable and may develop paddling convulsions, clonic-tonic muscle spasms, and an increased respiratory rate. They also may simply be found dead in the pasture. Rectal temperature is commonly normal. Convulsions may be triggered by any number of stimuli, from being chased by predators to acute changes in weather patterns. Lambs or kids with the milk replacer–associated form are usually anorexic and hyperexcitable and may salivate profusely.

Diagnosis.   Diagnosis is often based on signalment and history, as well as response to treatment. Serum magnesium levels less than 1.5 mg/dl may be indicative of this disease; levels less than 1 mg/dl should be considered diagnostic. Postmortem serum samples are of limited value. Magnesium concentrations in cerebrospinal fluid (for 12 hours after death), urine (for 24 hours after death), or anterior eye chamber fluid (for 48 hours after death) are good postmortem tests.

Treatment.   Treatment consists of the IV administration of 20% to 25% calcium borogluconate and 4% to 5% magnesium (50 ml). Oral calcium magnesium gel and subcutaneous injection of calcium magnesium salts are both beneficial to prevent relapse.

Prevention.   Because grass tetany results from a reduction in available magnesium, a number of methods can be used to increase consumption. Properly balanced fertilizers and magnesium compounds can be applied to the soil to increase plant concentrations of magnesium. These are helpful but not very economical because the primary problem with the occurrence of hypomagnesemia is reduced absorption by the animal rather than low plant concentrations. Therefore prevention is best accomplished by offering high-magnesium mineral supplements before the growth of lush spring forage and lambing or kidding. Most mineral supplements with high levels of magnesium are unpalatable; feeders should be checked frequently to ensure proper consumption. To enhance intake the keeper can mix magnesium oxide with molasses, corn, salt, or other feedstuffs. Daily consumption is important because magnesium in a readily usable form is poorly stored in the body. An average adult lactating ewe needs 7 to 9 g of magnesium oxide daily. An economical supplement is a 1:1 mix of trace-mineral salt and magnesium oxide, but this combination appears to be un-palatable. A more acceptable substitute may be equal parts of ground corn, trace-mineral salt, and magnesium oxide. Other palatable grains can be used in place of the corn. Legumes (e.g., alfalfa, clover, bird's foot, kudzu) are much better sources of both calcium and magnesium and their inclusion in a pasture helps reduce the incidence of hypomagnesemia.[4] Maintaining a high soil pH (greater than 5.5) enhances magnesium availability and intake by plants. The inclusion of vitamin D (5 to 10 IU/kg/day) in a milk replacer helps prevent hypomagnesemia in lambs or kids fed indoors.

FEEDING THE LAMB OR KID

Bottle Feeding

Rearing orphaned lambs or kids on milk replacer is quite expensive and labor intensive. If at all possible, keepers should attempt to graft the orphans onto another dam, rearing them on milk replacer only if this cannot be accomplished. Ideally, orphans need to consume small quantities of milk many times per day, which is generally not possible for most sheep and goat producers. Most producers feed "bottle babies" only one to three times each day. Many dairy kids or lambs are removed from their dams somewhere between birth and 72 hours of age and fed as orphans. The most economical way to raise orphans is to get them onto a dry concentrate feed as soon as possible.

The newborn needs to receive 10% to 20% of its body weight in colostrum, preferably within 3 to 12 hours after birth. If it is not available from the dam, frozen colostrum can be thawed and used. Colostrum absorption decreases rapidly from birth through 36 hours of age (see Chapters 6 and 14). Hemolytic crisis has been observed in some lambs fed cow colostrum. Still, cross-species colostrum is often better than no colostrum. Dairy cow colostrum is usually available, but is dilute in its immunoglobulin content. Any colostrum fed to an orphan should be free of caprine arthritis-encephalitis (CAE) and Johne's disease. If lambs or kids are unable to nurse, they need to be tubed.

After the initial amount of colostrum is fed, additional feeding should be withheld from newborns that are to be bottle-raised for as long as 5 hours. This encourages sucking, easing the transition and aiding in training to a bottle, nipple pail, or bucket. If the owner wishes to feed by hand, a lamb nipple attached to a soda bottle is a good system. The nipple should be placed in the mouth and the newborn's jaw moved in a chewing motion by the feeder. This usually stimulates the nursing reflex in all but very weak young. Lambs or kids left with their dams for more than 2 days require longer training to become accustomed to a bottle or pail. If a ewe or doe has too little milk to support more than one newborn, it is imperative that sufficient colostrum be given to all. The keeper should then leave the strongest, most vigorous newborn with the dam and raise the weakest artificially. Although immunoglobulin may not be absorbed after 12 to 36 hours, it is a rich source of vitamin A, energy, protein, and local gut-acting antibodies. It also acts as a laxative. If possible, colostrum should be fed for 2 to 3 days.

If lambs or kids are to be hand-fed, feeding 10% to 20% of their body weight in the form of good-quality milk replacer divided into four equal daily feedings is usually acceptable. Milk replacers for goats should be around 20% protein and 20% fat, with most of the protein supplied by an animal source (whey proteins). If the milk replacer appears brown, the protein sources may have been overheated, resulting in decreased digestibility. Antibiotics are commonly added to help reduce the incidence of bacterial respiratory and enteric diseases. Milk replacers should be fortified with vitamin A (20,000 to 30,000 IU/kg of dry matter), vitamin E (30 to 40 mg/kg of dry matter), and vitamin D (2500 to 3500 IU/kg of dry matter). Table 2-11 shows the composition of sheep and goat milk.[6] If lamb milk replacers are used for goats, they should be diluted because they contain more fat than naturally occurs in goat milk. Good-quality milk replacers designed for calves may be fed to goats and lambs in small quantities over numerous feedings (10% to 20% of body weight divided into four to six equal feedings). Whenever mixing milk replacers, the keeper should take care to ensure that the powder and milk are properly mixed into a suspension. Feeding small quantities over numerous feedings helps reduce the incidence of bloat. By the third week of life, some kids or lambs can be switched to a twice-daily feeding regimen. Because milk replacers are expensive, animals should be weaned as soon as possible. If lambs or kids are underfed or fed a poorly digestible replacer, they may become emaciated, weak, or comatose. Death is possible. Lambs or kids with this condition have lower than normal blood glucose, and necropsy reveals a body devoid of fat stores. The abomasums of starved neonates often become impacted with hair or poorly digestible items.

TABLE 2-11

COMPOSITION OF SHEEP AND GOAT MILK AS A PERCENTAGE OF DRY MATTER

ELEMENT	SHEEP MILK	GOAT MILK
Protein	32%	25%
Carbohydrate	25%	31%
Fat	38%	34%
Total solids as fed	19%	13%

From Naylor JM, Bell R: Raising the orphaned foal, *Vet Clin North Am (Equine Pract)* 1(1):173, 1985.

The most efficient and least labor-intensive system is to place the orphans on a self-feeder using refrigerated milk. This helps the orphans consume less milk and therefore nurse more frequently throughout a 24-hour period. In effect this regimen imitates the normal dam/newborn nursing regimen. Keeping the milk cold also may help prevent spoilage and lessen the extent to which the milk replacer separates out of suspension. In addition, kids or lambs using a self-feeder should have access to an extremely palatable dry diet. A mixture of corn, oats, alfalfa pellets, molasses, and soybean meal that provides 14% to 16% crude protein works well. Top-dressing the feed with a dry milk replacer also may stimulate early intake of the dry feed. Other extremely palatable ingredients to young ruminants are soybean hulls and various sources of bran, including wheat bran.

Creep Feeding

The term *creep feeding* refers to the use of supplemental feed for the nursing lamb or kid. The goals of a creep feeding program are to promote an adequate intake with a palatable feed, provide all necessary nutrients, and be as economical as possible. Both lambs and kids use feedstuffs more efficiently before weaning.

Lambs and kids will only nibble at the creep feed until they are 3 to 4 weeks old. Still, the creep feed should be made available as soon as possible to help the orphans get used to eating from one location and establish rumen function. The feeder should be placed in a dry, well-lit area where lambs or kids can easily gain access but still retain visual contact with their dams. A variety of methods can be employed to maximize the acceptance of the creep area. Some of these include hanging a light over the creep feeder, retaining one or two dams and their offspring in the area for a few days (with limited feed, of course), and putting all the animals in a small, confined space adjacent to the creep area.

Creep feeds need not be complex but they must be palatable because they are competing with milk. Pelleting or coarse grinding feeds usually increases intake. Fine grinding usually results in decreased intake as animals (particularly lambs) age. Pellets should be small enough for consumption. In goats, pellets larger than 5 to 7 mm may decrease intake. After the lambs or kids have begun to consume the creep feed, cheaper ingredients can be used to enhance the economics of the practice. However, until the animals reach 3 to 4 weeks of age, palatability is the key to successful creep feeding. If increased performance is to be attained from creep feeding lambs, they must consume more than 0.23 kg (0.5 lb) daily from 3 weeks of age to weaning. Enhanced performance may be attained if salt (0.5% of the creep feed), ammonium chloride (0.2 kg/440 kg feed, or 10 lb/ton), and vitamin E are added to most creep feeds. Some examples of creep feeds are shown in Table 2-12.

In general, creep feeding should provide an additional 0.5 kg of gain for each 1.8 to 3.2 kg (4 to 7 lb) of feed consumed. This efficiency varies from one set of conditions to another, but generally when feed costs are low and sale prices are high, creep feeding is usually profitable. It is less profitable when feed costs are high and sale prices are low. In the final analysis it is simply a matter of feed costs versus animal sale prices that determines the feasibility of creep feeding.

Weaning

Lambs and kids can be weaned as early as 3 or 4 weeks, but better results may occur if weaning is delayed until

TABLE 2-12

SAMPLE CREEP DIETS FOR LAMBS AND KIDS*

ELEMENT	SAMPLE 1	SAMPLE 2	SAMPLE 3	SAMPLE 4
Ground corn	33%	60%	63%	40%
Oats	—	—	—	11%
Soybean hulls	—	—	10%	—
Soybean meal	6%	8.5%	10%	6.5%
Alfalfa hay	55%	25%	—	35%
Bran	—	—	10%	—
Molasses	5%	5%	5%	6%
Trace mineral salt	0.5%	0.5%	0.5%	0.5%
Ammonium chloride	0.5%	0.5%	0.5%	0.5%
Limestone	—	0.5%	1%	0.5%

*Diets 1, 2, and 3 should be fed with an excellent-quality hay offered free choice. Diet 4 is a complete, pelleted feed.

8 to 12 weeks. Because of labor constraints, many keepers attempt to wean milk replacer–fed young as soon as possible. Kids of most meat and dairy breeds should weigh at least 9.1 to 11.4 kg (20 to 25 lb) and consume 0.23 kg (0.5 lb) of a 16% to 18% crude protein grain per day.

Because weaning is such a stressful event, the goal should be to get the lamb or kid accustomed to eating out of feedbunks and drinking from a water trough. The decision to wean lambs or kids depends on age, season of birth, whether they have been consuming creep feed, existing parasite or predator problems on the farm, market price, and available labor. Feedbunk location is important in helping newly weaned animals consume adequate amounts of dry matter. However, if excellent-quality forage is available, it can be used as the sole source of feed. A good strategy is to place the feedbunks perpendicular to the fence line so that the weanlings are forced to see and possibly investigate the feed as they walk (usually continually) the fence line. For the first 2 days of the weaning period, good-quality hay should be offered free choice. The weanlings should then be introduced to a concentrate feed offered at a level of about 1% of body weight per day. A lamb weighing 31.8 kg (70 lb) therefore consumes approximately 0.32 kg (0.75 lb) per day. After the lambs or kids have been introduced to the grain, the keeper can gradually increase the amount.

Some managers prefer to remove all grain supplements and place the dam on a poor-quality forage 1 week before weaning. This reduces milk production and decreases the incidence of mastitis. By 7 months, most dairy breed kids should weigh between 27.3 and 36.4 kg (60 to 80 lb). A good-quality mineral mixture should be offered free choice. The same guidelines described for mineral feeding of the male (50% dicalcium phosphate and 50% trace mineral salt) are applicable for weanlings.

Finishing

Finishing of lambs for slaughter can be accomplished in a variety of ways. There is no one perfect diet for finishing. Instead, each feeding facility accomplishes the goal by using feedstuffs that are available and economical to the area. Feedlots designed specifically for goats are not as common as those designed for lambs. Most goats are slaughtered off of forage-based diets with little use of concentrate feeding.

At slaughter the lamb should have approximately 0.23 to 0.46 cm of backfat. However, the amount of backfat often depends on specific market preferences. Slaughter weights have a wide range because of the variation in frame size among North American sheep, although they generally fall between slightly below 45.4 kg (100 lb) and 68 kg (150 lb). Ideally, the lambs should be marketed at the proper degree of finish, regardless of their weight.

Feeding beyond the lamb's ideal finish results in higher cost of gain because of decreased feed efficiency. Adding lean muscle is much more energy efficient than adding body fat. Blackfaced sheep and meat goat breeds generally finish at greater body weights.

If high-quality forage is available, lambs can be finished on it. This generally works best for smaller, younger lambs. Older, heavier lambs require some concentrate feeding. For example, a small-framed lamb born in January in the southeastern United States could be ready for slaughter in June having been grazed on only cool-season annual grasses (rye grass) or grass-legume pastures. However, a large-framed, spring-born lamb in the western United States may come off of range in the fall at 6 months weighing 31.8 to 41 kg (70 to 90 lb) and need a concentrate-based diet to be finished by 1 year.

Many lambs in North America are finished in a feedlot or dry lot. These lots vary in size and may be open areas, confinement barns, or a combination of both. An excellent feeding regimen is stepwise feeding whereby lambs (and occasionally kids) are given more grain as they get larger. By the end of the finishing period many are typically consuming about 80% concentrate and 20% roughage. However, when given free access to both roughage and concentrate, lambs consume about 60% to 70% concentrate and 30% to 40% roughage. A variety of cereal grains can be used by lambs, including corn, oats, barley, milo, and to some extent wheat. Amounts used are based on local economics. A protein supplement may be included depending on the amount of protein being provided by the roughage source. Alfalfa is commonly used as a roughage source because of its wide availability, and animals feeding on it may not need additional protein. Mineral and vitamin premixes also are added to some diets. Because the finishing period is usually accompanied by diets that emphasize grains, the nutritionist or clinician must be aware that excessive grain intake can predispose to urolithiasis, enterotoxemia, and bloat.

With the possible exception of sorghum, processing of grains does not appreciably increase lamb performance. Cracking, rolling, or flaking milo to break its hard seed coat increases its use by lambs. Feeding other grains whole may actually tend to decrease the incidence of acidosis and other digestive disturbances. Pelleting bulky rations may be of some benefit because of the increased level of consumption. The most important factor to consider with regard to pelleting or other processing is the potential for the lamb or kid to "sort" the feed and consume only a portion of the diet. For example, if the protein, mineral, and vitamin premix is a loose meal, cracking the grain may be beneficial in minimizing sorting, despite its lack of effect on use. Pelleted feeds help ensure a more uniform intake and are less dusty and easier to handle. However, they are more expensive and may increase the incidence of some diseases.

As stated earlier, goats are generally not finished under commercial settings. Most of the goats consumed in North America are slaughtered by the consumer; by small, local processing facilities; or in niche marketing systems. With some exceptions, goats tend to be sold in small groups over the course of the year. Because of this method of marketing, goats are generally kept on a forage-based diet rather than year-round feeding of grain. Still, some feedlots, or "grain on grass" operations do exist. If a group of kids is placed on a concentrate-based diet for finishing, the same basic principles discussed previously for lambs apply. Table 2-13 provides examples of growing and finishing diets for lambs and kids. Growing diets, which contain 14.5% protein and 68% TDN, are used for younger, lighter lambs and kids. Finishing diets, which contain 10% protein and 80% TDN, are more effectively fed to the older, heavier animals.

Regardless of the specie being fed, the introduction to and consumption of energy-dense diets in a feedlot setting is stressful and associated with many metabolic diseases. The nutritionist or clinician should ensure that animals being fed in the finishing stages be slowly introduced to these diets and vaccinated for *Clostridium perfringens C* and *D*, and possibly other diseases (e.g., contagious ecthyma, pasteurellosis) that are locally problematic. On arrival animals should be offered free access to a good-quality legume-grass hay, fresh clean water, and a mineral mixture. Animals should be introduced to the finishing diet slowly over a 2- to 4-week period. If males are fed, ammonium chloride or other urine acidifiers should be fed to prevent urolithiasis (see Chapter 10). The use of rumen buffers, antibiotics, ionophores (see the section on Feed Additives in this chapter), and free-choice hay are all effective in minimizing some production diseases.

FEEDING YEARLINGS

Females

Every sheep and goat enterprise is different in terms of overall goals. Some operations place importance on breeding ewes and does so that they have their first offspring by 1 year of age. Other farms or ranches may find it much more practical and economical to breed their animals to have their first offspring as 2-year-olds. A ewe's lifetime production can be as much as 20% greater if she is bred as a ewe lamb rather than as a yearling.[8]

If the goal is to have the females lamb or kid as yearlings, nutrition is crucial from weaning to breeding. In general, the female should obtain 65% of her projected mature weight by the time of breeding. In reality a range of weights probably exists within which small-framed sheep and goats may have acceptable conception rates at 55% to 60% of their projected mature weights, while some large-framed animals may need to be closer to 70% of their mature weights.

Depending on their weaning weights, most females need to gain between 0.11 and 0.23 kg (0.25 to 0.5 lb) per day from weaning until breeding. Under most situations this requires some supplemental energy or concentrate feeding. However, overfeeding young females can result in excessive fat deposition in the mammary glands and decreased lifetime milk production. After the females have been bred, moderate and steady weight gain is desirable until parturition, with a weight goal of 85% to 90% of the projected mature weight by 1 year of age.

If females are to be bred as yearlings, a moderate growth rate is most desirable. As long as a good, well-planned forage system is available, females can achieve desired weight gains with little or no grain supplementation. Sheep or goats that can successfully breed out of

---

TABLE 2-13

SAMPLE GROWER AND FINISHER DIETS FOR LAMBS AND KIDS

ELEMENT	GROWER 1	GROWER 2	GROWER 3	FINISHER 1*	FINISHER 2*	FINISHER 3*
Corn	33.5%	28.5%	32.1%	73.2%	76.0%	74.6%
Alfalfa	55%	—	—	20%	—	—
Grass hay	—	50%	—	—	17%	—
Cottonseed hulls	—	—	40%	—	—	14%
Soybean meal	5.5%	15%	21%	—	—	4%
Molasses	5%	5%	5%	5%	5%	5%
Trace mineral salt	0.5%	0.5%	0.5%	0.5%	0.5%	0.5%
Limestone	—	0.5%	0.9%	0.8%	1.0%	1.4%
NH$_4$Cl	0.5%	0.5%	0.5%	0.5%	0.5%	0.5%

*Finisher diets should contain enough limestone (or other calcium source) to provide a 2:1 calcium-phosphorus ratio in the diet.

season should be bred at 13 months so they can lamb or kid at 18 months. This requires less nutritional input than breeding 7-month-old females but still provides an acceptable generation interval for increased female productivity.

Regardless of the breeding system, animals should be weighed and body condition scored regularly whenever possible. If the body condition scores of the group begin to drop below 2.5, the keeper should offer supplemental energy; conversely, if the scores rise above 3.5, he or she should provide less energy. A good-quality mineral mixture as described for adult males is applicable for yearlings.

Males

Feeding developing males is quite straightforward. They should be developed using as much forage as possible, with just enough supplemental feeding to produce desirable gains (0.34 kg or 0.75 lb per day). This is easily accomplished with good genetics. Growing males should be offered a good-quality mineral mixture as described previously, with the keepers taking steps to prevent urolithiasis and other production-related diseases.

FEEDING SHOW ANIMALS

Lambs

All show animals should be offered a good-quality mineral mixture and given free access to fresh, clean water. Feeding show lambs should be as simple as possible while providing the desired rate of gain and appropriate "bloom." Ideally, the lamb should be fed 30% to 40% of its total daily intake as good-quality hay or forage; the remaining 60% to 70% of the diet should be in the form of a concentrate or grain mixture (Table 2-14). A lamb can eat as much as 3% to 4% of its body weight daily. At least 0.45 kg (1 lb) of hay per day should be fed with the

TABLE 2-14

CONCENTRATE MIXES FOR SHOW LAMBS*

ELEMENT	SAMPLE 1	SAMPLE 2
Corn	50%	45%
Oats	35%	—
Soybean hulls	—	40%
Soybean meal	10%	10%
Molasses	4%	4%
Mineral mix	1%	1%

*Animals should be introduced to high-grain diets slowly over 2 to 3 weeks.

concentrate. Lambs should be slowly exposed to the concentrate portions of the feed, taking 10 to 14 days to make the transition from little grain to the full amount. Feeds should never be switched abruptly and fresh clean water should always be offered free choice.

Mature Sheep

Mature show ewes and rams should consume approximately 1.36 to 2.27 kg (3 to 5 lb) of concentrate per day, depending on their size. They also should be offered good-quality hay free choice. The requirements for mature sheep are found in Table 2-7. Adult show animals should be maintained in good condition but should not be obese. A good exercise regimen is necessary to prevent overconditioning. Where possible, forcing animals to graze or walk some distance from grain to hay to water may prove valuable.

Show Goats

The feeding of young meat goats for show is similar to the feeding of show lambs discussed previously. The goal is to use a simple diet that provides the desired level of gain and degree of bloom. The same forages and concentrates discussed for lambs in Table 2-14 are appropriate for goats.

FEEDING FOR FIBER PRODUCTION

Sheep

Wool production is highly heritable; however, nutrition can affect wool growth and character. Within certain biologic limits, energy intake is directly proportional to wool production,[9] although separating protein effects from energy effects is difficult. As long as the minimal protein requirement is met, additional dietary protein does not appear to increase wool growth. Wool does contain an abundance of the sulfur-containing amino acid cystine. Therefore feedstuffs rich in sulfur-containing amino acids are important for optimizing wool growth.

In general, the effects of nutrition on wool production are associated with quantity rather than quality. Increased nutrient intake can increase wool production, within limits. However, quality can be affected during periods of severe nutrient deprivation. Under these conditions, fiber diameter is decreased. Extreme underfeeding can result in weak fiber with limited value.

The nutritional status of the ewe during gestation can influence the wool production of the subsequent offspring. Kelly et al[10] bisected embryos to produce clones that were then placed in ewes fed at maintenance or submaintenance energy and protein levels from day 50 to 140 of gestation. The lambs that were born to the ewes fed a submaintenance diet produced 0.136 kg (0.3 lb) less wool from 0.4 to 1.4 years of age. The wool from those lambs was coarser than that produced by lambs born to ewes fed at a maintenance level. These effects have been attributed to decreased hair follicle development in fetuses whose dams were fed deficient diets, and they continue for the rest of the offspring's life.

Goats

Angora goats produce large quantities of fiber per unit of body weight (Figure 2-5). The 2 to 3.6 kg (4.5 to 8 lb) of mohair produced per cutting can greatly increase nutritional demands. As with wool, mohair production can be improved with increased energy intake. However, protein appears to elicit more of a response on mohair growth than it does on wool growth. Cashmere appears to be only minimally affected by dietary manipulation. Increasing dietary protein above requirements increases mohair volume and diameter.[4] Angora does fed isocaloric diets containing either 12% or 19% protein had an increase in grease fleece weight and fiber diameter with the high-protein diet (approximately 0.57 kg or 1.25 lb).[8] Mohair also contains abundant amounts of sulfur, making sulfur-containing amino acids important in Angora goat nutrition. Recently, Qi et al[11] indicated that the NRC[6] may be erring on the low side in its recommendation of a 10:1 nitrogen-to-sulfur ratio for maximal mohair production, and that a ratio of 7.2:1 may be more useful. Therefore, if NPN is used as a protein source, sulfur supplementation is necessary.

Ranged Angora goats should receive nutritional supplementation during late gestation and early lactation. Salt-limited feeds can be used for both energy and protein under range conditions. Cottonseed or soybean meal (or other protein sources), corn, and salt (non-iodized, non-mineralized) can be added at a 1:3:1 ratio. The keeper should introduce the supplement slowly, adding more white salt if the animals are overconsuming and decreasing salt if they are underconsuming. This salt-limited feeding system can be an effective way to increase energy and protein intake for range-fed goats (and possibly sheep). Careful intake monitoring is important.

Adequate shelter should be provided to fiber-producing animals, particularly young animals and Angora goats, that have just been sheared. In early spring or late fall, animals may be susceptible to cold stress for as long as 4 weeks after shearing. The provision of shelters or wind breaks and an additional 0.23 to 4.5 kg (0.5 to 1 lb) per day of an energy supplement (cracked corn) above the normal feeding regimen can help minimize freezing and stress loss.

FEEDING GERIATRIC SHEEP OR GOATS

Pet sheep and goats can live much longer than animals in production units (Figure 2-6). Whenever feeding older sheep or goats, keepers should strive to maintain a proper body condition and weight. Body weight and condition loss are common problems among geriatrics. A complete physical examination, complete blood count, and serum chemistry analysis may be indicated to identify ongoing disease. Older animals may require special feeding because of dental disease, parasite damage to the bowel, and other general health problems. Good-quality hay, moistened pellets, lush forage, and palatable concentrates are often required for animals with dental disease (see Chapter 3).

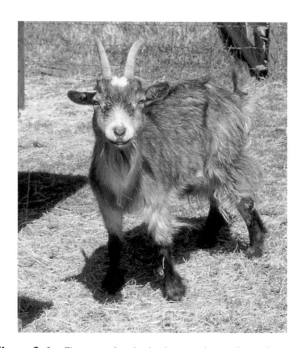

Figure 2-6   The care of geriatric sheep and goats is an often overlooked area of veterinary practice. Pet sheep or goats that receive proper care may live for more than 15 years. At the time of this writing, one author (Dr. Pugh) routinely treats goats and sheep in their late teens and early 20s, including this pygmy buck.

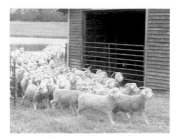

Figure 2-5   Angora goats are maintained on pastures and range. They tend to be used for brush control less commonly than other types of goats. However, if they are used for brush control, they may require supplemental sulfur because of excess tannin intake from some browse.

Allowing older animals access to feed, particularly if their social status has changed, and longer periods of non-competitive time to consume it helps maintain a good body condition score. Because many geriatric animals have arthritic conditions, minimizing excess body weight, properly trimming feet, and placing water and feed so animals are not forced to walk great distances are all valuable in case management. Diets designed for the geriatric horse can be used. However, if copper concentrations are greater than 10 ppm, these diets should not be fed to any sheep or to goats with a history of hepatic disease. If the animal has renal disease, the protein content of the diet should be maintained at 7% to 8%, and the calcium-to-phosphorus ratio should be kept at 1:1. A good-quality granular mineral mixture of equal parts dicalcium phosphate and trace mineral salt should be offered free choice. If older animals are losing weight, the keeper can slowly increase caloric intake by 7% to 10% in the form of fat. However, protein, fats, and copper should be restricted in animals with hepatic disease. Animals with hepatic or renal disease may benefit from the addition of B vitamins (orally or parenterally). If renal disease exists, the protein requirement should be met but not exceeded. If anorexia is a problem, varying the diet, offering lush grazing, and adding energy-dense feeds are useful strategies. Obviously, all husbandry practices that aid in overall health (e.g., proper shelter, deworming) enhance long-term survival.

REFERENCES

1. Russell A: Body condition scoring of sheep. In Boden E, editor: *Sheep and goat practice,* London, 1991, Bailliere Tindall.
2. Santucci PM et al: Body condition scoring of goats in extensive conditions. In Morand-Fehr P, editor: *Goat nutrition,* Wageningen, Netherlands, 1991, Pudoc.
3. Holland C, Kezar W: *Pioneer forage manual, a nutrition guide,* Des Moines, IA, 1995, Pioneer Hi-Bred International.
4. Bretzlaff K, Heinlein G, Huston E: Common nutritional problems feeding the sick goat. In Naylor JM, Ralston SL, editors: *Large animal clinical nutrition,* St Louis, 1991, Mosby.
5. *Nutrient requirements of sheep,* Washington, DC, 1985, National Academy Press.
6. *Nutrient requirements of goats: angora, dairy and meat goats in temperate and tropical countries,* Washington, DC, 1981, National Academy Press.
7. Naylor JM, Bell R: Raising the orphaned foal, *Vet Clin North Am (Equine Pract)* 1(1):173, 1985.
8. Sahlu T et al: Dietary protein level and ruminal degradability for mohair production in Angora goats, *J Anim Sci* 70:1526, 1992.
9. Allden WG: Under nutrition of the Merino sheep and its sequela: II the influence of finite periods of arrested growth on the subsequent wool growth, fleece development, and utilization of feed for wool production of lambs, *Austr J Ag Res* 19:639, 1968.
10. Kelly RW et al: Nutrition during fetal life alters annual wool production and quality in young Merino sheep, *Austr J Exp Agric* 36:259, 1996.
11. Qi K et al: Sulfate supplementation of Angora goats: metabolic and mohair responses, *J Anim Sci* 70:2828, 1992.

FURTHER READING

Ensminger ME, Oldfield JE, Heinemann WW: *Feeds and nutrition,* ed 2, Clovis, CA, 1990, Ensminger Publishing.
Naylor JM, Ralston SL: *Large animal clinical nutrition,* St Louis, 1991, Mosby.

PARENTERAL NUTRITION

Parenteral nutrition (PN) is the IV administration of energy, protein, fat, vitamins, and minerals for the nutritional support of animals. PN may be warranted in any state of debilitation where oral nutritional support is either contraindicated (e.g., enteritis, obstructions) or difficult to impossible (e.g., esophageal disease). Total parenteral nutrition (TPN) can be used to supply 100% of the animal's nutritional demands intravenously. Partial parenteral nutrition (PPN) may be used to supply a portion of the animal's nutritional demands if limited oral nutrition is feasible. TPN must include both carbohydrates and lipids as energy sources, as well as protein amino acid sources for body homeostasis and repair. Although TPN and PPN may be used in all ages of sheep and goats, cost often restricts its use to young animals or valuable adults. The duration for which the PN is to be used for nutritional support determines the components of the nutritional requirements that will be used. When instituting PN with an expected duration of less than 2 weeks, energy, protein, and some electrolytes are the most crucial components. However, in the rare event that PN is used for more than 2 weeks, the solutions must be balanced not only for energy, protein, and electrolytes, but also for micronutrients and vitamins.

As a general rule, all fluid deficits and electrolyte abnormalities should be corrected before the institution of either TPN or PPN.[1] Most PN solutions are hypertonic and their use may result in hyperglycemia, hyperosmolality, hyperlipemia, acidosis, electrolyte imbalances, or thrombophlebitis.[2] A Silastic or polyurethane catheter should be used to reduce the risk of thrombophlebitis.[2] Animals on PN are at high risk for sepsis and should be monitored closely for signs of sepsis (e.g., elevated body temperature, neutrophilia or left shift, hyperfibrinogenemia, hyperglycemia).[3] Strict attention should be paid to aseptic technique when mixing PN solutions and when working with IV lines containing PN solutions. Other complications of TPN include hypoglycemia, fatty liver, azotemia, dehydration, and anuria. The sheep or goat also should be monitored for derangements in serum electrolytes, alterations in acid/base status, increases in serum lipids, changes in blood glucose, and changes in blood urea nitrogen. In addition, urinary output should be monitored to ensure normal hydration and proper renal perfusion. Table 2-15 shows some serum chemistry changes that indicate improper PN supplementation.

TABLE 2-15

CHANGES IN SERUM CHEMISTRY VALUES INDICATIVE OF PROBLEMS WHEN USING PN

CONDITION	COMMENT
Hypoglycemia	Caloric needs not being met
Hyperglycemia	Sepsis or inappropriately high caloric content of PN fluid
Elevated BUN	Dehydration or calorie:NPN imbalance
Depressed BUN	Inadequate protein supplementation or hepatic disease
Elevated liver enzymes	Lipid content of solution exacerbating fatty liver or other hepatic disease

BOX 2-1

CALCULATION OF THE *DAILY ENERGY REQUIREMENT FOR SHEEP AND GOATS**

$$140 \text{ kcal/kg}^{0.75}/\text{day}$$
Calculate body weight in kg (lb $\div$ 2.2)
$$40 \text{ lb} \div 2.2 \text{ lb/kg} = 18.2 \text{ kg}$$
$$(140 \text{ kcal}) (18.2^{0.75})/\text{day} = 1233 \text{ kcal/day}$$

*This example uses a 40-lb animal. A calculator with an x^y function key is useful for this calculation.

As a general rule, the fluid requirement for most animals is 66 ml/kg per day. Of course, continuing fluid losses should be factored into replacement therapy. Occasionally a separate fluid line for electrolyte-fluid supplementation is needed when using PN, because concentrated electrolyte solutions may precipitate in PN solutions.

The authors of this chapter suggest that clinicians preparing PN solutions first calculate the animal's energy requirements. The caloric requirements for most animals can be calculated with the formula provided in Box 2-1. With respect to meeting the energy requirement, carbohydrates (50% dextrose solution) and fats (20% lipid solution) are the two sources generally used. Dextrose is the most commonly used carbohydrate source and has an energy value of 3.4 kcal/g. As a general rule, the maximum infusion rate of carbohydrates should not exceed 5 to 7 mg/kg per minute. Highly concentrated solutions should be administered through a central venous catheter because hypertonic PN solutions may result in phlebitis if small peripheral vessels are used. In neonates, rarely should a greater than 5% to 10% dextrose solution be given in peripheral veins. A 20% dextrose solution may be safely administered to adults via a jugular venous catheter. Unlike dextrose, lipids are isotonic and do not increase the osmolality of the TPN solution, yet they are very dense in energy. Lipids supply 9.1 kcal of energy per gram and can be infused at a rate of 2.5 to 3 g/kg per day. Usually, the clinician or nutritionist should try to supply 30% to 60% of the calories as lipids. If the clinician notes evidence of hepatic disease, he or she should use the low end of this lipid range (30%) and monitor serum sorbitol dehydrogenase closely. All the nutritional requirements cannot be met safely on the first day; instead, the caloric density and osmolality of the solution should be increased slowly over 2 to 3 days.[4] A polyionic IV fluid should be used during the acclimation period to maintain hydration.

To calculate the protein requirement for young lambs or kids, the authors of this chapter extrapolate from other species and use 2 to 3.75 g of amino acids per kg/day.[1,4] Throughout this discussion, values are given in kg of body weight of the animal being fed per day (kg/day). For adult animals, the authors again extrapolate from other species and use the requirement of 1 to 1.5 g of amino acids per kg/day.[1] The ratio of non-protein calories to grams of nitrogen should be maintained at 100:1 to 300:1.[4,5] Because protein is about 16% nitrogen, the grams of nitrogen can be calculated by dividing the number of grams of amino acids by 6.25[5]:

g amino acids $\div$ 6.25 = g nitrogen

For much of the rest of this discussion of PN, the authors use the example of supplying nutritional support through TPN for a 15-kg goat. This example can serve as a template for sheep and for animals of different weights. If the goat weighs 15 kg, the formula for energy requirement presented in Box 2-1 of 140 kcal/kg$^{0.75}$/day is solved as follows:

(140 kcal) (15 kg$^{0.75}$)/day = 1067 kcal/day

In this example, if the 15-kg goat needs 990 ml of fluid daily and the clinician decides to administer an amount 1.5 times greater than the maintenance amount to replace ongoing losses, the clinician should administer 1500 ml/day of fluid to the animal that is receiving nothing by mouth. As previously mentioned, unless a central venous line is used, the maximum dextrose concentration should not exceed 10%. Therefore 150 g of dextrose could be included in the daily 1500 ml to make 10% dextrose. This amount of dextrose supplies 510 kcal of energy per day **(150 g × 3.4 kcal/g = 510 kcal)**. In this example, 300 ml of a 50% dextrose solution supplies 150 g of dextrose **(150 g $\div$ 50 g/100 ml = 300 ml)**. Therefore 300 ml of 50% dextrose should be included in the daily 1500 ml of total fluid. However, 557 kcal of energy are still needed to meet the energy requirements:

1067 kcal − 510 kcal from dextrose
= 557 kcal of energy still needed per day

The clinician in this example can supply the remaining calories with 61.2 g of fat:

557 kcal needed ÷ 9.1 kcal/g = 61.2 g of fat

The maximum lipid utilization rate for this 15-kg animal is 45 g daily (3 g/kg/day × 15 kg = 45), but 61.2 g of fat are needed. Therefore it is impossible to meet the energy requirements by using a solution of less than 10% dextrose (which only supplies 510 kcal of energy) because enough lipid cannot be safely administered to make up the difference. If the dextrose concentration is increased to 15% (and a central venous catheter is used to avoid phlebitis), 1500 ml of a 15% dextrose solution supplies 765 kcal:

15 g/100 ml × 1500 ml = 225 g
225 g × 3.4 kcal/g = 765 kcal

The 765 kcal supplied by the 15% dextrose solution is in contrast to the 510 kcal of energy supplied by a 10% dextrose solution. If a 15% dextrose solution is used, only 302 kcal of energy are needed from fat **(1067 kcal required/day − 765 kcal supplied by the dextrose = 302 kcal needed from fat).** In this example, only 33 g of fat are now needed **(302 kcal ÷ 9.1 kcal/g = 33 g).** This is well within the daily fat utilization rate for this size animal (2.5 to 3 g/kg/day, or 45 g for the 15-kg animal).

The protein/amino acid (AA) requirement for a young goat is 2 to 3.75 g of AA/kg/day. For example, an 8.5% AA solution has approximately 1.3 g of nitrogen/100 ml. Using the base requirement of 2 g of AA/kg/day, a 15-kg goat needs 30 g of AA daily (2 g/kg/day × 15 kg). Approximately 353 ml/day of an 8.5% AA solution is required to provide 30 g of AA (30 g × 8.5 g/100 ml = 353 ml). The following formulas are used to calculate

whether this amount meets the non-protein calorie-nitrogen ratio of 100:1 to 300:1:

g of nitrogen = g of protein ÷ 6.25
Ratio = kcal ÷ g nitrogen

In this example, 30 g of protein ÷ 6.25 = 4.8 g of nitrogen. Because the non-protein calories from both carbohydrates and fats in this example are 1067, the ratio is 222:1 (1067 kcal ÷ 4.8 g of nitrogen = 222), which is in the range of 100:1 to 300:1 and therefore acceptable. A central venous catheter must be used when administering more than 1 to 1.5 g of protein/kg/day.

Although the plan is to administer 1500 ml of TPN solution per day, it may be more convenient or practical to mix the solution in 1-liter aliquots. Table 2-16 provides recipes. As previously mentioned, the clinician should begin PN with a solution containing only 25%[4] of the calculated amounts of dextrose, lipid, and amino acids and make up the difference in volume with a polyionic isotonic fluid (Table 2-16, column D). The energy and protein density should then be gradually increased over a period of 2 to 3 days (Table 2-16, column C). During this acclimation period the animal should be monitored closely for hyperglycemia or hypoglycemia, elevated blood urea nitrogen (BUN), acidosis, and electrolyte derangements. Monitoring these parameters while slowly increasing the energy and protein density of the TPN solution allows the clinician to adjust the protein, lipid, carbohydrate, and electrolyte concentration of the solution to the individual needs and tolerance of the animal. If the animal's blood work remains normal during the acclimation period, the full maintenance PN solution can be administered on the third or fourth day (Table 2-16, columns A and B). The sheep or goat also should be weighed daily to ensure that it maintains or gains weight. The transition back to enteral nutrition should be made gradually.[4]

Balanced polyionic isotonic electrolyte solutions are usually adequate to correct minor electrolyte derangements and mild acidosis or alkalosis. In the absence of

TABLE 2-16

RECIPES FOR PN SOLUTIONS FOR A 15-KG SHEEP OR GOAT (TO BE INFUSED AT THE RATE OF 1500 ML PER DAY)

INGREDIENT	A 1500 ML 100% MAINTENANCE*	B 1000 ML 100% MAINTENANCE	C 1000 ML 50% MAINTENANCE	D 1000 ML 50% MAINTENANCE
50% dextrose	450 ml	300 ml	150 ml	75 ml
8.5% amino acid†	350 ml	240 ml	120 ml	60 ml
20% lipid‡	165 ml	110 ml	55 ml	30 ml
Isotonic fluid	535 ml	350 ml	675 ml	835 ml

*Caloric and protein maintenance
†These volumes have been rounded to the nearest 10 ml for ease of measurement.
‡Because adding lipid directly to 50% dextrose can result in destruction of the lipid droplets, the lipid should be added last.

blood gas analysis, it is relatively safe to use total serum carbon dioxide (Tco_2) for evaluation of acid-base status if respiratory disease can be ruled out by thorough physical examination. Tco_2 accounts for 95% of serum HCO_3^- and therefore can be used if HCO_3^- or blood gas analysis is unavailable. If the potential exists for respiratory disease, complete blood gas analysis should be performed before the administration of alkalinizing agents.[6] Treatment of severe acidosis (Tco_2 less than 18 mmol/L) or alkalosis (Tco_2 greater than 31 mmol/L) may require specific fluid therapy. The fluid of choice to treat alkalosis is sodium chloride. Treatment of severe metabolic acidosis usually requires bicarbonate replacement therapy. The base deficit is calculated as follows[7]:

Base deficit = kg body weight

$$\times \text{ (normal } Tco_2 - \text{ patient } Tco_2) \times \text{ECV} - \text{cf}$$

where *ECV-cf* is the extracellular fluid volume correction factor (0.5 to 0.6 for neonates and 0.3 to 0.5 for adults).

To avoid the complications of bicarbonate therapy, the clinician may wish to correct only half of the base deficit initially and reevaluate the patient after initial volume and electrolyte replacement therapy. When possible, acid-base abnormalities should be corrected before the institution of TPN. If TPN is already underway, the clinician may choose to deliver bicarbonate therapy by a second IV line. The clinician or nutritionist should avoid adding more than 250 ml of 5% bicarbonate per liter of TPN solution to prevent the solution from becoming excessively hypertonic. As an example of base deficit replacement therapy, the authors will calculate bicarbonate replacement therapy for the same 15-kg goat if the Tco_2 is 15 mmol/L (which is the same as 15 mEq/L):

Base deficit = 15 kg $\times$ (24 − 15 mmol/L) $\times$ 0.5

$$= 67.5 \text{ mmol of } HCO_3^-$$

Bicarbonate is commonly supplied as a hypertonic 5% solution (1200 mmol/L). Isotonic bicarbonate (300 mmol/L) is a 1.3% solution that contains 150 mmol of HCO_3^- per liter (half of the 300 mmol/L). Therefore this 15-kg goat requires 450 ml of isotonic bicarbonate:

67.5 mmol deficit $\div$ 150 mmol/L

$$= 0.45 \text{ L, or 450 ml, of isotonic bicarbonate}$$

A simpler way to replace the deficit is to add enough 5% bicarbonate to the TPN to supply the 67.5 mmol deficit. Because 5% bicarbonate is 1200 mmol/L (half is Na and half is HCO_3^-), it contains 600 mmol/L, or 0.6 mmol/ml, of HCO_3^-. Therefore 112.5 ml is required to get the 67.5 mmol needed to replace the base deficit (67.5 mmol $\div$ 0.6 mmol/ml). As previously mentioned, the clinician may wish to replace only half of the deficit and then reevaluate the acid-base status. In this case 56 ml of 5% bicarbonate solution can be added to the TPN in place of 56 ml of polyionic fluid. The entire 56 ml could be included in 1 L of the TPN or it could be added at the rate of 37.5 ml per L of TPN so as to deliver the 56 ml of bicarbonate in the total daily 1500-ml fluid volume.

A similar formula has been used to calculate the deficit of other electrolytes such as potassium (K), chloride (Cl), and calcium (Ca):

Body deficit = kg body weight $\times$ (normal electrolyte value

$$- \text{ patient's electrolyte value)} \times \text{ECF} - \text{cf}$$

Acid-base status greatly affects the movement of potassium ions (K+) in and out of cells and the binding of Ca to albumin. Therefore correction of acid-base status often corrects minor imbalances of these electrolytes. Acidosis causes K+ to move extracellularly and increases serum K+, whereas alkalosis causes K+ to move intracellularly and decreases serum K+.[8] A pH change of 0.1 units results in a 0.6 mEq/L reciprocal change in K+.[8] Although the previous equation has been used to calculate K+ deficits, an accurate prediction of such a deficit is difficult because serum K+ depends on acid-base status.[5] Abomasal outflow obstruction results in hypochloremic, hypokalemic metabolic alkalosis.[8] In this case infusion of normal saline supplemented with K+ may be indicated. However, the infusion rate of K+ should not exceed 0.5 mEq/kg/hour.[9] Acidosis causes increased serum ionized calcium, whereas alkalosis causes decreased serum ionized calcium, which may cause an animal with normal total serum calcium to exhibit signs of hypocalcemia.[10] It is safest to administer K+ and calcium ions (Ca++) through an IV line containing only polyionic isotonic fluids so as not to cause precipitation of these cations in solution. Mineral supplementation is rarely necessary until after day 7 to 10 of PN. Minerals should be monitored with serum electrolyte analysis and supplemented if needed (Box 2-2). Both trauma and diarrhea may in-

---

BOX 2-2

GENERAL GUIDELINES ON MINERAL SUPPLEMENTATION*

Calcium	0.8 mEq ($\times$2 for growth or lactation)
Magnesium	0.33 mEq
Sodium	2.26 mEq
Phosphorus	3.6 mmol/day ($\times$2 for growth or lactation)
Zinc	0.6 mg
Iron	0.6 mg
Iodine	1.5 mcg

*When PPN or TPN are used for less than 7 days, mineral supplementation is rarely required. However, when PN is used for longer periods, close monitoring of serum electrolyte status may indicate a need for supplementation. All requirements are listed per kg of body weight per day.

BOX 2-3

ESTIMATES OF NUTRITIONAL REQUIREMENTS OF SOME VITAMINS FOR PN*

Vitamin A	25 IU
Vitamin D	6.6 IU
Vitamin E	224 mcg

*Vitamin supplementation is indicated if solutions are being administered for more than 7 days. All requirements are listed per kg of body weight per day.

crease loss of zinc (and possibly other nutrients). Vitamin supplementation (Box 2-3) also is not generally needed until after day 7 to 10 of PN, with the possible exception of the B vitamins, which may be of value if given every 2 to 3 days at labeled dosages from the onset of TPN. As a general rule, vitamin K (10 mg intramuscularly) can be given once a week.

REFERENCES

1. Spurlock SL, Ward MV: Parenteral nutrition in equine patients: principles and theory, *Compend Contin Educ Pract Vet* 13(3):461, 1991.
2. Chandler ML, Guilford WG, Payne-James J: Use of peripheral parenteral nutritional support in dogs and cats, *J Am Vet Med Assoc* 216(5):669, 2000.
3. Lippert AC, Fulton RB, Parr AM: A retrospective study of the use of total parenteral nutrition in dogs and cats, *J Vet Intern Med* 7:52, 1993.
4. Baker JC, Lippert AC: Total parenteral nutrition in the calf, *Compend Food Animal* 9(2):F71, 1987.
5. Spurlock SL, Furr M: Fluid therapy. In Koterba AM, Drummond WH, Kosch PC, editors: *Equine clinical neonatology*, Philadelphia, 1990, Lea and Febiger.
6. Constable PD: Clinical assessment of acid-base status, *Vet Clin North Am: Food Animal Pract* 15(3):447, 1999.
7. Berchtold J: Intravenous fluid therapy in calves, *Vet Clin North Am: Food Animal Pract* 15(3):505, 1999.
8. Sweeney RW: Treatment of potassium balance disorders, *Vet Clin North Am: Food Animal Pract* 15(3):609, 1999.
9. Tremblay RRM: Intravenous fluid therapy in calves, *Vet Clin North Am: Food Animal Pract* 6:77, 1990.
10. Goff JP: Treatment of calcium, phosphorus, and magnesium balance disorders, *Vet Clin North Am: Food Animal Pract* 15(3):619, 1999.

Chapter 3

Oral-Esophageal Diseases

CHRISTINE B. NAVARRE, MICHAEL Q. LOWDER, AND D.G. PUGH

Although few diseases affect the oral cavity and esophagus in sheep and goats, the ones that do usually result in depressed performance, weight loss, and occasionally death. Although exceptions exist, most problems of the oral cavity and esophagus are noninfectious diseases. The most common oral cavity abnormality that affects production is dental disease. Excessive dental wear and broken or missing teeth are common in geriatric animals or those living on range. Before beginning an oral-esophageal examination, the clinician should attain a complete history, perform a complete physical examination (including body condition scoring), and observe the animal grazing or eating grain, swallowing, and ruminating.

To perform a complete oral examination, the clinician should physically restrain or sedate the animal and place an oral speculum or gag in the mouth to enhance the visualization of the oral cavity. The clinician should note broken, worn, or missing teeth; ulceration, cracking, or swelling of the mucosa of the gums, dental pad, and tongue; and any fetid or abnormal odors. Incisor teeth in healthy adults should sit closely together. Grazing on rough, rocky pastures can wear grooves in the incisor teeth close to the gum margins.[1] The neck and throat areas should be palpated for swelling and other abnormalities. This chapter covers some of the diagnostic procedures, diseases, and treatments for problems of the mouth, its surrounding structures, and the esophagus.

DIAGNOSTIC PROCEDURES

Radiography

Radiography of the head and neck can be performed in sheep and goats using the same techniques used on other small animals. Fluoroscopy with contrast media may be needed to diagnose functional esophageal problems. A barium suspension (200 ml) or barium cream (100 ml) is recommended for adult sheep or goats.[2]

Endoscopy

Endoscopy can be useful for examining the pharynx and esophagus, as well as diagnosing pharyngeal abscesses, esophageal foreign bodies, and megaesophagus. Most flexible endoscopes used in large animal practice are too large for use in small ruminants, but endoscopes appropriate for small animals can be used. Sedation or general anesthesia is recommended to facilitate restraint. Passage of the endoscope through the nasal passages is preferred, but an endoscope with a small enough outside diameter is not always available. A speculum must be used if the endoscope is passed through the mouth to avoid damage to the endoscope from the teeth.

REFERENCES

1. Spence J, Aitchison G: Clinical aspects of dental disease in sheep. In Boden E, editor: *Sheep and goat practice*, London, 1991, Bailliere Tindall.
2. House JK et al: Ancillary tests for the assessment of the ruminant digestive system, *Vet Clin North Am: Food Animal Pract* 8(2):203, 1992.

DISEASES OF THE ORAL CAVITY

Normal Dental Anatomy

The normal dental formula of the permanent teeth for both sheep and goats is 2 (incisors 0/3, canines 0/1, premolars 3/3, molars 3/3) for a total of 32 teeth; the canine teeth function as fourth (lateral or corner) incisors (Figures 3-1 and 3-2).[1] The ages of permanent tooth eruption for sheep and goats are provided in Table 3-1;

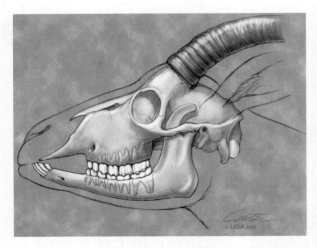

Figure 3-1 A lateral view showing the normal dentition of the goat. As the animal ages, excessive wear, wave mouth, tooth toss, and sharp points may all occur.

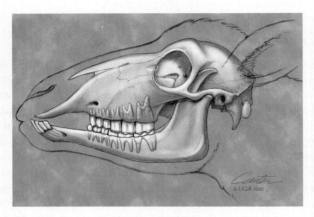

Figure 3-2 A lateral view showing the normal dentition of the sheep.

TABLE 3-1

AGES OF PERMANENT TOOTH ERUPTION IN SHEEP AND GOATS

PERMANENT TOOTH	AGE OF ERUPTION
Incisor 1	1 to 1.5 years
Incisor 2	1.5 to 2 years
Incisor 3	2.5 to 3 years
Incisor 4	3.5 to 4 years
Premolars	1.5 to 2 years
Molar 1	3 months
Molar 2	9 to 12 months
Molar 3	1.5 to 2 years

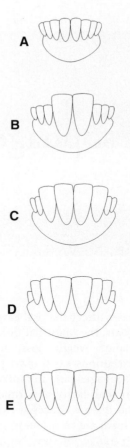

Figure 3-3 These frontal views of the incisors of sheep and goats show the small teeth characteristic of the pre-yearling animal (**A**), the two large permanent central incisors of the yearling (**B**), the dentition of 2- and 3-year-old animals (**C** and **D**), and the full dentition of the 4-year-old (**E**). Deciduous teeth are smaller than the permanent teeth that replace them.

the appearance of the incisors during the first few years of life is shown in Figure 3-3. Teeth should be white to translucent. The molars normally have sharpened points on the lateral or buccal aspect of the upper arcade and the medial or lingual aspect of the lower arcade. Unless these points are causing damage to the oral mucosa or tongue, they do not require routine removal by floating. Fluorine toxicity may result in soft, chalky areas on the teeth and/or irregular dental wear. Brown staining and tartar accumulation are common and rarely cause disease except when severe. Normal attrition is noted as a change in the shape of the incisors from rectangular to round; the teeth eventually become stubs and fall out.[2,3] The speed of this process is influenced mostly by diet, but soil type, malocclusions, and dental trauma also are contributing factors. Dental caries may be seen as holes in the teeth at the gum margin.[3] These are seen more commonly in lambs.[3] Grain-fed animals exhibit less dental attrition than those grazing on pastures on sandy to sandy loam soils. Animals grazing on sandy soils have more dental wear than those browsing or grazing lush forage pastures. Malocclusions, whether congenital or acquired (through trauma), usually result in excessive wear opposite to the site of the malocclusion.

Dental Attrition

Abnormal dental attrition occurs more commonly in sheep than in goats. The most common cause is the mastication of ingested sand and soil when forage length is short. Calcium-deficient, fluoride-toxic, or unbalanced diets also cause or contribute to this problem.[4,5] The highest incidence of dental attrition in sheep occurs in range ewes older than 4 years. Tooth loss can result in a 2-year decrease in the productive lives of sheep.[4] Most sheep and goats can accommodate the loss of an incisor, but molar loss is more serious because the molars are needed for chewing roughage.[7] Clinical signs of abnormal dental attrition include weight loss and worn, loose, or missing teeth.[4,6] A decrease in water intake can accompany dental disease as the teeth become sensitive to cold water. The clinician should examine the molars carefully and not rely just on the appearance of the incisors to diagnose this problem because molar attrition may be related more to weight loss than incisor attrition.[8] The authors of this chapter prefer to examine and visualize the upper molars directly; however, these teeth also may be palpable in some animals through the cheeks.[9] Managing grazing areas carefully, providing supplemental feed, ensuring the proper concentration of calcium in the diet, and paying attention to the calicum : phosphorus ratio all help prevent abnormal attrition. The inclusion of a trace mineral supplement also may be beneficial for dental health. However, keepers should take care when using salt or mineral blocks. Sheep and goats can break their teeth while trying to ingest adequate salt from salt blocks. The incidence of broken teeth may be reduced by providing salt in a "loose" or granular form.

Uneven molar wear can lead to wave mouth (Figure 3-4), and loss of molars can lead to accumulation of feed in the empty socket and overgrowth of the opposing tooth.[2] This condition may first be manifested as an increase in the incidence of pregnancy toxemia or excessive body condition score losses, as animals are unable to consume enough feedstuffs to meet requirements.[3] These problems occur more commonly in goats than in sheep. A foul odor from the mouth may be noted, along with signs of weight loss, quidding, and an abnormal head position (turning it to one side) when eating. In these cases an oral examination and floating the teeth may be necessary.

General Dental Care

Tooth disease caused by metabolic, nutritional, or toxic insults in sheep and goats probably occurs more commonly than noted in the scientific literature. The once-common practice of "trimming" or grinding sheep teeth

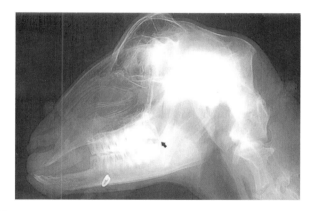

Figure 3-4 The *arrow* points to a large hook on the upper last molar. Note the way the hook protrudes into the lower mandible. This hook was associated with significant difficulty when chewing and weight loss in this animal.

has become controversial and has been outlawed in some countries.[8,10,11] The cutting or rasping of incisors to the point of exposing the pulp cavity may result in excessive pain or tooth abscesses and is of only limited benefit in improving production.[3] Dental care is commonly needed and may be most effective in the aged animal. Excessive enamel points that cause oral discomfort and ulceration and hooks or wave mouths can effectively be managed by floating the arcades. Wave or "sheer" mouth usually occurs in only a few animals in the flock.[3] Before floating, the clinician should flush the animal's mouth with water and administer mild sedation if necessary. Floating of the cheek teeth can be performed more efficiently using a full-mouth speculum (such as a Bailey mouth speculum or a pony or miniature horse full-mouth speculum) or a retractor to open the animal's mouth and allow inspection and visual guiding of the equipment. Miniature horse floats work well and provide an effective means for excessive tooth removal. Pneumatic horse floats work exceptionally well because the head is flat and small and the float has only a ¼ in reciprocating action. This small stroke distance is atraumatic to the oral mucosa. Individual sharp points can be cut with obstetrical wire or cutting pliers.[9] In cases of uncorrectable wave mouth or if an animal's teeth are worn away, a presoaked, well-balanced, pelleted diet may be fed as a mash.[7]

Periodontitis

Periodontitis is inflammation of the tissues around and supporting the teeth. It occurs mainly in sheep and is usually seen as a slight redness around some or all of the teeth. Periodontitis commonly causes loss of incisor teeth. The underlying etiology is unknown, but mechanical or chemical gingival trauma from poor feedstuffs, nutritional deficiencies, and bacterial plaque–induced gingivitis are implicated as causes of acute inflammation.

Bacteroides gingivalis and other bacteria also have been implicated as a cause of periodontal disease, although the etiology is still poorly understood. In severe cases edema may occur at the gingival surface.[3] If left untreated, gingivitis may progress to chronic inflammation and breakdown of the periodontal tissue.[1,4,12,13] This can result in the incisors becoming long and loose initially. As the condition progresses, the incisors, premolars, and molars begin to fall out.[1,4,12] Tooth root abscesses may also develop.[4] The gums or dental pads may be damaged in some animals. Malocclusion and gum recession or proliferation also may occur in some sheep and goats. However, ulcers caused by trauma usually heal without treatment.[3] Loss of body condition may or may not be evident, depending on the diet.

The use of periodontal disease (especially incisor loss alone) as a reason for culling is questionable.[1] Sheep with periodontitis or missing incisors may do well if hand fed (Figure 3-5). However, subclinical production losses may occur with periodontal disease[4] and often a loss of incisor teeth is concurrent with premolar and molar loss. Herd treatment with antibiotics may be impractical and is rarely effective from a therapeutic or economic standpoint.[1,3] Treatment of valuable individual animals with antimicrobials (oxytetracycline 20 mg/kg ever 48 hours for 2 to 3 treatments) and appropriate surgical techniques may be indicated. Until the exact causes and predisposing factors are known for periodontal disease, prevention includes optimizing nutrition.

Tooth Root Abscesses

Small ruminants with tooth root abscesses usually exhibit a localized bony enlargement of the maxilla in the area of the maxillary sinus or more commonly on the ventral surface of the mandible. Purulent drainage from the

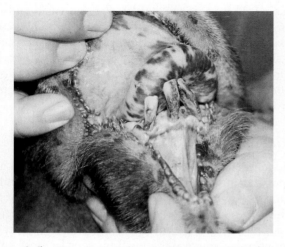

Figure 3-5   This more than 20-year-old ewe has missing incisors and periodontal disease. (Courtesy Dr. Cindy Wolf, St. Paul, Minnesota.)

swelling may be observed. Oral examination can reveal swelling of the gingiva around the affected tooth, tooth fractures, or normal findings. Radiographs may reveal boney lysis and periosteal reaction around the tooth roots.[14] Differential diagnoses include osteodystrophia fibrosa, lymphosarcoma, actinomycosis, trauma, and foreign body. Systemic administration of antimicrobials for 2 to 4 weeks may cure the problem, especially if the abscess is not open and draining and no obvious tooth abnormalities exist. Broad-spectrum antimicrobials (e.g., oxytetracycline, florfenicol) have been used with success by the authors of this chapter. If systemic administration of antimicrobials fails to correct the problem or if the condition is severe or the tooth is fractured below the gum line, the clinician should consider extraction.

Intraoral extraction can be performed in the small ruminant with a full-mouth speculum, dental picks, small (40-cm) molar forceps, and a fulcrum. A piece of wood or plastic (4 to 6 cm × 2 to 4 cm) can be used as a fulcrum. The gingiva is elevated away from the buccal and lingual sides of the affected tooth. Next, the clinician applies slow, steady pressure to the tooth in either the buccal or lingual direction for approximately 10 to 15 seconds and then moves the fulcrum in the opposite direction. After loosening the tooth, the clinician positions the fulcrum beside the head of the molar forceps, which is attached to the tooth. Downward pressure is slowly applied on the forceps until the tooth is extracted. Packing of the empty alveolus is usually not required, although flushing of the mouth twice daily for 3 to 5 days facilitates the healing process. A weak antiseptic or iodine solution can be used to flush the area. Animals with underlying or periapical infections may benefit from systemic administration of broad-spectrum antimicrobials (e.g., oxytetracycline). Comparison of preextraction and postextraction radiographs ensures complete tooth removal and helps the clinician determine whether postextraction curettage of the bony alveolus is required. In cases in which intraoral extraction is not indicated (e.g., if the tooth is fractured at the level of the gum), surgical repulsion is an option to be considered. A bacterial culture and sensitivity assay can be performed before or during surgery to ensure the use of the appropriate antimicrobials postoperatively. Pain medication should be administered as appropriate. Extraction of diseased teeth in sheep has been shown to increase production.[15]

Miscellaneous Tooth Abnormalities

Congenital absence of the lower incisors or premolars, persistent deciduous incisors, brachygnathism, and prognathism have all been reported in goats.[2,16] In sheep, persistent deciduous incisors, dentigerous cysts, brachygnathism, and prognathism are commonly seen dental abnormalities.[3,8,17,18] Most of these problems are not treatable, and animals should therefore be culled if health or production is depressed. Many pet animals with dental abnormalities lead full lives with special care, but because their pathologies may indicate genetic involvement, these animals should not be bred.

Actinobacillosis

Actinobacillosis is caused by the gram-negative rod *Actinobacillus lignieresii*. This organism normally resides in the mouth of ruminants and can gain entry to and infect the deeper soft tissues of the head after trauma. Actinobacillosis is reported in sheep, where it can cause granulomatous abscesses of the lips, parotid and submaxillary regions, or other areas of the head. Tongue lesions are not as common as in cattle.

Clinical signs.   The clinical signs depend on the site of infection but usually include weight loss if eating becomes difficult.[4,14,19] The drainage from the lesions may contain granules. Because the organism is a gram-negative rod, a Gram's stain of drainage can help differentiate this infection from caseous lymphadenitis.

Diagnosis.   Culture and biopsy of the lesions are needed for definitive diagnosis.[14]

Treatment.   Sodium iodide given intravenously (70 mg/kg as 10% to 20% solution) and repeated 1 week later is the treatment of choice. Treatment is usually successful and the prognosis is good, although regression of the lesion may be slow.[14] Refractory cases can be treated orally with organic iodides (ethylene diamine dihydroiodide [EDDI]) at 60 mg/kg/day for as long as 3 weeks.[14,19] Mild signs of iodism (e.g., epiphora, salivation, dandruff) are of no clinical significance, but the clinician should immediately discontinue treatment if more severe signs (e.g., coughing, inappetence, diarrhea) occur.

Actinomycosis

Actinomycosis (lumpy jaw) is caused by the organism *Actinomyces bovis*. This condition is uncommon in sheep as compared with cattle and has not been reported in goats. Actinomycosis must be considered as a differential diagnosis for tooth root abscesses in sheep because it also causes localized bony swellings on the mandible.

Treatment.   Treatment is the same as for actinobacillosis, although sulfadimethoxine (1 g/kg once a day) or isoniazid (15 mg/kg orally [PO]) also may be used. Any treatment should be continued for weeks to months.

Fractures of the Maxilla and Mandible

Fractures of the maxilla and mandible are usually traumatic in origin. However, tooth root abscesses and osteodystrophia fibrosa also may lead to pathologic fractures.[20] Fractures of the maxilla and mandible present acutely, with soft tissue swelling around the fracture and possibly bony crepitus. Animals are usually anorexic and may drool excessively. If the injury is discovered quickly, a fracture can be repaired with routine small animal orthopedic techniques. However, often these fractures go unnoticed and present as chronic healed fractures. If this occurs, mandibular fractures in particular may not heal in correct alignment, which can result in malocclusion. Chronic malocclusion can lead to uneven growth and wear of the teeth, interfering with prehension and mastication of food. Nondisplaced maxillary fractures may heal without fixation.

Pharyngeal Abscess

Pharyngeal trauma can lead to pharyngeal abscesses in sheep and goats.[21] The clinical signs include anorexia, excessive drooling, halitosis, swelling and pain in the pharyngeal area, and, in severe cases, dyspnea and bloat.[22] Affected animals may become dehydrated from decreased water intake and develop metabolic acidosis from loss of saliva. Sheep and goats are too small for the clinician to perform oral digital examination of the area. Radiography and endoscopy are needed to determine the extent and severity of the problem and assess for foreign bodies. The primary differential diagnosis in small ruminants is abscessation of the pharyngeal lymph nodes from caseous lymphadenitis. Pharyngeal abscesses associated with trauma are usually acute and accompanied by cellulitis and diffuse swelling of the entire pharyngeal area. In contrast, pharyngeal lymph node abscesses are chronic and produce localized swelling of the lymph nodes.

Administration of broad-spectrum antimicrobials and antiinflammatory drugs is indicated, as is intravenous fluid support. In refractory or severe cases or cases in which a foreign body is present, surgery may be indicated. If the original trauma occurred to the pharyngeal mucosa, the abscess should be drained into the pharynx, if possible. This procedure requires general anesthesia; endoscopy may provide better visualization of the area. A temporary tracheostomy may be necessary because these animals may experience short-term dyspnea after surgery.

Salivary Cysts

Salivary cysts occur in sheep and goats as discrete, fluctuant nodules on or behind the mandible. They can be differentiated from caseous lymphadenitis by needle aspiration. Fluid from a salivary cyst is clear and mucoid as opposed to the purulent fluid drained from an abscess.[14,21] Treatment is the same as for similar conditions in other species.

Bluetongue

Etiology and pathogenesis. Bluetongue is an acute viral disease caused by a ribonucleic acid (RNA) orbivirus that affects both domestic and wild ruminants. It is transmitted mainly by gnats of the genus *Culicoides*, although sexual and transplacental transmission can occur. Because of the vector transmission, the disease is more common in late summer and early fall.[4,23] Bluetongue virus (BTV) is endemic in many areas, particularly southern regions that are vector friendly. Cattle and other wild ruminants act as reservoirs; the virus can circulate in the blood of these animals for months to years, even though clinical disease is rare.[23,24] Many strains of the virus exist, and disease usually occurs when a new strain or an animal naive to the endemic strains is introduced.[4,23]

The incubation period of bluetongue in sheep is usually 7 to 10 days. The virus appears to cause a vasculitis resulting from infection of vascular endothelial cells. This vasculitis results in edema and necrosis of epithelial and mucosal surfaces. Teratogenic effects are caused by disruption of organogenesis by the virus in the developing fetus. The disease is most severe when previous exposure has occurred (sensitization). In cattle the disease operates through an immunoglobulin E (IgE) hypersensitivity reaction. Different breeds of sheep show differences in susceptibility to BTV—meat breeds are more susceptible than wool breeds and native African sheep are resistant to the disease. Feeder lambs are the most susceptible.

Clinical signs. Clinical signs are seen most commonly in sheep and all ages are susceptible. Goats are commonly infected with the virus but rarely show clinical signs.[2] Clinical signs result from generalized vasculitis and include a transient fever and edema of the muzzle, face, and ears. Profuse serous nasal discharge is seen initially; it later becomes mucopurulent, causing crusting around the nose. Oral mucous membranes are initially hyperemic. As the disease progresses, petechiae and ulcers develop, especially on the dental pad and commissures of the mouth. Cyanosis of the tongue is not common but does occur in some cases, hence the name *bluetongue*. Pulmonary edema develops and can result in secondary bacterial pneumonia. Lameness caused by coronitis and myositis, diarrhea (occasionally bloody), and wool breaks can all be seen in affected animals. Some animals may slough their hooves. The most dramatic clinicopathologic finding is severe leukopenia. Differential diagnoses include other vesicular diseases and photosensitization. The virus also is teratogenic and can cause abortions, stillbirths, and weak lambs.[4,23]

Diagnosis. Antibody tests of serum are not definitive because some antibodies persist for years after exposure and cross-reactivity with other orbiviruses can occur. In parts of the world where the disease is common, the diagnosis is usually based on clinical signs alone. The virus can be isolated from blood, semen, or tissues (spleen and brain from aborted fetuses). Viral isolation from blood obtained during the viremic, febrile state is the most definitive means of diagnosis. Serologic evaluation involves two types of viral antigen-group antigens called *P7* and *P2*. The former is found in all BTVs, whereas the latter determines the serotypes. Sera are commonly tested with complement fixation, agar gel immunodiffusion (AGID), or one of several enzyme-linked immunospecific assay (ELISA) tests. A competitive ELISA is considered the best serologic test for detection of group antibodies to BTV. A direct fluorescent antibody test also is available. Polymerase chain reaction (PCR)–based tests for bluetongue have recently become available and are extremely sensitive and specific. Other laboratory tests and observations that aid in diagnosis include leukopenia during the early febrile stage of the disease and an increase in serum creatinine kinase corresponding to the latter phase of muscle stiffness and lameness. Necropsy lesions are nonspecific. A definitive diagnosis of BTV requires virus isolation from blood or tissue from acutely infected animals (particularly the spleen) and aborted fetuses (especially the brain) or detection of RNA specific to BTV by PCR.[23]

Treatment. Treatment is supportive only. Broad-spectrum antimicrobials are indicated if secondary bacterial infections develop. Nonsteroidal antiinflammatory drugs are indicated for inflammation, fever, and pain. Nutritional and fluid support may be needed if affected animals cannot eat or drink.

Prevention. Prevention mainly involves controlling the *Culicoides* vector, but this can be difficult. Eliminating vector breeding grounds (mud with a high organic matter content) and housing animals at dusk and through the night (periods of peak gnat activity) may help.[4,23] Because of the complicated immunologic response to BTV, vaccine development is difficult.[25,26] Modified live virus (MLV) vaccines are available in some parts of the world. However, vaccines must contain the serotypes present in a particular location to be useful, and they are not without risks. The MLV vaccine can be teratogenic in early pregnancy, and there is a slight risk for abortion in late pregnancy, as well as infertility in breeding rams.[23] Sheep that have recovered from an attack of bluetongue are solidly resistant for months to infection by the same viral strain and to some different viral types. Active immunity in sheep requires both humoral and cellular immunity (see Chapters 6 and 18).

Contagious Ecthyma

Contagious ecthyma is a zoonotic disease of sheep and goats caused by a poxvirus. It also is commonly known as *contagious pustular dermatitis* or *sore mouth*. Young animals are most susceptible, but older naive animals also can be infected.

Clinical signs. Clinical signs include proliferative, crusting lesions, the majority of which occur on the mucocutaneous junctions of the mouth and nose. Lesions also may occur on other areas of the body, especially the udders of females nursing affected young.

Diagnosis. Diagnosis is usually made from physical examination findings, but virus identification in tissues can confirm the diagnosis. Very transient, early lesions are vesicular and need to be differentiated from other vesicular diseases.

Treatment. Nutritional and fluid support are important because affected animals are reluctant to eat and drink. Treatment of the lesions is usually not necessary unless secondary bacterial infection or maggot infestation occurs. Treatment does not speed the course of lesion regression, which is typically about 1 month. Crusts should not be removed; this action may delay healing, promote scarring, and increase the handler's chance of acquiring the disease. Animals usually make a full recovery.

Prevention. Prevention is best accomplished by maintaining a virus-free herd. However, this can be difficult because carrier animals may not show lesions. Keepers should carefully examine herd or flock additions for lesions. After a herd is infected, eliminating the disease is difficult because the virus is stable in crusts that have fallen from infected animals. A vaccine is available for herds or flocks in areas where sore mouth is endemic, but it is a live, virulent vaccine whose use is controlled in some areas by state regulatory officials.[27]

Other Viral Diseases

Other viral diseases that result in oral lesions, including foot and mouth disease (see Chapter 14) and vesicular stomatitis (see Chapter 14), are covered elsewhere in this book.

References

1. St-Jean G: Dental and periodontal diseases. In Smith BP, editor: *Large animal internal medicine*, ed 2, St Louis, 1996, Mosby.
2. Smith MC, Sherman DM: Digestive system. In Smith MC, Sherman DM, editors: *Goat medicine*, Philadelphia, 1994, Lea & Febiger.
3. Spence J, Atchison G: Clinical aspects of dental disease in sheep, *In Pract*, p 128, July 1986.
4. Kimberling CV: Diseases of the digestive system. In Kimberling CV, editor: *Jensen and Swift's diseases of sheep*, ed 3, Philadelphia, 1988, Lea & Febiger.
5. Sherman DM: Unexplained weight loss in sheep and goats. A guide to differential diagnosis, therapy, and management, *Vet Clin North Am: Large Animal Pract* 5:571, 1983.
6. Gnad DP et al: Diagnosing weight loss in sheep: a practical approach, *Comp Cont Ed Pract Vet* 22:S16, 2000.
7. Clarkson MJ, Winter AC: Teeth. In Clarkson MJ, Winter AC, editors: *A handbook for the sheep clinician*, Liverpool, 1997, University Press.
8. Barber DML, Waterhouse A: An evaluation of cutting of incisor teeth of ewes in an attempt to control premature tooth loss, *Vet Rec* 123:598, 1988.
9. Smith MC: Exotic diseases of small ruminants. Geriatric medicine for small ruminants, *Proc West Vet Conf*, p 144, 1998.
10. Denholm LJ, Vizard AL: Trimming the incisor teeth of sheep: another view, *Vet Rec* 119(8):182, 1986.
11. Spence JA, Hooper GE, Austin AR: Trimming incisor teeth of sheep, *Vet Rec* 118(5):617, 1986.
12. Spence JA, Atchison GU: Early tooth loss in sheep: a review, *Vet Ann* 25:125, 1985.
13. Cutress TW, Ludwig TG: Periodontal disease in sheep. 1. Review of the literature, *J Periodontol* 40:31, 1969.
14. Fubini SL, Campbell SG: External lumps on sheep and goats, *Vet Clin North Am: Large Animal Pract* 5:457, 1983.
15. Andrews AH: Clinical signs and treatment of aged sheep with loose mandibular or maxillary cheek teeth, *Vet Rec* 108:331, 1981.
16. Emele-Nwaubani JC, Ihemelandu EC: Anodontia of the incisor and canine teeth in a cryptorchid West African dwarf goat, *Trop Vet* 2:172, 1984.
17. Pearson EG: Diseases of the hepatobiliary system. In Smith BP, editor: *Large animal internal medicine*, ed 2, St Louis, 1996, Mosby.
18. Bruere AN et al: A syndrome of dental abnormalities of sheep, *New Zealand Vet J* 27:152, 1979.
19. Smith BP: Actinobacillosis. In Smith BP, editor: *Large animal internal medicine*, ed 2, St Louis, 1996, Mosby.
20. Andrews AH: Osteodystrophia fibrosa in young goats, *Vet Rec* 112:404, 1983.
21. Linklater KA, Smith MC: Conditions affecting the pharyngeal region and esophagus. In Linklater KA, Smith MC, editors: *Color atlas of diseases and disorders of the sheep and goat*, London, 1993, Wolfe Publishing.
22. Smith BP: Pharyngeal trauma/abscess. In Smith BP, editor: *Large animal internal medicine*, ed 2, St Louis, 1996, Mosby.
23. Michelsen PGE: Bluetongue. In Smith BP, editor: *Large animal internal medicine*, ed 2, St Louis, 1996, Mosby.
24. Katz J et al: Diagnostic analysis of the prolonged bluetongue virus RNA presence found in the blood of naturally infected cattle and experimentally infected sheep, *J Vet Diagn Invest* 6:139, 1994.
25. Campbell CH, Grubman MJ: Current knowledge on the biochemistry and immunology of bluetongue, *Prog Vet Microbiol Immun* 1:58, 1985.
26. Mahrt CR, Osburn BI: Experimental bluetongue virus infection of sheep; effect of previous vaccination: clinical and immunologic studies, *Am J Vet Res* 47:1191, 1986.
27. Michelsen PGE: Contagious ecthyma. In Smith BP, editor: *Large animal internal medicine*, ed 2, St Louis, 1996, Mosby.

DISEASES OF THE ESOPHAGUS

Esophageal Obstruction

Esophageal obstruction, or "choke," occurs sporadically when feedstuffs are swallowed that are too hard for proper mastication or too large to pass down the esophagus. Common feedstuffs that cause choke are sugar beets, corncobs, potatoes, turnips, apples, and pears.[1] Obstructing items usually lodge in the cervical portion of the esophagus but also may become stuck in the cardia.[2] Occasionally animals become choked after rapid ingestion of pelleted rations. This type of choke is usually transient and the animal is able to relieve it on its own. However, if esophageal spasm or swelling occurs, the condition may require treatment. Rarely, secondary esophageal obstruction may occur after the esophagus has previously ruptured.[3] The clinician should note that animals with either rabies or botulism may appear to have esophageal obstruction. Dental disease also may contribute to choke, and a thorough oral examination is indicated after the choke has been relieved.

Clinical signs. Animals that are choked are agitated and stand with the head and neck extended. Repeated coughing and retching motions occur, and saliva containing some feed particles may come from the mouth and nose. Prevention of normal eructation results in rumen tympany, which may cause death in untreated animals. Partial obstruction is usually not immediately life-threatening because bloat is less likely, but chronic loss of saliva can lead to dehydration and metabolic acidosis, pressure necrosis, and esophageal rupture.

Diagnosis. Diagnosis is by observation of clinical signs. The clinician may be able to palpate the offending object in the esophagus. However, the inability to palpate an esophageal obstruction does not preclude choke as a possible diagnosis. The clinician also may locate an obstruction while passing an esophageal tube.

Treatment. In cases of life-threatening bloat, rumen gas should be relieved first. This can be done by trocarization of the rumen through the left flank with a 14-gauge needle. After relieving the bloat, the clinician should attempt to remove the obstruction. If the obstruction is just behind the pharynx, forceps can be used to grasp and remove the object. If the obstruction is palpable in the cervical region, it can be manually massaged toward the pharynx and then removed. If the object is lodged in the chest, a well-lubricated stomach tube (10 to 15 mm outside diameter) can be used to try to push the object into the rumen. This should be done very gently to prevent esophageal rupture, especially in cases of chronic partial obstruction in which the esophagus may be very friable. In most cases, either mineral oil or obstetric lubricant is needed for lubrication of the tube and the obstructing object. Obstruction from pellets can be dislodged by gentle massage with a stomach tube, water, irrigation, or surfactant (e.g., dioctyl sodium sulfosuccinate [DSS]) (see Chapter 16). Heavy sedation or general anesthesia may be necessary for these procedures. Anesthesia or heavy sedation is essential in cases where mineral oil is used for lubrication because the animal's head must be kept in a lowered position to prevent aspiration. After relieving the obstruction, the clinician should observe the animal for signs of aspiration pneumonia and esophageal stricture. In cases of long-term choke or suspected esophageal damage, antibiotics (oxytetracycline 20 mg/kg every 48 to 72 hours or penicillin 20,000 IU/kg twice a day) and antiinflammatory drugs (flunixin meglumine 1 to 2 mg/kg) may be indicated to minimize long-term esophageal damage.

Prevention. The occurrence of choke is sporadic and sometimes unavoidable. Still, fencing off areas where choke-producing feedstuffs (e.g., apples) are located may minimize clinical cases. Placing large stones or bricks into feed bunks, providing adequate feed bunk space, and feeding multiple small grain meals may all slow feed intake, particularly if pelleted feeds are offered.

If choke is a recurrent problem in a particular animals, pellets or other dehydrated feedstuffs should be avoided. Affected animals may benefit from an oral examination and, where appropriate, dental care (e.g., floating).

Megaesophagus

Megaesophagus is an uncommon abnormality in sheep and goats, but it has been reported in Alpine and Nubian goats and Southdown sheep.[4,5] Esophageal infection with *Sarcocystis* species has been found on histopathology in some cases and therefore implicated as a cause. However, this organism is found routinely in the esophagi of normal animals. Regurgitation, vomiting, and swelling of the neck region are typical signs. No practical or effective treatment exists other than supportive care in most cases. If *Sarcocystis* is suspected, the clinician may give injectable folic acid inhibitors (e.g., trimethoprim-sulfadiazine 15 mg/kg once a day subcutaneously).

References

1. Matthews J: Abdominal distention. In Matthews J, editor: *Diseases of the goat,* ed 2, Oxford, England, 1999, Blackwell Science.
2. Kimberling CV: Diseases of the digestive system. In Kimberling CV, editor: *Jensen and Swift's diseases of sheep,* ed 3, Philadelphia, 1988, Lea & Febiger.
3. Fleming SA, Dallman MJ, Sedlacek DL: Esophageal obstruction as a sequela to ruptured esophagus in a goat, *J Am Vet Med Assoc* 195(11):1598, 1989.
4. Ramadan RO: Megaesophagus in a goat, *Agri-Pract* 14:26, 1993.
5. Braun U et al: Regurgitation due to megaesophagus in a ram, *Can Vet J* 31:391, 1990.

Chapter 4

Diseases of the Gastrointestinal System

CHRISTINE B. NAVARRE AND D.G. PUGH

The gastrointestinal system is, arguably, more prone to disease than any other part of the sheep or goat. Gastrointestinal parasitism alone is the most significant cause of production and animal losses in much of North America.[1,2] There is no substitute for a thorough physical examination when trying to determine the affected body systems of a sick animal; this is especially true in diseases of the gastrointestinal system. A complete physical examination should include palpation for body condition, assessment of abdominal shape and rumen motility, observation of the consistency of the stool, and evaluation for the presence of bloat. However, because rectal palpation cannot be performed in sheep and goats, diagnosis of disease in a particular segment of the gastrointestinal system can be difficult. Therefore, the clinician may have to perform ancillary diagnostic procedures to characterize gastrointestinal diseases properly.

DIAGNOSTIC PROCEDURES

Clinicopathologic Data

Clinicopathologic data consisting of a complete blood count (CBC), serum biochemical evaluation (SBE), and urinalysis can be helpful in differentiating gastrointestinal diseases, developing a prognosis and plan for treatment, and monitoring treatment. A CBC rarely identifies a specific disease, but it can be helpful in evaluating the severity of dehydration, anemia, and hypoproteinemia. The clinician must take care to interpret the packed cell volume (PCV) and total protein in light of the hydration status of the animal as noted on physical examination. An anemic or dehydrated hypoproteinemic animal may have normal PCV and total protein values. Both the CBC and SBE can be helpful in characterizing the presence and severity of an inflammatory disease process. Changes in the total and differential white blood cell count indicate

acute or chronic inflammation; increases in globulins or fibrinogen suggest a chronic inflammatory disease. Low protein levels, especially albumin, can point to chronic blood loss from intestinal parasitism or infiltrative bowel disease. Liver disease should be suspected if liver enzymes or bilirubin are elevated. However, liver enzymes can be normal in chronic liver disease. Also, albumin levels rarely drop in ruminants with liver disease, as they do in other species.[3] Changes in electrolytes can occur with gastrointestinal disease, especially if the animals are anorexic. Electrolyte measurements also are helpful in formulating a treatment plan. Hypochloremia and metabolic alkalosis occasionally occur in abomasal disease. A mild hypocalcemia may be encountered in some small ruminants with gastrointestinal atony. Because many animals with gastrointestinal disease are dehydrated and therefore azotemic and possibly hypoproteinemic, urinalysis is helpful to eliminate urinary disease as a cause of these pathologies.

Normal ranges for clinicopathologic values are included in this textbook (see Appendix III) and also have been published in several other textbooks.[4-7] However, clinicians would do well to learn the normal values, especially serum biochemistry values, established by the laboratory most commonly used for analysis.[7]

Rumen Fluid Analysis

Analysis of rumen fluid can help differentiate diseases of the forestomachs. An appropriately sized orogastric tube can be passed through the oral cavity for fluid collection (Figure 4-1). The clinician must properly restrain the animal, using a mouth speculum (Figure 4-2) to prevent tube chewing. If the tube is chewed, its roughened surface may damage the esophagus; parts of a broken tube can be swallowed. Rumen fluid also can be collected using percutaneous rumenocentesis[4,8-12] (Figure 4-3). A 16-gauge

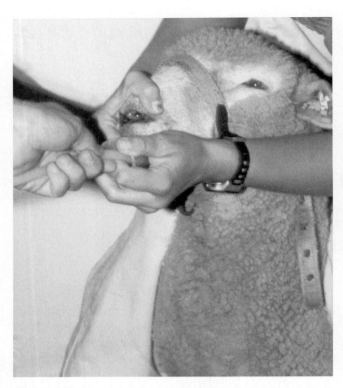

Figure 4-1 Passage of an orogastric tube through a mouth speculum. The tube should be lubricated and passed slowly down the esophagus.

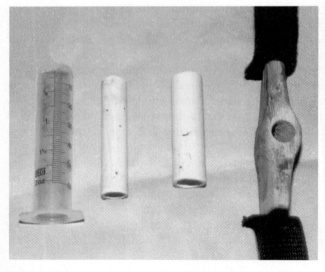

Figure 4-2 Mouth speculums for use in passing an orogastric tube. Various equipment designs can be used to protect the tube from being chewed.

needle can be inserted in the rumen through the abdominal wall caudal to the xyphoid and to the left of midline. The clinician then aspirates fluid with a syringe. Local anesthesia and sedation of the animal may be necessary. This technique avoids the saliva contamination that can

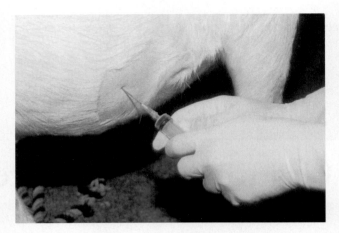

Figure 4-3 The site for performing a rumenocentesis. The area should be clipped, cleaned, and surgically prepared.

occur during collection with an orogastric tube, and it appears to be less stressful. Rumenocentesis presents a slight risk of peritonitis, but this risk can be minimized with proper restraint. Percutaneous rumenocentesis should not be performed on pregnant females.

After the fluid is collected, it can be analyzed for color, odor, pH, protozoal species and motility, methylene blue reduction time (MBR), Gram's staining characteristics, and chloride levels. Normal values are listed in Table 4-1. Anorexia may cause the fluid to appear darker, the pH to increase, and the number and motility of protozoa to decrease. A gray color, low pH, and dead or no protozoa are seen in rumen acidosis from grain overload. The MBR is prolonged with any type of indigestion. Large numbers of gram-positive rods (*Lactobacillus* species) also may be seen in rumen acidosis. Elevated rumen chloride indicates an abomasal or proximal small intestinal obstruction (either functional or mechanical).

Fecal Examination

The most important reason for examining feces in sheep and goats is to determine the presence and relative number of nematode parasites infesting an animal or flock. The quantitative technique for determining eggs per gram of feces (EPG) is shown in Box 4-1. Fecal EPG values of more than 500 to 1000 indicate serious infestation and the need for intervention.

Fecal occult blood testing and acid-fast staining of fecal smears also can be performed. Fecal occult blood tests can detect microscopic amounts of blood in the feces. However, they cannot indicate which part of the gastrointestinal tract is bleeding. Acid-fast stains of fecal smears that reveal clumps of acid-fast rods usually indicate infection with *Mycobacterium paratuberculosis* (Johne's disease). Generally, individual acid-fast rods found on fecal examination are nonpathogenic.

TABLE 4-1

NORMAL RUMEN FLUID CHARACTERISTICS OF SHEEP AND GOATS

CHARACTERISTIC	NORMAL VALUES
Color	Green
Odor	Aromatic
pH*	6.5 to 7.5
Protozoa†	Mixed sizes and species rapidly moving
Methylene blue reduction time‡	3 to 6 minutes
Gram's stain	Gram-negative rods predominate
Rumen chloride	Less than 25 to 30 mEq/L

From Nordlund KV, Garrett EF: Rumenocentesis: a technique for collecting rumen fluid for diagnosis of subacute rumen acidosis in dairy herds, *Bovine Pract* 28:109, 1994; Keefe GP, Ogilvie TH: Comparison of oro-ruminal probe and rumenocentesis for prediction of rumen pH in dairy cattle, *Proc 30th Ann Am Assoc Bovine Pract Conv*, p 168, 1997; Smith MC, Sherman DM: *Goat medicine,* Philadelphia, 1994, Lea & Febiger.
*Use pH paper with at least 0.5-unit gradations.
†Place a drop of fluid on a warm slide and cover with a coverslip. Examine under 100× magnification.
‡Mix one part 0.03% methylene blue to 20 parts rumen fluid. Measure time for blue color to clear to match a control tube of fluid.

Abdominocentesis

Abdominocentesis is useful in discerning the causes of fluid distention in the abdomen. Two methods can be used. The first technique involves tapping the lowest point of the abdomen slightly to the right of midline; it is useful in ruling out a ruptured bladder as the cause of general ascites (Figure 4-4).[4,13] The clinician should take care to avoid the prepuce in males. The second technique is useful if peritonitis is suspected. Because localized peritonitis is more common than generalized peritonitis, four sites are tapped.[14] The two cranial sites are slightly caudal to the xyphoid and medial to the milk veins on the left and right sides. The two caudal sites are slightly cranial to the mammary gland and to the left and right of midline. For either technique, manual restraint with sedation is recommended; the use of real-time ultrasonography may help locate fluid pockets. A 20-gauge needle or teat cannula can be used for fluid collection.[13] The clinician should prepare the site using sterile technique and provide local anesthesia when employing a teat cannula. Fluid should be collected in a small ethylenediamine tetra-acetic acid (EDTA) tube for analysis and a sterile tube for culture. Abdominal fluid can be difficult to obtain because of the small amounts normally present in

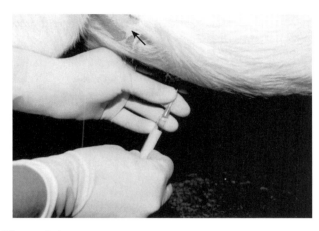

Figure 4-4 Ventral and caudal sites for performing abdominocentesis. The needle indicates the ventral site. The caudal site is the clipped area below the flank *(arrow)*.

BOX 4-1

McMaster's Quantitative Technique for Obtaining the Number of Nematode Eggs Per Gram of Feces

1. Weigh 2 g of feces and thoroughly mix with 28 ml of water. This is the preferred method. However, if a gram scale is not available, feces can be added to the 28 ml of water until the water level indicates 30 ml. This approximates 2 g of feces.
2. Remove 1 ml of well-mixed fecal-water suspension, add to 1 ml of Sheather's solution,* and mix well.
3. Fill both sides of a McMaster's chamber with the Sheather's solution–fecal-water mixture.
4. Allow to stand for 5 minutes.
5. Count ova inside of chamber lines on both sides. Multiply the number of ova by 100. This number approximates the number of eggs per gram of feces.

*Sheather's solution consists of 1470 ml distilled water, 5 lb sugar, and 30 ml liquid phenol. It is made by heating distilled water and sugar in the upper half of a double boiler until the sugar is dissolved, cooling, and then adding the phenol.

both sheep and goats. The clinician should minimize the ratio of EDTA to fluid because EDTA can falsely elevate protein levels. Using EDTA tubes made for small animals or shaking excess EDTA out of large tubes resolves this problem. Normal culture values are similar to those for cattle (clear, colorless to slightly yellow, 1 to 5 g/dl protein, less than 10,000 cells).[14] Cytologic examination is needed to characterize the cell population and assess for the presence of phagocytized bacteria.

Radiography

Radiography of the abdomen can be performed in small ruminants using small animal techniques. In adults, the rumen normally fills the entire abdomen. Radiography can detect gas distention of the small intestine, abdominal fluid, and foreign bodies.[14,15] Contrast techniques are useful for diagnosing atresia of the rectum or colon. Unlike in other small animals, contrast techniques are not practical for characterizing small intestinal problems in sheep and goats because the rumen dilutes and slows passage of the contrast media.[16]

Ultrasonography

Ultrasonography can be used to provide better characterization of abdominal distention, internal and external abdominal masses, and gross lesions of the liver. Ascites may be differentiated from fluid in the intestinal tract, and gas distention of the intestines can be differentiated from fluid distention. Normal ultrasonographic examination of the liver in sheep has been described.[17] The liver can be viewed on the right side from the seventh or eighth rib caudally to the thirteenth rib (Figures 4-5 and 4-6). Ultrasonography can be used to perform biopsies of organs or masses and to locate pockets of fluid.

Laparoscopy

Laparoscopy is more commonly used as a reproductive tool, but it also can be used diagnostically as an alternative to exploratory laparotomy in small ruminants.[18,19] General anesthesia is recommended. The technique for laparoscopic exploration of the abdomen used for cattle can be modified for use in sheep and goats.[20] The clinician inserts a cannula in the caudal abdomen and carefully inflates the abdomen with carbon dioxide (CO_2). With the animal restrained in dorsal recumbency and either sedated or anesthetized, the clinician places the cannula in the inguinal area as described for laparoscopic insemination in Chapter 6. Entrance on the right side allows visualization of most of the abdominal organs. The clinician should avoid the rumen when introducing the laparoscope into the abdomen. This procedure may be enhanced by lowering the head or rear of the animal, allowing better visualization of the entire abdomen. Animals should be properly ventilated during this procedure because inflation of the abdomen and lowering of the head can put pressure on the diaphragm.

Exploratory Laparotomy

Exploratory laparotomy can be a valuable diagnostic tool in evaluating gastrointestinal diseases when other tests indicate abdominal disease. In some cases, therapeutic surgical techniques can be performed at the same time. The technique of exploratory laparotomy used in cattle can be adopted for sheep and goats as long as the clinician keeps in mind that these animals are more likely to lie down during surgery and standing surgery should only rarely be attempted.[21] Small ruminants should be heavily sedated or placed under general anesthesia during this procedure. They may show signs of postoperative pain, anorexia, and depression and should be treated accordingly with a nonsteroidal antiinflammatory drug (NSAID) (flunixin meglumine 1.1 to 2.2 mg/kg intravenously [IV]).[14] The decision to use perioperative and postoperative antimicrobial agents should be based on the conditions under which the surgery is performed and the diagnosis made at surgery.

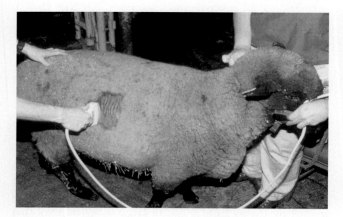

Figure 4-5 Demonstration of the site of liver ultrasonography. In sheep the area should be clipped, but in goats alcohol can be applied to the overlying hair and skin. If the area is clipped, the clinician should apply a bland coupling material (e.g., methyl cellulose, vegetable oil) between the skin and the transducer.

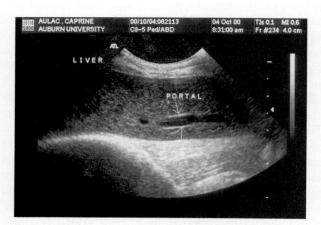

Figure 4-6 Normal ultrasonography of the liver in a goat. Note the degree of contrast. Liver abscesses, fibrosis, and fatty deposition can all be visualized.

Antimicrobial agents are not necessary for exploratory surgery performed aseptically, in a hospital setting, and without complications. However, they are indicated in field conditions, if infection is already present, and if the intestinal tract is opened. A combination of ceftiofur (1.1 to 2.2 mg/kg IV twice a day [BID]) and procaine penicillin G (22,000 IU/kg intramuscularly [IM] BID) can be administered until culture results indicate an absence of microbes.

Liver Biopsy

Liver biopsy in sheep and goats is performed using the same technique and instruments as in cattle.[12] However, sedation and ultrasound guidance are recommended.[22] The biopsy can be performed in the ninth to tenth intercostal space slightly above an imaginary line from the tuber coxae to the point of the elbow (Figure 4-7). The site should be surgically prepared, and a local anesthetic (2% lidocaine hydrochloride) infused subcutaneously. A small scalpel blade is used to make a stab incision through the skin. A 14-gauge, 11.5-cm liver biopsy instrument is inserted through the incision and the intercostal muscles and into the liver. The biopsy instrument should be directed toward the opposite elbow in most cases, but the use of real-time ultrasonography can help determine the direction and depth needed (2 to 4 cm). The clinician should avoid the vessels along the caudal border of the ribs. On reaching the liver, the clinician will note a slight increase in resistance. Samples can be submitted for culture (in a sterile plastic or glass vial or tube), histopathology (in formalin at a 10 : 1 ratio of formalin to tissue); and/or mineral analysis (in a plastic tube). When performing a liver biopsy for mineral analysis, the clinician should rinse the biopsy site with distilled and deionized water after sterile preparation to minimize sample contamination. Samples for mineral analysis should not be placed in formalin. The skin incision can be sutured,

stapled, or, if it is small enough, left alone to heal by second intention. The clinician or keeper should apply fly repellent to the area. The animal should have a history of *Clostridium* prophylaxis; if it does not, it should be vaccinated during or before the biopsy.

REFERENCES

1. *U.S. sheep health and management practices,* Fort Collins, CO, 1996, National Animal Health Monitoring System.
2. Pugh DG, Hilton CD, Mobini SM: Control programs for gastrointestinal nematodes in sheep and goats, *Comp Cont Ed Pract Vet* 20:5112, 1998.
3. Roussel AJ, Whitney MS, Cole DJ: Interpreting a bovine serum chemistry profile: Part 1, *Vet Med* 92(6):553, 1997.
4. Smith MC, Sherman DM: *Goat medicine,* Philadelphia, 1994, Lea & Febiger.
5. Howard JL, Smith RA: *Current veterinary therapy 4: food animal practice,* Philadelphia, 1999, WB Saunders.
6. Howard JL: *Current veterinary therapy 3: food animal practice,* Philadelphia, 1993, WB Saunders.
7. Keneko JJ: *Clinical biochemistry of domestic animals,* San Diego, CA, 1989, Academic Press.
8. Navarre CB et al: Analysis of gastric first compartment fluid collected via percutaneous centesis from healthy llamas, *J Am Vet Med Assoc* 214(6):812, 1999.
9. Nordlund KV, Garrett EF: Rumenocentesis: a technique for collecting rumen fluid for diagnosis of subacute rumen acidosis in dairy herds, *Bovine Pract* 28:109, 1994.
10. Keefe GP, Ogilvie TH: Comparison of oro-ruminal probe and rumenocentesis for prediction of rumen pH in dairy cattle, *Proc 30th Ann Am Assoc Bovine Pract Conv,* p 168, 1997.
11. VanMetre DC, Tyler JW, Stehman SM: Diagnosis of enteric disease in small ruminants, *Vet Clin North Am: Food Anim Pract* 16:87, 2000.
12. Smith MC: Commonly encountered diseases of goats, *Proceedings of the 1996 Symposium on the Health and Disease of Small Ruminants,* 1996, Kansas City, MO.
13. Matthews J: *Colic,* ed 2, Oxford, UK, 1999, Blackwell Science.
14. House JK et al: Ancillary tests for the assessment of the ruminant digestive system, *Vet Clin North Am: Food Anim Pract* 8(2):203, 1992.
15. Tanwar RK, Saxena AK: Radiographic detection of foreign bodies (goat), *Vet Med* 79:1195, 1984.
16. Cegarra IJ, Lewis RE: Contrast study of the gastrointestinal tract in the goat *(Capra hircus), Am J Vet Res* 38:1121, 1977.
17. Braun U, Hausammann K: Ultrasonographic examination of the liver in sheep, *Am J Vet Res* 53(2):198, 1992.
18. Gourley DD, Riese RL: Laparoscopic artificial insemination in sheep, *Vet Clin North Am: Food Anim Pract* 6:615, 1990.
19. Seeger KH, Klatt PR: Laparoscopy in the sheep and goat. In Harrison RM, Wildt DE, editors: *Animal laparoscopy,* Baltimore, 1990, Williams & Wilkins.
20. Anderson DE, Gaughan EM, St-Jean G: Normal laparoscopic anatomy of the bovine abdomen, *Am J Vet Res* 54:1170, 1993.
21. Hooper RN: Abdominal surgery in small ruminants, *Proceedings of the 1998 Symposium on the Health and Disease of Small Ruminants,* 1998, Las Vegas, NV.
22. Pearson EG: Diseases of the hepatobiliary system. In Smith BP, editor: *Large animal internal medicine,* St Louis, 1996, Mosby.

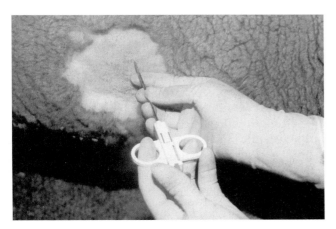

Figure 4-7   Liver biopsy. After the skin is clipped, anesthetized, and aseptically prepared, the surgeon makes a stab incision in the skin and introduces a 14-gauge biopsy needle.

DISEASES OF THE FORESTOMACHS

Bloat

Bloat is less common in small ruminants than in cattle, with goats having the condition less commonly than sheep. *Bloat* is the accumulation of either free gas or froth in the rumen, which causes rumen distention. The causes of bloat can be divided into three categories[1,2]:

1. Frothy bloat—caused by diets that promote the formation of stable froth
2. Free gas bloat—caused by diets that promote excessive free gas production
3. Free gas bloat—caused by failure to eructate

Pathogenesis. Frothy bloat is usually associated with the ingestion of legume forages or hay (particularly alfalfa) and with grazing on lush cereal grain pastures, but it also may occur with high-grain diets.[3] In the case of frothy bloat from a finely ground diet (usually corn), mucoprotein released from rumen protozoa stabilizes the foam at a low pH. In legume-associated frothy bloat, plant chloroplasts released into the rumen trap gas bubbles. Regardless of the form of frothy bloat, the small bubbles fill much of the rumen, preventing clearance of the rumen's cardia and resulting in a cessation of eructation. Free gas bloat also occurs with grain diets, especially if the animals are not adapted to the diet. Failure to eructate has a variety of causes. Physical obstructions of the esophagus such as choke or swollen mediastinal lymph nodes can cause free gas bloat. Any disease of the rumen wall can interfere with rumen contractions and eructation. Hypocalcemia, endotoxemia, pain, peritonitis, and some pharmaceutical agents (especially xylazine) can all interfere with rumen function and eructation.[1,2,4,5]

Clinical signs. Clinical signs of frothy bloat and free gas bloat from either food intake or physical obstruction of the esophagus are usually more severe and immediately life-threatening than bloat seen from rumen wall diseases and systemic influences. Abdominal enlargement occurs, particularly in the dorsal left paralumbar fossa. This may be subtle in sheep or Angora goats with full fleece. Signs of colic and anxiety are common. The rumen may be either hypomotile or hypermotile. Respiratory distress is evident, with some animals breathing through their mouths; death can ensue if the bloat is not treated.[3]

Diagnosis and treatment. This condition is a medical emergency, and therefore diagnosis and treatment should occur almost simultaneously. If the animal is not in immediate danger of dying, an orogastric tube can be passed. Most cases of free gas bloat are relieved with passage of the tube. A clinician should then take a thorough history and perform a complete physical examination to find the cause of the bloat. If the bloat is not relieved with an orogastric tube, the tube should be removed and examined for evidence of froth. Frothy bloat can be treated with poloxalene (44 mg/kg) or dioctyl sodium sulfosuccinate (DSS) (28 cc [1 oz]) delivered by orogastric tube. The froth encountered in frothy bloat caused by the ingestion of finely ground grain has a pH of less than 5.5. If frothy bloat occurs while animals are being fed concentrates, mineral oil (100 ml) may work better. Peanut oil (20 to 50 mg/kg), vegetable oil (100 to 200 ml), and hand soap (10 ml) also have been recommended in emergency situations.[3] If the animal is in severe respiratory distress, the clinician should insert a trocar or large needle into the rumen at the paralumbar fossa. If gas does not escape, or froth is seen coming out of the trocar, an emergency rumenotomy should be performed (see the Rumenotomy section of this chapter).[3] If several cases of bloat are encountered in a group of pastured animals, the entire group should be removed from the pasture and reintroduced slowly after gradual acclimation. If only one or two cases of bloat are encountered, the healthy animals can remain on the offending pasture, but grazing should be limited to ensure gradual acclimation.

Prevention. Prevention of frothy bloat involves limiting access to offending pastures or feedstuffs; providing supplemental feed and providing poloxalene in mineral supplements; and adding ionophores to the ration or supplement. When grazing or consuming legumes as "green-chop," animals should be introduced to the feed or pasture slowly, preferably over 2 to 3 weeks. Animals should be closely monitored after a frost and during the rapid growth phase of plants because legumes, particularly alfalfa, may be more likely to cause bloat at this time. Certain varieties of legumes that are designed for intensive grazing systems (e.g., Alfagraze) should be planted and managed in a manner that decreases the incidence of bloat (limited or creep grazing). Feeding dry, stemmy hay for 1 to 2 hours before allowing access to the legume pasture also may help minimize bloat. Grass-legume pastures in which legumes are limited to less than 50% of the forage are safer but can still pose a problem for animals that are selective grazers. Grazing legumes with high leaf tannin concentrations (e.g., arrowleaf clover, kudzu) is usually safer because tannins help break down rumen foam. The inclusion of poloxalene (10 to 20 mg/kg daily) in the feed or mineral supplement is useful in preventing frothy bloat. If poloxalene supplements are used, keepers should feed them for 1 to 2 weeks before moving animals onto a problem pasture.

Free gas bloat from concentrate feeds can be controlled by slow introduction to these feeds to allow for rumen adaptation and by the inclusion of ionophores in the diet.[1] Monensin (15 mg/head/day in ewes, 1 mg/kg/day in goats) and lasalocid (0.5 to 1 mg/kg/day in sheep and goats) both decrease the formation of free ruminal gas. By enhancing propionic acid formation, these drugs not only reduce the amount of methane produced in the rumen, they also improve the efficiency of nutrient assimilation from feedstuffs.

Bloat in lambs and kids can have the same causes as in adults but also can be caused by improper milk feeding. Overfeeding, feeding of large infrequent meals, and feeding spoiled or cold milk have all been associated with bloat in lambs and kids.[6] Rapid overdistention of the abomasum and improper chemical or physical composition of milk replacers inhibit rumen motility, leading to bloat. Even though the feeding of cold milk has been associated with bloat, the practice can be used effectively in orphan feeding programs. Lambs and kids tend to limit their intake of cold milk after they have become accustomed to cold milk in a free-choice feeding system. Milk is usually placed in the rumen when animals are tube-fed; this may result in milk spoilage.[1,6]

Simple Indigestion

Simple indigestion is a mild form of upset of the reticulo-rumen caused by a change in feeding routine. It can be caused by an alteration in the type of feed or in the amount of feed offered. The most common causes of simple indigestion are the addition of grain to the diet, an increase in the amount of grain fed, and an increase in the energy density of the diet. Examples of such dietary changes are replacing oats with corn or changing from whole to ground corn. If the changes are drastic, rumen acidosis can occur (see the following section). Other common causes are changes in hay or pasture, consumption of moldy hay, and ingestion of weeds and toxic plants after overgrazing or droughts. Clinical signs include mild anorexia that lasts for 1 to 2 days. Mild diarrhea and bloat also may occur. Rumen fluid pH can be unchanged, increased, or decreased depending on the inciting cause. Most animals improve with no treatment.[1]

Rumen Acidosis

Pathogenesis.   Rumen acidosis is caused by the rapid rumen fermentation of highly digestible carbohydrates that are ingested in excessive amounts. Although corn is commonly implicated, other cereal grains (oats, wheat, barley) may be involved, particularly if they are finely ground. The smaller the particle size, the more quickly rumen bacteria are able to ferment the carbohydrates contained in the feed. The common name of this condition is "grain overload," but breads, candy, apples and other fruits, beets, and potatoes also can cause this condi-

tion. Rumen acidosis usually occurs in animals that have been fed predominantly forage-based rations and are suddenly given access to large amounts of highly fermentable concentrates or concentrated forms of energy. It also can occur in animals that have been receiving concentrates previously, if the amount is suddenly and drastically increased; if access is denied for a time, then suddenly returned (e.g., during weather changes and alterations in water availability); or if ration mixing errors occur (e.g., leaving out monensin and rumen buffers)

As highly digestible carbohydrates are fermented, rumen pH drops. *Lactobacillus* species, which are lactic acid producers, proliferate in the acidic rumen environment and further lower rumen pH. As the rumen pH drops, rumen protozoa and many of the lactate users begin to die. Lactic acid production causes the osmotic pressure in the rumen to increase. Fluid is drawn from the systemic circulation into the rumen, resulting in dehydration and possibly hypovolemic shock. Lactate concentrations increase in the blood and may cause systemic lactic acidosis. The lactic acid in the rumen also is toxic to the rumen epithelium. Damage to the epithelium can result in leakage of bacteria and toxins into the portal and systemic circulation. Chronic sequelae to rumen acidosis include fungal rumenitis and occasionally liver abscesses.[1,7] Liver abscesses are less commonly encountered in sheep and goats than in cattle. Laminitis also can occur, but may be more of a problem in sheep than in goats.[8] The severity of the disease depends on the composition of the feed, particle size, amount of feed consumed, and the period of adaptation to the diet.

Clinical signs.   Clinical signs vary with the amount and type of feed ingested and the time since ingestion. Signs first appear 12 to 36 hours after ingestion of the offending feed; they vary from anorexia, depression, and weakness to a down animal suffering from severe circulatory shock. Dehydration is usually severe and evidence of toxemia is present (e.g., injected mucous membranes, increased scleral injection). Colic, bilateral ventral abdominal distention, rumen stasis, and a "splashy" feel to the rumen also may be present. Diarrhea can develop, adding to dehydration.[1,8,9] The diarrhea can range from a paste-like feces to very watery droppings with foam and occasionally pieces of grain easily recognized. Dehydration, lactic acidosis, and toxemia result in neurologic signs, including ataxia, head pressing, opisthotonos, and seizures. The body temperature is initially elevated but may drop as the condition worsens or the animal becomes toxic. Some animals develop polioencephalomalacia and appear blind.

Diagnosis.   The rumen fluid pH may fall below 5.5. The fluid itself is milky gray and particles of the inciting feed may be noticed. Protozoa are usually reduced in number or absent, and large gram-positive rods (*Lactobacillus* species) may be seen on Gram's stain.[9] Clinicopathology is consistent with dehydration (increased PCV and total protein, prerenal azotemia) and metabolic acidosis.[9] Liver enzymes (gamma-glutamyl transpeptidase [GGT], aspartate aminotransferase [AST], lactate dehydrogenase [LDH]) may be elevated on serum biochemical analysis.[1,10] The leukogram can vary from normal to a degenerative left shift, depending on the severity of the case. Urinalysis reveals an increased specific gravity.

Treatment. Treatment is aimed at correcting cardiovascular shock, dehydration, acidosis, and toxemia and removing or neutralizing the offending feedstuffs. IV fluids containing 5% sodium bicarbonate should be administered.[1,11] Oral fluids are contraindicated because they cannot be absorbed and may increase the rumen distention and discomfort of the animal. NSAIDs are indicated for toxemia (flunixin meglumine, 1.1 to 2.2 mg/kg IV).[1,11] Oral administration of magnesium hydroxide and magnesium oxide (1 g/kg) may neutralize the acidic pH and is sufficient in mild cases. However, if much of the feed is still in the rumen, these two alkalinizing agents will only work temporarily. Oral antibiotics have been recommended to kill rumen microflora and stop fermentation. However, the authors of this chapter feel they are contraindicated because the gram-negative anaerobes that need to flourish to reestablish normal rumen microflora are susceptible to most antimicrobials effective against *Lactobacillus* species. Removing the substrate for the *Lactobacillus* species is more effective. Because orogastric tubes with large enough bores to reflux feedstuffs are too large for sheep and goats, rumenotomy is indicated in severe cases to remove the feed (see the section on Rumenotomy in this chapter). After the rumen pH is corrected, transfaunation of the rumen microflora with about 1 qt of rumen fluid from a small ruminant is beneficial (Box 4-2). Thiamine supplementation (vitamin B_1, 5 mg/lb subcutaneously [SC] three times a day [TID] to four times a day [QID]) is indicated until rumen function returns.[11] In certain instances, calcium may be indicated and can be included in the IV fluids (calcium gluconate). The clinician should avoid mixing calcium salts and sodium bicarbonate. Bacterial leakage into the rumen wall, liver, and systemic circulation makes antimicrobial therapy necessary. The systemic antimicrobial agent of choice is penicillin (procaine penicillin G, 22,000 IU/kg IM BID) because anaerobes are the most likely offending organisms. If treated aggressively, the prognosis for immediate survival is good. Feed (grass hay only) and water should be limited until rumen contractions return to prevent overdistention of the rumen. The chronic sequelae discussed previously influence long-term survival.

Prevention. Prevention involves introducing concentrate feeds slowly to allow rumen microflora adaptation. Dietary change from a lower to a higher fermentable energy concentration should occur slowly and preferably over a 2- to 3-week period. In the case of animals being fed high-grain rations (e.g., club lambs, feedlot lambs, dairy goats), buffering agents can be added to the diet. Rumen buffers may improve milk production, increase feed intake, and increase rate of gain. The crude fiber content should comprise a minimum of 20% of the diet's total digestible nutrients (TDN). For example, the TDN is 75%, the minimum acceptable crude fiber is 15%. Crude fiber levels lower than this can be fed for short periods if the rumen is properly adapted, but problems may nevertheless occur. Sodium bicarbonate is probably the most commonly used buffer; it can be offered free choice or included in the diet as 1% of dry matter intake. Calcium carbonate or limestone (which both have low

---

BOX 4-2

COLLECTION, HANDLING, AND STORAGE OF RUMEN FLUID FOR TRANSFAUNATION

Collection	Collection is easiest from the rumen of a fistulated adult cow. If a fistulated cow is unavailable, fluid can be collected through a weighted orogastric tube. Alternatively, fluid can be collected from any normal ruminant at slaughter.
Handling	Rumen contents collected from a fistulated cow or at slaughter can be strained through gauze or cheesecloth to separate the fluid from the fibrous contents. Fluid collected through a weighted tube should be ready for storage.
Storage	Rumen fluid should ideally be administered immediately. However, it can be stored for 24 to 48 hours. The surface of the fluid should be covered with a layer of mineral oil to maintain an anaerobic environment and stored at refrigerator temperature. CAUTION: Do not store rumen fluid in a closed container because it may explode.

rumen solubility) and magnesium oxide (which has poor palatability) also can be included in the feed. Magnesium oxide should be limited to 0.5% to 0.8% of the dry matter intake.

Reticulitis/Rumenitis/Parakeratosis

Pathogenesis. Reticulitis and rumenitis can result from chemical or mechanical damage to the mucosal lining of the reticulorumen. The most common cause of chemical damage is rumen acidosis. However, ingestion of caustic toxins also can damage the mucosa. Mechanical damage can occur from ingested foreign bodies or the formation of rumen bezoars. In cattle, some viruses such as the ones that cause bovine virus diarrhea and infectious bovine rhinotracheitis can infect the rumen wall. Similar viruses have yet to be identified in sheep and goats. After the mucosa has been damaged, secondary infection by bacteria or fungi can occur.[12] Previous treatment with oral antibiotics may predispose to fungal infections of the rumen wall, especially if the mucosa is already damaged. Actinobacillosis, actinomycosis, and tuberculosis rarely affect the rumen wall. Tumors of the rumen wall also have been reported.[1,13] Not all of these causes of reticulitis and rumenitis have been reported in sheep and goats, but all are potential problems.

Clinical signs. The clinical signs of these diseases are vague. Anorexia and forestomach hypomotility may be the only clinical signs.

Diagnosis. Confirming a diagnosis also may prove difficult. Samples of rumen fluid may only show changes associated with anorexia (alkaline pH, decreased numbers and motility of protozoa, prolonged MBR time; see Table 4-1 for normal values). Occasionally fungal organisms may be seen on Diff Quik stained slides of rumen fluid. In these cases a diagnosis of fungal rumenitis should be made. An exploratory laparotomy and rumenotomy may be required to diagnose foreign bodies or masses. Rumen parakeratosis is characterized by dark, thickened, and clumped rumen papillae. It is seen mainly in feedlot lambs that consume finely ground or pelleted rations.[14] The parakeratotic rumen papillae are fragile and predisposed to damage, which can increase the chances of rumenitis.[1]

Treatment and prevention. Treatment depends on the inciting cause. Dietary changes should be made to decrease energy density and increase fiber intake. Mild rumenitis may improve with time and supportive care (transfaunation, fluid support, high-quality feed). Fungal rumenitis can be treated with thiabendazole (25 mg/kg orally).[15] Severe changes may lead to scarring and permanent impairment of rumen function.

DISEASES OF THE RETICULORUMEN

Traumatic Reticuloperitonitis

Traumatic reticuloperitonitis is not as common in small ruminants as in cattle, but it has been reported. Goats are affected more commonly than sheep. This is probably because of the dietary habits of small ruminants; they tend to be selective grazers and do not "vacuum" the ground as cattle do. Offending foreign bodies that cause traumatic reticuloperitonitis include pieces of wire and needles.[16,17] The clinical signs are identical to those in cattle and may include anorexia, depression, colic, signs of heart failure, and evidence of draining tracts from the chest cavity. Treatment is usually difficult.

Rumen Impaction

Rumen impaction can occur after dehydration, blockage of the omasal orifice by a foreign body, sand ingestion, or consumption of diets high in fiber and low in digestibility.[18] Clinical signs are nonspecific, but the firm rumen can usually be palpated in the left flank. The feces may be scant and dry. Oral fluids containing magnesium sulfate (60 g) may loosen impactions, but a rumenotomy is required in severe cases.[18]

Rumenotomy

To reduce rumen fill, sheep or goats should ideally have feed withheld for 24 hours before rumenotomy. However, this is usually impossible because in most cases rumenotomy is an emergency procedure. The perioperative administration of antimicrobial agents is essential because even with meticulous technique some contamination of the incision site and possibly the peritoneal cavity is inevitable. Because the rumen microflora is predominantly composed of anaerobic bacteria, penicillin (22,000 IU/kg) is the antimicrobial agent of choice and should be administered 2 to 4 hours before surgery. If the rumenotomy is being performed in an emergency situation, penicillin salts (potassium or sodium) that can be given IV provide therapeutic concentrations more rapidly than procaine penicillin. NSAIDs (flunixin meglumine, 1.1 to 2.2 mg/kg IV) also are recommended before surgery. If necessary, treatment of cardiovascular shock and dehydration with IV fluids also should begin before surgery and continue until the animal is rehydrated and in stable condition (see Appendix II).

General anesthesia is recommended, but heavy sedation and local anesthetic infiltration of the incision site can be efficiently used (see Chapter 16). The clinician should clip and surgically prepare a square area from 5 cm in front of the last rib to the tuber coxae, and from the dorsal midline to the lower abdomen, encompassing the entire left paralumbar fossa.

The surgeon makes a skin incision approximately 5 cm longer than the width of the hand 5 cm caudal and parallel to the last rib. The incision is continued through the muscle layers into the abdomen. Because the abdominal wall is relatively thin, the surgeon should take care not to enter the rumen or bowel. The surgeon grasps the rumen wall and pulls it through the incision; suturing it to the skin with a simple continuous circular pattern around the entire incision. This forms a seal that minimizes rumen content contamination of the deep layers of the incision and peritoneal cavity. The rumen wall is then incised inside the circle of sutures. The incision in the rumen wall should be large enough for the surgeon to put his or her hand inside the rumen without traumatizing the rumen wall.

After the rumen has been explored and emptied and the primary reason for doing the procedure has been completed, the surgeon closes the rumen wall in a continuous inverting pattern (Cushing, Lembert, or Guard's rumen stitch) with absorbable suture (0 catgut). The area should be rinsed with copious amounts of sterile isotonic fluids, and a new set of sterile instruments, sterile gloves, and surgical attire should be used for the remainder of the surgery. The surgeon then removes the suture securing the rumen to the skin and rinses the area again before performing routine closure of the abdominal muscles and subcutaneous layers with absorbable suture (0 catgut) in simple continuous patterns, taking care to close dead space between layers. The skin is closed with a continuous pattern (Ford interlocking) using a nonabsorbable suture material.

The sheep or goat should be observed closely by the clinician for signs of complications, including peritonitis, incisional dehiscence, incisional hematoma, abscess, and hernia formation. Penicillin therapy (procaine penicillin G, 22,000 IU/kg BID) should continue for at least 5 days. The skin sutures can be removed 10 to 14 days after surgery.

REFERENCES

1. Garry FB: Indigestion in ruminants. In Smith BP, editor: *Large animal internal medicine*, ed 2, St Louis, 1996, Mosby.
2. Guard C: Bloat or ruminal tympany. In Smith BP, editor: *Large animal internal medicine*, ed 2, St Louis 1996, Mosby.
3. Matthews J: *Diseases of the goat*, ed 2, Oxford, UK, 1999, Blackwell Science.
4. Brikas P, Tsiamitas C, Wyburn RS: On the effect of xylazine on forestomach motility in sheep, *J Vet Med* 33:174, 1986.
5. van Miert ASJPAM, van Duin CTM, Anika SM: Anorexia during febrile conditions in dwarf goats: the effect of diazepam, flurbiprofen and naloxone, *Vet Quart* 8:266, 1986.
6. Chennells D: Bloat in kids, *Goat Vet Soc J* 2:16, 1981.
7. Nour MSM, Abusamra MT, Hago BED: Experimentally induced lactic acidosis in Nubian goats: clinical, biochemical, and pathological investigations, *Sm Rumin Res* 31(1):7, 1999.
8. VanMetre DC, Tyler JW, Stehman SM: Diagnosis of enteric disease in small ruminants, *Vet Clin North Am: Food Anim Pract* 16:87, 2000.
9. Braun U, Rihs T, Schefer U: Ruminal lactic acidosis in sheep and goats, *Vet Rec* 130(16):343, 1992.
10. Lal SB et al: Biochemical alterations in serum and cerebrospinal fluid in experimental acidosis in goats, *Res Vet Sci* 50(2):208, 1991.
11. Smith MC: Commonly encountered diseases of goats, *Proceedings of the 1996 Symposium on the Health and Disease of Small Ruminants*, 1996, Kansas City, MO.
12. Perez V et al: Generalized aspergillosis in dairy sheep, *J Vet Med* 46(9):613, 1999.
13. Norval M et al: Rumen papillomas in sheep, *Vet Microbiol* 10(3):219, 1985.
14. Kutas F, Galfi P, Neogrady S: Effect of monensin on development of ruminal parakeratosis in fattening lambs, *Zentralblatt fur Veterinarmedizin* 30(7):506, 1983.
15. Kersting KW, Thompson JR: Lactic acidosis. In Howard JL, Smith RA, editors: *Current veterinary therapy 4: food animal practice*, Philadelphia, 1999, WB Saunders.
16. Sharma KB, Ranka AK: Foreign body syndrome in goats—a report of five cases, *Indian Vet J* 55(5):413, 1978.
17. Maddy KT: Traumatic gastritis in sheep and goats, *J Am Vet Med Assoc*, p 124, Feb 1954.
18. Smith MC, Sherman DM: *Goat medicine*, Philadelphia, 1994, Lea & Febiger.

DISEASES OF THE ABOMASUM

Abomasitis

Abomasitis and abomasal ulcers in adult sheep and goats are associated with rumen acidosis or chronic rumenitis but also can be caused by infections.[1-4] Finely ground feeds, pelleted rations, systemic stress, and feeding lush forages have all been implicated. Anecdotal associations with mineral deficiency (copper) have gone unproved.

Clinical signs and diagnosis. This disease often goes unnoticed in mild cases, and the most common signs are anorexia and colic. No definitive antemortem diagnostic tests are available. Fecal occult blood is often absent. Occasionally dark stool, altered appetite (wood chewing), and bruxism are seen. Therefore other causes of colic should be eliminated. Diagnosis is based on clinical signs.

Treatment. Effective therapy can be difficult. Oral medications such as coating agents must first pass through the rumen, and therefore arrive at the abomasum diluted. IV (not oral) ranitidine (15 mg/kg once a day [SID]) may be beneficial.[5] Herd problems of rumen acidosis may be addressed with buffers in the feed.

Abomasal Hemorrhage

A syndrome of abomasal hemorrhage, bloat, and ulceration is seen in lambs and kids 2 to 10 weeks of age. *Sarcina*-like bacteria, *Clostridium falax*, *Clostridium sordelli*, and *Clostridium septicum* have been isolated from many of these cases.[6-9] *C. septicum* infections of the abomasum are commonly called *braxy*.[1] The feeding of milk replacer free choice, iron deficiency, and bezoars have been implicated as predisposing factors.[10,11]

Clinical signs.   The signs of this syndrome are severe, acute abdominal distention; colic; and death.[6-9]

Diagnosis and treatment.   The diagnosis of this condition is by postmortem examination. Treatment in suspected antemortem cases is unsuccessful.

Prevention.   Adding formalin to milk replacers and vaccinating for clostridial diseases may decrease the occurrence of this disease.[10,12] Lambs or kids on problem farms can be vaccinated for *Clostridium* species during the first week of life with multivalent bacterins.

Abomasal Impaction

Similar to rumen impaction, abomasal impaction usually occurs when poor-quality roughage is fed, but it also can be seen with foreign body obstruction of the pylorus.[4,13,14] Goats appear to be more commonly affected than sheep, and Boer goats are more commonly affected than Angora goats.[15] Pregnant animals may be more prone to this condition.

Clinical signs and diagnosis.   Affected animals are usually anorexic. They have mild distention of the ventral abdomen, and in some cases the firm abomasum can be palpated through the abdominal wall on the right side.[16] Weight loss may be apparent. Clinicopathologic evaluation may be normal, or mild hypochloremic metabolic alkalosis may be present, with elevated rumen chloride concentrations (more than 50 mEq/L).[16]

Treatment.   Diet changes and mineral oil by mouth (PO) are the most commonly employed treatments. Abomasotomy can be attempted, but it has rarely been reported in small ruminants and does not usually improve the animals' long-term prognosis. When attempting abomasotomy, the clinician should perform the procedure with the animal in dorsal recumbency and under general anesthesia. The abomasum can best be visualized through an incision parallel and to the right of midline, caudal to the xyphoid process. The prognosis is poor.[13]

Prevention.   Dietary manipulation to improve feed or forage quality is the best mode of prevention.

Abomasal Emptying Defect

Abomasal emptying defect is a disease that presents similarly to abomasal impaction but is recognized only in Suffolk sheep. The underlying cause is unknown.

Unlike abomasal impaction, this disease is associated with concentrate feeding and often occurs around lambing time. The clinical signs are chronic weight loss, abdominal distention, and anorexia. Clinical pathology and rumen chloride levels are the same as described for abomasal impaction. On necropsy the abomasum is greatly distended, and the contents may be liquid or dry. Treatment with laxatives, cathartics, motility modifiers, and abomasotomy has been mostly unsuccessful.[17-19]

Azalea, Laurel, and Rhododendron Toxicity

Members of the azalea, laurel, and rhododendron plant group produce andromedotoxins that alter sodium metabolism, resulting in prolonged nerve depolarization. These plants are cardiotoxic, but affected animals generally exhibit acute gastrointestinal upset. These evergreen shrubs produce thick, dark green leaves. They also have five-lobed, white to pink, saucer-shaped flowers that bloom around July. Some of these plants are grown as ornamental shrubbery around homes, whereas others grow wild along streams, cliffs, and rocky slopes. They can be short or tall (as large as 10 m) and can form thickets. All parts of these plants are toxic.

Clinical signs.   Animals browsing a new area, those fed clippings from trimmed azalea hedges, and underfed, hungry animals given access to these plants are likely candidates for intoxication. Animals that ingest as few as two or three leaves may show signs of salivation, grinding teeth, nasal discharge, colic, epiphora, and acute digestive upset within 6 hours of ingestion. As the intoxication progresses, animals become depressed and exhibit projectile vomiting, frequent defecation, and a slowed pulse. Terminally intoxicated animals become paralyzed and comatose. Some sheep and goats develop aspiration pneumonia secondary to intoxication.

Diagnosis.   The diagnosis of this condition is usually based on clinical signs coupled with a history of ingestion of one of these plants and/or the discovery of these plants in the gastrointestinal tract.

Treatment.   Intoxicated animals may recover in 1 to 2 days without any therapy if the offending plants are removed from the diet. However, the administration of charcoal (2 to 9 g/kg PO), atropine (0.06 to 0.1 mg/kg IV), other antiarrhythmic drugs, and IV fluids all may be indicated. To manage the aspiration pneumonia, the administration of antibiotics (penicillin 22,000 units/kg BID IM) and oral magnesium hydroxide also may be beneficial. Obviously, any existing dehydration should be corrected (see Appendix II).

Prevention.   Mountainous or hilly areas should be fenced. Feeding shrubbery clippings is discouraged.

REFERENCES

1. Kimberling CV: *Jensen and Swift's diseases of sheep,* ed 3, Philadelphia, 1988, Lea & Febiger.
2. Matthews J: *Diseases of the goat,* ed 2, Oxford, UK, 1999, Blackwell Science.
3. Gundula A, Shirley H: Two cases of phycomycotic ulceration in sheep, *Vet Rec* 77:675, 1965.
4. Linklater KA, Smith MC: *Color atlas of diseases and disorders of the sheep and goat,* London, 1993, Wolfe Publishing.
5. Duran SH et al: pH changes in abomasal fluid of sheep treated with intravenous and oral ranitidine, *Proceedings of the Eleventh ACVIM Forum,* Washington, DC, 1993, American College of Veterinary Internal Medicine.
6. DeBey BM, Blanchard PC, Durfee PT: Abomasal bloat associated with *Sarcina*-like bacteria in goat kids, *J Am Vet Med Assoc* 209(8):1468, 1996.
7. Vatn S, Tranulis MA, Hofshagen M: *Sarcina*-like bacteria, *Clostridium falax* and *Clostridium sordelli* in lambs with abomasal bloat, haemorrhage and ulcers, *J Comp Path* 122(2/3):193, 2000.
8. Ellis TM, Rowe JB, Lloyd JM: Acute abomasitis due to *Clostridium septicum* infection in experimental sheep, *Aust Vet J* 60(10):308, 1983.
9. Eustis SL, Bergeland ME: Suppurative abomasitis associated with *Clostridium septicum* infection, *J Am Vet Med Assoc* 178(7):732, 1981.
10. Vatn S, Ulvund MJ: Abomasal bloat, haemorrhage and ulcers in young Norwegian lambs, *Vet Rec* 146(2):35, 2000.
11. Vatn S, Torsteinbo WO: Effects of iron dextran injections on the incidence of abomasal bloat, clinical pathology and growth rates in lambs, *Vet Rec* 146:462, 2000.
12. Gorrill AO, Nicholson JWG, MacIntyre TM: Effects of formalin added to milk replacers on growth, feed intake, digestion and incidence of abomasal bloat in lambs, *Can J Anim Sci* 55(4):557, 1975.
13. Bath GF, Bergh T: A specific form of abomasal phytobezoar in goats and sheep, *J South African Vet Med Assoc* 50(2):69, 1979.
14. Smith MC, Sherman DM: *Goat medicine,* Philadelphia, 1994, Lea & Febiger.
15. Bath GF: Abomasal phytobezoariasis of goats and sheep, *J South African Vet Med Assoc* 49:133, 1979.
16. Kline EE et al: Abomasal impaction in sheep, *Vet Rec* 113(8):177, 1983.
17. Guard C: Abomasal dilation and emptying defect of Suffolk sheep. In Smith BP, editor: *Large animal internal medicine,* ed 2, St Louis, 1996, Mosby.
18. Rings DM et al: Abomasal emptying defect in Suffolk sheep, *J Am Vet Med Assoc* 185(12):1520, 1984.
19. Ruegg PL, George LW, East NE: Abomasal dilation and emptying defect in a flock of Suffolk ewes, *J Am Vet Med Assoc* 193(12):1534, 1988.

DISEASES OF THE INTESTINES

Diarrhea in Lambs and Kids

Diarrhea in lambs and kids is a complex, multifactorial disease involving the animal, the environment, nutrition, and infectious agents. Decades of research have been devoted to the study of the pathophysiology of infectious diarrhea of calves; the pathology in lambs and kids is quite similar. Despite improvements in management practices and prevention and treatment strategies, diarrhea is still the most common and costly disease affecting neonatal ruminants.[1-4]

Some general preventive measures (e.g., improved sanitation) decrease disease no matter the cause. However, specific control measures such as vaccination require the definition of a specific cause of diarrhea. Table 4-2 lists the agents most likely to cause diarrhea in lambs and kids, tissues or other samples required for diagnosis, and commonly employed test methods. The color and consistency of the feces and any gross lesions can appear similar no matter the cause. Therefore laboratory identification of infectious agents and tissue histopathology are key to establishing a diagnosis. Because autolysis and secondary bacterial invasion of the gut begins within minutes of death, necropsy samples taken immediately from euthanized lambs and kids yield the most reliable diagnostic material. Mixed infections with two or more pathogens are common, and pathogens that are a problem on a farm change from year to year.[3,5,6] In some cases an underlying nutritional deficiency or excess may occur concurrently with an infectious agent. Therefore the clinician should be careful to take a variety of samples to ensure that all pathogens and predisposing factors involved are recognized; continued reevaluation of the causes of diarrhea is crucial. Examination of several cases, with a focus on those in the acute phases, is important. Although examination of antemortem fecal samples can be diagnostic, laboratory testing of tissue samples may yield better results. Treatment and preventive measures specific to a particular disease are discussed with that disease in the following paragraphs. General supportive treatment and control measures are covered at the end of this section.

Causes of Diarrhea in Neonatal Lambs and Kids

Four major pathogens cause diarrhea in lambs and kids during the first month of life: enterotoxigenic *Escherichia coli* (ETEC), rotavirus, *Cryptosporidium* species, and *Salmonella* species. The relative prevalence of these infectious agents varies greatly among studies. This variance most likely results from differences in location, season, diagnostic techniques, and the occurrence of mixed infections. Other, less common causes of diarrhea in neonates are *Giardia* infections and nutritional diarrhea. Figure 4-8 shows the ages at which diarrhea is expected with certain infections.

Enterotoxigenic *Escherichia coli*

Pathogenesis. ETEC employs two virulence factors to cause disease. The first is the ability to attach and colonize the intestinal villi, which is accomplished via fimbria or pili. The most important fimbria in lambs are K99 and F41.[7,8] The fimbrial antigens can be recognized from samples sent to most diagnostic laboratories and are im-

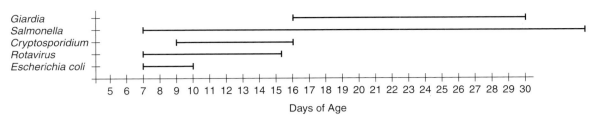

Figure 4-8 Ages at which infectious agents cause diarrhea in lambs and kids.

TABLE 4-2

DIAGNOSTIC SAMPLES AND TESTING METHODS REQUIRED FOR DIFFERENTIATION OF THE MOST COMMON CAUSES OF INFECTIOUS DIARRHEA OF LAMBS AND KIDS

CAUSATIVE AGENT	SAMPLE REQUIRED	TEST METHOD*
Escherichia coli	2 to 3 g feces	Culture and serotyping for K99 and F41
	Formalin-fixed small intestine	Histopathology
Rotavirus	2 to 3 g feces or colonic contents	EM, ELISA, VI, CF, PCR
	Formalin-fixed small and large intestine	Histopathology
	Frozen small and large intestine	VI, FA, IP
Cryptosporidia	2 to 3 g feces	FA, fecal flotation
	Air-dried fecal smear	Acid-fast stain
	Formalin-fixed small and large intestine	Histopathology
Salmonella	2 to 3 g feces	Culture, PCR
	Formalin-fixed small and large intestine	Histopathology
	Frozen small and large intestine and mesenteric lymph nodes	Culture
Giardia	Wet mount of feces	Iodine staining
	Feces	ELISA, FA
Clostridium perfringens	Frozen small intestinal contents and abomasum, small and large intestine	Culture, toxin identification
	Formalin-fixed abomasum and small and large intestine	Histopathology
Coccidia	2 to 3 g feces	Fecal flotation
	Formalin-fixed small and large intestine	Histopathology

From Rings DM, Rings MB: Managing *Cryptosporidium* and *Giardia* infections in domestic ruminants, *Vet Med* 91(12):1125, 1996; Cohen ND et al: Comparison of polymerase chain reaction and microbiological culture for detection of salmonella in equine feces and environmental samples, *Am J Vet Res* 57:780, 1996; Drolet R, Fairbrother JM, Vaillancourt D: Attaching and effacing *Escherichia coli* in a goat with diarrhea, *Can Vet J* 35(2):122, 1994.
*EM, Electron microscopy; *ELISA*, enzyme-linked immunospecific assay; *VI*, virus isolation; *CF*, complement luxation; *PCR*, polymerase chain reaction; *FA*, fluorescent antibody; *IP*, immunoperoxidase.

portant in diagnosing this agent as a cause of diarrhea. After the organism attaches to the villi, it produces the second virulence factor, enterotoxin. Enterotoxin interferes with the normal physiology of the gut, with resultant diarrhea.[8] Calves have an age-associated resistance, most likely related to the blocking of fimbrial attachment to the gut, so ETEC occurs mainly in calves less than a week old.[9,10] The mode of infection is fecal-oral.

Clinical signs. ETEC is seen in lambs and kids less than 10 days of age but is most common at 1 to 4 days of age, so age-related resistance also may occur in these animals.[3,7] It usually presents as an outbreak in lambs and kids between 12 and 48 hours of age. Because ETEC causes a "secretory" diarrhea, bicarbonate loss in the diarrhea leads to severe acidosis, with lambs and kids quickly becoming dehydrated and recumbent. However, many infected animals die before developing diarrhea. Affected neonates are depressed, stop nursing, and may show excessive salivation. Fluid sequestration in the abomasum causes a "splashing" sound on movement. This condition results in high mortality if animals are not treated promptly.[7]

Diagnosis. Fecal culture and serotyping for the K99 and F41 fimbrial antigens are the basis for diagnosis. Because many nonpathogenic *E. coli* are normal gut inhabitants, simply culturing this organism is usually insignificant.[8] Occasionally the bacteria do not express the fimbrial antigens in culture, so ETEC cannot be ruled out if the culture is negative for K99 and F41.[11] Histologic evidence of colonization of the small intestine can support a diagnosis.

Treatment. Supportive care consisting of fluid therapy with either oral, IV, or SC administration of a polyionic solution is the mainstay of therapy. The use of oral antimicrobial agents is controversial. Although antibiotics may kill the ETEC, they also may interfere with normal gut flora. If fluid support is provided, the diarrhea usually subsides without antibiotic treatment. Still, oral neomycin (10 to 12 mg/kg BID) or trimethoprim sulfa (30 mg/kg PO) and systemic ampicillin (10 to 20 mg/kg IM BID) or amoxicillin (10 to 20 mg/kg IM TID) may be beneficial. NSAIDs are indicated to decrease inflammation of the gut and provide some analgesia. The use of flunixin meglumine (1 to 2 mg/kg IM) has been shown to decrease fecal output in ETEC infections in calves[12] and appears to be beneficial in lambs.

Prevention. It is recommended that clinicians vaccinate ewes and does with bovine ETEC vaccine before they give birth to increase passive immunity.[3,4,8] Monoclonal and polyclonal antibody products for calves may be beneficial during an outbreak if it can be given to lambs or kids within the first 12 hours of life. The use of neomycin (10 to 12 mg/kg PO BID) in lambs that appear normal may help stop the progression of an outbreak. Shearing ewes prepartum to minimize fecal ingestion by neonates and ensuring that newborns ingest adequate colostrum both help decrease the incidence of this disease. Making sure that ewes and does give birth at a 2.5 to 3.5 body condition score increases the chance of adequate colostrum manufacture by the dam.

Rotavirus

Pathogenesis. Lambs and kids are infected with group B rotaviruses, whereas most other animals and human beings are infected with group A rotaviruses.[13] Rotaviruses infect villus tip cells of the small intestine, which results in villus atrophy and malabsorptive diarrhea.[14]

Clinical signs. Rotavirus generally causes diarrhea in lambs and kids 2 to 14 days old, but older animals also can be affected. Young animals can become very depressed and dehydrated.[3,13,15,16]

Diagnosis. Detection of the organism by electron microscopy of fecal or colonic samples or by immunologic

techniques on feces or tissue sections is the basis of diagnosis.[13,16] Because these organisms are sloughed with the villus tip cells they infect, and viral antigens are complexed with the lambs' and kids' antibodies, tissue samples from acutely infected animals are best.[17] Rotavirus has been detected in animals without diarrhea, so other causes of diarrhea should be investigated as well.[4,5]

Treatment and prevention. Rotavirus is treated with supportive care. Prevention by vaccination of ewes and does with bovine rotavirus vaccines before they give birth is recommended to increase passive immunity.[3,4,8]

Cryptosporidiosis

Pathogenesis. *Cryptosporidium parvum* is a protozoa that can cause a malabsorptive diarrhea similar to that seen with rotavirus infection. Unlike other protozoal agents such as the one that causes coccidiosis, cryptosporidia do not require fecal excretion for sporulation to infective stages.[18] They sporulate in the gut and about 20% become immediately infectious to other villus tip cells without ever leaving the intestines. This method of autoinfection can result in severe disease that can be sustained for long periods. Because some of the oocysts also are immediately infectious when they are shed in feces, spread of infection can occur quickly.

Clinical signs. Cryptosporidia can cause diarrhea in lambs and kids 5 to 10 days of age.[4,19,20] Affected animals are often active, alert, and nursing. The diarrhea is usually very liquid and yellow. Diarrhea can vary from mild and self-limiting to severe, especially with mixed infections.[4,5,19,21] Relapses are quite common, and this organism usually occurs as a component of mixed infections.

Diagnosis. Acid-fast staining of air-dried fecal smears is a quick and easy method of diagnosis. Examination under 40× to 100× magnification reveals round protozoa that have taken up the red color of the carbol fuchsin portions of the stain on a green background (Figure 4-9). Although they can be diagnosed by fecal flotation, their very small size (4-6 μm) makes this method difficult and subject to false negative results.[22,23] Both immunologic and polymerase chain reaction (PCR) techniques have been developed to improve detection limits.[22,24] Cryptosporidia also can be identified with histology. Cryptosporidiosis is a zoonotic disease, and people can easily become infected from handling infected animals or feces.[18]

Prevention. No consistently effective treatment for cryptosporidiosis in ruminants has been identified. Anecdotal reports suggest that decoquinate and monensin sodium may be useful in control of cryptosporosis. Decoquinate (2.5 mg/kg PO) may be very useful in prevention of cryptospirosis in goats and possibly kids. During an

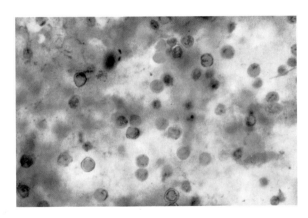

Figure 4-9   Red-staining *Cryptosporidium* on a blue-green background in a fecal smear prepared with an acid-fast stain. This protozoal parasite induces villous atrophy and decreased digestion.

outbreak affected animals should be isolated from the rest of the flock. No new animals should be added to a pen in which the disease has been diagnosed. Keepers should depopulate pens in which the disease has been diagnosed and attempt to clean the environment. Cryptosporidiosis can be particularly difficult to control because of the organisms' persistence in the environment and resistance to most chemical disinfectants. However, ammonia (5% to 10%) and formalin (10%) seem to be most effective.[19,25] Feeders should be constructed to minimize fecal contamination. Studies are currently underway to develop a vaccine for cryptosporidiosis in cattle. Early results are favorable, and this may prove the best way to control the disease in the future.[26] This is potentially a zoonotic disease, and therefore clinicians and keepers should exercise great caution when handling affected animals.

Salmonellosis

Pathogenesis.   The bacterial genus *Salmonella* has thousands of serotypes, and all potentially cause diarrhea in animals. *Salmonella* can cause diarrhea in lambs and kids of any age.[3,4] The microbes produce enterotoxins, are invasive, and cause severe inflammatory disease and necrosis of the lining of the small and large intestines.

Clinical signs.   Animals less than 1 week old are more likely to die acutely without clinical signs, whereas animals older than 1 week are more likely to have diarrhea.[4,7,27] An acute onset of fever, depression, tenesmus, and shock is occasionally observed. *Salmonella*-induced diarrhea is more likely to contain blood.[4] This also is a zoonotic disease that warrants protective measures.

Diagnosis.   A diagnosis of this condition is based on culture of the organism in feces or tissues and histologic examination of the small and large intestine.[28] More sensitive PCR techniques for identifying *Salmonella* species in feces are being developed.[29] The diarrhea may occa-

sionally contain fibrin, but many animals die before this is observed. Clinicians may note leukopenia or leukocytosis in the CBC results.

Treatment.   Therapy for *Salmonella*-induced diarrhea involves supportive care and possibly parenteral antimicrobial therapy. The use of antimicrobial agents is controversial and probably does not influence the gastrointestinal infection. However, because this is an invasive organism, parenteral use of antimicrobial agents may be beneficial in preventing septicemia. Antimicrobial susceptibility patterns are difficult to predict for *Salmonella* species, so antimicrobial therapy should be based on culture and sensitivity results. Ceftiofur sodium (1.1 to 2.2 mg/kg IM BID) or trimethoprim sulfadiazine (15 mg/kg SC SID) can be administered until antimicrobial sensitivity results are known.

Prevention.   Latent carriers of *Salmonella* can potentially shed organisms to other animals, particularly when they are stressed.[4] Newly introduced animals should be isolated for 1 month, and fecal culture should be considered.[4] Bleach is an effective disinfectant to use during an outbreak. Identification of carrier animals by fecal culture is recommended for herd problems. Vaccine efficacy is questionable, and to date its effects have not been thoroughly evaluated in sheep and goats.

GIARDIA: *Giardia*-induced diarrhea is more commonly seen in but not limited to 2- to 4-week-old lambs and kids.[4,30] The diarrhea is usually transient, but infected animals can continue to shed cysts for many weeks, even when they are clinically normal.[22,31,32] Therefore simply finding the agent in feces does not mean it is the cause of diarrhea, especially in older animals. However, these animals may be a source of infection for other animals and possibly humans.[22,30] Iodine-stained wet mounts of feces or tissue is the classic method of diagnosing giardiasis, but more sensitive immunologic techniques are now available.[22,30] Infected animals can be treated effectively with fenbendazole (5 to 10 mg/kg BID for 3 days or SID for 5 days).[22] *Giardia* has historically been treated with metronidazole (50 mg/kg PO SID for 5 days). However, use of this drug class in food animals is currently illegal in the United States. This is potentially a zoonotic condition.

Nutritional Diarrhea

Infectious agents are not the only cause of diarrhea in neonates. Nutritional problems can result in diarrhea, but these causes are overshadowed in the literature because the resulting diarrhea is usually mild and subsides without treatment. Nutritional diarrhea is most common in orphaned animals as a result of keepers offering poor-quality milk replacers, making mixing errors, or feeding large amounts infrequently (see Chapter 2). Diarrhea resulting from consumption of lush pasture or high-energy rations is a common occurrence. In most cases such diarrhea is self-limiting. The incidence of this form of gastric upset can be minimized by a slow introduction (over 2 to 3 weeks) to energy-dense diets.

Calves with infectious diarrhea that develop maldigestion or malabsorption can have secondary nutritional diarrhea from an inability to digest carbohydrates (lactose, xylose).[33,34] This has been reported in goats, and also is probably a cause of diarrhea in lambs.[35] Diarrhea resulting from primary lactose deficiency also has been reported in calves.[36] Calves on poor-quality milk replacers can develop an overgrowth of normal enteric *E. coli*, resulting in diarrhea.[37] If lactose intolerance is suspected, decreasing the amount of lactose fed and using commercially available lactose enzymes may alleviate signs.

CAUSES OF DIARRHEA IN OLDER LAMBS AND KIDS

The most common cause of diarrhea in older lambs and kids is nematode infestation. This condition is discussed later in this chapter in the section on causes of adult diarrhea. Other major causes of diarrhea in older lambs and kids are *C. perfringens* and coccidiosis.

Clostridium perfringens

C. perfringens types A, B, C, and D can all cause diarrhea in lambs and kids, but type D is the most common agent.[4,7,38]

Pathogenesis. The disease occurs in peracute, acute, and chronic forms and is commonly called *enterotoxemia* or *overeating disease.* In the case of type C infection, a beta-toxin can cause acute hemorrhagic enteritis. Type C infection is seen mostly in lambs or kids younger than 3 weeks of age. An epsilon-toxin is responsible for pathology in type D infections. Enterotoxemia is usually seen in rapidly growing feedlot lambs on high concentrate rations. It also is associated with other feeding changes, including changes in type of pasture. However, it occasionally occurs with no reported dietary changes, particularly in goats.[4,7,39] This disease usually occurs in the fastest-growing and most well-conditioned animals. It can occur in vaccinated herds (again, more commonly in goats) so it should not be ruled out if a history of previous vaccination is present.[4]

Clinical signs. The peracute form of clostridial infection is characterized by the rapid onset of severe depression; abdominal pain; profuse, bloody diarrhea; and neurologic signs. Death occurs within hours of the onset of signs. Sudden death may occur without signs of diarrhea. The onset of neurologic signs followed by sudden death is more common in sheep, whereas goats are more likely to show signs of diarrhea before death.[4] Similar but less severe signs are seen in the acute form of the disease. The chronic form occurs more commonly in goats.[4,39]

Diagnosis. Antemortem diagnosis is based on clinical signs. At necropsy, *C. perfringens* can be cultured from intestinal tissue samples. However, the significance of a positive culture can be difficult to interpret because these organisms can be present in the gut normally and then proliferate after death. Histologic examination of sections of the gut can be helpful. Identification of the toxins (namely the epsilon-toxin) in intestinal contents is required for a definitive diagnosis.[4,7] Because the toxin degrades within several hours of death, not finding the toxin does not preclude enterotoxemia as a diagnosis.[38]

Treatment. Treatment is rarely effective but consists mainly of aggressive supportive care. *C. perfringens* type D antitoxins (15 to 20 ml SC) can be administered to animals during an outbreak of enterotoxemia if clinical signs are noted before death. The antitoxin may be more effectively used as a preventive in the face of an outbreak. During an outbreak any animals that have not been vaccinated should be given the antitoxin and vaccinated with the toxoid simultaneously; those previously vaccinated should receive a booster vaccination.

Prevention. Routine vaccination should start at 4 to 6 weeks of age and be followed by a booster 3 to 4 weeks later. However, on farms where the disease has become endemic, lambs or kids can be vaccinated and given antitoxin during the first week of life. Yearly vaccination, preferably a few weeks before the ewes and dams give birth increases colostral immunity in neonates and improves prevention programs. Goats may not respond as well to vaccination as sheep, so biannual or triannual vaccination is recommended, especially in problem herds.[4,38] Vaccination with only *C. perfringens* types C and D and tetanus is superior to the use of more polyvalent clostridial vaccines.[4] Reducing the energy density of the diet and avoiding sudden dietary changes or alterations of the feeding routine are crucial to prevention. Reducing internal parasites, particularly tapeworms, may further reduce the incidence of these disorders.

Coccidiosis

Pathogenesis. Coccidiosis is a protozoan parasitic disease that is a common cause of diarrhea in lambs and kids. It also may cause subclinical production losses.[19] Clinical disease is often seen when some form of stress (e.g., dietary change, weather changes, parturition, weaning) is occurring on the farm or in the flock. *Eimeria* species cause the disease in sheep and goats; each is infested with its own host-specific species. Unlike *Cryptosporidium*, which can be shed in feces in the infective stage, coccidia must sporulate outside the host to become infective. Sporulation occurs under moderate temperatures and high moisture conditions. The nonsporulated and sporulated oocysts can survive a wide range of temperatures and may survive for years under certain conditions.

Clinical signs.   Lambs and kids are most susceptible to the problem at approximately 1 to 4 months of age, although younger animals may become infected. Clinical disease is common after the stress of weaning, feed changes, or shipping. Crowded conditions result in excessive manure and urine contamination, which is ideal for the buildup and sporulation of the oocysts. Under these conditions, animals may be exposed to high numbers of infective organisms and develop diarrhea. The diarrhea in lambs and kids is *usually* not bloody, but it can contain blood or mucus and be very watery. Anorexia, dehydration, weakness, rough hair coat, and death all may occur.[19] Weight loss is common, and constant straining can result in rectal prolapse. In severe cases the disease becomes protracted because of necrosis of the mucosal lining. Even if these animals are treated appropriately, the diarrhea continues until the intestinal mucosa heals, which can take several days to weeks. Permanent scarring can result in chronic poor development, even if the diarrhea subsides.[19,40-42]

Diagnosis.   Acute coccidiosis can be easily diagnosed from a direct smear or flotation of feces (Figure 4-10). In the chronic stages, most of the organisms have been shed and very low numbers are seen on fecal examination. Because normal animals can shed small numbers of pathogenic species or large numbers of nonpathogenic species, interpretation of fecal examinations in the chronic stages of coccidiosis or in animals with diarrhea from other causes can be difficult.[40-42] In these cases the clinician should rule out other diseases before making a diagnosis of coccidiosis. Blood analysis may show both anemia and hypoproteinemia.

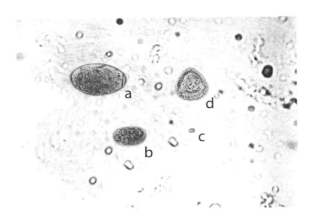

Figure 4-10   Parasites found on fecal examination. Trichostrongylid-type eggs (HOTC complex) *(b)*, Coccidia *(c)*, and tapeworm "eggs" *(d)* may be identified with flotation techniques. *Fasciola hepatica (a)* eggs are found with sedimentation techniques.

Treatment.   Treatment of affected animals with clinical signs includes supportive care and administration of coccidiostats. All animals in the group should be treated during an outbreak. The use of coccidiostats has little effect on the existing infection, but it does prevent the spread of the disease from continued exposure to infective organisms.[40] Many coccidiostats inhibit coccidia development and prevent disease if given prophylactically.[40] They are of little value if they are given after the onset of clinical disease. Sulfa drugs appear to be clinically beneficial, but they may simply decrease secondary or concurrent bacteria-induced diarrhea.[40] Because coccidia develop some resistance to coccidiostats, these drugs should be administered only before stressful events (e.g., shipping, weaning, parturition).[40] The drugs listed in Table 4-3 and trimethoprim sulfa (15 mg/kg orally SID for 5 days) are approved for use in the United States.[7,41]

Prevention.   Control involves improved sanitation and possibly the use of coccidiostats. Preventing overcrowding decreases the buildup of manure and infective oocysts. Exposure to sunlight and desiccation are two of the most effective means of killing the organisms. Minimizing stress and optimizing nutritional intake also are important. Coccidiostats available in the United States are shown in Table 4-3 and Appendix I. To avoid toxicity in growing animals, the clinician or keeper must carefully adjust dosages to the changing levels of feed intake as animals grow. All agents except amprolium should be fed for at least 4 weeks.[19,40] This allows exposure and subsequent development of immunity to occur while preventing the detrimental effects of clinical disease. However, coccidia can become resistant to coccidiostats; fecal samples should be periodically evaluated after prolonged use of a particular product. Anecdotal reports suggest amprolium resistance may occur on some farms. Moreover, if amprolium is offered with a creep feed rich in thiamine, its ability to act as a thiamine antagonist may be compromised. Year-round use of coccidiostats increases the potential for resistance. Therefore they should be fed only during times of expected risk.[40] The inclusion of lasalocid (1 kg of 6% premix) or decoquinate (1 kg of 13% premix) in 22 kg of trace mineralized salt fed as the only source of salt for 30 days prepartum can reduce the number of oocysts shed in ewe or dam feces. This practice can reduce the coccidia contamination of pasture and thereby remove a source of infection for kids and lambs. The benefits of administering lasalocid and monensin beyond coccidia control include increased feed efficiency, enhanced growth rate, and decreased incidence of free gas bloat. However, if coccidiostats are included in either mineral or feed supplements, inconsistent or depressed intake may result in subtherapeutic drug dosing.

Lambs are resistant to infection in the first few weeks of life. Exposure to the protozoa during this time confers immunity and resistance to later infections.[40,42]

TABLE 4-3

COCCIDIOSTATS USED FOR TREATMENT AND PREVENTION OF COCCIDIOSIS IN SMALL RUMINANTS*

COCCIDIOSTAT	DOSE	COMMENTS
Lasalocid	20 to 30 g per ton of feed; 0.5 to 1 mg/kg body weight per head per day in feed or salt	Approved for use in sheep in the United States
Decoquinate	0.5 mg/kg body weight per head per day in feed or salt	Approved for use in goats in the United States
Monensin	10 to 30 g per ton of feed	Approved for use in goats in the United States; may be most effective choice for goats
Amprolium	50 mg/kg body weight per head per day for 21 days (NOTE: This dose is five times the recommended calf dose)	Not approved for use in small ruminants in the United States; comes in liquid and crumble form; can potentially cause polioencephalomalacia at high doses and with prolonged administration
Sulfaquinoxaline	13 mg/kg body weight per head per day as 0.015% solution in water for 3 to 5 days	Approved for use in sheep in the United States
Sulfamethazine	119 to 238 mg/kg body weight per head per day in sheep; 50 g per ton of feed in goats	Not approved for use in small ruminants in the United States
Salinomycin	382 g per ton of feed in goats	Not approved for use in small ruminants in the United States

From Foreyt WJ: Coccidiosis and cryptosporidiosis in sheep and goats, *Vet Clin North Am: Food Anim Pract* 6(3):655, 1990; Craig TM: Coccidiosis in small ruminants, *Proceedings of the Small Ruminants for the Mixed Animal Practitioner, Western Veterinary Conference,* 1998, Las Vegas, NV. Smith MC: Parasitic diseases of goats, *Proceedings of the 1996 Symposium on the Health and Disease of Small Ruminants,* 1996, Nashville, TN.
*Not approved for dairy animals in the United States.

MISCELLANEOUS CAUSES OF DIARRHEA IN KIDS AND LAMBS

Adenovirus, caprine herpesvirus, coronavirus, *Campylobacter jejuni, Yersinia* species, and *Strongyloides papillosus* can cause diarrhea in lambs and kids of various ages.[2,4,6] Enterohemorrhagic *E. coli* (EHEC) and enteropathogenic *E. coli* (EPEC) also have been isolated in the feces of kids with diarrhea.[43,44] These *E. coli* types are K99- and F41-negative. Culture and serotyping of these organisms from feces and tissue samples with typical histopathologic lesions is diagnostic. Although ETEC is not zoonotic, EHEC and EPEC can potentially affect humans.

TREATMENT OF LAMBS AND KIDS WITH DIARRHEA

Although some causes of diarrhea have specific treatments, many animals need to be treated for dehydration and metabolic acidosis regardless of the inciting cause. Animals with only mild diarrhea, especially mild nutritional diarrhea, may not require therapy unless they become dehydrated. If kids or lambs become less than 8% dehydrated and are only mildly depressed but still willing to nurse, they can be treated with oral electrolytes designed

for calves. Fluids can be administered by bottle or by tube if the animal will not nurse. The keeper or clinician should carefully adjust the amount of fluids for lambs and kids (250 to 500 ml, or 8 to 16 oz, as opposed to 4 L in a calf). Because most electrolyte solutions designed for calves contain glucose, after they have been mixed they should be refrigerated and any leftovers discarded within 24 hours. IV fluids may be needed to treat more severe dehydration. If the lamb or kid is too weak to stand, IV fluids are indicated. Isotonic fluids containing electrolytes should be given to replenish losses. Glucose can be added to fluids to make a 1% to 2.5% solution. Sodium bicarbonate also may be administered, especially if the dehydration is severe. A rule of thumb is to give one fourth of the calculated fluid need (see Appendix II) as isotonic bicarbonate (1.3%). Extra potassium (10 to 20 mEq/L) can be added to fluids because most animals are severely dehydrated from diarrhea and depleted in potassium, even though their blood potassium levels may be elevated. If extra potassium is added, acidosis must be corrected concurrently. After correcting the dehydration, the keeper or clinician can offer oral electrolyte-enriched fluids to replace ongoing losses caused by continued diarrhea.

Removing milk or milk replacer from the diet is not recommended. Young animals need nutrients, and even high-energy, glucose-containing electrolyte solutions are no substitute for milk. Animals should continue to receive milk replacer in normal amounts or be allowed to nurse; they can be supplemented with oral electrolytes if necessary. Animals being hand fed should be offered small amounts frequently to help minimize problems. Electrolytes should never be mixed with milk, but should instead be given in separate feedings. If lactose deficiency is suspected, lactase drops or capsules (available in health food stores) can be added to milk or milk replacer.[35]

NSAIDs (flunixin meglumine, 1.1 to 2.2 mg/kg IV; ketoprofen, 2.2 to 4.4 mg/kg IV) are beneficial, especially if toxemia is involved, as in ETEC, enterotoxemia, and salmonellosis. It is the authors' opinion that antimicrobial agents should be reserved for proven outbreaks of salmonellosis and for animals with other causes of diarrhea that do not respond to fluid therapy and NSAIDs; these drugs should only be administered parenterally. The use of oral coating agents and antacids is popular, but it has not been shown to be beneficial and is not therapeutically logical in light of the pathogenesis of these diseases. Probiotics may be beneficial in reestablishing the normal flora of the small intestine. The authors' rule of thumb is that nothing should be given orally except milk, oral electrolytes, and probiotics.

GENERAL CONTROL MEASURES FOR INFECTIOUS DIARRHEA

Ensuring adequate intake of high-quality colostrum and minimizing stress are important for prevention of all neonatal diseases. A normal lamb or kid will stand and nurse within 45 minutes to 1 hour of birth. The ingestion of colostrum within 2 to 3 hours is essential in preventing hypothermia and hypoglycemia and decreasing the incidence of various diseases. Lambs or kids born as twins or triplets, weak or injured neonates, those born during severe weather, those born from a dam with dystocia, and those delivered by Cesarean section are all candidates for colostrum supplementation. If supplemental colostrum is provided, it should be good-quality colostrum from females that have tested negative for Johne's disease, ovine progressive pneumonia (OPP), and caprine arthritis-encephalitis (CAE). Mixing colostrum from several cows decreases the incidence of the "cow colostrum–associated" hemolytic disease sometimes seen in lambs. If the lamb or kid is unable to nurse, it should be tube fed 50 ml/kg of colostrum. The veterinarian or animal handler can sit comfortably holding the lamb or kid in sternal recumbency in the lap. A 12 to 14 French soft feeding tube is then lubricated, inserted into the side of the mouth, and passed slowly. If the tube is placed in the trachea, the lamb or kid will become uncomfortable and may shake and cough. The tube may be palpated on the left side of the throat. After the tube has been slowly passed to the thoracic inlet, colostrum can be administered by gravity flow (see Chapter 6).

Prepartum shearing of the dam may decrease the ingestion of feces by lambs. Good sanitation of lambing and kidding areas is paramount in management programs that stress prevention. The presence of organic matter interferes with the effectiveness of many disinfectants, so removal and proper disposal of feces, carcasses, and placentas are essential. When disposing of waste material containing either *Cryptosporidium* or *Giardia*, the keeper should be careful to avoid contaminating water sources. Infected animals should be isolated to prevent spread of the infection throughout the flock. In general, infected animals should remain in the environment where the infection was first diagnosed, because it is already contaminated. Removing pregnant ewes or dams to a clean area before lambing or kidding helps minimize the continued spread of disease. If possible, lambs and kids already born but not showing clinical signs should be removed to a third area. If "safe" pastures are maintained for internal nematode control, they are ideal for use in an emergency situation to control these diseases. Although some animals may appear normal, they may be incubating and possibly shedding the infective agents of a disease. If such animals are moved with pregnant females, they can be a source of contamination in a clean area. If healthy lambs and kids cannot be moved to a third, relatively safe area, they should be left with the clinically infected animals because they have already been exposed.

References

1. Sherman DM: Causes of kid morbidity and mortality: an overview, *Proceedings of the Fourth International Conference on Goats,* Brasilia, Brazil, 1987, EMBRAPA-DDT.
2. Vickers MC: Enteric infections in young goats and their control, *Proceedings of the Sixteenth Seminar, Sheep and Beef Cattle Society,* Palmerston North, New Zealand, 1986.
3. Blackwell TE: Enteritis and diarrhea, *Vet Clin North Am: Large Anim Pract* 5(3):557, 1983.
4. Smith MC, Sherman DM: *Goat medicine,* Philadelphia, 1994, Lea & Febiger.
5. Nagy B et al: Infectious gastrointestinal diseases of young goats, *Proceedings of the Fourth International Conference on Goats,* Brasilia, Brazil, 1987, EMBRAPA-DDT.
6. Nagy B et al: Occurrence of cryptosporidia, rotaviruses, coronavirus-like particles and K99+ *Escherichia coli* in goat kids and lambs, *Proceedings of the Third International Symposium on Veterinary Laboratory Diagnostics,* Ames, Iowa, 1983.
7. Kimberling CV: *Jensen and Swift's diseases of sheep,* ed 3, Philadelphia, 1988, Lea & Febiger.
8. Hodgson JC: Escherichia coli *in domestic animals and humans,* Wallingford, UK, 1994, Cab International.
9. Runnels PL, Moon HW, Schneider RA: Development of resistance with host age to adhesion of K99+ *Escherichia coli* to isolated intestinal epithelial cells, *Infect Immun* 28(1):298, 1980.
10. Zeman DH, Thomson JU, Francis DH: Diagnosis, treatment, and management of enteric colibacillosis, *Vet Med* 84(8):794, 1989.

11. Schultheiss P: Diarrheal disease in calves, *Large Anim Vet* 47(2):24, 1992.
12. Roussel AJ et al: Effect of flunixin meglumine on *Escherichia coli* heat stable enterotoxin-induced diarrhea in calves, *Am J Vet Res* 49(8):1431, 1988.
13. Theil KW et al: Group B rotavirus associated with an outbreak of neonatal lamb diarrhea, *J Vet Diagn Invest* 7(1):148, 1995.
14. Babiuk LA, Sabara M, Hudson GR: Rotavirus and coronavirus infections in animals. In Karger S, editor: *Infection and immunity in farm animals*, Switzerland, 1985, Basel.
15. Theil KW, Lance SE, McCloskey CM: Rotaviruses associated with neonatal lamb diarrhea in two Wyoming shed-lambing operations, *J Vet Diagn Invest* 8(2):245, 1996.
16. Munoz M et al: Rotavirus excretion by kids in a naturally infected goat herd, *Sm Rum Res* 14(1):83, 1994.
17. Heath SE: Neonatal diarrhea in calves: diagnosis and intervention in problem herds, *Comp Cont Ed Pract Vet* 14(7):995, 1992.
18. Moore JA, Blagburn BL, Lindsay DS: Cryptosporidiosis in animals including humans, *Comp Cont Ed Pract Vet* 10(3):275, 1988.
19. Foreyt WJ: Coccidiosis and cryptosporidiosis in sheep and goats, *Vet Clin North Am: Food Anim Pract* 6(3):655, 1990.
20. Berg IE, Peterson AC, Freeman TP: Ovine cryptosporidiosis, *J Am Vet Med Assoc* 173(12):1586, 1978.
21. Sanford SE et al: Cryptosporidiosis, rotaviral, and combined cryptosporidial and rotaviral infections in goat kids, *Can Vet J* 32(10):626, 1991.
22. Rings DM, Rings MB: Managing *Cryptosporidium* and *Giardia* infections in domestic ruminants, *Vet Med* 91(12):1125, 1996.
23. Corwin RM: Cryptosporidiosis: a coccidiosis of calves, *Comp Cont Ed Pract Vet* 14(7):1005, 1992.
24. Webster KA et al: Detection of *Cryptosporidium parvum* oocysts in feces: comparison of conventional coproscopical methods and the polymerase chain reaction, *Vet Parasit* 61(1/2):5, 1996.
25. Campbell I et al: Effect of disinfectants on survival of *Cryptosporidium* oocysts, *Vet Rec* 111(18):414, 1982.
26. Perryman LE et al: Protection of calves against cryptosporidiosis with immune bovine colostrum induced by a *Cryptosporidium parvum* recombinant protein, *Vaccine* 17(17):2142, 1999.
27. Bulgin MS, Anderson BC: Salmonellosis in goats, *J Am Vet Med Assoc* 178(7):720, 1981.
28. House JD, Smith BP: Current strategies for managing salmonella infections in cattle, *Vet Med* 93:756, 1998.
29. Cohen ND et al: Comparison of polymerase chain reaction and microbiological culture for detection of salmonella in equine feces and environmental samples, *Am J Vet Res* 57:780, 1996.
30. Kirkpatrick CE: Giardiasis in large animals, *Comp Cont Ed Pract Vet* 11(1):80, 1989.
31. Koudela B, Vitovec J: Experimental giardiasis in goat kids, *Vet Parasit* 74(1):9, 1998.
32. Olsen ME et al: Effects of giardiasis on production in a domestic ruminant (lamb) model, *Am J Vet Res* 56(1):1470, 1995.
33. Nappert G et al: Determination of lactose and xylose malabsorption in preruminant diarrhetic calves, *Can J Vet Res* 57(8):152, 1993.
34. Naylor JM: Neonatal ruminant diarrhea. In Smith BP, editor: *Large animal internal medicine*, ed 2, St Louis, 1996, Mosby.
35. Weese JS, Kenney DG, O'Connor A: Secondary lactose intolerance in a neonatal goat, *J Am Vet Med Assoc* 217(3):372, 2000.
36. Olchowy TWJ et al: Lactose intolerance in a calf, *J Vet Int Med* 7(1):12, 1993.
37. Roy JHB: *The calf,* ed 4, London, 1980, Butterworth.
38. Uzal FA, Kelly WR: Enterotoxemia in goats, *Vet Res Commun* 20:481, 1996.
39. Songer JG: Clostridial diseases of small ruminants, *Vet Res* 29:219, 1998.
40. Craig TM: Coccidiosis in small ruminants, *Proceedings of the Small Ruminants for the Mixed Animal Practitioner, Western Veterinary Conference,* 1998, Las Vegas, NV.
41. Smith MC: Parasitic diseases of goats, *Proceedings of the 1996 Symposium on the Health and Disease of Small Ruminants,* 1996, Nashville, TN.
42. Clarkson MJ, Winter AC: *A handbook for the sheep clinician,* ed 5, Liverpool, UK, 1997, University Press.
43. Duhamel GE, Moxley RA, Maddox CW: Enteric infection of a goat with enterohemorrhagic *Escherichia coli* (0103:H2), *J Vet Diagn Invest* 4(2):197, 1992.
44. Drolet R, Fairbrother JM, Vaillancourt D: Attaching and effacing *Escherichia coli* in a goat with diarrhea, *Can Vet J* 35(2):122, 1994.

DIARRHEA IN ADULT SHEEP AND GOATS

The differential diagnosis list for acute and chronic diarrhea in small ruminants is very long.[1] The most common cause of diarrhea in adult sheep and goats is parasitism; another major cause is Johne's disease. Both of these diseases are discussed in the following sections. Other causes of acute diarrhea include rumen acidosis, peritonitis, endotoxemia, and ingestion of toxins. The list of toxins that cause diarrhea also is very long, and often the diarrhea is not the primary clinical sign. Some of the more common toxins that produce diarrhea are arsenic, toxic amounts of salt, levamisole, copper, oak, selenium, and pyrrolizidine alkaloids.[1] *Salmonella* species and chronic enterotoxemia can cause diarrhea in adult animals. Coccidiosis can occur in adults under severe stress or in animals that possess limited immunity because of lack of exposure. Hepatic and renal disease and copper deficiency are sometimes accompanied by chronic diarrhea, but weight loss is a more common sign in adults.

INTESTINAL PARASITISM

Nematode Infestation

Etiology and pathogenesis. Sheep and goats are infested with many of the same gastrointestinal nematode parasites as cattle, but these parasites tend to either be species-specific or have some amount of host specificity. Sheep and goats are susceptible to the same nematodes and tend to share resistance to those that infect cattle and horses. The major gastrointestinal nematodes that parasitize pastured sheep and goats are *Haemonchus, Ostertagia, Trichostrongylus, Cooperia, Nematodirus, Oesophagostomum,* and *Bunostomum* species. The acronym *HOTC* comes from the first letter of each of the first four genera of parasites listed. The specific parasites that produce disease vary from flock to flock. Climate usually determines which parasites are of clinical significance on a farm, and the weather determines when the parasites will be transmitted and infective. In much of the United States, *Haemonchus* is the most significant parasite with respect to both clinical disease and anthelmintic resistance. Most of these parasites affect the abomasum or small intestine of young, recently weaned animals and occasionally adult animals. Sheep (and, to a lesser extent, goats) that are older than 18 months may be less susceptible. Overcrowding and overgrazing with concurrent pasture mismanagement and malnutrition usually increase susceptibility to these parasites. Inadequate nutrient or protein intake may result in greater susceptibility.[2]

The life cycle appears to be similar in most of these parasite species. Adults lay eggs that are passed in the feces; except for *Nematodirus* species, the eggs hatch under favorable environmental conditions. The larvae go through several free-living developmental stages becoming infective. When the infective larvae are ingested by the host, the parasite completes its life cycle as an adult. *Trichuris* eggs are the infective stage and can survive for extended periods in dry lots or barns.[4] However, *Trichuris* is associated with minimal pathology. During dry environmental conditions, fecal pellets tend to trap the nematode larvae, whereas in wet conditions, larvae are released onto the pasture. Therefore drought conditions followed by rain can result in devastatingly high rates of pasture contamination as larvae that have remained in fecal pellets are released.[2]

Very high environmental temperatures result in shorter survivability of some stages of infective larvae. Most of the larvae have adapted the ability to over-winter, but can survive only for short periods outside the host during spring. *Nematodirus* is an exception in that the developmental stages leading to infective larvae occur while the microbe is still encapsulated in the egg. However, compared with other species of parasite, *Nematodirus* is of minor importance. *Nematodirus battus* may pose a threat to young, newly weaned and therefore immunologically naive grazing lambs. The hookworm *Bunostomum* also is different, as it may infect the host by either oral ingestion or percutaneous penetration. With the exception of the small intestinal parasite *Strongyloides*, lambs or kids fed indoors or in dry pens tend to be free of parasites.

Clinical signs. All intestinal nematode infections produce similar signs, although infection with the more rarely encountered *Bunostomum* may perhaps result in more profound anemia. If they infest the animal in sufficient numbers, all nematodes may cause poor growth, decreased feed conversion, decreased milk production, weight loss, diarrhea, anemia, ventral edema (bottle jaw), midline edema, and death. Again, all these parasites can potentially result in disease, but *Haemonchus* is the most devastating, particularly in more temperate regions.[2]

Diagnosis. Antemortem diagnosis of nematode infestation is made by examining the feces for nematode eggs. Although a direct fecal smear can be examined, the mere presence of parasite eggs is not helpful in determining the parasite load of an animal or animals. Quantifying of the EPG of feces is the best way of estimating parasite loads. The quantitative McMaster's technique for determining the EPG of feces is shown in Box 4-1. Common nematode eggs are shown in Figure 4-10.

Treatment and control program. After taking a thorough history of the previous parasite control program used on a farm and determining its effectiveness, the clinician can design and implement a new control program.[2,3] However, before deciding to implement a deworming program, the clinician should decide which parasites are in need of control and whether control of these parasites is cost effective in a particular flock. Whenever possible, a dewormer that can reduce EPG counts on the farm by 90% should be identified and used for at least a year. Of all the parasite prevention programs, strategic deworming or a combination of strategic and tactical programs appear to produce the best results.[2,4,5]

Strategic deworming is used when most of the parasites are inside the animals and not on the pasture.[2] In northern climates, strategic deworming can best be carried out during the winter, when the nematode parasites are in a hypobiotic state. When environmental conditions are inhospitable for the survival of the infective larvae, some of the most pathogenic nematodes (e.g., *Haemonchus)* may become hypobiotic; that is, they assume a state of arrested development. They may then mature to the adult stage when environmental conditions become conducive for the survival of their eggs or larvae. Preventing or decreasing the numbers of maturing adults by killing the larvae before the periparturient rise in parasite egg production and pasture contamination is an excellent management tool.[4,6,7] Unfortunately, in warmer, more temperate to subtropical environments, this method is less effective because larvae can survive the environment for longer periods. The addition of a protein supplement overlapping the expected periparturient rise has been shown to decrease the number of parasite eggs shed around the time of parturition. However, the cost of the protein supplement may outweigh its benefits.[8]

A strategic program entails the use of an anthelmintic agent that is capable of killing encysted larvae. Animals are then moved to parasite-free or safe pastures—areas in which the level of parasite contamination is too low to result in infection of grazing animals. Examples of safe pastures include pastures where sheep or goats have not grazed for 3 to 6 months in the spring or fall, respectively (and depending on the climate); pastures used for hay production; new pastures (i.e., those used for corn, cotton, or other crops); and pastures grazed by horses or cattle. The use of safe pastures is paramount in any deworming program. Rotating pastures after less than 3 months during the warm part of the year or less than 6 months during cooler months is ineffective.[3] However, if pastures are tilled and replanted, by the time new grazeable forage is available, infective parasite larvae will be dead or significantly decreased.[3]

An alternative to pasture rotation is to perform an initial strategic deworming before lambing or kidding and follow it with two to four more dewormings at 3-week intervals throughout the lambing and kidding period.[9-11] Treating lambs or kids at weaning and moving them to a safe pasture is a form of strategic deworming.[4] In lambs or kids to be sold at an early age, the administration of a single anthelmintic treatment followed by a move to a safe pasture may be all that is required. A "double treat and move" system is required for lambs kept for 12 to 18 weeks after weaning, particularly during the summer.[12,13] This form of strategic deworming requires two treatments 6 to 8 weeks apart as well as two safe pastures. In northern climates where animals are moved to a dry lot or barn for the winter, a strategic anthelmintic administration as animals are moved off pasture can help reduce the parasite burden through the winter.[14] If this deworming is followed by minimal or no exposure to grazing areas and another dewormer is administered before the spring rise in fecal egg counts, the total parasite burden on spring pasture can be drastically reduced, effectively controlling parasites until summer or fall.

Tactical deworming programs are used to remove parasites from their hosts before they enter their reproductive phase and can contaminate the pasture.[4] An example of tactical deworming is treating animals 10 to 14 days after a rain, particularly if the rain has followed a drought. Parasite transmission is worse in most flocks during this time as pastures become heavily contaminated. McMaster's counts of more than 1000 EPG in the spring or more than 2000 EPG in the fall warrant tactical deworming.[2,4,7]

Opportunistic deworming and salvage deworming are usually less effective in long-term flock management. Many times salvage deworming programs are used to save the lives of heavily parasitized animals.[4] If animals are dewormed only after showing signs of parasitism (e.g., bottle jaw, anemia), animal and flock productivity have already been depressed. Deworming during handling for other procedures (e.g., castration, vaccination, shearing) is an example of an opportunistic program. It is convenient but is not conducive to long-term flock health. Flock work should be scheduled around parasite management programs, not vice versa.[2,14]

Suppressive deworming programs entail the use of anthelmintics at regular intervals, usually every 2 to 4 weeks. Suppressive programs are labor-intensive, tend to be very expensive, fail to identify animals with superior immunity to parasites, and ultimately result in anthelmintic resistance despite initial effectiveness.[2,4]

As a general rule, the more frequently deworming occurs, the more quickly resistance is attained to anthelmintics. After deworming, only resistant parasites remain to infect the animal and they are able to reproduce freely, resulting in proliferation of resistant strains.[2,4] Using drugs that remain in tissues at inappropriately low concentrations and treating and retaining immunocompromised animals encourage the development of anthelmintic resistance. Practices that ensure adequate dosages, proper treatment techniques, and appropriate types of anthelmintics should be emphasized.[2,13]

The clinician should do everything in his or her power to minimize the incidence of anthelmintic resistance, both through their own actions and by counseling owners in proper use of deworming drugs. The product development market for anthelmintics is the cattle industry. The small sheep and goat markets simply use drugs made available for cattle. Because most available anthelmintics are highly effective in controlling parasites, anthelmintic resistance in sheep and goats must be avoided. The anthelmintics that have been used previously on a flock, the route of administration (e.g., PO, SC, IM, pour-on), and the length of use should be determined. Few dewormers are approved for use in sheep and goats, but many approved for use in cattle and horses may be effective.[2,7] If sheep graze with goats that harbor anthelmintic-resistant parasites, the sheep also may become infected.[4] However, if sheep are allowed to graze while the goats browse and the two groups rarely mingle, less parasite movement will occur between these species.

Resistance to macrolides (e.g., ivermectin, doramectin, moxidectin) does occur. Resistant worms are generally not very tolerant of cold temperatures and therefore resistance to this drug class in northern environments is not as large a problem as it is in more temperate or subtropical zones.[15] Although moxidectin is not approved for use in sheep and goats in the United States, it has been shown to be effective in cases where ivermectin resistance is encountered.[2] Still, this drug should be avoided until all other anthelmintics have failed. Craig[3,4] has suggested that clinicians refrain from injecting or using pour-on macrolide preparations designed for cattle in small ruminants. This practice may enhance the development of resistant strains of some internal parasites because of inappropriately low drug absorption (with pour-on use) or long-term subtherapeutic levels (with injection).[4]

If resistance to tetrahydropyrimidines (e.g., morantel, pyrantel) occurs in a flock, levamisole also may be ineffective. Morantel and levamisole resistance in parasites appears to be sex-linked. Therefore if animals are not exposed to these drugs for several years, reversion to susceptibility can occur.[3,4]

If resistance to one of the benzimidazole dewormers has been documented in a flock, some resistance to all members of that class is likely.[4] Benzimidazole-resistant *Haemonchus* species appear to be more virulent, produce more eggs, cause greater environmental contamination, and survive in the environment as free-living larvae for longer periods. Benzimidazole-resistant parasites apparently do not revert to susceptible forms, even over long periods. Therefore the clinician or keeper should exercise caution to minimize resistance.[4] Benzimidazole efficacy can be improved by increasing dosages, dividing dosages into two treatments administered at 12-hour intervals, and instituting pretreatment fasting.[2]

If resistance to numerous classes of anthelmintics occurs on a farm, combining two of the resistant classes of dewormers (fenbendazole and levamisole) has proven effective.[16] When using combined dewormers, the clinician should administer the full therapeutic dosage of each. Anthelmintics are metabolized at different rates by sheep and goats. Goats may require larger dosages of some dewormers than sheep.[7] Craig[4] has suggested that if no dose rate is known for a particular anthelmintic for sheep or goats, the animals should be treated at twice the suggested cow dosage. Pour-on anthelmintics designed for cattle tend to be of limited value when used topically on either goats or sheep.[2] A list of dewormers useful in sheep and goats is listed in Table 17-3. To maximize a parasite control program, anthelmintics that appear effective should be used for only 1 year before a new class of deworming drug is used. More frequent rotation (after less than 1 year) of anthelmintic agents hastens resistance and should be avoided whenever possible.

Whenever a flock is dewormed, animals should be treated based on the heaviest animal in the group and not on the group's average weight. Underdosing can hasten the formation of parasitic resistance and therefore should be avoided.[4] Holding the sheep or goats in a dry lot overnight or feeding only dry hay for 12 to 24 hours before and 12 hours after deworming appears to improve the efficacy of some orally administered anthelmintic agents (benzimidazole). Limiting feed intake before deworming slows the rate of passage of ingesta through the bowel, enhancing drug effectiveness.[2,13,14] Feed should never be withheld from sick or debilitated animals or late-term females.[2,13,14] Most dewormers may effectively control adult or larval parasites but are ineffective against eggs. Therefore animals should be kept on a dry lot for as long as 3 days after deworming, then moved to a safe pasture. Use of this procedure minimizes parasite egg contamination of the new pasture because most of the egg-contaminated feces is voided within 72 hours of deworming. If more than one dosage appears on the drug label, the larvacidal dose should be used (fenbendazole at 10 mg/kg rather than 5 mg/kg).[2]

Anthelmintic effectiveness can be determined by comparing a McMaster's fecal EPG on the day of deworming with one taken 7 to 14 days later. If less than a 90% drop in EPG is found, anthelmintic resistance exists and the animals should be switched to another class of dewormer.[2] Although it is a controversial method, the authors have used this technique to identify anthelmintic

effectiveness for many years and on many farms and ranches.[2,14] The authors randomly collect feces from 5% to 10% (or a minimum of 10 animals) of the sheep or goats on the farm. A composite sample is prepared by combining equal amounts of stool from all animals. Craig[3] has suggested that combining stool samples from many animals alters the accuracy of the tests because great individual variation in fecal egg counts occurs among animals. Composite egg counts more accurately reflect parasite burdens in groups of young animals, and individual fecal examinations are more accurate in adults.[2,4] Still, the authors prefer to use composite samples unless obvious differences in stool character or body condition score exist among the sampled animals. Anthelmintic resistance can be minimized by using drugs that reduce fecal egg counts by 90%. Pre- and post-deworming changes in EPG should be evaluated yearly or whenever resistance is suspected.[4] In vitro methods of assessing flock parasite resistance also are available at some diagnostic laboratories. In most in vitro tests, larvae are hatched from collected feces and the sensitivity of different anthelmintics is determined by larval exposure. These tests are very accurate but tend to be quite expensive.

The most effective method to prevent anthelmintic resistance is to not use deworming drugs at all.[4] One of the most overlooked management procedures is the identification and selection of parasite-resistant sheep and goats.[2] Some breeds or familial lines within breeds have excellent parasite resistance (e.g., Gulf Coast Native and Barbados sheep, some strains of Spanish, Pygmy, and Tennessee myotonic-fainting goats).[2] One study[17] comparing Boer-crossed goats with non-Boer crosses found that the Boer crosses had significantly more parasite infestations. Only a small number of flock members contribute the greatest amount of environmental parasite contamination because susceptible animals shed the most eggs in their feces. Animals with the lowest EPG in a flock may be those that possess the most parasite resistance.[4] Salvage deworming programs should generally be avoided, but they may be used as aggressive selection criteria. That is, animals that do well with little or no deworming, particularly those grazing heavily contaminated pastures, should be identified and retained in the breeding flock. Those that become infected should be dewormed to salvage them or save their lives and then sold when possible. Proper record keeping and identification of all animals is paramount in selecting for parasite resistance.[2,14] This aggressive approach can yield excellent results if it is carefully implemented, but devastating losses can occur if it is poorly managed.

When introducing new animals to a flock, keepers should have biosecurity programs in place to limit the introduction of new or potentially anthelmintic-resistant parasites. New flock additions should be kept in a dry lot for 3 weeks and dewormed at least twice with two different classes of dewormers during this period. The effectiveness of the anthelmintic agent used should be determined by fecal examination before the animal is allowed contact with the rest of the flock.[2]

Other nontraditional chemical methods of parasite control are used by some owners. Some appear to be worthless (e.g., diatomaceous earth), but others (e.g., nematophagous fungi, herbal dewormers) may prove effective in some situations.

Cestode Infestation

Pathogenesis. The most common gastrointestinal tapeworm of sheep and goats seen in North America belongs to the genus *Moniezia*. Cestodes (tapeworms) are usually of more concern to owners than clinicians, who generally consider them only incidental low-grade pathogens, particularly in adult animals. Still, several 10- to 20-foot-long tapeworms can compete with the host for nutrients, hinder normal gut motility, and excrete some toxic wastes into the host's gastrointestinal tract. Mature tapeworm eggs are passed in the feces individually or protected in proglottides, which are usually visible to the owner. The eggs embryonate and infect a mite, a small pasture-living arthropod that serves as the intermediate host. A sheep or goat ingests the mite while grazing, allowing the tapeworm to complete its life cycle.

Clinical signs. Tapeworms may rarely cause disease in lambs and kids less than 6 months of age. Anecdotal reports suggest a cause-effect relationship between heavy tapeworm infestation and an increased incidence of *C. perfringens* enteritis, digestive disturbances (e.g., diarrhea, constipation), poor condition, and anemia. Ulceration at the site of attachment may be seen on necropsy. Rarely species of *Trypanosoma*, the fringed tapeworm, may cause liver condemnation.

Diagnosis and treatment. A presumptive diagnosis can be made by finding proglottides in the stool, eggs on direct smears, or eggs on fecal flotations (see Figure 4-10). Treatment with albendazole (15 mg/kg), fenbendazole (20 to 25 mg/kg), or praziquantel (10 to 15 mg/kg) may be effective either with a single treatment or with daily therapy (e.g., fenbendazole daily for 3 to 5 days). Because of the free-living nature of the arthropod intermediate host, animals are readily reinfected after treatment, which may give rise to the false assumption that the therapy was ineffective. Again, tapeworm infestation *may* result in disease, but often it is easier to blame the tapeworm segment seen in the stool as a cause of disease than to implicate the unseen thousands of HOTC complex parasites in the abomasum and small intestine of the animal.[3,14]

Johne's Disease

Johne's disease (also called *paratuberculosis*) is a chronic wasting and diarrheal disease caused by the bacteria *My-cobacterium avium* subspecies *paratuberculosis*. Transmission of the organism is primarily by the fecal-oral route. Young animals are more susceptible to infection than adults. It can be transmitted through milk and placenta.

Pathogenesis. Bacterial shedding in feces and milk and transplacental transmission is more common in animals showing clinical signs.[18-20] Therefore the offspring of infected animals and especially the offspring of animals showing clinical signs are most likely to acquire the infection. After an animal is exposed, it will either clear the organism or develop a chronic, persistent infection. The infection is most commonly isolated to the ileal regions of the small intestine, where it causes granulomatous thickening of the intestine and subsequent malabsorptive diarrhea. Infected animals may be asymptomatic for years.

Clinical signs. Morbidity rates are low (approximately 5%), but for every animal with clinical signs, several exist in the subclinical state, and may be a source of both horizontal and vertical transmission.[18] Both sheep and goats appear to remain asymptomatic until 2 to 7 years of age. The most consistent clinical sign in sheep and goats is chronic weight loss. Chronic diarrhea occurs in approximately 20% of cases.[18] Signs may appear with or be exacerbated by stress, especially after parturition.[18,19] Hypoproteinemia and chronic mild anemia are the only consistent clinicopathologic findings. Because of their low protein levels, infected animals can develop submandibular edema.

Diagnosis. Diagnosis is by culture of the organism from feces. Unfortunately, this testing takes between 8 and 14 weeks, but it can detect 40% to 60% of clinically infected goats. Sheep strains of Johne's disease and some goat variant strains seem to be more difficult to culture in media used to identify cattle strains of the disease. Therefore fecal culture in sheep and goats appears to be of limited benefit.[19,20] A relatively inexpensive and easily performed method of identifying approximately 50% of all clinically infected animals is acid-fast staining of fecal smears.[18,19] A PCR test of feces also is available, but its sensitivity is lower than that of fecal culture. Good diagnostic results can be obtained with serologic testing for antibodies (e.g., agar gel immunodiffusion [AGID], enzyme-linked immunospecific assay [ELISA], complement fixation) in animals showing clinical signs. The specificity of all the serologic tests is greater than 95% in sheep and goats with signs of clinical disease, although the sensitivity is not as high.[19-21] Therefore a positive serologic test in an animal showing clinical signs indicates that the animal has Johne's disease. However, the disease cannot be ruled out with a negative test. Sheep and goats appear to respond differently in regard to the formation of antibodies. Sheep tend to develop antibodies in the later stages of the disease, whereas antibodies may be detected much earlier in the goat. The AGID test appears to be the best serologic test currently available.[22,23] The ELISA and complement fixation tests can cross-react with *Corynebacterium pseudotuberculosis,* making them of limited value in flocks with caseous lymphadenitis infections.[19,24] Necropsy diagnosis is based on the finding of thickened, corrugated intestines, especially in the area of the ileum. Acid-fast staining of impression smears (taken from the ileum and ileocecal lymph nodes) can help yield a quick diagnosis. The staining of numerous clumps of acid-fast rods is highly suggestive of Johne's disease.

Prevention. Johne's disease has no effective treatment, so prevention and control are imperative. However, preventing the introduction of Johne's disease into a herd can be difficult. Because animals with subclinical infection may not shed the organism or may shed only small quantities of it, fecal culture is helpful only if a positive culture is obtained. The sensitivity of serologic tests of animals with subclinical disease is low and variable among flocks.[19,20] Negative test results in subclinically infected animals are common. However, the specificity of serologic tests remains high, and therefore a positive test is a valid reason to not purchase an animal.[19] Because Johne's disease also occurs in cattle, supplemental colostrum supplies should come only from dairy herds with no history of Johne's disease.

After Johne's disease is diagnosed in a herd, several control measures can be taken. Sanitation is important because the organism is highly resistant in the environment (able to survive more than 1 year under most conditions).[20] Reduced stocking rates, frequent cleaning of pens, and use of automatic waterers decrease fecal transmission. Keepers should cull the offspring of infected animals. Culling animals based on the results of AGID tests or fecal culture of the flock is recommended. Animals should be tested at least once a year. More frequent testing as resources allow speeds the identification of infected animals. A vaccine for cattle is only available in some locales and clinicians or keepers may require official permission to use it. Vaccine use does not eliminate infection, but it can decrease herd prevalence, delay the onset of clinical signs, and decrease cross-transmission by infective bacterial shedding in the feces.

REFERENCES

1. Smith BP: Alterations in alimentary and hepatic function. In Smith BP, editor: *Large animal internal medicine,* ed 2, St Louis, 1996, Mosby.
2. Pugh DG, Mobini SM, Hilton CD: Control programs for gastrointestinal nematodes in sheep and goats, *Comp Cont Ed Pract Vet* 20(4 suppl.):S112, 1998.
3. Craig TM: Epidemiology of internal parasites: effects of climate and host reproductive cycles on parasite survival, *Proceedings of the Small Ruminants for the Mixed Animal Practitioner, Western Veterinary Conference,* 1998, Las Vegas, NV.
4. Craig TM: Anthelmintic resistance: the selection and successful breeding of superior parasites, *Proceedings of the Small Ruminants for the Mixed Animal Practitioner, Western Veterinary Conference,* 1998, Las Vegas, NV.
5. Menzies P: Control and prevention of specific diseases of sheep and goats, *Proceedings of the Symposium on Health and Disease of Small Ruminants,* Nashville, TN, 1996, American Association of Small Ruminant Practitioners.
6. Herd RP: Control of periparturient rise in worm egg counts of lambing ewes, *J Am Vet Med Assoc* 182:375, 1983.
7. Bretzlaff K: Production medicine and health programs for goats. In Howard JL, editor: *Current veterinary therapy in food animal practice 2,* Philadelphia, 1986, WB Saunders.
8. Donaldson J: The effects of dietary protein on establishment and maturation of nematode populations in adult sheep. In Barrel GK, editor: *Sustainable control of internal parasites in ruminants,* Christchurch, UK, 1997, Lincoln University.
9. Herd RP: Nematode infections—cattle, sheep, goats, swine. In Howard JL, editor: *Current veterinary therapy in food animal practice 2,* Philadelphia, 1986, WB Saunders.
10. Miller JE: Parasites affecting goats in the Southeast, *Proceedings of Goat Production and Marketing Opportunities in the South,* 1995, Fort Valley, GA.
11. Uriarte J, Valderrabano J: Grazing management strategies for the control of parasitic diseases in intensive sheep production systems, *Vet Parasit* 37:342, 1990.
12. Smith MC, Sherman DM: *Goat medicine,* Philadelphia, 1994, Lea & Febiger.
13. Herd RP, Zajac AM: Helminth parasites of the gastrointestinal tract. Nematode infections in cattle, sheep, goats, and swine. In Howard JL, Smith RA, editors: *Current veterinary therapy 4,* Philadelphia, 1998, WB Saunders.
14. Pugh DG, Navarre CB: Parasite control programs in sheep and goats, *Vet Clin North Am: Food Anim Pract,* 17(2):, 2001.
15. Wescott RB, Foreyt WJ: Epidemiology and control of trematodes in small ruminants, *Vet Clin North Am: Food Anim Pract* 2:373, 1986.
16. Miller DK, Craig TM: Use of anthelmintic combinations against multiple resistant *Haemonchus contortus* in Angora goats, *Small Rum Res* 19:281, 1996.
17. Hollis A et al: Preliminary investigation of anthelmintic efficacy against GI nematodes of goats and susceptibility of goat kids to gastrointestinal nematode infection, *Proceedings of the ARD Symposium,* 2000, Fort Valley, GA.
18. Greig A: Johne's disease in sheep and goats, *In Pract* 22(3):146, 2000.
19. Smith MC: Paratuberculosis in small ruminants, *Proceedings of the Small Ruminants for the Mixed Animal Practitioner, Western Veterinary Conference,* 1998, Las Vegas, NV.
20. Stehman SM: Paratuberculosis in small ruminants, deer, and South American camelids, *Vet Clin North Am: Food Anim Pract* 12(2):441, 1996.
21. Clarke CJ et al: Comparison of the absorbed ELISA and agar gel immunodiffusion test with clinicopathologic findings in ovine clinical paratuberculosis, *Vet Rec* 139(29):618, 1996.
22. Thomas GW: Paratuberculosis in a large goat herd, *Vet Rec* 113(20):464, 1983.
23. Shulaw WP et al: Serodiagnosis of paratuberculosis in sheep by use of agar gel immunodiffusion, *Am J Vet Res* 54(1):13, 1993.
24. Pepin M, Marly J, Pardon P: *Corynebacterium pseudotuberculosis* infection in sheep and the complement fixation test for paratuberculosis, *Vet Rec* 120(10):236, 1987.

INTESTINAL OBSTRUCTION

Any cause of intestinal obstruction that occurs in other ruminants may occur in sheep and goats. Most of these diseases produce abdominal discomfort and occasionally abdominal distention. Diagnosis can be difficult because rectal palpation cannot be performed on small ruminants. Abdominal radiographs and ultrasonography may help differentiate these diseases, but exploratory surgery may be required to obtain a definitive diagnosis and select appropriate treatment.

Intussusception

Intussusception is more common in young animals, but it can occur in adults. It occurs when one segment of the intestine telescopes into an adjacent segment. Any portion of the intestine can intussuscept, but the ileum and ileocecal junction are the most common areas involved. When intussusception occurs, the lumen of the intestine narrows to the point of obstruction. The initiating cause is not always known.[1,2] It is associated with an intestinal mass in adults and enteritis in young animals.[1] *Oesophagostomum* infestations have been implicated as a cause in sheep.[1]

Clinical signs. The initial complaint is colic (manifested as kicking at the abdomen, repeated rising and lying down, and vocalization) followed by low-grade pain. True colic signs are variable in lambs and kids. In some cases, after the initial colic episode subsides, animals show no evidence of pain until the abdomen becomes distended. The time between the initial intussusception and abdominal distention depends on where the blockage occurs. Intussusception of the ileal area may take several days to cause bilaterally symmetric abdominal distention. Fecal output is scant, and what little there is may be dark or tarry, or may contain mucus. Dehydration becomes evident, hypochloremic metabolic alkalosis may develop and rumen chloride levels may increase with obstructions of the duodenum.

Diagnosis. Abdominocentesis may yield fluid compatible with a transudate (increased protein concentration and leukocyte numbers).[1] Radiography and ultrasonography reveal fluid-distended intestinal loops. Occasionally the intussusception itself can be visualized with ultrasonography or palpable through the abdominal wall. If the disease is not treated, intestinal rupture and peritonitis can occur.

Treatment. Surgical correction is required. If the intussusception is corrected early, the prognosis is good in the absence of peritonitis. Fluid support is needed to correct dehydration and metabolic abnormalities. Fluids should be administered IV until rumen function returns. Ringer's solution with added calcium (approximately 25 ml calcium borogluconate per liter) and potassium (10 to 20 mEq/L) is a good choice for fluid therapy.

Foreign Body Obstruction

Ingested foreign bodies or bezoars can obstruct portions of the intestines.[3,4] The signs are similar to those of obstruction caused by intussusception and depend on the part of the intestine that is blocked. In some cases the obstructing body can be seen with radiography or ultrasonography. Surgical removal is required for treatment.

Cecal Volvulus and Torsion of the Root of the Mesentery

Cecal volvulus and torsion of the root of the mesentery occur sporadically in sheep and goats.[1,3] Extreme abdominal pain, rapid abdominal distention, and circulatory collapse are typical signs. Immediate surgical correction and circulatory support are needed.

Intestinal Atresia

Atresia of the colon, rectum, and anus can all occur as congenital problems. The clinical sign of progressive abdominal distention usually is noted in the first week of life. Atresia of the anus can be diagnosed on physical examination, but atresia of the colon and rectum may require contrast radiography for a definitive diagnosis. Surgical establishment of anal patency can be performed for atresia ani. A permanent colostomy may be required for atresia of the colon and rectum. Atresia of the anus and rectum are considered heritable in cattle.[1] In the authors' experience, atresia ani is more common in sheep than in goats.

If surgical correction of atresia ani is attempted, the animal should be neutered or kept out of the breeding program because of the potential genetic basis for this condition. Occasionally a slight bulge in the skin may occur where the anus should be located, especially in male lambs. Ultrasonography can be used to locate a feces-filled rectum. For surgical correction, the clinician should locate the area where the anus should be, prepare it with sterile technique, and infiltrate it with a local anesthetic. The surgeon then makes a circumferential incision to remove the overlying skin covering the rectum. An alternative is to make an X-shaped incision into the rectum. Treated animals should be given mineral oil, DSS, or stool softeners as needed.

Intestinal Ileus

Ileus of the small intestine is a pseudo-obstruction that occurs when there is an absence of intestinal motility. The animal's failure to pass ingesta leads to signs similar to intussusception. The cause of ileus is usually unclear, but it often occurs secondary to systemic diseases. The same elements that cause rumen stasis may potentially result in intestinal stasis and ileus. Symptomatic treatment with NSAIDs for pain and inflammation and fluids for dehydration is usually curative.[1] However, if signs persist, surgical exploration is indicated to rule out true obstructive diseases.

Peritonitis

Pathogenesis.   Infection of the peritoneal lining of the abdominal cavity may lead to septic peritonitis. Common causes include uterine tears; rupture of the rumen or abomasum secondary to rumenitis, abomasitis, or abomasal ulcers; trocarization of the rumen for bloat; and rupture of the intestine secondary to obstruction.

Clinical signs.   Signs depend on the severity of the condition. Abdominal discomfort and distention, dehydration, injected mucous membranes, depression, and death can all occur in cases of peritonitis. The presence of a fever is variable, both heart rate and respiration rate are usually elevated, and respiratory effort may be guarded. Animals may be febrile early, but have a normal to low body temperature as the condition progresses.

Diagnosis.   Abdominal ultrasound can be useful in locating pockets of fluid for abdominocentesis, which usually yields fluid with increased protein concentration and leukocyte numbers. On occasion, intracellular bacteria are observed on cytologic examination. The presence of extracellular bacteria is not diagnostic because accidental enterocentesis can occur. Culture of abdominal fluid and subsequent antimicrobial sensitivity tests are indicated for the implementation of proper treatment. The causative organisms vary depending on the source of the bacteria. Rumen bacteria are typically gram-negative anaerobes, and *E. coli* and other enteric bacteria are common if the intestine is the source of infection. Exploratory surgery may be required to diagnose a gastrointestinal rupture. The CBC can be normal but often shows an inflammatory leukogram and, in severe cases, a degenerative left shift.

Treatment.   Treatment includes the prescription of appropriate antimicrobial agents, the administration of NSAIDs for pain and endotoxemia, and fluid support for dehydration. The prognosis is guarded, especially if an intestinal rupture has occurred.

Rectal Prolapse

Pathogenesis, clinical signs, and diagnosis.   Rectal prolapse is more common in sheep than in goats. This evagination of the rectal mucosa and rectal structures (and possibly the descending colon) is usually associated with excessive straining. Straining is seen in lambs with diarrhea caused by coccidiosis, *Salmonella*, or dietary imbalances, in ewes or ewe lambs with vaginal prolapse, in males with urolithiasis, and in animals grazing lush forage (particularly legumes such as alfalfa and clover). It also can occur secondary to chronic coughing, short tail docking, and the use of growth implants.[5-7] Rabies also can cause chronic straining and rectal prolapse.[5-9] Regardless of the cause, after the rectal mucosa becomes everted and exposed, irritation of the mucosa causes further straining, which exacerbates the problem. Venous drainage of the prolapse may be compromised, but the arterial supply usually remains intact and contributes to the swelling. Rectal prolapses are graded as Type I to IV, based on the portion of rectum and distal colon that is everted.[5] A description of these grades in shown in Table 4-4.

Treatment.   Correction may be cost prohibitive for feedlot lambs, and immediate slaughter is recommended. In more valuable animals, very mild, early cases can be treated with frequent application of hemorrhoidal ointment designed for humans and manual replacement of the prolapsed mucosa into the anus. The authors try to avoid applying purse-string sutures in the anus because they tend to serve as a nidus and result in further straining. However, if less aggressive therapies do not relieve the problem in 24 hours, a purse-string suture may become necessary, particularly in Type I and II prolapse. In all cases and modes of treatment, restricting feed for 24 to 48 hours and administering mineral oil is recommended. Dusty feedstuffs (concentrates, pellets, hay) should be avoided because they may contribute to coughing, which exacerbates this condition. Adding molasses to feeds and lightly wetting hay may help reduce problems with dust.

Purse-string suture is easily performed. The prolapsed tissue and perineal area are washed with mild soap and lubricated with petroleum jelly or hemorrhoidal ointment before the prolapse is replaced.[5,9] After replacing the prolapsed mucosa, the clinician inserts a tubular object (syringe case, wooden dowel, gloved finger) into the rectum. He or she then places a purse-string suture of nonabsorbable suture material (3-5 nylon) in the skin around the anus, tightens it around the tubular object, and ties it off. The suture should be placed around the anus using a cutting needle, and entering and exiting at the 12 o'clock position. Tying the knot above the anus ensures that less fecal soiling of the suture will occur. The clinician should tie the suture in a bow knot to allow easy identification over the next few days and then remove the tubular object. The suture should be tight enough to prevent prolapse but loose enough to allow feces to pass. The clinician should regularly reevaluate the animal and if possible loosen the purse-string suture at 24-hour intervals until no tension exists. After a full day of no

TABLE 4-4

GRADES OF RECTAL PROLAPSE

TYPE	DESCRIPTION	COMMENTS
Type I	Small, circular amount of submucosal swelling protrudes through anus; probing reveals a pocket or fornix just inside anus	Good prognosis if there is no damage to mucosa; purse-string suture, iodine injection, submucosal resection
Type II	Slightly more circular submucosal and mucosal swelling, possibly containing retroperitoneal rectal tissue from anus; probing reveals a pocket just inside anus	Good prognosis if treated quickly and no mucosal damage; purse-string suture, iodine injection, submucosal resection, rectal amputation
Type III	Complete prolapse containing part of the retroperitoneal structures of the rectum and the descending colon; probing reveals a fornix just inside anus; the affected portion of the descending colon does not prolapse through the anus	If there is vascular injury to the descending colon, prognosis is guarded to poor; submucosal resection or rectal amputation are the methods of choice
Type IV	The descending colon appears as a tube, and has intussuscepted through the rectum and anus; unlike the previous types, in this case a probe or finger can be inserted into the prolapse through the anal sphincter for a distance of 5 to 10 cm	If there is vascular injury to the descending colon, prognosis is poor; abdominal exploration may be required to determine the extent of damage to the descending colon

From Hooper RN: General surgical techniques for small ruminants: Part II, *Small Ruminants for the Mixed Animal Practitioner, Western Veterinary Conference*, 1998, Las Vegas, NV.

tension, the suture can be removed. If animals continue to strain, an epidural anesthetic can be administered. Petroleum jelly and hemorrhoid gels should be placed on the anus daily.[5,9]

The **injection of counterirritants** around the rectum (1 ml or less of Lugol's iodine) either alone or in conjunction with anal purse-string suturing is a quick and inexpensive treatment.[5,6,9] The clinician inserts an 18-gauge needle (5 cm) deeply into the skin around the anus at 12, 3, and 9 o'clock. An injection at the 6 o'clock position should be avoided because swelling around the urethra can result in obstruction.

For more severe cases, submucosal resection or rectal amputation of tissue may be necessary.[5,9] Rectal amputation can be performed with a prolapse ring or suture technique.[7] **Prolapse ring** usage is a salvage technique. The clinician inserts the prolapse ring into the rectum and places an elastrator band or suture around the area to be amputated to induce vascular compromise and necrosis of tissue. If a ligature is used, it should be tightened to allow purchase on the tube or ring. A fibrosis is induced just proximal to the band or suture, and mucosa subsequently grow across the areas.[5] Strictures, peritonitis, and abscesses are possible complications, but this technique may be useful as a field procedure.

Submucosal resection can be performed under epidural analgesia after the prolapse and the perineal area have been surgically prepared. The clinician places two spinal needles (9 to 10 cm) at 90-degree angles to each other 2 to 4 mm distal to the anal sphincter and through the entire prolapse.[5]

A circular incision is made 2 to 4 mm distal to the spinal needles through the mucosa and around the outside of the anus. Another circular incision is made just distal to the caudal extent of the prolapse into the point where the mucosa reflects on itself on the innerside of the prolapse. The clinician connects these two incisions with a longitudinal incision parallel to the prolapse and dissects the mucosa between the circumferential incisions.[5] The mucosal edges are then sutured with a simple interrupted pattern using a suitable absorbable suture material. After completely suturing the mucosal surfaces, the clinician removes the two spinal needles and places a purse-string suture in the anal sphincter. Placement of the suture and follow-up care are the same as described for the purse-string suture technique. Submucosal resection decreases the incidence of both peritonitis and stricture formation compared with other surgical techniques, but it is expensive.[5]

In all of these techniques, a caudal epidural anesthetic (2% lidocaine, 0.5 ml per 45 kg) is recommended to decrease straining and ease pain from the procedures.[6,7] A xylazine epidural (0.01 to 0.03 mg/kg as sufficient [QS] to 2 ml with 2% lidocaine) may give longer relief (approximately 4 to 6 hours) from straining than lidocaine. An alcohol epidural also may prevent straining for extended periods. Either isopropyl alcohol or ethanol can be used to demyelinate the motor and sensory nerves.[5] This type of anesthesia can be permanent and therefore should be used only for animals intended for slaughter. Because of the potential for some loss of sciatic nerve function, the clinician should perform a test injection of a local anesthetic (2% lidocaine) before using alcohol. If the epidural appears effective and no ataxia or muscle weakness of the rear limbs occurs, the clinician can inject a mixture of equal parts of lidocaine and alcohol into the sites where the test epidural was performed. Possible problems with alcohol epidural anesthesia include injection site necrosis, sciatic nerve dysfunction, and the inability to void feces.[5]

Regardless of the type of epidural used, the clinician clips, washes, and dries the area before placing a small needle (20- to 21-gauge [2.6 cm]) in the most cranial yet moveable intracaudal vertebral space—usually C1 to C2 or C2 to C3. The needle is placed on the dorsal midline, with the needle 90 degrees to the skin and the hub moved slightly caudal, and then slowly advanced.

*R*EFERENCES

1. Guard C: Obstructive intestinal diseases. In Smith BP, editor: *Large animal internal medicine,* ed 2, St Louis, 1996, Mosby.
2. Mitchell WC: Intussusception in goats, *Agri-Practice,* p 1918, Dec 1983.
3. Smith MC, Sherman DM: *Goat medicine,* Philadelphia, 1994, Lea & Febiger.
4. Sherman DM: Duodenal obstruction by a phytobezoar in a goat, *J Am Vet Med Assoc* 178:139, 1981.
5. Hooper RN: General surgical techniques for small ruminants: Part II, *Proceedings of the Small Ruminants for the Mixed Animal Practitioner, Western Veterinary Conference,* 1998, Las Vegas, NV.
6. Pipkin AB: Rectal prolapse in ruminants and horses. In Smith BP, editor: *Large animal internal medicine,* ed 2, St Louis, 1996, Mosby.
7. Kimberling CV: *Jensen and Swift's diseases of sheep,* ed 3, Philadelphia, 1988, Lea & Febiger.
8. Welker B, Modransky P: Rectal prolapse in food animals. Part 1: cause and conservative management, *Comp Cont Ed Pract Vet* 13:1869, 1991.
9. Welker B, Modransky P: Rectal prolapse in food animals. Part II: surgical options, *Comp Cont Ed Pract Vet* 14:554, 1992.

DISEASES OF THE LIVER

Liver Abscesses

Liver abscesses usually occur as a result of chronic rumenitis in cattle, but they are rare in sheep and goats. They can occur in feedlot lambs and kids and other animals fed rations high in grain. In lambs and kids, septicemia or extension of an umbilical vein infection can cause liver abscesses.[1] In most cases, however, liver abscesses are an incidental finding. Weight loss, anorexia, depression, and decreased production (growth, milk) may occur. In adults, *Corynebacterium pseudotuberculosis* is the most common cause. *Actinomyces pyogenes* and *Fusobacterium necrophorum* also are cultured from abscesses.[1-3]

Liver enzymes may or may not be elevated. Diagnostic ultrasonography of the liver may help detect abscesses, especially if they are numerous and widespread. However, no specific treatment or control measure is available. Many of the preventive protocols used for feeder cattle apply to the control of abscesses in sheep and goats. These include slowly introducing concentrates into the diet, offering long-stemmed hay free choice, and including rumen buffers (alkalinizing agents) and antimicrobial agents in the feed.

Pregnancy Toxemia/Fatty Liver Syndrome

Pathogenesis. Fatty liver occurs in conjunction with pregnancy toxemia in ewes and does during the last month of gestation. It is most common in thin or obese ewes or does with a single large fetus, twins, or triplets.[1] During late gestation, particularly in obese females, the abdominal space is filled with accumulated fat and an ever-expanding uterus. Because of the lack of rumen space, these females have difficulty consuming enough feedstuffs to satisfy energy requirements. In most management systems, late gestation occurs during the winter months, when less pasture is available and poorer-quality feedstuffs are offered. Energy requirements for ewes and does carrying twins or triplets is greatly increased during the final 2 months of gestation because 70% to 80% of fetal growth occurs during this time. Ewes with twins require 180% more energy, and those with triplets need 200% to 250% more dietary energy. Pregnancy toxemia also occurs in association with anorexia caused by other diseases (foot rot, OPP, CAE) or sudden stresses (feed or weather changes, predator attacks, hauling). Whatever the initiating cause, a period of anorexia and lack of sufficient energy intake result in a negative energy balance. These animals begin to mobilize body stores of fat and transport them to the liver. In the liver, fat is catabolized to glycerol and free fatty acids (FFAs). FFAs can be used in the citric acid cycle (Krebs cycle) as an energy source, but not in the direct formation of glucose. Anorexic animals have less ruminal substrate available for production of the glucose precursor propionic acid. However, oxaloacetate, which is an integral part of the citric acid cycle, is removed from the cycle and converted into glucose. Depletion of oxaloacetate inhibits the normal citric acid cycle's function, inhibiting the use of FFAs. As the pool of FFAs increases, they are converted to ketone bodies or repackaged into lipoproteins. Because ruminants are not efficient at transporting lipoproteins out of the liver and back to the adipose stores, the lipoproteins overwhelm the liver's ability to handle this massive buildup, resulting in a fatty liver. Because less substrate is available for glucose formation, more oxaloacetate is "cannibalized" from the citric acid cycle, further inhibiting the body's ability to use FFAs. This in turn causes the continued accumulation of ketone bodies. Hypoglycemia, hyperketonemia, and potentially uremia and death can occur.

Clinical signs. Animals suffering from fatty liver or pregnancy toxemia become anorexic and depressed, display altered behavior, and become recumbent. Some are constipated, grind their teeth, have a ketone smell to their breath, and suffer from dystocia. Neurologic signs include blindness, circling, incoordination, star-gazing, tremors, and convulsions.[4,5] Death can occur if the condition is left untreated. In the case of in-utero fetal death, maternal septicemia-endotoxemia and death are common sequelae.

Diagnosis. Diagnosis is based on clinical signs, the presence of multiple fetuses, and typical clinicopathologic findings. CBC results may be normal or show an eosinophilia, neutropenia, and lymphocytosis. These animals may or may not be hypoglycemic, but ketoacidosis, hypocalcemia, and hypokalemia are common.[2,4] Liver enzymes are usually within normal limits but occasionally may be increased. Azotemia, both from dehydration and secondary renal disease, is a common finding, and a fatal uremia may occur. Blood concentrations of ß-hydroxybutyric acid greater than 7 mmol/L are consistent with pregnancy toxemia. Urinalysis will be positive for both ketones and protein. Urine is collected from sheep by holding the nares and from does by frightening them and then allowing them a perceived escape when they stop, squat, and void. Although not commonly performed, liver biopsy can help determine the extent of fatty infiltration. This syndrome must be differentiated from hypocalcemia, hypomagnesemia, polioencephalomalacia, encephalitis, lead toxicity, and cerebral abscesses.

Treatment. Very early cases (before the animal exhibits recumbency) may be treated with oral or IV glucose. A balanced electrolyte solution with extra calcium (25 ml of a 23% calcium borogluconate per liter), potassium (10 to 20 mEq/L), and 5% dextrose is needed. In some cases, sodium bicarbonate is valuable in treating acidosis (see Appendix II). Energy intake must be increased, and propylene glycol can be administered (15 to 30 ml every 12 hours) as a glucose precursor. Rumen transfaunation and supplementation with vitamin B complex (including vitamin B_{12}, biotin, niacin, and thiamine) also are recommended. After females become recumbent, treatment must be very aggressive. Removal of the fetuses is crucial in these cases. Chemically inducing parturition (by administering 2.5 to 10 mg of prostaglandin $F_{2\alpha}$ or 0.75 μg/45 kg of cloprostenol in does and 15 to 20 mg of dexamethasone in ewes) and giving the ewe or doe medical support (fluids, B vitamins, glucose) while waiting is a useful protocol in some cases. Unfortunately, during the time before parturition, endotoxemia from dead fetuses further compromises the female. For this reason, the authors recommend immediate Cesarean section on depressed moribund animals (see Chapters 6 and 16). The owner should be forewarned of the poor prognosis for animals already in a moribund state. Fluid support during and after surgery is crucial.

Regardless of the therapeutic plan, the animal should be offered a palatable, energy-rich, highly digestible feedstuff. The keeper and clinician should take care to minimize the risk of a confounding disease during convalescence (e.g., lactic acidosis, polioencephalomalacia).

Prevention. Fatty liver and pregnancy toxemia can be prevented through proper nutrition. Maintaining animals in proper body condition throughout the year and making sure energy and protein levels are adequate in late gestation (see Chapter 2) are two key preventive measures.[2,4] The owner/manager should be taught to assess body condition in individual animals and should maintain emergency stores of feed in case of severe weather or natural disasters. The requirement for energy may be one and a half to two times maintenance for single fetuses and two to three times maintenance for multiple fetuses. Prevention of concurrent disease that may further increase energy demands or cause anorexia (e.g., intestinal parasitism, foot rot) is crucial. The keeper should take care to increase the grain portion of the diet slowly because anorexia from rumen upset can lead to this disease.[2] Ewes should be offered 0.5 to 1 kg of a cereal grain (corn, oats, barley, or a combination) every day during the final months of gestation; does can be offered ½ to 1 kg of grain. Keepers should maintain ewes and does at a body condition score of 2.5 to 3 (see Chapter 2) throughout gestation and evaluate the animals' energy every 2 to 4 weeks.

Ultrasonography can help identify females with multiple fetuses. These animals should be separated into groups and fed accordingly. Ultrasonographic determination of fetal numbers is best accomplished between days 45 and 90 after breeding with a 3.5 mHz transducer; a 5 mHz transducer produces better results between days 45 to 50. Either type of transducer may be of value and these windows of time may be expanded by the ability of the operator (see Chapter 6). Determination of fetal numbers may be enhanced by shearing the hair or fiber in front of the udder, applying a coupling substance to the skin, and viewing as much of the abdomen as possible, building a mental image of its structures and the number of fetuses while systematically moving from one side of the posterior abdomen to the other.

Keepers and clinicians should ensure that ewes are healthy and free of chronic diseases (e.g., OPP, CAE, foot rot, chronic parasitism) and that a good-quality trace mineral salt mixture is available free choice. The addition of lasalocid (0.5 to 1 mg/kg/day) or monensin (1 mg/kg/day) to the feed or mineral mixture enhances the formation of the glucose precursor propionic acid and improves the efficiency of feed use. However, monensin should be used with caution because toxicity may occur; the agent should comprise no more than 30 ppm of the complete diet. The inclusion of niacin (1 g/head/day) in a feed supplement or mineral mixture helps prevent pregnancy toxemia. Supplementation with lasalocid, monensin, or niacin should begin 2 to 4 weeks before the females give birth.

Shearing in the last trimester also is recommended in ewes.[5] Many sheep producers routinely clip the wool around the vulva. If complete body shearing is performed, the incidence of fatty liver or pregnancy toxemia may be decreased. Sheared sheep require less energy to walk and graze. Sheared ewes also tend to shiver on cold days, exercising the enzyme systems that promote the more efficient use of FFAs as energy substrate. These ewes tend to seek shelter during cold weather, which may decrease lamb losses resulting from hypothermia. Obviously, if ewes are to be shorn, keepers should make adequate shelter available.

Keepers should avoid hauling or moving females during late gestation. Proper predator control measures should be maintained. Good hoof care programs should be in place on farms or ranches where grazing is the predominant form of nutrient intake. Sheep and goats should have their teeth checked to ensure good dentition before the breeding season. Animals with poor teeth should be culled.

Measuring serum β-hydroxybutyric acid concentrations is useful in assessing energy status in ewes. Values of 0.8 to 1.6 mmol/L suggest a negative energy balance. Keepers should take steps to correct the problem by feeding better-quality, more digestible feedstuffs.

White Liver Disease

White liver disease is a form of fatty liver disease reported only in Angora and Angora-cross goats and sheep. It is associated with cobalt deficiency.

Pathogenesis.   Cobalt is needed by rumen microflora to produce cyanocobalamin, or vitamin B_{12}, which is a coenzyme for methylmalonyl-CoA mutase. In turn, this enzyme is needed to convert propionate to glucose through the Krebs cycle. Cobalt deficiency leads to the accumulation of methylmalonyl-CoA, or methylmalonic acid, which is converted to branched chain fatty acids that accumulate in the liver.[2,6] High-grain diets that are fermented to propionate coupled with deficient or marginal cobalt intake may predispose to this condition.[2,6] White liver disease has not been reported in the United States, but ill thrift from cobalt deficiency has been observed. It is therefore possible that the disease goes unrecognized.[1]

Clinical signs.   Signs are most commonly seen in young animals, and include ill thrift, anorexia, and diar-

rhea; sheep may exhibit photosensitization. Clinicopathologic findings include a macrocytic, normochromic anemia and hypoproteinemia.[1,2]

Diagnosis.   Abnormal serum or liver concentrations of vitamin B_{12} or liver cobalt are the basis of diagnosis. Liver cobalt concentrations on a dry matter basis of 0.08 ± 0.02 ppm were reported in goats with white liver disease, compared with 0.53 ± 0.11 ppm in controls.[6]

Treatment and prevention.   Sheep can be treated with oral cobalt (1 mg/head/day) or vitamin B_{12} injections. The condition can be prevented by including cobalt in the ration by feeding a good-quality trace mineral salt.[2]

Liver Flukes

Both *Fasciola hepatica* and *Fascioloides magna* can infest sheep and goats. The disease occurs along the Gulf Coast and in the Pacific Northwest and Great Lakes areas.

Pathogenesis.   The life cycles of *F. hepatica* and *F. magna* are similar in that each requires an aquatic snail as an intermediate host. Fluke eggs that are passed in animal stool hatch in water to form miracidia, which penetrate the intermediate host. The miracidia develop through several intermediate hosts to form cercariae, which emerge from the intermediate hosts to encyst as infective metacercariae on forage. Sheep or goats accidentally ingest the metacercariae, which then encyst in the small intestine. They can migrate into the liver in approximately 6 weeks and may begin to lay eggs within 3 months after infection. *F. hepatica* is capable of laying eggs in sheep for several years. The flukes also can migrate into the bile ducts or through hepatic tissue, leaving large anaerobic tracts and producing acute or chronic disease.[7] Sheep and goats are definitive hosts for *F. hepatica*, whereas only some species of deer and elk are definitive hosts for *F. magna*. *F. magna*, unlike *F. hepatica*, never matures and continues to migrate, causing severe damage and death.[7,8] *F. magna* does not complete its life cycle in sheep or goats. The most serious complication of acute liver fluke infestation is black disease *(Clostridium novyi)*, which presents as sudden death.

Clinical signs.   *F. hepatica* infestation usually causes acute disease in sheep and goats but can present as a chronic condition. Chronic disease is the result of the mature flukes in the bile ducts and is manifested in depressed growth and milk production. Acute disease occurs when large numbers of immature flukes migrate at once, particularly in animals with limited immunity to flukes. Signs include anorexia, depression, weakness, dyspnea, anemia, ascites, colic-like signs, dry feces, and sudden death. The clinical signs are identical to those of nematode infestations (i.e., chronic weight loss, ill thrift, diarrhea, anemia, hypoproteinemia). Similar but more severe signs occur with *F. magna* infection, which is usually fatal.[2,5,8]

Diagnosis. Antemortem diagnosis of fluke infestation can be difficult. Finding eggs in feces is diagnostic for *F. hepatica*. Eggs are only produced by adults and not in great numbers, so a negative fecal test cannot preclude acute or chronic fascioliasis. Fluke eggs do not float in routine fecal flotation methods used for nematode diagnosis; a sedimentation technique should be used for suspected fluke infestations. To perform a sedimentation test, the clinician mixes 2 to 3 g of feces with 200 ml of tap water and strains the mixture through a tea strainer into a beaker. The sediment can be examined 15 minutes later under a dissecting microscope. Eggs are light yellow to golden and have an operculum at one end (see Figure 4-10). *F. magna* does not mature, so eggs are not produced and fecal examination is of no value. Most fluke infestations are discovered by finding the flukes at necropsy or slaughter. An ELISA test may be available in the future.[2,5,8] CBCs of affected animals may indicate eosinophilia and anemia. Increased liver enzymes and hypoalbuminemia also are occasional findings.

Treatment. Because antemortem diagnosis is difficult, the clinician should institute fluke treatment after ruling out other differential diagnoses if the possibility of fascioliasis exists. If fascioliasis is diagnosed at necropsy, the remaining animals in the herd should be treated. Because flukicides available in the United States are highly effective only against mature flukes, the timing of treatment is important. In the southern portions of North America the snails are ingested in the spring and the flukes migrate in the summer and mature in the fall. In cooler, northern climates, snails may remain active during summer, so flukes can mature in the fall and into the winter. Clinicians should begin treatment in the southern United States in the late summer or early fall. A single treatment in late winter or early spring is commonly used in the northern climates of North America. Albendazole (15-20 mg/kg orally) and clorsulon (7 mg/kg orally, 2 mg/kg SC) are very effective against adult *F. hepatica*.[2,9,10] Clorsulon has no efficacy against nematode parasites but is highly efficacious against both adult and late-stage immature flukes. Albendazole (15 mg/kg orally) is somewhat useful in controlling *F. magna* at 8 weeks after infestation, and clorsulon is effective only at very high dosages.[11-13] Unfortunately, neither agent can kill 100% of *F. magna*, and only a few remaining flukes can be fatal.

Prevention. Control of fluke infestations is difficult, although timely treatment of animals can decrease infections in successive years. Decreasing exposure is the key to control. Eliminating the snail is impractical, but fencing off low-lying areas may prevent ingestion. Depending on local fluke life cycles, keepers should avoid grazing animals on areas with high fluke populations during peak infection times. Areas where water stands or flows over grazing pastures, streams, and irrigation ditches (particularly those with clay soil) are high-risk zones.

Cysticercosis

Cysticercus tenuicollis is the larval stage of the dog tapeworm *Taenia hydatigena*, of which sheep and goats are intermediate hosts. The larval stage migrates through the liver, then attaches to the liver or other abdominal organs and causes black, winding tracts and cysts in the liver. Acute disease occurs only with large numbers of cysticerci and is characterized by depression and weakness resulting from liver damage. The chronic cystic stage is usually asymptomatic. No treatment is available and control is problematic because it requires treating infestation in dogs and preventing contact with dogs.[1,2,5]

Copper Toxicosis

Pathogenesis. Copper (Cu) toxicosis is more common in sheep than in goats. Goats appear closer to cattle than sheep in their ability to store and handle Cu and resist toxicosis. Toxicity results from chronic accumulation in the liver from the ingestion of excess Cu in relation to molybdenum (Mo) or sulfate in the diet. In sheep, a Cu-to-Mo ratio greater than 10:1 leads to the accumulation of excess Cu. The most common sources of excess Cu in sheep and goats are trace mineral mixtures and feeds formulated for cattle or horses. Clinical signs are often absent during the chronic accumulation phase. Acute disease is seen when Cu is suddenly released from the liver in large amounts. Stress usually precipitates this acute phase. Acute release and subsequent high blood Cu concentrations cause an acute hemolytic crisis, resulting in anemia, hemoglobinuria, and acute renal failure. Existing hepatic disease (such as that caused by liver flukes) may predispose animals to this condition. Some breeds seem to be prone to Cu absorption and storage problems (Merino sheep), whereas others tend to be more resistant and prone to deficiency (pygmy goats) (see Chapters 2 and 3).

Clinical signs. Anorexia, depression, diarrhea, and weakness are all signs of Cu toxicity. Many affected animals are found dead with hemolysis and icterus. Signs of abdominal pain and diarrhea are sometimes present. Port wine–colored urine is evidence of hemoglobinuria. Hemoglobinemia produces icterus of the mucosal membranes and fever.

Diagnosis.   On clinicopathologic examination, anemia, hemoglobinemia, hyperbilirubinemia, increased liver enzymes, and azotemia are present. Urinalysis reveals hemoglobinuria and isosthenuria. The combination of azotemia and isosthenuria indicates acute renal failure. Definitive diagnosis of acute disease requires measurement of Cu concentrations in serum. Normal blood Cu concentrations are approximately 50 to 200 μg/dl in sheep and goats.[2,5,14] These concentrations increase 10- to 20-fold with an acute hemolytic crisis.[5] On necropsy, kidney Cu concentrations are the most diagnostic because liver concentrations may be normal from release into the bloodstream. Generally kidney concentrations greater than 100 ppm and liver concentrations greater than 350 ppm on a dry matter basis are diagnostic.[2,5] If tissue copper is reported in wet weight, the conversion to dry tissue weight can be estimated by multiplying the tissue concentration by a factor of 3.5

Treatment.   Treatment of acutely affected animals is often futile. It consists of supportive therapy for the acute renal failure and anemia and attempts to lower liver Cu stores. Fluid therapy for the acute renal failure (see Appendix II) is of therapeutic value, and a blood transfusion may be needed if the PCV drops precipitously. Ammonium tetrathiomolybdate (1.7 mg/kg IV or 3.4 mg/kg SC on alternate days for three treatments) is the most economical agent for treatment for acute cases. In valuable animals, D-penicillamine (26 to 50 mg/kg BID or 52 mg/kg SID PO for 6 days) increases urinary Cu excretion. Trientine is used in human beings, but has shown variable results in sheep.[15] Treatment of the remainder of the flock should include the administration of ammonium molybdate (50 to 500 mg/head/day PO) and sodium thiosulfate (300 to 1000 mg/head/day PO) for 3 weeks.[15] Stress should be minimized, so keepers and clinicians should delay routine maintenance procedures such as deworming and hoof trimming until after treatment. The offending source of Cu should be eliminated.

Prevention.   Avoiding high dietary Cu (more than 10 ppm), a high Cu-to-Mo ratio (greater than 10:1) in the feed, Cu-containing foot baths, and other sources of Cu is crucial. Including supplemental Mo in the diet to lower the Cu-to-Mo ratio to 6:1 to 8:1 is beneficial. This requires 2 to 6 ppm of Mo in many instances. Often too much emphasis is placed on the trace mineral component of the diet. The clinician should be aware that even if no Cu is added to the trace mineral mixture and the element does not appear on the product label, the mineral mixture may still contain Cu. Many components of mineral mixes are contaminated with Cu (zinc sulfate may contain 400 ppm of Cu, dicalcium phosphate may contain more than 30 ppm of Cu). Therefore the clinician needs to perform a dietary analysis to find and correct the problem.

Toxic Hepatitis

Pathogenesis.   The liver is vulnerable to toxic insult because one of its major functions is detoxification. The most common plants that are gastrointestinal and liver toxins are shown in Table 4-5. Clinical signs depend on the cause. Acute, severe toxicity is more common with chemical toxicosis, whereas plant toxins usually cause chronic disease. A thorough history is important and in many cases inspection of the animals' environment is required.

Clinical signs.   The clinical signs of toxic hepatitis can be vague. Animals may only show anorexia and depression. Icterus is more common with hemolytic diseases and is not always seen with liver disease. Photosensitivity is a common clinical feature in ruminants and hepatoencephalopathy also can occur.

Diagnosis.   Clinicopathologic data are more helpful in diagnosing acute toxicity. Serum AST and LDH levels can increase with hepatocellular necrosis but are not liver-specific, so muscle injury and disease must be ruled out. These enzymes also increase if serum is not separated from a blood clot in a timely fashion.[1] Increased levels of alkaline phosphatase (AP) and GGT indicate biliary stasis. AP also is not liver-specific, but increased serum levels of GGT are very specific for liver disease. GGT also increases in some hepatocellular diseases, so testing for its normal concentrations is important.[15] Unfortunately, all of these enzymes can be normal with liver disease, especially if it is chronic. Hyperbilirubinemia, hypoglycemia, low blood urea nitrogen (BUN), and hypoalbuminemia are not always evident as classically taught. If hepatoencephalopathy is suspected, blood ammonia concentrations may be elevated. Blood ammonia analysis may be impractical in the field because the blood should be kept on ice, and the test should be performed within 30 minutes of collection. To enhance the accuracy of blood ammonia analysis, the clinician should collect blood from a normal control animal for comparison. Ammonia concentrations three times those of the control animal are diagnostic.[16] Liver biopsy remains the most valuable tool in diagnosing liver disease. Although clotting dysfunction may occur in liver disease, it is an uncommon complication in ruminants and should not discourage the clinician from performing a liver biopsy.

Treatment.   If the intoxication is caught in the acute stage, activated charcoal (500 g per adult animal) can be given. Supportive care, especially fluid support with dextrose solutions, is the mainstay of therapy. Low-protein diets may suppress ammonia production temporarily, but they can be detrimental over time depending on the production status of the animal. If photosensitization occurs, animals should be housed indoors if possible, and broad-

TABLE 4-5

PLANTS CAUSING GASTROINTESTINAL OR HEPATIC DISEASE

PLANT	COMMENTS	SIGNS
Cocklebur	Erect annual herbage in sandy soils, flood plains, and overgrazed pastures; seeds are toxic	Within hours to days of ingestion—anorexia, vomiting, colic, dyspnea, gastroenteritis, chronic hepatitis, hepatic damage, death
Senico-groundsel, Crotalaria, heliotropism, amsinckia (fiddleneck), echium	Pyrrolizidine alkaloid; excreted in milk and urine and can cross placenta; young more susceptible	Dullness, weakness, weight loss, icterus, fibrosis, hepatocytomegaly, bile duct proliferation, photosensitivity; subcutaneous edema, diarrhea
Lantana	Found in sandy, tropical areas; berries, leaves, and hay are toxic	Chronic toxicity—slow hepatic failure; icterus, photosensitization, weakness, bloody diarrhea, cholestasis, hepatic toxicity
Sneezeweed, bitterweed, rubberweed	Grows in overgrazed pastures; all parts of plant are toxic	Acute toxicity—gastrointestinal upset, depression, serous nasal discharge, salivation, bloat; chronic toxicity—vomiting, bittermilk lesions, hepatic and renal congestion, gastric edema, aspiration pneumonia; pulmonary edema
Cabbage, kale, rape, mustard, wild mushroom	Remove from diet; add iodine to diet (for goiter)	Gastroenteritis, hepatic necrosis, photosensitization, goiter, hemolysis
Horsebrush	Stop grazing, keep animals indoors	Bighead, itching, uneasiness, inflamed eyes, blindness, serum discharge from scabs; degenerative changes in liver and elevated liver enzymes
Clover (crimson, red, subterranean burclover)		Photosensitization
St. John's wort	Perennial herb; grows along roadsides and in overgrazed fields; remove from diet and keep animals in shade	Increased respiration, diarrhea, pruritus, dermatitis, diarrhea, death

spectrum (systemic or topical) antibiotics may be necessary to control secondary bacterial dermatitis. Corticosteroids (dexamethasone 0.1 to 1 mg/kg IV or IM) may be indicated in early cases of photosensitization to decrease inflammation. Neurologic signs can be controlled with phenobarbital (initial dose: 10 to 20 mg/kg IV diluted in saline and administered over 30 minutes; subsequent doses: 1 to 9 mg/kg IV diluted in saline, as needed up to TID). Diazepam (Valium) is contraindicated in hepatoencephalopathy because it may worsen signs.[17]

Miscellaneous Liver Diseases

Congenital hyperbilirubinemia, or black liver disease, occurs in mutant Corriedale sheep (Dublin-Johnson syndrome).[1] This is a genetically recessive condition. It is characterized by an abnormality in the excretion of conjugated bilirubin and phylloerythrin and is often seen in animals consuming green forage. Clinical signs include anorexia, photodermatitis, and icterus. Liver biopsy of affected animals reveals dark to black granules in otherwise normal hepatocytes. The syndrome first manifests itself in lambs around 5 months of age.[18]

A similar condition occurs in Southdown lambs around 6 months of age (Gilbert's syndrome). This too is a recessive condition that causes decreased hepatic uptake of phylloerythrin and bilirubin, with concurrent renal failure.[18] Signs include icterus, photodermatitis, and ulceration around the ears and mouth. A liver biopsy reveals normal hepatic tissue. In both of these conditions, animals should be kept out of sunlight and fed minimal

TABLE 4-5

PLANTS CAUSING GASTROINTESTINAL OR HEPATIC DISEASE—cont'd

PLANT	COMMENTS	SIGNS
Blue-green algae	Toxic after a bloom	Vomiting, diarrhea, liver failure, photosensitization; necropsy findings include swollen bloody liver, edema around gallbladder, centrolumbar apoptosis, and necrosis
Pokeweed		Vomiting, cramps, diarrhea, weakness, dyspnea, prostration, tremors, convulsions
Gossypol (cottonseed)	Toxicity seen in younger pre-ruminants	Poor performance, convulsions, cardiac toxicity
Rhubarb	Contains oxalic acid	Gastrointestinal toxicity
Oak	Acorns and oak buds are most toxic	Abdominal pain, pseudomembranes in gastrointestinal tract, bloody diarrhea, depression, renal toxicity
Castor bean	Beans most toxic	Gastrointestinal irritation, bloody diarrhea, central nervous system disturbances
Mistletoe	Berries not toxic	Nausea, diarrhea
Others:		
English ivy		
Sesbania		
Narcissus		
Elderberry		
Spurge		
Buckwheat		
St. Anne's lace		
Milkweed		
Parsley, giant hogweed		

amounts of green forage. Obviously, affected animals should be neutered or culled.

Various tumors of the liver, including fibrosarcoma, lymphosarcoma, and cholangiocellular carcinoma, have been reported.[17,18] The use of ultrasonography and ultrasound-guided liver biopsy may aid in diagnosis.

REFERENCES

1. Fetcher A: Liver diseases of sheep and goats, *Vet Clin North Am: Large Anim Pract* 5:525, 1983.
2. Smith MC, Sherman DM: *Goat medicine,* Philadelphia, 1994, Lea & Febiger.
3. Santa Rosa J et al: A retrospective study of hepatic abscesses in goats: pathological and microbiological findings, *Br Vet J* 145(1):73, 1989.
4. Parson EG, Maas J: Hepatic lipidosis. In Smith BP, editor: *Large animal internal medicine,* ed 2, St Louis, 1996, Mosby.
5. Kimberling CV: *Jensen and Swift's diseases of sheep,* ed 3, Philadelphia, 1988, Lea & Febiger.
6. Johnson EH et al: Hepatic lipidosis associated with cobalt deficiency in Omani goats, *Vet Res Commun* 23(4):215, 1999.
7. Craig TM: Epidemiology of internal parasites: effects of climate and host reproductive cycle on parasite survival, *Proceedings of the Small Ruminants for the Mixed Animal Practitioner, Western Veterinary Conference,* 1998, Las Vegas, NV.
8. Wescott RB, Foreyt WJ: Epidemiology and control of trematodes in small ruminants, *Vet Clin North Am: Food Anim Pract* 2:373, 1986.
9. Foreyt WJ: Efficacy and safety of albendazole against experimentally induced *Fasciola hepatica* infections in goats, *Vet Parasit* 26(1-2):261, 1988.
10. Rehbein S, Visser S: Efficacy of an injectable ivermectin/clorsulon combination against *Fasciola hepatica* in sheep, *Vet Rec* 145(16):468, 1999.

11. Foreyt WJ, Foreyt KM: Albendazole treatment of experimentally induced *Fascioloides magna* infection in goats, *Agri-Practice*, p 1441, Sept 1980.

12. Conboy GA, Stromberg BE, Schlotthauer JC: Efficacy of clorsulon against *Fascioloides magna* infection in sheep, *J Am Vet Med Assoc* 192(7):910, 1988.

13. Foreyt WJ: Evaluation of clorsulon against *Fascioloides magna* in cattle and sheep, *Am J Vet Res* 49(7):1004, 1988.

14. Kaneko JJ: *Clinical biochemistry of domestic animals*, ed 4, San Diego, CA, 1989, Academic Press.

15. Plumlee KH: Metals and other inorganic compounds. In Smith BP, editor: *Large animal internal medicine*, St Louis, 1996, Mosby.

16. Roussel AJ, Whitney MS, Cole DJ: Interpreting a bovine serum chemistry profile: Part I, *Vet Med*, 92:553, 1997.

17. Divers TJ: Therapy of liver failure. In Smith BP, editor: *Large animal internal medicine*, St Louis, 1996, Mosby.

18. Ogilvie TH: *Large animal internal medicine*, Baltimore, 1998, Williams & Wilkins.

PATHOLOGY OF THE UMBILICUS

Umbilical Hernia

The umbilicus is an opening in the ventral abdominal wall that allows passage of the umbilical vessels and allantoic stalks. This opening should close within a few day of birth. The failure of this opening to close properly is termed *umbilical hernia*. The hernial sac has an inner peritoneal layer and an outer layer of skin. These hernias are probably of genetic origin but may occur as sequelae to umbilical remnant infection. The opening in the abdominal wall is perceived as a ring on palpation. If the clinician can insert more than one finger into the hernial ring or if the hernia persists for more than 3 to 4 weeks, surgical intervention is indicated.

Penning. Clamps or rubber bands may be of value for closing small hernias (those less than 4 cm in diameter). The clinician should either lightly sedate the animal or infiltrate the skin around the hernia with a local anesthetic (2% lidocaine). The animal should be placed on its back and held by a technician-helper. Any viscera prolapsing into the hernial sac should be replaced into the abdomen. The clinician then inserts two metal pins (baby diaper pins can be used) through the skin and on opposite sides of the hernial ring, just on the edge of the linea alba. The pins should be placed deep enough to sit next to the abdominal wall. Slight tension is placed on the skin in the center of the umbilical sac, pulling it away from the abdomen. When the clinician is confident that all viscera have been cleared from the hernial sac, he or she places an elastrator band between the pins and the abdominal wall. This results in ischemic necrosis of the skin. The skin will slough and the abdominal defect will heal in 7 to 14 days. Lambs should be given tetanus prophylaxis. This procedure and other clamping techniques are useful in females and some males. However, urine scalding of the skin may occur in some males. Clinicians should closely monitor animals that have undergone clamping.

Surgical resection. In cases in which the hernial ring is larger than 5 cm, surgical intervention should be carried out. Animals can be sedated and then infiltrated with a local anesthetic or placed under general anesthesia. The area around the hernia is clipped and surgically prepared. The clinician opens the hernial sac and introduces a finger into the abdomen to ensure that no viscera have adhered to the inner lining of the ring and that no enlarged or infected umbilical remnants are present. He or she then carefully excises the ring and closes the defect in the abdominal wall. This closure can be made by simply opposing the abdominal wall with a horizontal mattress pattern stitch (absorbable suture). An alternate closure of the abdominal wall is to suture the peritoneal lining in a separate pattern and close the abdominal wall defect so one side of the defect is pulled to overlap the other side. The upper free edge is sutured to the opposite wall with a near-far-far-near pattern. The authors choose not to employ surgical techniques that slow this procedure. The subcutaneous tissue can be closed with simple interrupted pattern using absorbable suture and the skin should be closed with whatever pattern the clinician prefers. Animals should be given tetanus prophylaxis and antibiotics. They should be closely monitored for signs of sepsis and surgical failure. Exercise should be limited for 7 to 14 days after surgery.

Umbilical Infections

Infections of the umbilical arteries (omphaloarteritis) and veins (omphalophlebitis) and urachal disease can occur because of failure or partial failure of passive transfer of colostral antibodies and subsequent sepsis. Contamination of the umbilicus, retracting of these structures after stretching and breaking, and chemical damage (from strong tincture of iodine) to the amniotic remnants are other possible causes.[1,2,3] Dipping the umbilicus with iodine or iodine-chloriodine substances is a common practice. Aggressive use of these chemicals may precipitate serious inflammation of the cord. Excessive torsion of the umbilical cord, distention of the proximal urachus, and some genetic factors may all be associated with patent urachus, which also may occur as a sequela to omphaloarteritis or omphalophlebitis.

Clinical signs and diagnosis. The clinical signs include umbilical swelling, pain, and occasionally drainage or discharge of the umbilical stump. Palpation and transabdominal ultrasonographic evaluation reveal an enlarged cord-like structure ascending from the umbilicus cranially (umbilical vein) or caudally (urachus or umbilical artery). Ultrasonographic evaluation may indicate an abscess or thickened tissue. Patent urachus is associated with dermatitis, urine scalding of the ventral abdomen, and urine dribbling. If the urachus becomes infected it may leak urine intraperitoneally or subcutaneously. Both of these developments may be identified with abdominal palpation, ballottement, ultrasonographic evaluation, and, when indicated, paracentesis.[1] The CBC may indicate neutrophilia. Blood culture is indicated if sepsis occurs simultaneously. Occasionally infection of the internal structures may occur with no outward umbilical swelling. Deep abdominal palpation and/or the use of real-time ultrasound are necessary to attain a diagnosis. Animals with umbilical infections also may have signs of septicemia, anorexia, depression, joint distention, and fever.

Treatment.   If a patent urachus occurs without inflammation of the associated tissues, it can be cauterized daily with iodine or silver nitrate. However, if it remains patent for more than 5 days, it should be surgically closed. The animal should be placed under general anesthesia (see Chapter 16). The area around the umbilicus should be clipped and surgically prepared, and the animal should be placed on a broad-spectrum antimicrobial agent 2 to 4 hours before surgery. The clinician opens the abdomen lateral to the umbilicus and digitally explores the adjacent area for adhesion formation. The urachus should be identified and followed to the urinary bladder. After this, the clinician should amputate the urachal attachment to the bladder and close the bladder with a double-layered inverting pattern (Cushing). The abdominal wall, subcutaneous tissue, and skin are closed as described for umbilical hernia repair.

On occasion some cases of omphalophlebitis-omphaloarteritis can be treated medically. Prolonged antibiotic therapy with a broad-spectrum antimicrobial agent (ceftiofur 2.2 mg/kg SID or oxytetracycline 20 mg/kg SC every 72 hours) may be attempted. However, if medical therapy is ineffective, the infected umbilical remnants should be marsupialized or excised. The authors prefer more aggressive, surgical removal of the umbilical remnants. As with urachal surgery, the abdomen should be opened lateral to the umbilicus. Depending on the severity of infection and the amount of tissue involved, the clinician may need to perform extensive dissection of necrotic tissue and possibly intestinal resection.[3]

If the infection of the umbilical vein extends to and involves the liver, marsupialization of the umbilical vein is an effective method of therapy.[2,3] The clinician can pull the vein to the most cranial portion of the abdominal incision and suture it to the muscle layers and skin before closing the abdomen as described for umbilical hernia repair. However, a preferable method is to close the abdominal wall, pull the transected umbilical vein through, and suture it to a separate stab incision. This may help minimize the incidence of abdominal wall herniation. Only monofilament, absorbable, non-gut suture material should be used.[3] The venous stump should be flushed daily with antiseptic solution (1% chlorhexidine, 0.1% povidone iodine), and the animal should be maintained on antibiotics for more than 14 days. The venous stump usually closes within a month.[3]

Prevention.   Umbilical infections can be prevented or drastically reduced by ensuring adequate intake of good-quality colostrum. Lambs and kids also should be only minimally stressed (particularly during the first 2 to 3 days of life) to enhance colostral absorption. In some management scenarios, proper dipping of the navel with non-caustic materials also helps reduce the incidence of this disease.

REFERENCES

1. Lofstedt J: Neonatal conditions, with emphasis on equine neonate. In Ogilvie TM, editor: *Large animal internal medicine,* Baltimore, 1998, Williams & Wilkins.
2. Rings DM: Umbilical hernia, umbilical abscess, and auricle fistula, *Vet Clin North Am: Food Anim Pract* 11:137, 1995.
3. Hooper RN: General surgical techniques for small ruminants: Part II, *Proceedings of the Small Ruminants for the Mixed Animal Practitioner, Western Veterinary Conference,* 1998, Las Vegas, NV.

Chapter 5

Diseases of the Respiratory System

ELLEN B. BELKNAP

EVALUATION OF THE RESPIRATORY SYSTEM

History

While watching and assessing the patient, the clinician should obtain a thorough history, including the duration of any problems, exposure to other animals, recent movement, previous vaccinations and treatments, responses to treatment,[1] and number of animals affected. Given appropriate attention, the history alone may pinpoint the diagnosis.[2,3]

Physical Examination

Watching the animal from a distance is crucial to evaluating the respiratory system as part of the physical examination. The animal's attitude and appearance give clues to its health. The clinician can make a more accurate assessment of the animal's resting respiratory rates and better evaluate the breathing pattern by observing from a distance. A clinician may note stridor (inspiratory dyspnea) before even seeing the animal, whereas an exaggerated expiratory effort may imply lower respiratory disease. Any nasal discharge should be noted. The clinician should observe other animals in the herd to assess whether any others are displaying clinical signs of disease, respiratory or otherwise. Close attention should be given to the inspection of the nose, oral cavity, nasal cavity and sinuses, larynx, trachea, and thorax. Observation, palpation, percussion, and auscultation all may be employed in this inspection.

Auscultation

Sheep and goats have 13 ribs, which are used by clinicians to define the lung borders. That is, the cranial ventral border is found at the sixth rib, the middle of the thorax is at the seventh rib, and the caudal border is at the eleventh rib. Auscultation is much easier in goats than in sheep, but by taking the time to part the wool for greater contact, a skilled clinician can achieve good auscultation in both species. Eliminating as much excess noise in the barn as possible produces better results with this diagnostic tool. Normal breath sounds are loudest over the trachea and base of the lung, but upper respiratory conditions often result in more abnormal sounds in the trachea. In addition, abnormal sounds may be referred from disease within the thorax. However, by localizing the site of maximal loudness, the clinician can assign the origin of the abnormal noise to the upper or lower respiratory tract. Normal breath sounds are loudest on inspiration because it is an active process compared with passive expiration. Abnormal sounds include *crackles*, which are caused by the opening of closed airways, and *wheezes*, which are whistling, squeaking sounds caused by the vibration of airway walls or narrowed airways with air going through them.[4,5] The clinician should perform deep palpation over the trachea to assess whether a cough can be elicited and characterized. The thorax also may be percussed, although this is more difficult in sheep than in goats. Pleural friction sounds, which are caused by the rubbing of altered pleural surfaces, may occur during both inspiration and expiration, but they are rarely auscultated.

Diagnostics

Complete blood count. A complete blood count (CBC) with a fibrinogen concentration may be useful in evaluating the type of disease process and the severity of inflammation. Sheep and goats typically do not experience dramatic increases in white blood cell counts during bacterial infections, but counts greater than 20,000 cells/μl are usually significant. During acute inflammatory or infectious processes, a left shift of neutrophils may be observed; such a shift is classified as *regenerative* when mature neutrophilia coexists and as *degenerative* with concurrent neutropenia. An understanding of this response can be helpful in monitoring the progression of the condition, especially in cases of septicemia with a degenerative left shift. Neutropenia is rare in goats. Fibrinogen responses in ruminants are dramatic and may be the only observable abnormalities in some inflammatory conditions.

Thoracocentesis. Thoracocentesis is indicated in animals with pleural effusion. The use of real-time ultrasonography may help guide needle placement, but simply inserting the needle into the seventh intercostal space at the costochondral junction level or higher usually works well. After clipping and surgically preparing the site and infusing a local anesthetic, the clinician should insert the biopsy needle (18-gauge, 3 to 10 cm) just off the cranial border of the rib to avoid intercostal vessels and nerves.

Nasal swab. Collecting a nasal swab specimen for virus isolation is useful if no animals are available for necropsy. Either a Dacron- or cotton-tipped swab may be used. The clinician should wipe the external nares with a paper towel before inserting the swab and rotating it fairly vigorously to obtain mucosal cells. The swab should be broken above the tissue culture media so as to not contaminate the media. Most diagnostic laboratories provide veterinarians with viral transport media that can be kept frozen until needed. Most transport media are supplemented with antibiotics, but this should not preclude clean technique by the clinician attempting virus isolation.

Tracheal sampling. The clinician may use either a transtracheal wash or an endoscope-collected sample to culture pathogens from the lower respiratory tract. A small endoscope (8 to 9 mm) may be passed through the nasal passages of adult small ruminants. If this is not possible, the endoscope can be passed orally with the aid of a wooden mouth speculum and mild sedation. Transtracheal fluid collection may be performed by clipping and aseptically scrubbing the middle third of the neck, infiltrating the skin and subcutaneous tissue with local anesthetic (2% lidocaine, 0.5 ml), and making a stab incision with a scalpel throughout the skin and subcutaneous tissue. The clinician then inserts a 14-gauge needle or trocar through the trachea and sterilely passes tubing (220 polyethylene [PE]) to a point just past the tracheal bifurcation. Endoscopic visualization of the PE tubing and pockets of fluid can enhance sample collection. The clinician should inject sterile isotonic solution (20 ml) through the tubing and immediately retrieve the fluid with continuous suction. If little fluid is collected, the PE tubing may be advanced and the procedure repeated.

Radiographs. Radiography is a helpful diagnostic indicator that, along with the evaluation of clinical signs, can be used to determine the efficacy of therapy. For example, the discovery of pulmonary abscesses during radiography warrants a graver prognosis and may indicate the necessity of a change of therapy. Skull radiographs may be indicated for intranasal masses, pharyngeal swellings, nasal foreign bodies, and cases of severe sinusitis. Many of the techniques used for other small animals can be applied to sheep and goats.

Sinus centesis. Sinus centesis may be diagnostic as well as therapeutic. The clinician clips and aseptically prepares the area, infiltrates the skin and subcutaneous tissue with a local anesthetic (2% lidocaine, 0.5 ml), and then makes a stab incision with a sterile scalpel blade. Alternatively, a Steinmann pin can be used to drill a small hole. Samples should be appropriately taken for cytology or culture and lavage should be performed using either PE tubing or a "tom cat" catheter (if future treatments are required).

Ultrasound. Examination of the chest with real-time ultrasonography is helpful to evaluate the presence and extent of pleural effusion, pleural fibrin deposits and adhesions, atelectasis, consolidation, and some abscesses. Ultrasound also may be used as a guide in thoracocentesis and lung biopsy. Goats are better subjects than sheep for ultrasonography because they typically have less body fat (Figure 5-1). During real-time ultrasonography the pleura and superficial lung surfaces may be visualized. Moreover, consolidated lung parenchyma provides a better acoustic medium and is often well visualized. Pulmonary abscesses that extend to the surface of the lung may be detected by ultrasonography (Figure 5-2). Diagnostic ultrasonography is more sensitive than radiography in detecting small amounts of pleural fluid. As the echogenicity of the fluid increases, the cellular and protein content of the fluid also increases.

Blood gas analysis. Depending on the age of the animal, an arterial blood gas sample may be taken from the femoral, auricular, or brachial artery using a heparinized syringe.[2] The sample should be sealed with a tube stopper after the air has been evacuated from the syringe. Analysis of the sample may determine whether ventilatory assistance is required. Hypoxemia (PaO_2 less than 85 mm Hg) may result from hypoventilation, diffusion impairment, ventilation-perfusion mismatch, or right-to-left shunting of blood. Not all animals will benefit from the administration of oxygen or assisted ventilation, so it is important that the clinician interpret the blood gas results accurately and use them in conjunction with other diagnostic tests to determine appropriate treatment.

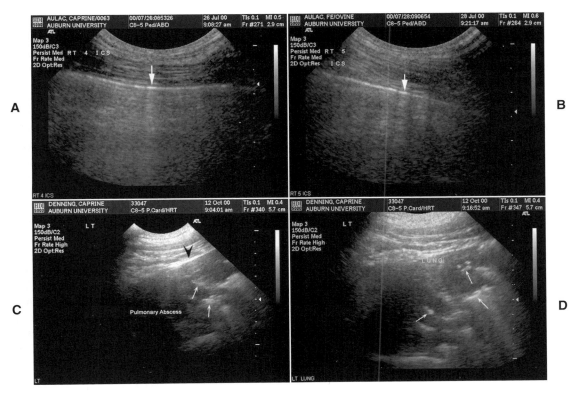

Figure 5-1   Ultrasound image of a normal caprine thorax **(A)**, a normal ovine thorax **(B)**, and a caprine thorax with pneumonia **(C** and **D)** using a 3 MHz probe. Dorsal is to the right and ventral is to the left in the ultrasounds. The *arrows* point to the pleural surface. (Courtesy Dr. Margaret Blaik, Auburn, Alabama.)

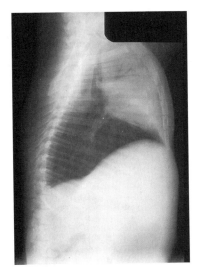

Figure 5-2   Radiograph of a kid with bronchopneumonia. Note the air bronchograms.

Lung biopsy.   Obtaining a percutaneous lung biopsy is not without risks, but it may be beneficial in establishing a diagnosis. As with thoracocentesis, the clinician clips and aseptically prepares the skin over the seventh intercostal space and anesthetizes the skin and subcutaneous tissue (2% lidocaine, 0.5 to 1.0 ml subcutaneously [SC]).

An ultrasound-guided biopsy at the ninth intercostal space, approximately 11 cm ventral to the dorsal midline, may be attempted.[6] The clinician then makes a small stab incision through the anesthetized area using a sterile scalpel blade, advances a sterile biopsy instrument (14-gauge), and collects the sample. The procedure can be performed safely with experience and may help differentiate inflammatory, allergic, emphysematous, edematous, and neoplastic changes.[7]

REFERENCES

1. De Las HM et al: Evidence for a type D-like retrovirus in enzootic nasal tumour of sheep, *Vet Rec* 132:441, 1993.
2. Pringle JK: Ancillary testing for the ruminant respiratory system, *Vet Clin North Am* 8(2):243, 1992.
3. Pringle JK: Assessment of the ruminant respiratory system, *Vet Clin North Am* 8(2):233, 1992.
4. Curtis RA et al: Lung sounds in cattle, horses, sheep and goats, *Can Vet J* 27:170, 1986.
5. Kotlikoff MI, Gillespie JR: Lung sounds in veterinary medicine. Part I. Terminology and mechanisms of sound production, *Comp Cont Ed Pract Vet* 5(8):634, 1983.
6. Braun U et al: Ultrasound-guided percutaneous lung biopsy in sheep, *Vet Rec* 146:528, 2000.
7. Braun U et al: Percutaneous lung biopsy in cattle, *J Am Vet Med Assoc* 215:679, 1999.

UPPER RESPIRATORY DISEASES

Enzootic Nasal Tumor

Pathogenesis. Enzootic nasal tumors of sheep and goats may be unilateral or bilateral conditions; they cause progressive inspiratory dyspnea.[1] The tumors originate from the olfactory mucosa of the ethmoid or nasal turbinates, and their etiology is thought to be associated with a type D/B retrovirus.[2,3] Enzootic tumors have been experimentally transmitted from sheep to sheep and goat to goat.[4] Their incidence is sporadic but because they occur in related flocks they do indicate an enzootic problem.[5] Sheep and goats as young as 15 and 7 months, respectively, have been diagnosed with these tumors.[1,6]

Clinical signs. Affected animals present with copious seromucous to mucopurulent nasal discharge and stridor. Exercise intolerance, facial asymmetry, anorexia, head shaking, sneezing, decreased air flow, exophthalmos, and open-mouth breathing have all been reported.[6] The tumor is locally invasive, obliterating the airway, but is rarely metastatic (Figure 5-3). Erosion of maxillary and other skull bones and invasion of the orbit may occur occasionally.[1] Initially, the lesions are small nodules, but they grow into mucoid, nodular cystic masses that can occlude the caudal nasal cavity and sometimes the pharynx or larynx.[5] Inflammatory polyps may be present in the adjacent nasal cavity.[3]

Diagnosis. A preliminary diagnosis of a nasal mass is made by observation of clinical signs along with percussion of the sinuses. Endoscopy or radiography may be helpful in defining the mass, but only biopsy can confirm the diagnosis of an enzootic tumor. Histologically, these tumors are classified as *adenomas, adenopapillomas,* and *adenocarcinomas.* In goats the tumor tends to originate from the serous gland cells, whereas in sheep the tumor is thought to arise from Bowman's gland.[1]

Treatment. Treatment, if warranted, is surgical removal. The surgeon makes an I-shaped incision over the dorsal midline of the dorsum of the face and reflects the skin flaps. The surgeon then makes another I-shaped incision into the nasal bones, reflects the nasal bones with the periosteum, and removes the nasal septum.[7] The mass can then be easily accessed and removed. Gauze soaked in 1:100,000 epinephrine is used to assist hemostasis. This procedure can be accompanied by significant blood loss, so a donor animal should be available. Without treatment, most affected animals die within 90 days of the onset of clinical signs.[5,6]

Oestrus ovis Infestation

Pathogenesis. The adult *Oestrus ovis* fly deposits larvae around the animal's nostrils. The larvae then migrate up the nasal passage into the dorsal turbinates and sinuses, where they develop for weeks to months before coming out to pupate on the ground. Few or no signs are associated with initial infestation, but infestation with subsequent generations of flies produces excessive clinical signs, probably as a result of a hypersensitivity reaction.

Clinical signs. The animal may develop a secondary bacterial infection and possibly sinusitis. Irritation from the adult fly can result in shaking of the head, rubbing of the nose, and stomping of the feet—all of which decrease grazing time. Infestation of the nasal cavity with the larval (bot) stage irritates the tissues, causing rhinitis, sneezing, mucopurulent nasal discharge, stridor, and decreased airflow (Figure 5-4).[8] Both sheep and goats may be affected, although goats usually acquire the infection from sheep and have milder clinical signs. Occasionally, secondary interstitial pneumonia will develop.

Diagnosis. Endoscopy is helpful in making a diagnosis, and radiographs may demonstrate mineralized bots. The copious nasal discharge of affected animals contains numerous eosinophils and mast cells.

Treatment. Ivermectin (200 μg/kg SC) is used in the late summer to prevent the buildup of heavy infestations

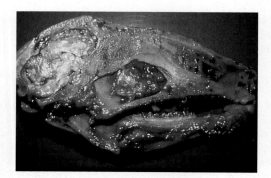

Figure 5-3 Nasal adenocarcinoma. Note the dark mass at the nares.

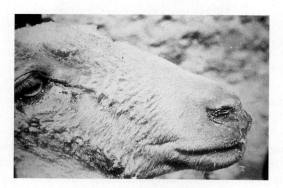

Figure 5-4 A ewe with an *Oestrus ovis* infestation. Notice the nasal discharge.

and again in the winter to kill overwintering larvae. Antibiotics may be of some value in treating secondary pneumonia, but clearing the nasal passages of the bots is usually all that is required.

Sinusitis

Pathogenesis. Inflammation of the paranasal sinuses is an infrequent finding in sheep and goats, but it should be considered in cases of obvious drainage from previous dehorning sites or facial deformity and swelling. Most often, the frontal and maxillary sinuses are involved. Frontal sinus infections usually occur in animals with a history (weeks to months) of dehorning, whereas maxillary sinusitis is most commonly observed secondary to tooth problems. Inflammation of both sinuses may occur as a sequela to nasal bot infestation, nasal adenocarcinoma or other neoplasia, facial fractures, and horn injuries.

Clinical signs. Clinical signs include drainage from a dehorning site, facial asymmetry or bulging, softening of facial bones, nasal discharge, unequal airflow from nostrils, foul odor, head shaking or rubbing, head and neck extension, and head resting or head pressing.[9] Nonspecific signs include pyrexia, lethargy, and anorexia. Neurologic signs may be present in chronic cases and the animal may hold its head at an abnormal angle or squint its eyes.

Diagnosis. Diagnosis is usually made by clinical signs, but radiographs or sinus centesis may be helpful. Percussion over the affected sinus to detect resonance also may aid diagnosis. An oral examination is useful to define lesions of the teeth or pharyngeal abnormalities. Culture and sensitivity of the purulent material may assist in treatment.

Treatment. Lavaging the affected sinus daily with a 0.1% chlorhexidine in saline solution using a teat cannula or French catheter may be helpful. If the animal has systemic signs, the clinician may administer procaine penicillin G (22,000 IU/kg twice a day [BID]), flunixin meglumine (1.1 mg/kg intravenously [IV] or intramuscularly [IM] BID), or ketoprofen (3.0 mg/kg IV or IM once a day [SID]). Even though the two sinuses usually communicate, the frontal sinus of the mature sheep or goat is very compartmentalized, making treatment difficult. For this reason the clinician may need to drill numerous holes into the sinus. The clinician should pack gauze or other material into the sockets of extracted teeth to avoid food material contamination. Treatment may take as long as 2 weeks to heal the animal. In severe cases the sinus infection may extend into the calvaria and result in meningitis. Bandaging the heads of sheep and goats after dehorning may help prevent sinusitis. The

bandages should be removed in 5 to 7 days, depending on the size of the dehorning site and the cleanliness of the bandage.

Pharyngitis

Pathogenesis. Inflammation of the pharyngeal area usually results from trauma caused by dosing equipment, rough feed, or foreign objects. Continued use of older plastic balling guns, specula, and stomach tubes allows the sheep or goat to chew and make the surface even more traumatic. Foreign objects that cause swelling include antibiotic or anthelmintic boluses, wire, and plant awns. Common organisms associated with disease include *Actinomyces pyogenes, Fusobacterium necrophorum,* and *Corynebacterium pseudotuberculosis.* Mild lesions may resolve on their own. More severe lesions may progress to abscesses, granulomas, and severe cellulitis (phlegmon).

Clinical signs. Clinical signs include coughing, obviously painful swallowing, nasal discharge, and anorexia or only wanting to drink. The animal's breath may have a foul odor and the animal may stand with its head and neck extended. Drooling, fever, dehydration, and aspiration pneumonia also may be noted. Stridor may be pronounced with more obstructive lesions. Depending on the amount of swelling, the pharynx may be occluded. Visual inspection of the oral cavity is difficult, but the clinician may be able to note hyperemia, swelling, exudate, food material, and possibly foreign bodies.

Diagnosis. External palpation of the pharyngeal area generally induces coughing and a painful response. Culture of purulent drainage or abscesses can be done, although contamination is difficult to avoid. Radiography or endoscopy may be required to diagnose the lesion definitively.

Treatment. Treatment may include use of nonsteroidal antiinflammatory drugs (NSAIDs) and broad-spectrum antibiotics. Tube feeding and oral administration of antibiotics should be avoided. A temporary rumen fistula is sometimes placed to ensure adequate nutrition. Pharyngeal abscesses may be drained into the pharyngeal area and, if possible, flushed with a dilute Betadine (0.1% to 0.2%) in saline solution.

Retropharyngeal Abscesses

Abscesses of the retropharyngeal lymph nodes may occur secondary to pharyngeal pathology or result from infection with *Corynebacterium pseudotuberculosis.* Stridor, coughing, and difficulty swallowing may be observed. These abscesses are usually not lanced or lavaged because of the potential to spread the organism. Surgical removal is possible but difficult because of the importance of avoiding the jugular vein, carotid artery, and vagus nerve. Moreover, reports have described a false carotid aneurysm in sheep resulting in severe inspiratory dyspnea.[10]

Necrotic Laryngitis

Necrotic lesions of the larynx may be caused by *Fusobacterium necrophorum*. The organism is ubiquitous, but requires a perforated mucous membrane to gain entrance to the laryngeal tissue and produce inflammation and necrosis of the larynx. Clinical signs include a moist, painful cough; inspiratory dyspnea; difficulty swallowing; and salivation. Although necrotic laryngitis is a common problem in calves, it is not frequently seen in sheep and goats. It is more common in animals that are housed indoors or kept in crowded feedlots.

Laryngeal Chondritis

Laryngeal chondritis has been described in Texel sheep.[11,12] Affected animals exhibit increased upper respiratory noise, dyspnea, and some cyanosis. Endoscopy is helpful to observe edema and suppuration of the arytenoid cartilage. It is thought that the short head characteristic of this breed may predispose to the disease. The treatment is the same as for affected horses—removal of the affected laryngeal cartilage.

Tracheal Collapse

Usually considered a congenital defect, tracheal collapse is characterized by stridor, exercise intolerance, and coughing. In a case reported in a 4-month-old goat, the kid was smaller than its litter mates but displayed no signs at rest.[13] A tentative diagnosis may be made by observing the clinical signs and palpating a collapsed trachea, but radiographs or endoscopy may be necessary for confirmation in some cases. Surgical correction is possible with the use of prosthetic tracheal rings.[14]

References

1. De Las HM, Garcia de Jalon JA, Sharp JM: Pathology of enzootic intranasal tumor in thirty-eight goats, *Vet Path* 28:474, 1991.
2. De Las HM et al: Evidence for a type D-like retrovirus in enzootic nasal tumour of sheep, *Vet Rec* 132:441, 1993.
3. DeMartini JC, York DF: Retrovirus-associated neoplasms of the respiratory system of sheep and goats, *Vet Clin North Am* 13:55, 1997.
4. De Las HM et al: Experimental transmission of enzootic intranasal tumors of goats, *Vet Path* 32:19, 1995.
5. McKinnon AO et al: Enzootic nasal adenocarcinoma of sheep in Canada, *Can Vet J* 23:88, 1982.
6. Rings DM, Rojko J: Naturally occurring nasal obstructions in 11 sheep, *Cornell Vet* 75:269, 1985.
7. Trent AM, Smart ME, Fretz PB: Surgical management of nasal adenocarcinoma in sheep, *J Am Vet Med Assoc* 193:227, 1988.
8. Baker JC: Ruminant respiratory system. In Smith BP, editor: *Large animal internal medicine*, Philadelphia, 1996, WB Saunders.
9. Ward JL, Rebhun WC: Chronic frontal sinusitis in dairy cattle: 12 cases (1978-1989), *J Am Vet Med Assoc* 201:326, 1992.
10. Rings DM, Constable P, Biller DS: False carotid aneurysm in a sheep, *J Am Vet Med Assoc* 189:799, 1986.
11. Johnson R et al: Nasal squamous-cell carcinoma in a sheep, *Mod Vet Pract* 63:897, 1982.
12. Lane JG et al: Laryngeal chondritis in Texel sheep, *Vet Rec* 121:81, 1987.
13. Jackson PG et al: Tracheal collapse in a goat, *Vet Rec* 119:160, 1986.
14. Scarratt WK, Bradley RL, Booth LC: Collapsed trachea in two calves, *Comp Cont Ed Pract Vet* 7:S49, 1985.

TYPICAL PNEUMONIAS

Pasteurellosis

The pneumonic form of pasteurellosis is the most common and is regarded as one of the most important infectious bacterial diseases of sheep and goats.[1-3] *Pasteurella haemolytica* is a normal inhabitant of the upper respiratory tracts of sheep and goats. Most cases of pasteurellosis are caused by *P. haemolytica* type A, but *P. multocida* also has been implicated.[4] *P. haemolytica* has two biotypes, A and T, that differ morphologically, biochemically, biologically, and serologically. Colonies of biotype A are usually small and gray, whereas biotype T colonies are larger (2 mm in diameter) and have brown centers[5]; both are gram-negative coccobacilli. Biotype A is responsible for pneumonic pasteurellosis and also may cause septicemia in young lambs. Serotype A2 is the most common isolate in ovine pneumonic pasteurellosis.[6,7] Biotype T has been isolated from cases of pneumonia and septicemia in older lambs.[8] On the basis of surface antigens the biotypes are divided into 17 different serotypes.[9]

Pathogenesis. *P. haemolytica* produces a number of virulence factors, including lipopolysaccharide (LPS), or endotoxin, which is considered of primary importance in inducing early pulmonary pathophysiologic changes and stimulating immune responses in vaccines.[10] Stress in the form of transport, bad weather, poor ventilation, nutritional imbalances, parasitism, confinement, handling, and weaning may be involved in the etiology of pneumonic pasteurellosis. Predisposing agents include parainfluenza-3, adenovirus type 6, respiratory syncytial virus, *Chlamydia, Bordetella parapertussis*, and *Mycoplasma ovipneumoniae*.[11] Stress and either viral-viral or viral-bacterial synergism work in concert to overwhelm the host's defense mechanisms, allowing secondary or opportunistic invaders (e.g. *Pasteurella*) to enter the respiratory tract.

Experimental inoculation of lambs with *P. haemolytica* alone or in combination with adenovirus type 6 of P13 may cause severe respiratory disease.[8-10,12] Combined infections may result in early death or slow resolution of lesions. More consistent results are obtained when *P. haemolytica* is administered 6 to 8 days after the virus.[12] *P. haemolytica* alone may cause an acute serofibrinous pneumonia and pleuritis resulting in death or rapid recovery depending on the severity of the serofibrinous pneumonia.[9] Intratracheal injection of LPS from *P. haemolytica* A1 results in an acute fibrinopurulent pneumonia, indicating that LPS contributes to the pathogenesis of *P. haemolytica* infection in the lungs.[10] The use of dexamethasone alone to mimic stress was insufficient to produce infection or pneumonic lesions without another form of stress (e.g., transport) on an animal that was previously experimentally challenged intranasally with *P. haemolytica* A2.[13]

Inoculation of goats with *P. haemolytica* either IV or by an intratracheal route resulted in consolidated pulmonary lesions and some fibrinous lesions.[14] Certain unknown factors may be involved in the predilection of *P. haemolytica* to colonize the lungs because IV inoculation of other gram-negative organisms in cattle does not result in pulmonary deposition.[15] Although *P. haemolytica* has been isolated from tonsillar tissue in cattle and sheep, intratonsillary inoculation of *P. haemolytica* does not result in pulmonary lesions.[14]

Clinical signs.   Septicemia (Figure 5-5), arthritis, and otitis media may occur secondarily to the pneumonia. Outbreaks can occur, usually involving one particular serotype, in any age, breed, or sex. Springtime outbreaks are most often associated with severe weather and generally involve nursing lambs 2 weeks to 2 months of age and some ewes. In the fall, outbreaks generally occur in 5- to 7-month-old lambs after shipment to feedlots. Morbidity rates may reach 50%, but mortality rates are generally low. Transmission is by inhalation of droplets from carriers or direct contact. Nursing lambs may be infected by ewes with *P. haemolytica* mastitis. Goats are susceptible to pneumonic pasteurellosis under natural conditions.[16] One study[7] found that of all the pneumonic lesions of goats discovered at necropsy, 20% were caused by *P. multocida*.

The first sign of pneumonia may be sudden death. Other early clinical signs include fever (105° to 108° F), depression, anorexia, weight loss, isolation from the flock, mucopurulent nasal discharge or lacrimation, tachypnea, coughing, and increased lung sounds (crackles and wheezes). The disease course is usually 12 hours to 3 days, with recovery occurring in 14 to 20 days. Outbreaks may last 1 month. Chronically affected lambs and kids have reduced lung capacity, reduced weight gain, and decreased feed efficiency; death is possible.[8]

Diagnosis.   Necropsy of affected animals reveals a secondary fibrinopurulent pleuropneumonia (Figure 5-6), with excess serous fluid often present in the pleural and

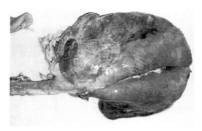

Figure 5-5   A set of lungs and liver from an animal with septicemic pasteurellosis.

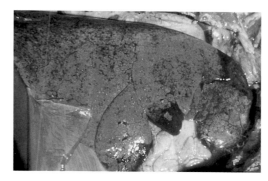

Figure 5-6   A set of lungs with *Pasteurella* pneumonia.

peritoneal cavities. Lesions within the lungs consist of areas of consolidation with one or more foci of necrosis surrounded by hemorrhage.[9] Hydropericardium can sometimes be seen. Histopathologic examination may reveal pneumonitis with multifocal areas of acute fibrinopurulent bronchopneumonia, coagulative necrosis, and fibrinous pleuritis.[8] Often areas of necrosis are surrounded by masses of basophilic spindle-shaped leukocytes called *oat cells;* their presence is considered by some to be pathognomonic for pasteurellosis. A tentative diagnosis can be made with a history of stress, clinical signs of acute bronchopneumonia, and the presence of gross lesions at necropsy. Isolation of *P. haemolytica* is confirmatory.[13]

Treatment.   Most cases respond to treatment with long-acting oxytetracycline (20 mg/kg SC every 48 to 72 hours).[8] Medication of entire flocks is achieved by administering sulfonamides in the drinking water or orally (200 mg/kg/day followed by 66 mg/kg daily for 4 days). Ampicillin and penicillin have been reported to be effective. Tylosin (10 to 20 mg/kg), ceftiofur (2.2 to 4.4 mg/kg IM or IV every 24 hours), and florfenicol (20 mg/kg IM every 48 hours) may be used as well. Tilmicosin (10 mg/kg SC) can be effective in some sheep but should be avoided in goats.[17]

Prevention.   Pneumonia can be prevented by minimizing stress and instituting vaccination programs. Susceptibility to bacterial infections is at its highest 7 days after viral respiratory infection because viral lung titers are declining, pulmonary antiviral antibody titers are peaking, alveolar macrophages contain peak levels of viral antigen, and the antibacterial activity of the macrophages is severely impaired.[18] Vaccinating with a modified live virus (MLV) product for bovine herpesvirus 1 (BHV1), parainfluenza-3 (PI3), and bovine respiratory syncytial virus (BRSV) before shipping to the feedlot may decrease mortality compared with nonvaccinated lambs.[19] Additional vaccination with a *Hemophilus somnus* bacterin does not appear to increase the level of protection afforded by the MLV vaccine alone. A vaccination study evaluating the efficacy of a killed *P. haemolytica* serotype A1 and A2 vaccine resulted in an outbreak of primarily pneumonic *P. multocida*, suggesting that vaccines for pasteurellosis need to contain antigens affording cross-protection against both species and numerous serotypes.[20,21]

A later study evaluated a vaccine containing whole cell antigens of *P. haemolytica* A1 and another containing *P. haemolytica* A1 cell surface and leukotoxin antigens. Neither agent provided any clear evidence of a lower rate of pneumonia compared with nonvaccinated control lambs.[20,22] Another study found that the most widespread serotype (A2) is not very immunogenic in lambs.[2,23] The only *Pasteurella* species vaccines available for use in sheep and goats are the whole cell bacterins, which are generally considered ineffective.

Stress can be induced by many risk factors. Minimizing climatic changes, reducing overcrowding, decreasing transportation, minimizing improper ventilation, and eliminating major fluctuations in diet can all help decrease risk factors known to place more stress on the respiratory system.

ACUTE RESPIRATORY VIRUSES

In all acute respiratory viral pneumonias, therapy should be directed at preventing or treating secondary bacterial pathogens and providing supportive measures to help decrease the debilitating effects of these diseases.

Parainfluenza Type 3

PI3, which is a member of the paramyxovirus family, is a ribonucleic acid (RNA) virus. The one serotype of PI3 that infects sheep is related to but distinct from the PI3 that infects cattle and human beings.[19] Most infections are inapparent because more than 70% of sheep are seropositive for PI3,[24] but outbreaks have been reported with high rates of morbidity. Although respiratory syncytial virus (RSV) and adenoviruses may predispose to pneumonic pasteurellosis, PI3 appears to be more important.[25]

Clinical signs. Clinical signs include frequent coughing, serous nasal discharge, and occasional ocular discharge. Body temperature is usually not elevated. The disease is more common in lambs younger than 1 year.

Diagnosis. Diagnosis of PI3 infection is made by isolating the virus from nasal swabs from animals that have been infected for less than 1 week or by measuring serologic responses.

Prevention. Protection against experimental and natural cases of pneumonic pasteurellosis by use of a live intranasal PI3 vaccine has been demonstrated.[26-30]

Adenovirus

The adenoviruses are deoxyribonucleic acid (DNA) viruses. Many different antigenic types exist in ruminants.[24] Depending on which of the six serotypes is causing infection, seroprevalence of a flock may range from approximately 7% to 83%.[24,31,32] Although adenovirus has been isolated from sheep with respiratory disease, the importance of the virus is not completely under-stood. However, it is thought to cause mild respiratory disease that increases in severity with concurrent *P. haemolytica* infections.[26,33] The virus is most often isolated from young lambs with respiratory and enteric disease.[33]

Clinical signs. Clinical signs are mild and include pyrexia, anorexia, sneezing, serous nasal discharge, and pneumonia. Experimental challenge with adenovirus may result in a proliferative bronchiolitis and an anteroventral bronchopneumonia.

Diagnosis. Diagnosis of adenovirus infection is by virus isolation from nasal swabs or paired serologic testing, if available.

Prevention. No vaccines are used for this virus in the United States.

Respiratory Syncytial Virus

BRSV, a pneumovirus of the family *Paramyxoviridae*, is an important respiratory virus of cattle that also has been implicated in cases of respiratory disease in sheep and goats. The importance of RSV as a primary cause of respiratory disease in sheep and goats is equivocal and many researchers believe it is of greater importance as a predisposing pathogen to secondary bacterial pneumonia. Questions remain about possible interspecies transmission. Prevalence studies have reported 42% of 447 free-ranging bighorn sheep and 52.5% of 378 ewes to be seropositive to BRSV.[24,34]

Recent studies have suggested the existence of two ruminant subgroups of RSV, with one subgroup representing RSV isolated from calves and goats and the other representing RSV obtained from sheep.[35] Radiolabeled probes based on differences in the G glycoprotein genes were used to characterize the genetic heterogenicity of the various ruminant RSV isolates by the ribonuclease protection assay. Previous reports had suggested that some ovine RSV isolates should be considered distinct RSVs based on reverse transcriptase polymerase chain reaction (RT-PCR) and DNA hybridization using primers and a probe to the fusion (F) protein messenger RNA (mRNA) of BRSV.[36] An RSV-specific whole virus enzyme-linked immunospecific assay (ELISA) and a peptide-based ELISA were used to demonstrate anti-RSV activity in the majority of sera from sheep, goats, cattle, and human beings, whereas antibodies specific to BRSV were found in all cattle and the majority of goats tested.[37] The role of maternal antibodies in ruminant RSV infections is controversial, with some demonstrating a protective effect and others apparently predisposing to clinical disease and viral shedding.[38]

Experiments have shown that the ovine isolate of RSV, when inoculated in a challenge model, causes mild primary pneumonia in lambs, with lung lesions similar to those described in naturally occurring epizootic pneumonia in sheep.[38,39] Pulmonary lesions in lambs experimentally infected with BRSV are not as pronounced, with less peribronchial and perivascular lymphoid accumulation and collapse of airways.[40-42] The loss of cilia and cell necrosis identified in experimental disease in lambs are thought to lead to decreased efficiency of mucociliary clearance and predispose to secondary bacterial pneumonia.[43] Other studies have reported a synergistic effect of RSV and *P. haemolytica* in experimental challenges in lambs.[44-46] Experimental infection of lambs with BRSV and RSV-specific antibodies did not influence the severity and duration of clinical disease, titer of virus shed, or humoral and cellular immune responses compared with single inoculation with BRSV, although the duration of viral shedding was prolonged.[47] The virus has been reported as causing acute respiratory disease with a high rate of mortality in goats,[48] although most keepers report mild respiratory disease unless the condition is complicated by *P. haemolytica* A.[49]

Clinical signs. Clinical signs observed in goats with RSV include anorexia, pyrexia, conjunctivitis, cough, tachypnea, and tachycardia. Auscultation may reveal increased bronchial sounds and possible crackles. Friction rubs may be auscultated in cases of mixed infection.

Diagnosis. Necropsy of affected animals may reveal diffuse interstitial pneumonia and firm, edematous lungs. The presence of syncytial cells on histopathologic examination is characteristic of RSV infection. Immunoperoxidase staining of tissues may indicate RSV antigen in the epithelial cells of the alveolar and bronchial walls and in syncytial and alveolar lumens.[49]

Prevention. To date no RSV vaccines have been marketed for sheep and goats. Identification of viral subgroups is important for vaccine development so that all subgroups may be included for protection against all possible strains an animal may encounter.

Ovine and Caprine Herpesvirus

Caprine herpesvirus (CHV) has been isolated in lung and nasal swabs of goats during outbreaks of pneumonia in which *P. haemolytica* also was isolated.[50] The specific role of CHV in caprine or ovine pneumonia has been questioned, although some reports describe it as a cause of rhinitis, vulvovaginitis, and abortion in adult goats.[51,52] Both BHV1 and CHV can infect cattle and goats, but their pathogenicity is restricted to the natural host.[51] Previous reports evaluating herpesvirus isolates taken from sheep and goats with various problems determined by restriction endonuclease analysis and radioimmunoprecipitation that the isolates were more closely related to BHV1 than CHV.[53] Experimental challenge with CHV induced a clinical rhinitis with histopathologic lesions of tracheitis. However, none of the challenged goats became severely ill.[54] Although it may not lead to serious disease, CHV can proliferate in the upper respiratory tracts of goats.[54] Ovine herpesvirus-1 has been isolated from cases of ovine pneumonia.[55] Lambs inoculated experimentally with CHV developed subclinical pneumonia with interstitial changes in the lungs; after a later administration of corticosteroids, the virus was re-isolated, indicating that the virus may go into a latent state.[56] These authors propose that CHV may be associated with ovine pulmonary carcinoma.

Mycoplasma Pneumonia of Sheep

Mycoplasma pneumonia also is known as *enzootic pneumonia, chronic nonprogressive pneumonia,* and *atypical pneumonia.* Typically, *Mycoplasma ovipneumoniae* is thought to be the primary organism, with *P. haemolytica* A, other *Mycoplasma* organisms, and *Chlamydia psittaci ovis* being secondary invaders.[2,57]

Pathogenesis. As with the bovine respiratory disease complex, stress and minor viral pathogens may predispose to *Mycoplasma* pneumonia. The disease occurs in intensively reared lambs that live in areas with poor ventilation and in assembled groups of lambs in feedlots; it most commonly develops as maternal antibody levels wane. Reservoirs such as older animals and convalescent adults infect lambs mainly after weaning. Encapsulation allows the organism to evade the host's immune response and promotes long-term colonization of the upper respiratory tract.[58] Goats also may be affected.[59] Transmission is by the respiratory route (contact or aerosol) and results in ciliostasis and production of an exudate that allows bacterial colonization of the lungs (e.g., with *P. haemolytica*).[57]

The *Mycoplasma* component of the disease is thought to restrict the lethality of the *Pasteurella.*

Clinical signs. The disease is mild and is characterized by chronic coughing and dyspnea on exertion. Mucopurulent nasal discharge, fever, and depression may be observed when *Pasteurella* is involved. Productivity is usually decreased. High morbidity and low mortality rates are generally associated with this nonprogressive, often subclinical, condition.[60]

Diagnosis. Diagnosis is based on the presence of mild, chronic pneumonia in lambs younger than 1 year. Lesions at necropsy include consolidation of the cranial lobes (and occasionally the anterior border of caudal lobes) with pleuritis. Consolidated areas may be gray to red-brown with red atelectatic areas and firm, gray-white nodules on the cut surface. An interstitial, cuffing-type pneumonia with nodular lymphoid hyperplasia, bronchiolar epithelial hyperplasia, and mononuclear lymphocytic cuffs around bronchioles and blood vessels is seen on histopathologic examination. Alveoli contain exudate consisting mostly of macrophages and few neutrophils. A characteristic feature is the presence of nodular hyaline "scars" in the bronchiolar walls. Pleuritis may occasionally occur with this disease. The characteristic lesions seen on necropsy and histopathology confirm the diagnosis. An immunoperoxidase staining of formalin-fixed, paraffin-embedded sections for detection of either antigen has been described.[61] Culture of the organism in broth media is diagnostic, as is detection of antibodies by an ELISA.[62,63] However, cross-reactivity among different *Mycoplasma* species has created concern about the ELISA's specificity.[64]

Treatment. Treatment with oxytetracycline (20 mg/kg SC every 48 to 72 hours), tilmicosin (10 mg/kg SC), and florfenicol (20 mg/kg IM every 48 hours) can be effective in eliminating the infection. Some *in vitro* studies also indicate that enrofloxacin may be effective.[65]

Prevention. Prevention and control rely on reducing the density of housed lambs, ensuring adequate ventilation, and separating batches of assembled lambs. No vaccine is available.

M. ovipneumoniae and *Mycoplasma arginini* have been isolated from young lambs with a chronic "coughing syndrome." It is thought that failure of the immune response and chronic persistence of *M. ovipneumoniae* may play a role in this condition.[66] A large number of lambs with the disease had autoantibodies in their serum that reacted with cilia of the upper respiratory tract.[66] A syndrome of severe paroxysmal cough leading to rectal prolapse and poor weight gain is widespread in the midwestern United States; it produces variable severity and morbidity.[64]

Mycoplasma Pneumonia in Goats

The most important *Mycoplasma* groups that infect ruminants in known as the *Mycoplasma mycoides* cluster. It consists of *M. mycoides* subspecies *mycoides* small colony, *M. mycoides* subspecies *mycoides* large colony, *M. capricolum* subspecies *capripneumoniae, M. mycoides* subspecies *mycoides, M. mycoides* subspecies *capri, M. capricolum* subspecies *capricolum,* and bovine serogroup 7.[67] Differentiation between members of this cluster by conventional methods can be difficult, and specific diagnosis may rely on PCR.[68] Immunohistochemical methods using monoclonal antibodies are useful for diagnosing specific strains of the *M. mycoides* cluster.[69,70] Greater success in isolating the organism is attained in more acute cases, whereas chronic infections result in less successful isolation.[71] ELISA is reported to be useful for diagnosis.[72] Neither *M. mycoides* subspecies *capri* or *M. capricolum* subspecies *capricolum* occur in the United States.

M. mycoides subspecies *mycoides* large colony (Mmm) was first reported on the East Coast of the United States in 1969[73] and is now prevalent throughout the country.[74,75] It has been isolated in several countries in ovine and caprine species and is associated with low mortality rates.[76]

Pathogenesis. Asymptomatic lactating does act as carriers, shedding the organism in their milk.[75] In one outbreak, as many as 1×10^7 to 1×10^8 colony-forming units of the organism were shed in each milliliter of colostrum or milk, resulting in the death of 200 kids.[76] The organism is transmitted orally to the kids through the ingestion of contaminated milk or colostrum. Transmission among adults is thought to involve the external auditory meatus, which has been determined to be a source of numerous *Mycoplasma* organisms, of which Mmm was the predominant isolate.[74] Ear mites (*Psoroptes* species) are thought to serve as vectors for *Mycoplasma* organisms.[77] Experimentally, infected fleas of the order *Siphonaptera* have been reported to transmit Mmm to susceptible kids. *M. mycoides* subspecies *mycoides* small colony, the causative organism of contagious bovine pleuropneumonia, has been isolated from the milk of goats showing clinical signs of pneumonia.[78] Interstitial pneumonia lesions were observed on necropsy, with primary lesions occurring at the apical, cardiac, and diaphragmatic lobes. Hypertrophy of the mesenteric lymph nodes was evident. Experimental studies demonstrate the hematogenous spread of the organism and the severe pathogenicity of Mmm (regardless of the route of inoculation), suggesting that natural infection may occur by any route. Occasionally, *M. capri* has been isolated from cases of caprine pneumonia, although its significance is uncertain.[71,79] Experimental inoculation of goats with *M. capri* isolates from natural pneumonia and pleuropneumonia cases resulted in severe respiratory disease and death.[28] Experimental inoculation of kids with *M. capricolum* subspecies *capricolum* resulted in diffuse interstitial pneumonia, congestion, and edema, but no signs of pleuropneumonia.[29] *M. capri*, *M. capricolum* subspecies *capricolum*, and Mmm were administered by different routes to 12 kids, and although the former two organisms are not present in the United States at this time, all three produced mycoplasmosis and severe lesions detectable by immunohistochemistry; *Mycoplasma* antigens were established as the cause.[80,81]

Clinical signs. Adult goats typically display fever, pleuropneumonia, mastitis, and polyarthritis, whereas common signs in kids include septicemia, meningitis, and arthritis.[82,83] One outbreak was characterized by increased cases of mastitis and increased morbidity and mortality of kids up to 2 months of age. Affected kids suffered from pyrexia and acute death, neurologic disease and death, or pyrexia and pneumonia, with most dying within 3 to 5 days of respiratory signs.[61] Pyrexia, leukopenia, and coagulopathies are observed with septicemia in goats.[82] In herds with endemic infection, the primary complaint may be of increased kid morbidity with pneumonia and polyarthritis. Milking herd exposure may result from the purchase of an infected doe and may produce mastitis and abortions before the kids exhibit problems.[84]

Diagnosis. Diagnosis is made by the discovery of lesions at necropsy. These include acute fibrinous pneumonia and pleuritis, suppurative polyarthritis, periarthritis, osteomyelitis, myocarditis, renal infarction, and lymphadenitis.[71]

Treatment. Treatment may help decrease clinical signs of the disease, but the prognosis is poor and treatment may not eliminate the carrier state. Recovered animals generally continue shedding the organism for life. The *Mycoplasma* organisms are generally sensitive to tetracyclines (oxytetracycline 10 mg/kg IV BID or long-acting oxytetracycline 20 mg/kg SC or IM every 48 to 72 hours) and macrolides (20 mg/kg IM BID), but not beta-lactams.

Prevention. Maintenance of a closed herd is the simplest way to avoid introducing *Mycoplasma* into a flock or herd.[85,86] After it is present in a herd, preventive practices should focus on milking practices and management of kids. Routine culturing of milk to identify infected does is imperative to prevent further infection. Initially, bimonthly cultures should be taken from each doe until no new cases are discovered for two consecutive cultures. After that, monthly samples can be taken for 2 to 3 months, followed by pooled samples for 6 months. Tank samples should be collected and frozen weekly; the keeper or clinician should investigate any increase in somatic cell counts or California mastitis test (CMT)

results. Infected does may be culled or isolated and milked separately or last. In clinically normal carrier does, environmental stress (weather changes) appears to be an important factor in the predisposition to clinical disease. Kids born to infected does should be separated immediately after birth, fed heat-treated colostrum, and then fed pasteurized goat milk, cow milk, or milk replacer. Transmission also may occur among does at milking; therefore teat dipping of does and the wearing of gloves by milkers are essential. Milkers should use individual paper towels to dry teats. A killed vaccine has been reported to prevent experimental infection.[87] In the midst of an outbreak the use of chlortetracycline or tetracycline as a feed supplement may minimize the spread of the disease.

Contagious Caprine Pleuropneumonia

The causative organism of contagious caprine pleuropneumonia (CCPP) is the F38 biotype of *Mycoplasma*, recently reclassified as *M. capricolum* subspecies *capripneumoniae*.[67,88-90] This specific *Mycoplasma* is very contagious in housed goats. Morbidity is usually 100% and mortality may range from 60% to 100%. Only goats are naturally infected.

Clinical signs. Clinical signs include pyrexia, cough, dyspnea with accompanying grunting, wide-based forelimb stance, anorexia, and listlessness. Death may occur within 2 days.[91]

Diagnosis. On necropsy the lung lobes (unilateral or bilateral) are enlarged, firm, and variegated with red, yellow, white, and gray foci.[92] A fibrinous pleuritis and pleural effusion are generally present, with occasional pericarditis.[71] Although it is occasionally seen in North America, the disease is prevalent in Africa, Asia, and eastern Europe. In North America the disease is inappropriately diagnosed as other mycoplasmal pneumonias of the goat. A latex agglutination test has been developed to diagnose CCPP in the field, whereas conventional methods or PCR and restriction enzyme analysis may be used in the laboratory.[93,94]

Treatment. Treatment early in the course of the disease consists of the administration of tylosin (20 mg/kg IM every 12 hours), enrofloxacin (5 mg/kg IV or IM SID), lincomycin (10 to 20 mg/kg IM every 12 to 24 hours), or tetracycline (20 mg/kg SC every 48 to 72 hours).[95] Goats that survive the acute phase may have chronic lesions, but a carrier state does not appear to exist among long-term survivors.[96]

Prevention. Prevention may be afforded through the use of vaccines and the maintenance of closed herds.[97,98] In the midst of an outbreak, the use of chlortetracycline or tetracycline as a feed supplement may help minimize the spread of the disease.

Chlamydia

Pneumonia caused by *Chlamydia psittaci*, an obligate intracellular bacterium, is relatively rare in sheep and goats.[99] Its occurrence is generally linked to animals that have or have had polyarthritis or abortions. The incidence of pneumonia caused by *Chlamydia* in goats was found to be only 6.4% (14 of 218) in a study from India.[79] In calves, chlamydial infection is reported to enhance the severity of *P. haemolytica*.[100]

Clinical signs. Clinical signs may include depression, pyrexia, a dry hacking cough, nasal discharge, dyspnea, and diarrhea.[101] *Chlamydia* may be identified by observing the organism in stained impression smears or fixed tissue sections by indirect immunofluorescence, Gimenez stain, or yolk sac inoculation and isolation.[33,102] Antibody titers to *Chlamydia* may be assessed by either an ELISA or a complement fixation test. Indirect immunofluorescence also may be used to identify the organism.

Diagnosis. Reported lesions include consolidation of cranial lobes with interstitial changes and intracytoplasmic elementary bodies within alveolar macrophages observed on histopathologic examination. Edematous septa and thickened bronchioles that yield a turbid exudate when compressed also have been described.[101]

Treatment. In most cases, chlamydial infections respond to treatment with oxytetracycline (20 mg/kg SC or IM every 48 to 72 hours). In the midst of an outbreak the use of tetracycline or chlortetracycline in the diet of normal, unaffected animals may be beneficial.

Ovine Pulmonary Carcinoma

Sheep pulmonary adenomatosis (SPA), ovine pulmonary carcinoma (OPC), or jaagsiekte are contagious, slow, viral infections that affect the respiratory system. Susceptibility seems to be age-related, with neonates and lambs younger than 10 weeks being more likely to develop OPC.[103,104] Incidence of the natural disease is low in goats, although OPC has been experimentally transmitted in kids.[105] The disease is found as a sporadic or endemic condition in sheep or goats of all continents of the world except Australia.[105,106] Lung fluid and nasal exudate of affected sheep contain high concentrations of the infectious virus. Viruses from lung wash fluid from a sheep with jaagsiekte were purified and sequenced, revealing that the capsid sequence is most related to a type D retrovirus and the envelope region is most related to a type B retrovirus. Reports indicate that the disease coexists with ovine progressive pneumonia in some animals.[103]

Clinical signs. Clinical signs are usually seen in 2- to 4-year-old sheep, although the virus may infect younger sheep. Progressive respiratory distress and weight loss are the common clinical signs.[107] When infected sheep are forced to exert themselves, auscultation of the respiratory tract reveals harsh respiratory sounds on inspiration and expiration and occasionally crackles and wheezes. Tachypnea is a consistent finding, whereas coughing is inconsistent. Lowering the head or raising of the rear limbs of the sheep usually produces a flow of accumulated fluid from the nostrils. Most animals are not febrile and continue to eat unless a secondary bacterial pneumonia exists. The course of the disease is progressive and death usually occurs within weeks or months of the appearance of clinical signs.[108]

Diagnosis. Necropsy of animals with OPC, SPA, or jaagsiekte reveals heavy lungs that exude clear fluid from the cut surface and clear, foamy fluid from the trachea.[109] Large, firm, gray masses may be identified in the cranioventral lobes, with smaller ones in the caudodorsal lobes.[110] The OPC tumor is well-differentiated and arises from alveolar type II or nonciliated bronchiolar cells.[108] Metastasis may occur to the bronchial or mediastinal lymph nodes in as many as 10% of cases.[108,109]

Prevention. No treatment or vaccine exists for this disease. Eradication efforts in some countries are based on extensive slaughtering of large numbers of animals because of the lack of an antemortem diagnostic test. Nevertheless, sheep can still spread the virus to others through nasal or lung fluid. After a diagnostic test for use on lung or nasal fluid is developed, prevention or even eradication of this disease may be possible.

Ovine Progressive Pneumonia

Ovine progressive pneumonia (OPP), as it is called in the United States, or maedi, as it is called in Europe, is a chronic progressive pneumonia or atypical pneumonia of sheep that is caused by a nononcogenic, single-stranded RNA lentivirus of the family *Retroviridae*. Economically, OPP is one of the most important diseases affecting sheep in North America. Losses resulting from sick animals, reduced production, and decreased sales can all be attributed to ovine lentivirus (OvLV) infection. However, one report demonstrated that subclinical infection with OvLV had no apparent negative effect on the number of lambs produced or grease fleece weight compared with seronegative sheep in the same flock,[111] and another reported no difference in milk production between seropositive and seronegative ewes with regard to OvLV.[112] Nevertheless, flocks that have eradicated OvLV report fewer ewe losses, increased weaning weights, no indurative mastitis, and a lower incidence of pregnancy toxemia.[47] Although the results of studies of indirect losses are variable, it seems likely that the degree of economic loss caused by OvLV infection is associated with the level of sheep production, breed type, local husbandry practices, and flock variations. Therefore generalizations about the appearance and behavior of flocks with seropositive ewes are not useful or accurate.[113,114]

Pathogenesis. The OvLV persists within infected monocytes and macrophages[115,116] and may exist in a latent state for an undetermined period. It infects goats infrequently.[117] OvLV is closely related to the caprine arthritis-encephalitis (CAE) virus. Because of its long incubation period (2 to 4 years), the disease is usually seen in older ewes. The seroprevalence of OvLV varies from as low as 0.5% of 2040 sheep in west Texas to as high as 49% of sheep in the Rocky Mountain region; seroprevalence progressively increases with age.[118,119] Direct or colostral or milk transmission are the most likely routes, whereas vertical transmission is rarely observed.[120,121] A recent report indicates that OvLV may be present in semen contaminated by leukocytes.[122] Blood has not been demonstrated to be a source of transmission. Animals frequently become infected as lambs, with the outcome of infection influenced by viral phenotype, infectious dose, colostral antibodies, age, and host genetic factors.[113,123] OvLV has a strong ability to mutate and the resultant antigenic drift produces new strains of the virus. This accounts for the different patterns of disease associated with different strains of OvLV.[113] Close confinement and the duration of exposure also play significant roles in transmission. Many sheep remain asymptomatic carriers for life.[124] In flocks with both infected and uninfected ewes, approximately 40% of the offspring of infected ewes and 20% of the offspring of uninfected ewes become seropositive within 1 year.[125]

After sheep have become infected, they remain infected and persistently viremic, even though they may produce antibodies. The virus localizes in the lungs, central nervous system (CNS), and hematopoietic tissue. In the lung, OvLV stimulates reticular cells and lymphocytes to proliferate, causing thickening of the interalveolar septa and producing adenomatosis of the alveolar lining. Regional lymphadenopathy also is common. In addition, indurative lymphocytic mastitis, proliferative arthritis, and (less frequently) nonsuppurative encephalitis may be caused by OvLV.

Clinical signs. Clinical signs of OvLV often appear after periods of stress, exertion, or inclement weather. The clinical course is characterized by an insidious, slowly progressive malaise resulting in chronic degenerative disease.[126] Initially the sheep become listless; progressive emaciation (thin ewe syndrome) and dyspnea, especially after exercise, occur later. Despite this the sheep maintain their appetites and normal temperatures in the absence of secondary bacterial pneumonia, although they may exhibit tachypnea (80 to 120 breaths per minute).

Nasal discharge and coughing may be observed, but auscultation of lungs is usually not remarkable. As the disease progresses, affected animals demonstrate open-mouth breathing, flaring of the nostrils, forced expirations, and more coughing. The signs may last 3 to 6 months or persist for years. Chronic nonsuppurative arthritis, vasculitis, mastitis, encephalitis, and rarely posterior paresis may be observed.[127,128] The indurative mastitis ("hardbag") is characterized by a large (symmetric or asymmetric), hard udder with no abnormal secretions. Ataxia, stumbling, and unilateral proprioceptive deficits may be the first signs noticed with posterior neurologic manifestations. These signs can slowly progress over weeks to months to rear limb paralysis or quadriplegia.[114,128] A moderate, hypochromic anemia and leukocytosis may be observed, as well as hypergammaglobulinemia in advanced disease.[109,128] After signs appear, the mortality rate is 100%, with the animals dying or being culled within a year.[128]

Diagnosis. Diagnosis is by use of an ELISA employing a recombinant transmembrane envelope protein.[129] This test is more sensitive than the commonly used agar gel immunodiffusion (AGID) and more economical than the whole-virus ELISA or Western blot.[130] PCR testing is a more sensitive and economical way to detect viral nucleic acids than actual virus isolation.[131] In addition, PCR can be used to test kids before maternal antibody levels decline. Sensitivity of the AGID and PCR are about 95% to 96%, with both missing a few positive animals. For eradication purposes the use of both tests is recommended, as is repeating tests two or three times over several months. Necropsy of dead ewes reveals large (two to three times normal weight), heavy lungs, possibly with vertical rib impressions because of their swelling (Figure 5-7). The lungs are firm, do not collapse after removal, and are gray-blue or gray-yellow. Evidence of secondary bacterial pneumonia may be present. The tracheobronchial and mediastinal lymph nodes are greatly enlarged, bulge on cut surfaces, and have a gray-white color.[109] Arthritis commonly affects the appendicular joints, with extensive proliferation of the synovium, fibro-

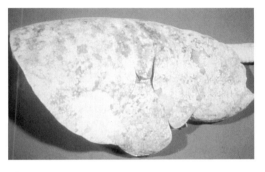

Figure 5-7 A set of lungs of a sheep with ovine progressive pneumonia. Note the distended appearance.

sis of the joint capsule, and degeneration of the articular cartilage and bone.[132] Gross examination of the spinal cord and brain is generally normal. Histopathologic examination is distinct, with a chronic diffuse interstitial pneumonia, hyperplasia of lymphoid cells around airways and blood vessels, and accumulation of mononuclear cells in the interstitium. Lymphocytic meningitis, choroiditis, and leukoencephalitis have been reported in some sheep.[133,134]

Prevention. Control of the disease can be difficult. Closing the flock, testing, and culling can eliminate the virus from a flock within several years. Seropositive animals and offspring less than 1 year old can be removed from the premises and raised in a separate facility. Feeding OvLV-free colostrum or milk replacer or grafting to seronegative ewes may be an alternative. The keeper or clinician should test the flock twice annually until two consecutive negative herd tests are obtained; positive animals should be culled. The size of the flock may help determine the most effective approach. After a flock is established as negative for OvLV, all additions must test negative before joining the flock. Antibody titers may be low just before and after parturition because of the sequestering of antibodies in colostrum. A vaccine will most likely never be available because of the mutagenic properties of the virus. Management of the disease must be directed toward decreasing transmission and reducing the prevalence of seropositive animals within a flock.

References

1. Martin WB: Respiratory infections of sheep, *Comp Immun Micro Infect Dis* 19:171, 1996.
2. Jones GE, Gilmour JS: Non-progressive (atypical) pneumonia. In Jones GE, Gilmour JS, editors: *Diseases of sheep*, Oxford, UK, 1991, Blackwell Scientific.
3. Kanwar NS et al: Pneumonic pasteurellosis in goats, *Ind J Comp Micro Immun Infect Dis* 19:99, 1998.
4. Cutlip RC, Brogden KA, Lehmkhul HD: Changes in the lungs of lambs after intratracheal injection of lipopolysaccharide from *Pasteurella haemolytica* A1, *J Comp Path* 118:163, 1998.
5. Porter JF et al: Predisposition of specific pathogen-free lambs to *Pasteurella haemolytica* pneumonia by *Bordetella parapertussis* infection, *J Comp Path* 112:381, 1995.
6. Young JD, Griffith JW: Spontaneous *Pasteurella* pneumonia in adult laboratory goats complicated by superinfection with *Corynebacterium pseudotuberculosis* and *Muellerius capillaris*, *Lab Anim Sci* 35:409, 1985.
7. Sharma RK et al: Serotyping of *Pasteurella multocida* associated with caprine pneumonia, *Ind J Anim Health* 15:81, 1989.
8. Brogden KA, Lehmkuhl HD, Cutlip RC: *Pasteurella haemolytica* complicated respiratory infections in sheep and goats, *Vet Res* 29:233, 1998.
9. Cutlip RC et al: Lesions in lambs experimentally infected with ovine adenovirus serotype 6 and *Pasteurella haemolytica*, *J Vet Diagn Invest* 8:296, 1996.
10. Cutlip RC, Brogden KA, Lehmkuhl HD: Changes in the lungs of lambs after intratracheal injection of lipopolysaccharide from *Pasteurella haemolytica* A1, *J Comp Path* 118:163, 1998.
11. Porter JF et al: Predisposition of specific pathogen-free lambs to *Pasteurella haemolytica* pneumonia by *Bordetella parapertussis* infection, *J Comp Path* 112:381, 1995.
12. Davies DH, Herceg M, Thurley DC: Experimental infection of lambs with an adenovirus followed by *Pasteurella haemolytica*, *Vet Micro* 7:369, 1982.
13. Zamri-Saad M et al: Experimental infection of dexamethasone treated goats with *Pasteurella haemolytica* A2, *Brit Vet J* 147:565, 1991.
14. Debey BM et al: A comparison of the intratracheal intravenous and intratonsillar routes of inoculation of goats with *Pasteurella haemolytica*, *Vet Res Commun* 16:247, 1992.
15. Thomas LH et al: Evidence that blood-borne infection is involved in the pathogenesis of bovine pneumonic pasteurellosis, *Vet Path* 26:253, 1989.
16. Young JD, Griffith JW: Spontaneous *Pasteurella* pneumonia in adult laboratory goats complicated by superinfection with *Corynebacterium pseudotuberculosis* and *Muellerius capillaris*, *Lab Anim Sci* 35:409, 1985.
17. Sargison ND, Scott PR: Evaluation of antibiotic treatment of respiratory disease, including suspected septicemic pasteurellosis in five-week-old lambs, *Agri-Pract* 16:25, 1995.
18. Jakab GJ: Viral-bacterial interactions in pulmonary infection, *Adv Vet Sci Comp Med* 26:155, 1982.
19. Hansen DE, McCoy RD, Armstrong DA: Six vaccination trials in feedlot lambs for the control of lamb respiratory disease complex, *Agri-Pract* 16:19, 1995.
20. Black H, Donachie W, Duganzich D: An outbreak of *Pasteurella multocida* pneumonia in lambs during a field trial of a vaccine against *Pasteurella haemolytica*, *N Z Vet J* 45:58, 1997.
21. Chandrasekaran S et al: Evaluation of combined *Pasteurella* vaccines in control of sheep pneumonia, *Br Vet J* 147:437, 1991.
22. Black H, Duganzich D: A field evaluation of the efficacy of two vaccines against ovine pneumonic pasteurellosis, *N Z Vet J* 43:60, 1995.
23. Gilmour NJ et al: Experimental immunization of lambs against pneumonic pasteurellosis, *Res Vet Sci* 35:80, 1983.
24. Goyal SM et al: Prevalence of antibodies to seven viruses in a flock of ewes in Minnesota, *Am J Vet Res* 49:464, 1988.
25. Malone FE: Health problems associated with intensification of sheep, *Irish Vet J* 46:91, 1993.
26. Davies RL, Arkinsaw S, Selander RK: Evolutionary genetics of *Pasteurella haemolytica* isolates recovered from cattle and sheep, *Infect & Immun* 65:3585, 1997.
27. Davies DH, McCarthy AR, Penwarden RA: The effect of vaccination of lambs with live parainfluenza virus type 3 on pneumonia produced by parainfluenza virus type 3 and *Pasteurella haemolytica*, *N Z Vet J* 28:201, 1980.
28. Davies DH et al: Vaccination against ovine pneumonia: a progress report, *N Z Vet J* 31:87, 1983.
29. Salsbury DM: Control of respiratory disease and border disease of sheep, *Vet Med* 80:401, 1984.
30. Rodger JL: Parainfluenza 3 vaccination of sheep, *Vet Rec* 125:453, 1989.
31. Adair BM, McFerran JB: Survey for antibodies in respiratory syncytial viruses in two groups of sheep in Northern Ireland, *Vet Rec* 115:403, 1984.

32. Lehmkuhl HD, Cutlip RC, Brogden KA: Seroepidemiologic survey for adenovirus infection in lambs, *Am J Vet Res* 54:1277, 1993.

33. Baker JC: Ruminant respiratory system. In Smith BP, editor: *Large animal internal medicine*, St Louis, 1996, Mosby.

34. Dunbar MR et al: Seroprevalence of respiratory syncytial virus in free-ranging bighorn sheep, *J Am Vet Med Assoc* 187:1173, 1985.

35. Alansari H et al: Analysis of ruminant respiratory syncytial virus isolates by RNAse protection of the G glycoprotein transcripts, *J Vet Diagn Invest* 11:215, 1999.

36. Oberst RD et al: Characteristic differences in reverse transcription-polymerase chain reaction products of ovine, bovine, and human respiratory syncytial viruses, *J Vet Diagn Invest* 5:322, 1993.

37. van der Poel WH et al: Bovine respiratory syncytial virus antibodies in non-bovine species, *Arch Virol* 140:1549, 1995.

38. Bryson DG et al: Studies on the pathogenesis and interspecies transmission of respiratory syncytial virus isolated from sheep, *Am J Vet Res* 49:1424, 1988.

39. Sharma R, Woldehiwet Z: Pathogenesis of bovine respiratory syncytial virus in experimentally infected lambs, *Vet Micro* 23:267, 1990.

40. Trigo FJ et al: Pathogenesis of experimental bovine respiratory syncytial virus infection in sheep, *Am J Vet Res* 45:1663, 1984.

41. Lehmkuhl HD, Cutlip RC: Experimentally induced respiratory syncytial viral infection in lambs, *Am J Vet Res* 40:512, 1979.

42. Lehmkuhl HD, Cutlip RC: Experimental respiratory syncytial virus infection in feeder-age lambs, *Am J Vet Res* 40:1729, 1979.

43. Masot AJ et al: Pathological study of experimentally induced bovine respiratory syncytial viral infection in lambs, *J Vet Med Series B* 43:233, 1996.

44. Trigo FJ et al: Interaction of bovine respiratory syncytial virus and *Pasteurella haemolytica* in the ovine lung, *Am J Vet Res* 45:1671, 1984.

45. Al Darraji AM et al: Experimental infection of lambs with bovine respiratory syncytial virus and *Pasteurella haemolytica*: clinical and microbiologic studies, *Am J Vet Res* 43:236, 1982.

46. Sharma AK, Kharole MU: Pneumonic pasteurellosis in sheep, *Livestock Adv* 18:31, 1993.

47. Keles I, Woldehiwet Z, Murray RD: The effects of virus-specific antibodies on the replication of bovine respiratory syncytial virus in vitro and on clinical disease and immune responses in lambs, *Vet Immunol Immunopath* 62:221, 1998.

48. Sharma SN et al: Syncytia and giant cell pneumonic lesions in goat, *Ind J Vet Path* 20:48, 1996.

49. Redondo E et al: Spontaneous bovine respiratory syncytial virus infection in goats: pathological findings, *J Vet Med Series B* 41:27, 1994.

50. Buddle BM et al: A caprine pneumonia outbreak associated with caprine herpesvirus and *Pasteurella haemolytica* respiratory infections, *N Z Vet J* 38:28, 1990.

51. Engels M, Ackerman M: The pathogenesis of ruminant herpesviruses, *Proceedings of the Symposium on IBR and other ruminant herpesvirus infections*, ed 12, New York, 1995, Elsevier.

52. Berrios PE, McKercher DG, Knight HD: Pathogenicity of a caprine herpesvirus, *Am J Vet Res* 36:1763, 1975.

53. Whetstone CA, Evermann JF: Characterization of bovine herpesviruses isolated from six sheep and four goats by restriction endonuclease analysis and radioimmunoprecipitation, *Am J Vet Res* 49:781, 1988.

54. Buddle BM et al: Experimental respiratory infection of goats with caprine herpesvirus and *Pasteurella haemolytica*, *N Z Vet J* 38:22, 1990.

55. Maizan M et al: Isolation of parainfluenza type 3 and ovine herpes type 1 viruses associated with respiratory disease complex in sheep, *J Vet Malaysia* 6:43, 1994.

56. Scott FM et al: Infection of specific-pathogen free lambs with a herpesvirus isolated from pulmonary adenomatosis, *Arch Virol* 80:147, 1984.

57. Alley MR, Ionas G, Clarke JK: Chronic non-progressive pneumonia of sheep in New Zealand —A review of the role of *Mycoplasma ovipneumoniae*, *N Z Vet J* 47(15):155, 1999.

58. Niang M et al: Demonstration of a capsule on *Mycoplasma ovipneumoniae*, *Am J Vet Res* 59:557, 1998.

59. Martrenchar A, Bouchel D, Zoyem N: Isolation and experimental studies of *Mycoplasma mycoides* subsp. *mycoides* LC and *Mycoplasma ovipneumoniae* in goats in northern Cameroon, *Small Rum Res* 16:179, 1995.

60. Bouljihad M, Leipold HW: Preliminary pathologic observations of sheep with chronic non-progressive pneumonia, *Agri-Pract* 16:25, 1995.

61. Haziroglu R et al: Detection of *Mycoplasma ovipneumoniae* and *Pasteurella haemolytica* antigens by an immunoperoxidase technique in pneumonic ovine lungs, *Vet Path* 33:74, 1996.

62. Thirkell D et al: The humoral immune response of lambs experimentally infected with *Mycoplasma ovipneumoniae*, *Vet Micro* 24:143, 1990.

63. Clarke JK, Brown VG, Alley MR: Isolation and identification of mycoplasmas from the respiratory tract of sheep in New Zealand, *N Z Vet J* 22:117, 1974.

64. Niang M et al: Differential serologic response to *Mycoplasma ovipneumoniae* and *Mycoplasma argini* in lambs affected with chronic respiratory disease, *J Vet Diagn Invest* 11:34, 1999.

65. Eissa SI, El-Shater SA, Dardeer MAA: Efficacy of quinolones and aminoglycosides against bovine and ovine mycoplasma, *Egypt J Agric Res* 77(15):1361, 1999.

66. Niang M et al: Occurrence of autoantibodies to cilia in lambs with a 'coughing syndrome', *Vet Immunol Immunopath* 64:191, 1998.

67. Leach RH, Erno H, Macowan KJ: Proposal for designation of F38-type caprine mycoplasmas as *Mycoplasma capricolum* subsp. *capripneumoniae* subsp. *nov.* and consequent obligatory relegation of strains currently classified as *Mycoplasma capricolum* to an additional new subspecies, *M. capricolum* subsp. *capricolum* subsp. *nov*, *Int J Sys Bacteriol* 43(15):603, 1993.

68. Hotzel H, Sachse K, Pfutzner H: A PCR scheme for differentiation of organisms belonging to the *Mycoplasma mycoides* cluster, *Vet Micro* 49:31, 1996.

69. Rodriguez F et al: An immunohistochemical method of detecting *Mycoplasma* species antigens by use of monoclonal antibodies on paraffin sections of pneumonic bovine and caprine lungs, *J Vet Med* 43:429, 1996.

70. Rodriguez JL et al: A pathological and immunohistochemical study of goat kids undergoing septicaemic disease caused by *Mycoplasma capricolum* subsp. *capricolum*, *Mycoplasma mycoides* subsp. *capri* and *Mycoplasma mycoides* subsp. *mycoides* (large colony type), *J Vet Med Series B* 45:141, 1998.

71. Ross RF: Mycoplasma—animal pathogens. In Kahane I, Adoni A, editors: *Rapid diagnosis of Mycoplasma*, New York, 1993, Plenum Press.

72. Levisohn S, Davidson IC, Rapport E: Application of an ELISA test for diagnosis of caprine mycoplasmosis, *IOM Letters* 1:499, 1990.

73. Jonas AM, Barber TL: *Mycoplasma mycoides* var, *capri* isolated from a goat in Connecticut, *J Infect Dis* 119:126, 1969.

74. Damassa AJ: Prevalence of mycoplasmas and mites in the external auditory meatus of goats, *Calif Vet* 12(15):10, 1983.

75. East NE et al: Milkborne outbreak of *Mycoplasma mycoides* subspecies *mycoides* infection in a commercial goat dairy, *J Am Vet Med Assoc* 182:1338, 1983.

76. Rodriguez JL et al: High mortality in goats associated with the isolation of a strain of *Mycoplasma mycoides* subsp. *mycoides* (large colony type), *J Vet Med Series B* 42:587, 1995.

77. Cottew GS, Yeats FR: Mycoplasmas and mites in the ears of clinically normal goats, *Aust Vet J* 59:77, 1982.

78. Nayak NC, Bhowmik MK: Pathogenicity of *Mycoplasma mycoides* subsp. *mycoides* (large colony type) for goat kids, *Small Rum Res* 5:155, 1991.

79. Rahman T, Singh B: Clinicopathological features of pulmonary mycoplasma in goats, *Ind Vet J* 67:915, 1990.

80. Gutierriz C et al: Clinico-pathological and haematological findings in goat kids experimentally infected simultaneously with *Mycoplasma mycoides* subsp. *capri* and *Mycoplasma mycoides* subsp. *mycoides* (large colony-type), *Small Rum Res* 31:187, 1999.

81. Brandao E: Isolation and identification of *Mycoplasma mycoides* subspecies *mycoides* SC strains in sheep and goats, *Vet Rec* 136:98, 1995.

82. Rosendal S, Erno H, Wyand DS: *Mycoplasma mycoides* subspecies *mycoides* as a cause of polyarthritis in goats, *J Am Vet Med Assoc* 175:378, 1979.

83. Rodriguez JL et al: Clinicopathological and haematological study of experimentally infected goat kids with *Mycoplasma capricolum* subsp. *capricolum*, *J Appl Anim Res* 2:169, 1999.

84. East NE: Common infectious conditions, *Small Ruminants for the Mixed Animal Practitioner, Western Veterinary Conference*, 1998, Las Vegas, NV.

85. Butler AB, Anderson KL, Lyman RL: Mycoplasmal polyarthritis and septicemia in a goat herd, *Large Anim Pract* 15:23, 1998.

86. Blackwell TE et al: Differences in signs and lesions in sheep and goats with enterotoxemia induced by intraduodenal infusion of *Clostridium perfringens* type D, *Am J Vet Res* 52:1147, 1991.

87. Bar-Moshe B, Rapoport E, Brenner J: Vaccination trials against *Mycoplasma mycoides* subsp. *mycoides* (large colony-type) infection in goats, *Isr J Med Sci* 20:972, 1984.

88. Boermans HJ, Ruegg PL, Leach M: Ethylene glycol toxicosis in a pygmy goat, *J Am Vet Med Assoc* 193:694, 1988.

89. McMartin DA, Macowan KJ, Swift LL: A century of classical contagious caprine pleuropneumonia: from original description to aetiology, *Br Vet J* 136:507, 1980.

90. Macowan KJ, Minette JE: The role of *Mycoplasma* strain F38 in contagious caprine pleuropneumonia (CCCP) in Kenya, *Vet Rec* 101:380, 1977.

91. Darzi MM et al: The pathogenicity and pathogenesis of *Mycoplasma capricolum* subsp. *capripneumoniae* (F38) in the caprine mammary gland, *Vet Res Commun* 22:155, 1998.

92. Smith MC: Exotic diseases of small ruminants, *Small Ruminants for the Mixed Animal Practitioner, Western Veterinary Conference*, 1998, Las Vegas, NV.

93. Rurangirwa FR et al: A latex agglutination test for field diagnosis of contagious caprine pleuropneumonia, *Vet Rec* 121:191, 1987.

94. Johansson KE, Persson A, Persson M: Diagnosis of contagious caprine and contagious bovine pleuropneumonia by PCR and restriction enzyme analysis. Towards livestock disease diagnosis and control in the 21st century, *Proceedings of an International symposium on Diagnosis and Control of Livestock Diseases Using Nuclear and Related Techniques*, Vienna, Austria, 1998, International Atomic Energy Agency.

95. Shaheen M, Haque Shaheen M, Haque S: Therapeutic efficacy of tiamulin hydrogen fumarate, enrofloxacin, oxytetracycline and lincomycin in caprine mycoplasmal pneumonia, *Ind J Vet Med* 19(15):74, 1999.

96. Wesonga HO et al: Late lesions of experimental contagious caprine pleuropneumonia caused by *Mycoplasma capricolum* ssp. *capripneumoniae*, *J Vet Med* 45(15):105, 1998.

97. Sikdar A, Sirvastava NC, Uppal PK: Development of a killed vaccine against caprine pleuropneumonia: preliminary investigation in goats, *Ind Vet J* 70(15):600, 1993.

98. Rurangirwa FR et al: An inactivated vaccine for contagious caprine pleuropneumonia, *Vet Rec* 121:397, 1987.

99. Kimberling CV: *Jensen and Swift's diseases of sheep*, Philadelphia, 1988, Lea & Febiger.

100. Polataz JL, Christensen NR: Bovine respiratory infections. I. Psittacosis-lymphogranuloma venereum group of viruses as etiologic agents, *J Am Vet Med Assoc* 134(15):222, 1959.

101. Smith JA: The interstitial pneumonias. In Smith BP, editor: *Large animal internal medicine*, St Louis, 1996, Mosby.

102. Perez-Martinez JA, Storz J: Chlamydial infections in cattle. Part I, *Mod Vet Pract* 66(15):517, 1985.

103. Rosadio RH et al: Lesions and retroviruses associated with naturally occurring ovine pulmonary carcinoma (sheep pulmonary adenomatosis), *Vet Path* 25:58, 1988.

104. Rosadio RH et al: Retrovirus-associated ovine pulmonary carcinoma (sheep pulmonary adenomatosis) and lymphoid interstitial pneumonia. I. Lesion development and age susceptibility, *Vet Path* 25:475, 1988.

105. Tustin RC et al: Experimental transmission of jaagsiekte (ovine pulmonary adenomatosis) to goats, *Onderstepoort J Vet Res* 55:27, 1988.

106. Verwoerd DW, Tustin RC, Payne AL: Jaagsiekte: an infectious pulmonary adenomatosis of sheep. In Olsen RG, Krakowka S, Blacksee JR, editors: *Comparative pathobiology of viral diseases*, Boca Raton, FL, 1985, CRC Press.

107. Martin WB: Respiratory infections of sheep, *Comp Immun Micro Infect Dis* 19:171, 1996.

108. DeMartini JC, Rosadio RH, Lairmore MD: The etiology and pathogenesis of ovine pulmonary carcinoma (sheep pulmonary adenomatosis), *Vet Micro* 17:219, 1988.

109. Lofstedt J: Progressive viral pneumonias of sheep and goats. In Smith BP, editor: *Large animal internal medicine*, St Louis, 1996, Mosby.

110. DeMartini JC, York DF: Retrovirus-associated neoplasms of the respiratory system of sheep and goats, *Vet Clin North Am* 13:55, 1997.

111. Snowder GD et al: Prevalence and effect of subclinical ovine progressive pneumonia virus infection on ewe wool and lamb production, *J Am Vet Med Assoc* 197:475, 1990.

112. Snowder GD et al: Effect of ovine progressive pneumonia on ewe milk production, *J Anim Sci* 76(suppl. 2):171, 1989.

113. Brodie SJ, Snowder GD, DeMartini JC: Ovine progressive pneumonia: advances and prospects for control, *Sheep Res J* 8:116, 1992.

114. Watt NJ, Scott PR, Gessert M: Maedi visna ovine progressive pneumonia virus infection: a comparative study of the disease in the United Kingdom and the United States, *Agri-Pract* 16:29, 1995.

115. Knowles DP et al: Evaluation of agar gel immunodiffusion serology using caprine and ovine lentiviral antigens for detection of antibody to caprine arthritis-encephalitis virus, *J Clin Micro* 32:243, 1994.

116. Cheevers WP, McGuire TC: The lentiviruses: maedi/visna, caprine arthritis-encephalitis, and equine infectious anemia, *Adv Virus Res* 34:189, 1988.

117. Cutlip RC et al: Seroprevalence of ovine progressive pneumonia virus in various domestic and wild animal species, and species susceptibility to the virus, *Am J Vet Res* 52:189, 1991.

118. de la Concha-Bermejillo A et al: Seroprevalence of ovine progressive pneumonia in Texas, *Sheep and Goat Res J* 14(15):127, 1998.

119. Cutlip RC et al: Seroprevalence of ovine progressive pneumonia virus in sheep in the United States as assessed by analyses of voluntarily submitted samples, *Am J Vet Res* 53:976, 1992.

120. Brodie SJ et al: Maternal factors associated with prenatal transmission of ovine lentivirus, *J Infect Dis* 169:653, 1994.

121. Cutlip RC et al: Effects on ovine fetuses of exposure to ovine progressive pneumonia virus, *Am J Vet Res* 43:82, 1982.

122. de la Concha-Bermejillo A et al: Venereal shedding of ovine lentivirus in infected rams, *Am J Vet Res* 57:684, 1996.

123. de la Concha-Bermejillo A et al: Pathologic responses of lambs to experimental inoculation with *Acholeplasma laidlawii, J Vet Diagn Invest* 8:115, 1996.

124. Froeling J: Review and case report on ovine progressive pneumonia, *Agri-Pract* 13:35, 1992.

125. Smith C: Ovine lentivirus: a real or imagined threat, *J Am Vet Med Assoc* 200:139, 1991.

126. DeMartini JC et al: Pathogenesis of lymphoid interstitial pneumonia in natural and experimental ovine lentivirus infection, *Clin Infect Dis* 17(suppl. 1):S236, 1993.

127. Cutlip RC et al: Mastitis associated with ovine progressive pneumonia virus infection in sheep, *Am J Vet Res* 46:326, 1975.

128. Knowles DP, McGuire TC, Cheever WP: Ovine progressive pneumonia (visna/maedi). In Knowles DP, McGuire TC, Cheever WP, editors: *Veterinary diagnostic virology: a practitioner's guide,* St Louis, 1992, Mosby.

129. Kwang J et al: Evaluation of an ELISA for detection of ovine progressive pneumonia antibodies using a recombinant transmembrane envelope protein, *J Vet Diagn Invest* 5:189, 1993.

130. Kwang J, Cutlip RC: Detection of antibodies to ovine lentivirus using a recombinant antigen derived from the env gene[+], *Biochem Biophys Res Commun* 183:1040, 1992.

131. Barlough J et al: Double-nested polymerase chain reaction for detection of caprine arthritis-encephalitis virus proviral DNA in blood, milk, and tissues of infected goats, *J Virol Meth* 50:101, 1994.

132. Cutlip RC et al: Ovine progressive pneumonia (maedi-visna) in sheep, *Vet Micro* 17:237, 1988.

133. Cutlip RC, Jackson TA, Lehmkuhl HD: Lesions of ovine progressive pneumonia: interstitial pneumonitis and encephalitis, *Am J Vet Res* 40:1370, 1979.

134. Brodie SJ et al: Current concepts in the epizootiology, diagnosis, and economic importance of ovine progressive pneumonia in North America: a review, *Small Rum Res* 27:1, 1997.

ATYPICAL PNEUMONIAS

Verminous Pneumonia

Of the parasites known to cause bronchitis in sheep and goats, *Dictyocaulus filaria* is the most pathogenic, *Muellerius capillaris* (Figure 5-8) is the most common and least pathogenic, and *Protostrongylus rufescens* is intermediate in pathogenicity.

Dictyocaulus usually appears as a full infection of 2- to 18-month-old sheep. These animals generally have chronic fever, cough, nasal discharge, tachypnea, anorexia, and weight loss. At necropsy the parasites may be observed in the bronchi, especially in the diaphragmatic lobes (Figure 5-9). Pulmonary edema, emphysema, and atelectatic and pus-filled lobules also may be evident.

P. rufescens can cause serious disease in domestic sheep, although infestation is rarely reported in North America.[1] The life cycle requires an intermediate host of either a snail or slug, and the adult nematodes live in the bronchioles. The first-stage larvae are best diagnosed in fecal samples by use of the Baermann technique, but they also may be found in nasal secretions. Clinical signs in a recent report

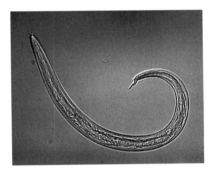

Figure 5-8   A light micrograph of first-stage larvae of *Muellerius capillaris* recovered by the Baermann technique. (Courtesy Dr. Byron L. Blagburn, Auburn, Alabama.)

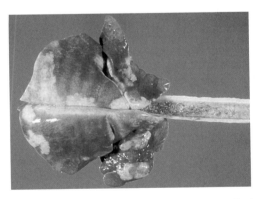

Figure 5-9   A set of lungs infested with *Dictyocaulus filaria*. Note the larvae in the trachea. (Courtesy Dr. Byron L. Blagburn, Auburn, Alabama.)

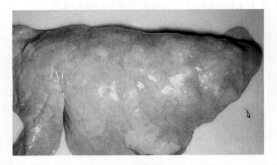

Figure 5-10 A set of lungs infested with *Muellerius capillaris.* Note the light-colored, raised nodules over the dorsal aspect of the caudal lobes. (Courtesy Dr. Byron L. Blagburn, Auburn, Alabama.)

included diarrhea, weight loss, mucopurulent nasal discharge, tachypnea, and increased respiratory sounds.[1]

M. capillaris causes few clinical signs. However, necropsy of infected animals reveals gray or greenish subpleural granulomas in the caudal lobes. Goats are reported to have widespread interstitial pneumonia without nodular lesions (Figure 5-10).[2,3] *M. capillaris* may predispose animals to secondary infections and reduce general health.[2,4]

Treatment. Treatment is with either ivermectin (200 μg/kg SC) or fenbendazole (7.5 mg/kg by mouth [PO]). Refractory cases of *M. capillaris* may require larger doses of either fenbendazole (15 mg/kg at 35-day intervals to 30 mg/kg at 30-day intervals) or ivermectin (300 μg/kg) because immature stages of *Muellerius* may survive lower doses or single treatments.[5,6] Larval stages of *M. capillaris* may survive in the pasture from one season to the next, so goats may be reinfected.[7]

Prevention. Prevention by eliminating the intermediate host mollusk is helpful, but most difficult.

Aspiration Pneumonia

Pathogenesis. Aspiration pneumonia is caused by the entry of foreign material into the lower respiratory tract, resulting in pulmonary necrosis. This condition usually results from errors when using stomach tubes or drenching equipment. It also may be a sequela to neurogenic or pathologic damage of the pharynx, cleft palate, or anesthesia (see Chapter 16).

Clinical signs. Clinical signs depend on the amount of material that enters the respiratory tract. Large quantities of fluid often produce sudden death from asphyxia. Coughing; shallow, rapid respirations; and frothing from the nose and mouth may be observed before the animal collapses and dies. Gurgling or fluid sounds may be auscultated over the trachea. Aspiration of smaller volumes of

foreign material result in dyspnea, abnormal lung sounds such as crackles and wheezes, signs of septicemia, foul breath odor (which initially may smell like the fluid aspirated), and nasal discharge that may contain some of the aspirated material. A gangrenous pneumonia generally develops and most affected animals die within a week.

Diagnosis. The diagnosis is based on clinical signs and history. Radiographs may demonstrate a severe cranioventral bronchopneumonia. A CBC demonstrates acute inflammation with leukopenia, left shift of neutrophils, and elevated fibrinogen. Sampling of tracheal fluid may reveal numerous cell types and debris, with culture of the fluid revealing a mixture of organisms including *Corynebacterium, Fusobacterium, Bacteroides, Escherichia coli, Klebsiella, Pseudomonas, Staphylococcus aureus,* and *Streptococcus.* Necropsy of dead animals verifies the presumptive diagnosis, revealing cranioventral pneumonia, food material in the airways, gangrenous lesions, and possibly pleuritis.

Treatment. The treatment is lengthy and requires broad-spectrum antibiotics (penicillin, tetracycline, florfenicol), NSAIDs, and supportive care. Nasal oxygen may be beneficial.

Prevention. Most cases can be avoided with preventative measures. Especially with extremely sick animals the clinician should ascertain the correct placement of the stomach tube by blowing into it while another person auscultates over the left paralumbar fossa. When drenching animals, clinicians and keepers should avoid holding the head too high or administering liquid too fast. The overzealous use of fluids in treating choke cases should be avoided. Specific neurologic diseases such as lead toxicity and rabies may all result in aspiration pneumonia or metabolic disturbances such as hypocalcemia. Withholding water and food for an appropriate period before anesthesia is crucial; also, maintaining recumbent animals in a sternal position helps prevent the aspiration of foreign materials (see Chapter 16).

PLANT TOXICITIES

Atypical Interstitial Pneumonia

Ingestion of *Perilla* mint *(Perilla frutescens),* a common weed in the Southeastern United States, results in respiratory toxicity. This weed, also known as *purple mint, wild coleus,* and *beefsteak plant,* has a pneumotoxin in its leaves and seeds. The plant is purple-tinged at maturity and has square stems; the flower and seed stage (occurring from August to October) is the most toxic. After being absorbed by the rumen, the toxin is thought to be metabolized by a mixed function oxidase system, resulting in toxic intermediates that damage type I pneumocytes and bronchiolar epithelial cells. This causes hyaline membrane formation and proliferation of type II pneumocytes, leading to adenomatosis.

Clinical signs. The clinical signs of toxicity include an acute onset of dyspnea and tachypnea, extension of the head and neck, open-mouth breathing, frothing at the mouth, and sudden death. Exertion may exacerbate signs and precipitate death.[8]

Diagnosis. Necropsy reveals distended lungs (some with rib impressions) that fail to collapse on opening of the chest. The lungs are wet, heavy, emphysematous, and edematous; emphysematous bullae and froth in the airways are often observed (Figure 5-11). Histopathologic examination reveals interstitial edema and emphysema, congestion, and alveolar epithelial hyperplasia.[8]

Treatment. Treatment is supportive and relies on minimizing stress.

    Moldy sweet potato ingestion can result in a similar condition. 4-Ipomeanol is a furanoterpene mycotoxin produced by *Fusarium solani* growing on moldy sweet potatoes. The pathogenesis, clinical signs, lesions, and treatment are similar to that for *Perilla* mint.

    Ingestion of **Brassica** species plants (rape, kale, turnip tops, beet tops) also may result in atypical interstitial pneumonia. These plants contain large amounts of D,L-tryptophan, which is converted in the rumen to 3-methyl indole, which is absorbed and metabolized by a mixed function oxidase system in the respiratory tract, producing toxic intermediates. Increased rates of morbidity and mortality are observed. Clinical signs and treatment are similar to those for intoxication with moldy sweet potato and *Perilla* mint.

Hydrogen Cyanide Toxicity

Hydrocyanic acid (HCN) toxicity is caused by the ingestion of plants containing cyanogenetic glycosides. Damage to the plant (wilt, frost, drought) results in the release of cyanide, which blocks cellular respiration by deactivating the cytochrome oxidase enzyme of oxidative transport. As a result, blood in the affected animals is bright red because hemoglobin cannot release oxygen to the tissues. This only occurs when the detoxification capabilities of the liver and kidney are exceeded. All livestock are susceptible to the effects of HCN, but sheep and cattle are at the greatest risk.[9]

Clinical signs. Clinical signs include dyspnea, salivation, anxiety, staggering, tremors, and terminal convulsions. Sudden death is common in affected animals.

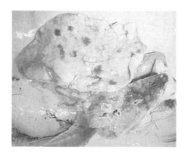

Figure 5-11 *Perilla* mint toxicity. Interstitial pneumonia in sheep. Note the distended appearance of the lungs.

Diagnosis. The diagnosis is made by observation of clinical signs and a history of access to toxic plants. The diagnosis may be confirmed by identifying 1.4 and 10 μg of HCN/g of liver and rumen contents, respectively.[10] Rapid intake of 2 to 4 mg HCN/kg of body weight is generally lethal.[10]

Treatment. Treatment includes administration of sodium nitrate (16 mg/kg IV) followed by methylene blue or sodium thiosulfate (30 to 40 mg/kg IV). The drugs must be given soon and may need to be repeated.

Nitrate-Nitrite Toxicity

Pathogenesis. Nitrate toxicity may be observed in both sheep and goats because of the conversion of nitrate to nitrite in the rumen. Nitrite binds to iron ions (Fe 2+), and hemoglobin is converted into methemoglobin, which has a greatly decreased ability to transport oxygen. This results in hypoxia. When levels of methemoglobin exceed 30%, the blood appears brown.

Clinical signs. Clinical signs include dyspnea, tachypnea, weakness, exercise intolerance, and sudden death. Spontaneous recovery may be observed in mildly affected sheep and goats.

Diagnosis. Diagnosis is confirmed by assessing the nitrite levels of the blood, urine, or aqueous humor. High nitrate levels in feed or water also may be diagnostic.

Treatment. Treatment is with methylene blue (1 to 2 mg/kg of a 1% solution IV every 6 to 8 hours).

Prevention. Keepers can prevent nitrate-nitrite toxicity by ensuring that nitrate comprises no more than 0.6% of the diet.[11] Drought, recent fertilization, and retarded growth of plants increase the risk of nitrate toxicity.

OTHER DISEASES CAUSING RESPIRATORY SIGNS

Caprine Arthritis-Encephalitis

CAE virus (CAEV) causes a persistent lentiviral infection of goats that produces several progressive, debilitating diseases. It is caused by a C-type retrovirus of the subfamily *Lentivirinae,* as is OPP. The most common route of transmission for CAEV is by a kid ingesting milk or colostrum from an infected doe. Horizontal transmission also may occur, but only after prolonged contact. The virus infects mononuclear cells, which are then infected for life.

Although the most common manifestation of CAEV infection is arthritis, an interstitial pneumonia has been reported in infected kids and adults. It produces chronic pneumonia, weight loss, and dyspnea.[12] Lesions occur predominantly in the caudal or cranioventral lobes. The lesions of CAEV interstitial pneumonia closely resemble those of OPP. Experimentally, the chronic interstitial lesions have not been reproduced with inoculation of CAEV.

Other causes of pneumonia should be considered because numerous agents may be responsible for the clinical presentation. Serologic testing using either an AGID or ELISA test may help identify the cause of infection. Using the AGID test in conjunction with PCR testing is best for eradication and control purposes.[12a] Virus isolation is not routinely performed, but histopathologic examination of tissues may provide a diagnosis. No treatment or vaccine is available for CAEV. Prevention is crucial for maintaining CAEV-negative herds. Separation and testing of new animals before mixing with the preexisting population are important, as is routine testing of animals to decrease the incidence of seroconversion. Kids from infected or suspicious does should be removed at birth and fed heat-treated colostrum, cow colostrum, and pasteurized milk until they are weaned (see Chapters 9 and 14).[13]

Tuberculosis

Pathogenesis. Tuberculosis is a more serious problem in goats than in sheep. *Mycobacterium bovis* is widespread in some goat flocks but is reported rarely in sheep.[14,15] Close proximity to infected cattle herds and wildlife is thought to play a role in increased prevalence. Occasionally *M. avium* or *M. tuberculosis* may produce disease.[16] Spread of the organism is usually by respiratory secretions, feces, milk, urine, vaginal discharge, semen, and draining lymph nodes.[17] The route of entry in ruminants is the respiratory tract. The organism then invades local lymph nodes, where it causes necrosis surrounded by a granuloma. The abdominal cavity is sometimes involved, suggesting ingestion as a possible route of infection, possibly as a result of the coughing and subsequent swallowing of lung fluid.[14]

Clinical signs. Clinical signs include weight loss and mild signs of respiratory disease because the primary focus of the disease is generally the lung. A deep, moist, chronic cough may be heard in the early stages, with tachypnea, dyspnea, and abnormal lung sounds identified in the latter stages. Enlarged local lymph nodes may contribute to stridor, dysphagia, and bloat.

Diagnosis. Necropsy lesions include granulomatous lymph nodes that are more prevalent in the respiratory nodes but also occur in the liver and mesenteric lymph nodes. The granulomas are encapsulated and filled with yellow to orange, creamy to caseous, purulent material and gritty foci. Histologically, lesions consist of central calcification and caseation surrounded by zones of epithelioid cells and Langhans' giant cells enclosed in fibrous capsules.[14] Acid-fast organisms may be present. These lesions should be differentiated from those of caseous lymphadenitis.

Prevention. Suspected cases should be tested by intradermal skin testing with 0.1 ml of mammalian tuberculin purified protein derivative injected in the caudal tail fold; the injections are assessed in 66 to 78 hours as negative, suspect, or reactor. Keepers should have suspect animals further tested by federal veterinarians using the comparative cervical test. Depending on governmental regulations, reactors are quarantined, appropriately identified, and sent to an approved slaughter plant or disposed of under regulatory supervision.[16] False positive results may occur as a result of concurrent *M. paratuberculosis, M. avium,* or *M. tuberculosis* infection. When all animals older than 12 months have tested negative consecutively two times annually, they should be declared free of tuberculosis.

Caseous Lymphadenitis

Caseous lymphadenitis is a chronic insidious disease of sheep and goats caused by a gram-positive rod, *Corynebacterium pseudotuberculosis,* often found in manure, soil, on the skin, and in infected organs.[18,19] The organism has two subspecies, one responsible for caseous lymphadenitis in small ruminants and the other causing ulcerative lymphadenitis in horses and cattle. Although the disease is of great importance economically to the sheep and goat industry because of carcass condemnation, it is known primarily for causing a peripheral lymphadenopathy. Prevalence rates may reach 50% to 60% or greater.[20] The organism most often gains entrance to the body through contamination of superficial wounds or mucous membranes or indirectly through fomites such as shearing blades, feeders, grooming equipment, and bedding. Transmission also may occur by inhalation or ingestion. The organism may survive in the environment for long periods. After it gains entrance to the body, the organism follows lymphatic vessels and migrates to regional lymph nodes, where it may then disseminate to other parts of the body.

Clinical signs.   When the infection affects the respiratory system, clinical signs include weight loss, dyspnea, tachypnea, and a chronic cough.[21]

Diagnosis.   Pulmonary radiographs may reveal one or more masses, but a definitive diagnosis may be obtained by culture of a transtracheal wash. In the authors' and others' experiences, serologic tests using a synergistic hemolysis inhibition method are not reliable.[22] Various ELISA tests have been developed with varying specificities and sensitivities, yet few laboratories run these tests routinely.[23] Involvement of the mandibular, retropharyngeal, prescapular, prefemoral, and supramammary lymph nodes is common. In the thoracic cavity, abscesses occur in the lung parenchyma, mediastinal lymph nodes, and bronchial lymph nodes. The number of lung abscesses may range from a few to 20 or 30.[20] Lymph nodes in the abdominal viscera and skeletal tissue are less likely to be involved.[24] Involvement of internal nodes is more likely in older animals because morbidity rates increase with age; as much as 70% of an infected flock may be infected.[25] Internal involvement is thought to contribute to the "thin ewe" or "fading goat" syndromes[20,26] (see Chapter 14).

Prevention.   Identification of affected animals should result in culling and a greater attempt to identify affected individuals and prevent contamination of others and the environment. Good hygienic practices during lambing or kidding, docking, and shearing may all help to prevent exposure to the organism.[19] Vaccination has produced equivocal results but may reduce the number of lesions and the severity of the disease. Anecdotal reports suggest reactions may be encountered when using sheep vaccines for caseous lymphadenitis in goats.

Diaphragmatic Hernia

Herniation may be congenital or acquired. In ruminants the reticulum usually herniates through the diaphragm after parturition, breeding (males), or a traumatic incident. Increased intraabdominal pressure may be responsible for the herniation in cases that have no association with a foreign body.[27] Affected animals may demonstrate signs of dyspnea, weakness, and possibly weight loss.[27] Radiography can be helpful in diagnosing suspected cases. If diagnosed early, surgical correction may be curative. Surgical approaches are similar to those used in other species.

Neoplasia

Although they are uncommon, lymphosarcomas, pleural mesotheliomas, adenocarcinomas, and squamous cell tumors may be identified in the respiratory tracts of sheep and goats.[28] OPC has been discussed previously in this chapter. Thoracocentesis and radiography can be used for preliminary diagnosis of pulmonary tumors; the diagnosis is confirmed at necropsy.

Coccidioidomycosis

The agent that causes coccidioidomycosis, *Coccidioides immitis,* is a soil fungus whose spores may infect sheep and goats through inhalation and possibly ingestion or cutaneous abrasion. The disease is not contagious but is enzootic in the southwestern United States. The disease manifests as chronic weight loss and a persistent cough. Affected sheep are febrile and have abscesses in peripheral lymph nodes.[29] Necropsy of affected animals reveals granulomas with creamy purulent material, most commonly in the bronchial and mediastinal lymph nodes. Intradermal and complement fixation tests use coccidioidin, an extract of the fungus, for diagnosis. Culture or histopathologic examination and identification of the spherules also are diagnostic. No effective treatment is available.

Pneumocystis carinii Pneumonia

Pneumonia and sudden death in goats has been reported to be caused by the sporozoan *Pneumocystis carinii.*[30] Affected animals generally have had a history of chronic disease that allowed them to become immunocompromised and infected.

Clinical signs.   Clinical signs include fever, weight loss, tachypnea, mucopurulent nasal discharge, chronic cough, weakness, tachycardia, and death. The diagnosis is made by observing the organisms in tracheal wash fluid silver-stained sections from lung biopsy. A diffuse and locally extensive interstitial pneumonia is observed on necropsy. The clinician should rule out caseous lymphadenitis and tuberculosis in affected animals. Treatment of animals is generally not effective.

Pneumothorax

Although it is uncommon in sheep and goats, pneumothorax should be considered in animals with inspiratory dyspnea and an abdominal component to breathing. Rupture of an emphysematous bulla as a result of persistent coughing or straining may produce this condition. Animals with these clinical signs and a history of attack by predators also may exhibit subcutaneous emphysema and bite wounds. Usually the mediastinum is complete in sheep and goats, so this condition presents unilaterally, thus enhancing survival. Reduced lung sounds are auscultated on the affected side and a difference in resonance is noted between sides on percussion. Radiographs may confirm the diagnosis. Removal of air through a one-way suction catheter results in substantial improvement of the case. Because pleuritis is a possible complication, these animals should receive antibiotics for at least 1 week.

Pleuritis

Pleuritis is rare in sheep and goats and almost always occurs as a sequela to another disease process such as pasteurellosis, extension of peritonitis, liver abscesses, tuberculosis, traumatic injuries to the chest, hypoproteinemia, and septicemia.

Clinical signs. Clinical signs attributable to pleuritis include weight loss, decreased milk production, fever, depression, reluctance to move, extended head and neck, dyspnea, restricted respiratory movements, soft and suppressed cough, pain on percussion of the chest with an identifiable fluid line, and friction rubs or silence on auscultation because of increased fluid in the pleural space.

Diagnosis. Clinical diagnosis may be enhanced by a CBC indicating anemia of chronic disease or an acute inflammatory response with hyperfibrinogenemia. Hyperglobulinemia may occur in more chronic cases. Ultrasound of the chest or thoracocentesis can confirm the diagnosis.

Treatment. If possible, the clinician should drain and culture fluid from the pleural space. If the protein level is less than 2.5 g/dl or the cell count is less than 3000 cells/mm^3 in the pleural fluid, a transudate is present, most likely caused by hypoproteinemia, right heart failure, neoplasia, or acorn toxicity. The clinician should therefore treat the underlying problem. Broad-spectrum antibiotics, analgesics, and supportive care are indicated. However, the prognosis is generally guarded.

Acknowledgments

Special thanks to Rachel Eddleman and Carolyn Zorn of Auburn University, Auburn, Alabama, for technical assistance.

References

1. Mansfield LS et al: Lungworm infection in a sheep flock in Maryland, *J Am Vet Med Assoc* 202:601, 1993.
2. Nimmo JS: Case report: six cases of verminous pneumonia (*Muellerius* sp.) in goats, *Can Vet J* 21:49, 1979.
3. Kanwar NS, Paliwal OP, Ram K: Verminous pneumonia in goats, *J Vet Parasitol* 12:139, 1998.
4. Kazacos KR et al: Fenbendazole for the treatment of pulmonary and gastrointestinal helminths in pygmy goats, *J Am Vet Med Assoc* 179:1255, 1981.
5. McCraw BM, Menzies PI: Treatment of goats infected with the lungworm *Muellerius capillaris*, *Can Vet J* 27:287, 1986.
6. Bliss EL, Greiner EC: Efficacy of fenbendazole and cambendazole against *Muellerius capillaris* in dairy goats, *Am J Vet Res* 46:1923, 1985.
7. Helle O: The efficacy of fenbendazole and albendazole against the lungworm *Muellerius capillaris* in goats, *Vet Parasitol* 22:293, 1986.
8. Smith JA: The interstitial pneumonias. In Smith BP, editor: *Large animal internal medicine*, St Louis, 1996, Mosby.
9. Galey FD: Disorders caused by toxicants. In Smith BP, editor: *Large animal internal medicine*, St Louis, 1996, Mosby.
10. Diseases of the respiratory system. In Kimberling CV, editor: *Jensen and Swift's diseases of sheep*, Philadelphia, 1988, Lea & Febiger.
11. Radostits OM et al: *Veterinary medicine*, Philadelphia, 2000, WB Saunders.
12. Ellis TM, Robinson WF, Wilcox GE: The pathology and aetiology of lung lesions in goats infected with caprine arthritis-encephalitis virus, *Aust Vet J* 65:69, 1988.
12a. James K. Collins, personal communication, June 2000.
13. Rowe JD, East N: Risk factors for transmission and methods for control of caprine arthritis-encephalitis virus infection, *Vet Clin North Am* 13(15):35, 1997.
14. Davidson RM, Alley MR, Beatson NS: Tuberculosis in a flock of sheep, *N Z Vet J* 29:1, 1981.
15. Cordes DO et al: Observations on tuberculosis caused by *Mycobacterium bovis* in sheep, *N Z Vet J* 29:60, 1981.
16. Gutierrez M, Garcia Marin JF: *Cryptococcus neoformans* and *Mycobacterium bovis* causing granulomatous pneumonia in a goat, *Vet Pathol* 36:445, 1999.
17. Baker JC: Ruminant respiratory system. In Smith BP, editor: *Large animal internal medicine*, St Louis, 1996, Mosby.
18. DeMartini JC et al: Pathogenesis of lymphoid interstitial pneumonia in natural and experimental ovine lentivirus infection, *Clin Infect Dis* 17(suppl. 1):S236, 1993.
19. Ellis JA: Ovine caseous lymphadenitis, *Comp Cont Ed Pract Vet* 5:S505, 1983.
20. Pugh DG: Caseous lymphadenitis in small ruminants, *Prac North Am Vet Conf* 11:982, 1997.
21. Jones SL, Schumacher J: What is your diagnosis? Mineralized retropharyngeal mass (3 × 5 cm) compressing the pharynx ventrally, *J Am Vet Med Assoc* 197:395, 1990.
22. Brown CC et al: Serodiagnosis of inapparent caseous lymphadenitis in goats and sheep, using the synergistic hemolysis-inhibition test, *Am J Vet Res* 47:1461, 1986.
23. Ter Laak EA et al: Double-antibody sandwich enzyme-linked immunosorbent assay and immunoblot analysis used for control of caseous lymphadenitis in goats and sheep, *Am J Vet Res* 53:1125, 1992.
24. Stoops SG, Renshaw HW, Thilsted JP: Ovine caseous lymphadenitis: disease prevalence, lesion distribution, and thoracic manifestations in a population of mature culled sheep from western United States, *Am J Vet Res* 45:557, 1984.
25. East NE: Common infectious conditions, *Small Ruminants for the Mixed Animal Practioner, Western Veterinary Conference*, 1998, Las Vegas, NV.
26. Ashfaq MK, Campbell SG: Experimentally induced caseous lymphadenitis in goats, *Am J Vet Res* 41:1978, 1980.
27. Ahmed SS, El Hamamsy H: Diaphragmatic hernia in a sheep, *Vet Rec* 115:441, 1984.
28. McCullagh KA, Mews AR, Pinsent PJN: Diffuse pleural mesothelioma in a goat, *Vet Pathol* 16(15):119, 1979.
29. Radostits OM et al: Diseases caused by algae and fungi. In Radostits M et al, editors: *Veterinary medicine*, Philadelphia, 2000, WB Saunders.
30. King JM: Sudden death in sheep and goats, *Vet Clin North Am* 5(15):704, 1983.

Chapter 6

*T*heriogenology of Sheep and Goats

SEYEDMEHDI MOBINI, ALAN M. HEATH, AND D.G. PUGH

Sheep and goats are very fertile animals. On a percent body weight basis, very few species rival the testicular size of the ram or buck. The ewe and doe also have reproductive potential far superior to that of most other domestic animals. Before beginning an examination of the reproductive system, the clinician should examine the animal as a whole. The old saying, "Sex (reproductive potential) is a luxury" is true. Animals need to be productive (i.e., healthy) before they are able to be "reproductive." The examining clinician also should understand the animal's utility. A single range ewe usually does not undergo the same sort of reproductive manipulation performed on a donor animal used in an embryo transfer program. Reproductive medicine, or theriogenology, of sheep and goats is covered in this chapter. In some portions of the chapter sheep and goats are discussed separately, but when applicable the two species are discussed together.

MALE REPRODUCTION

Anatomy and Physiology of the Male

The anatomy of the reproductive organs of the ram and buck is similar to that of other ruminants. The penile urethra is surrounded by the corpus spongiosum penis (CSP) throughout its length. The urethra terminates as a vermiform appendage. Blood enters the CSP proximally and exits through two exhaust veins located on the free portion of the penis. Contractions of the urethralis and bulbospongiosus muscles force blood rhythmically through the CSP, producing the characteristic pulses of urine observed during normal micturition. The most prominent structure of the penis is the corpus cavernosum penis (CCP). It consists of cavernous space supported by fibrous trabeculae. This cavernous tissue is located on the dorsal surface and partially surrounds the CSP. At its origin in the pelvis the CCP is composed of two crura that join before leaving the pelvis. The entire penis is surrounded by the tunica albuginea. The two paired retractor penis muscles arise from the coccygeal vertebrae and pass around the anus to become two distinct muscles that attach to the ventrolateral surface of the penis at the distal bend of the sigmoid flexure. The penis is normally held in a S-shaped bend (sigmoid flexure) except during erection and ejaculation by the retractor penis muscles[1] (Figure 6-1).

The testicles are suspended away from the body by the pendulous scrotum. The scrotum is composed of undulating epidermis that may or may not be covered by wool, depending on the breed and husbandry practices. A rich plexus of blood vessels, lymphatics, and sweat glands lies beneath the skin. The dartos, a smooth muscle layer, is connected to the vaginal tunics of the testicle by the scrotal fascia. The scrotal fascia is the connective tissue that is typically broken down when the clinician separates the skin from the testicle during routine castration. The vaginal tunics are outcroppings of the peritoneum and form a protective covering over the testicles. The space between the two layers of vaginal tunic (parietal and visceral) as it reflects around the testicle normally contains a small amount of peritoneal fluid. The scrotal septum, composed primarily of the dartos muscle, divides the scrotum into two halves.[2]

The testicle itself is surrounded by a thick fibrous connective tissue known as the *tunica albuginea.* The parenchyma of the testicle is composed of seminiferous tubules that contain the germ cells and their supporting cells (Sertoli cells). The seminiferous tubules drain into the rete testes, which in turn is drained by 10 to 12 efferent ducts. These ducts drain into the head of the epididymis, which is located on the dorsal craniolateral aspect of the testicle. The body of the epididymis curves around the lateral portion of the testes and ends caudomedially as the tail. The tubular structure is reflected dor-

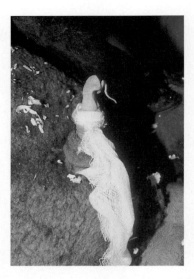

Figure 6-1 Gauze strip wrapped around the penis at the junction of the free portion of the penis and the prepuce to prevent retraction into the sheath. Note the prominent villiform appendage.

sally and becomes the vas deferens.[2] Rams and bucks have a full complement of accessory sex glands. The small bulbourethral glands are located caudally in the pelvic cavity on either side of the pelvic urethra; they can be palpated rectally. They also have lobulated vesicular glands, disseminate prostates, and a widening of the vas deferens known as the ampulla.[3] Spermatogenesis requires about 49 to 60 days from the start of germ cell division until the sperm are released from the seminiferous tubules. Another 10 days to 2 weeks are required for the sperm to pass from the seminiferous tubules through the epididymis.[4]

Puberty and Seasonality

Ram. Puberty typically occurs in the ram at 6 months. It is defined as the point at which the ram develops an interest in sexual activity and produces spermatozoa in sufficient numbers to achieve pregnancy in ewes. The exact age of puberty depends somewhat on breed and time of birth. Rams born early in the spring are older at puberty than late-born lambs. Moreover, rams that are periodically exposed to cycling ewes tend to reach puberty earlier.[5] Rams are seasonal breeders; the sperm quality, daily sperm output, and sexual activity are modulated by the increased periods of darkness that typically occur in the fall (Northern Hemisphere). This seasonality in the ram also is manifested by an increase in the testicular circumference.[6] Melatonin is secreted from the pineal gland during the dark hours. The increase in this hormone that occurs as day length shortens is responsible for many of the physiologic mechanisms associated with the ram in transition from the non-breeding to the breeding season.[6] Manipulation of light-dark intervals and the use of mela-

tonin can alter the breeding season of rams, but the practicality of these procedures is debatable.[7]

A change in the sexual attitude of the ram toward the ewe as day length decreases defines the onset of the breeding season. He becomes more sexually interested in the female, and courtship behavior occurs more frequently. Rams display a typical flehmen response to females in estrus after sniffing the vulva region and urine from the estrus female. He often strikes out at the female with one front leg before mounting her.[6] The physiologic changes in testicular size, mating behavior, and semen quality are caused by the activation of the hypothalamus and a decrease in the effectiveness of testosterone on the negative inhibition of gonadotropin-releasing hormone (GnRH). Significant differences are seen between the breeding and the non-breeding season with respect to the pattern of GnRH and luteinizing hormone (LH) pulses and the response of the pituitary gland to GnRH.

Buck. Breed, age, and nutrition contribute to the onset of sexual maturity in the buck.[8] The age at puberty depends on the breed, varying from 2 to 3 months in pygmy breeds to 4 to 5 months in Nubian and Boer bucks. Most breeds of goats raised in the temperate environment of the Northern Hemisphere possess sperm in the ejaculate at 4 to 5 months. However, at this age their semen quality is poor and they are not suitable for breeding.[9] Nubian and Boer bucks begin exhibiting libido at 10 to 12 weeks and start producing quality semen at about 8 months.[8,9] Natural adhesions of the urethral process and glans penis to the prepuce make the immature buck incapable of copulation. This attachment begins to separate at 3 months, and fertile mating is possible at 4 to 5 months.[8,9] Fast-growing, well-fed, and well-managed kids are able to breed sooner than starved males of equal age.

Whether bucks are truly seasonal breeders is controversial. Many bucks have depressed libido, reduced pheromones, decreased scrotal circumference (SC), lower semen freezability, and a larger number of abnormal spermatozoa outside of the breeding season. All these changes reflect lower levels of LH and testosterone. LH and testosterone concentration, libido, and odor presence in the buck peaks in the fall.[10,11] Sexual behavior of the buck includes actively seeking does in estrus, courtship (kicking, pawing, muzzling, grunting, and flehmen), mounting, intromission, and ejaculation. Ejaculation occurs spontaneously and is characterized by a strong pelvic thrust with a rapid backward movement of the head.[9] After ejaculation the buck dismounts and shows no sexual arousal for a few minutes to several hours.

References

1. Beckett SD, Wolfe DF: Anatomy of the penis, prepuce, and sheath. In Wolfe DF, Moll HD, editors: *Large animal urogenital surgery*, ed 2, Baltimore, 1998, Williams & Wilkins.

2. Heath AM, Purohit RC: Anatomy of the scrotum, testes, epididymis, and spermatic cord (bulls, rams, and bucks). In Wolfe DF, Moll HD, editors: *Large animal urogenital surgery*, ed 2, Baltimore, 1998, Williams & Wilkins.

3. Ashdown RR, Hancock JL: Functional anatomy of male reproduction. In Hafez ESE, editor: *Reproduction in farm animals*, ed 4, Philadelphia, 1980, Lea and Febiger.

4. Pineda MH, Faulkner LC: The biology of sex. In McDonald LE, editor: *Veterinary endocrinology and reproduction*, ed 3, Philadelphia, 1980, Lea and Febiger.

5. Price EO, Borgwardt R, Dally MR: Heterosexual experience differentially affects the expression of sexual behavior in 6- and 8-month old ram lambs, *Appl Anim Behav Sci* 46:193, 1996.

6. Fitzgerald J: Applied reproductive physiology of the ram. In Youngquist RS, editor: *Current therapy in large animal theriogenology*, Philadelphia, 1997, WB Saunders.

7. Nett TM: Controlling seasonal reproduction: emphasis on the male, *Proceedings of the Society for Theriogenology*, 1991, Nashville, TN.

8. Smith MC, Sherman DM: *Goat medicine*, Philadelphia, 1994, Lea and Febiger.

9. Goyal HO, Memon MA: Clinical reproductive anatomy and physiology of the buck. In Youngquist RS, editor: *Current therapy in large animal theriogenology*, Philadelphia, 1997, WB Saunders.

10. Hill J: Goat reproductive management, *Proceedings of the Symposium on Health and Diseases of Small Ruminants*, Nashville, TN, 1996, American Association of Small Ruminant Practice.

11. Wilddeus S: Reproductive management for meat goat production, *Proceedings of the Southeast Region Meat Goat Producers Symposium*, Tallahassee, FL, 1998, Florida A & M University.

SELECTION AND MANAGEMENT

Ram

A ram with good-quality semen, adequate testicular size, and good libido can breed 100 ewes in a 17-day breeding season.[1] However, most producers in North America use 3 to 3.5 rams per 100 ewes. Yearlings and mature rams can be expected to service 35 to 50 ewes, whereas ram lambs should only be expected to service 15 to 25 ewes.[2] Adjustments should be made for multiple sire breeding units. It is desirable to always have more than three rams to a multiple sire unit because this tends to alleviate some of the territorial fighting among rams.

Libido serving capacity and testing can provide useful information regarding how many ewes a ram can be expected to service or even if a ram should be retained.[3] Serving capacity tests are performed to measure how many times a ram services ewes during a defined period. One report suggests that the test serving pen should be approximately 3 m by 5 m and in clear view of rams that are to be tested.[4] However, larger or smaller pens may be used. Typically the ram is placed in a pen with two to four cycling, unrestrained ewes for a period of 20 to 40 minutes. The keeper monitors and records all sexual behavior, with emphasis on the number of breedings. Such tests are the most reliable predictor of an animal's libido. Ewes used for libido tests may be synchronized to estrus, or ovariectomized and administered estrogen. Compared with low-libido rams, rams that are identified as high-performing or having a high degree of libido have a higher lambing percentage and more live lambs born per exposed ewe. Serving capacity tests also may be used to determine proper ram-to-ewe stocking ratios.[1,6] These tests of flock reproduction can produce a shorter, more uniform lambing season.[3] Adult rams achieving four to six or more breedings during 30 minutes are preferred. Rams achieving two or three breedings during 30 minutes are acceptable. Rams that appear sexually inactive can be tested twice. If they still appear to be sexually inactive, the keeper can paint the rumps of the tested ewes with different colors of ink and leave the rams overnight in the pen with them. The next day the keepers should examine the rams' chests for the colored ink.[5] Still, fertility is maximized if only acceptable groups of rams are kept for breeding.

Selection of rams from high-producing ewes as measured by the number of lambs born, the weight of lambs weaned, and a history of having lambs early in the season also may have a positive relationship with fertility.[7] It appears that rams born co-twin to male siblings have higher serving capacities than those born co-twin to females.[8] Rams also should be selected for structural soundness and for the genetics they can pass on to their offspring because they contribute approximately 60% to 80% of the genetics of the average flock.[1] Rams should be maintained on a good nutritional, vaccination, and deworming program. Their body condition scores before breeding season should be 3.5 to 4. Obesity minimizes willingness to breed. Rams should be sheared and their feet trimmed before breeding season. During breeding season, free access to shelter or shady areas should be provided to minimize heat stress–associated infertility. Special care should be taken during the initial examination of rams to eliminate those that have diseases of the reproductive tract.

Buck

A number of breeds of goats are well established in North America. Some of the dairy breeds are Alpine, Nubian, Saanen, Toggenburg, and Lamancha. Angora and cashmere are the predominant fiber-producing goat breeds. Meat goat breeds include Spanish (brush goat), Tennessee stiff-legged, pygmy, Boer, Kiko, and Genemaster. Bucks are chosen based on individual performance or progeny testing for traits such as milk production, meat traits, adaptability, and twinning rate. Prolific bucks are preferred. Birth, weaning, and yearling information is valuable in establishing the superiority or inferiority of a potential sire. Selection for growth rate and meat production should be a high priority for meat goats. Bucks should have good conformation and be large and muscular. Selection based on testicle size is important; bucks with the largest testicles usually produce the highest-quality sperm.

The same serving capacity tests used for rams are applicable to bucks. Bucks with apparent defects in posture and genital tract abnormalities should be avoided. Because the intersex condition has been linked to the polled gene, the use of phenotypic polled bucks should be avoided. Changing bucks every 2 years prevents loss of vigor and reduces inbreeding in the herd. Bucks should be kept separate from does in a group on pasture or in single housing. They should be introduced with females only during the established mating season, after which their job for the year is finished. Bucks require proper nutrition, routine foot care, vaccination, deworming, and exercise.

BREEDING SOUNDNESS EXAMINATION IN THE RAM

A breeding soundness examination (BSE) should be performed on all rams before the beginning of the breeding season. With the ram being expected to breed as many as 100 ewes during a season, his individual worth far outweighs the cost of a BSE. A proper BSE consists of a thorough physical examination with special attention to the scrotum and testicles, as well as an evaluation of the semen quality. Most BSEs do not routinely include an evaluation of the ram's libido or his physical ability to make intromission. The veterinarian should communicate clearly with the client regarding the limitations of the BSE performed and the need for some sort of libido testing. This testing can often be accomplished by directly observing the animal in the first part of the breeding season. Large sheep producers may be encouraged to keep an extra 10% more rams that have been deemed satisfactory according to a veterinary examination to ensure adequate ram power.

Physical Examination

A complete physical examination should be performed on all rams, with particular emphasis on the eyes and feet. The ram can be restrained by placing him on his rump in a sitting position. The scrotum should be palpated to ensure that both testicles are present, approximately equal in size, and of firm consistency; the clinician should note any localized swellings or areas of induration. The head and tail of the epididymis is palpated for swelling, pain, and signs of inflammation. Epididymitis is a relatively common problem in rams. Any ram exhibiting signs of epididymitis should be considered infected with *Brucella ovis* until proven otherwise. The clinician should examine the spermatic cord for deformities in the vascular plexus and vas deferens. The penis can usually be

extended by pressing down around the external preputial orifice and grasping the protruding penis with a gauze pad. Occasionally the sigmoid flexure may need to be straightened to assist in extending the penis. The clinician should carefully examine the penis for evidence of active lesions or old scars. The penis can be held in extension by wrapping a strip of gauze around the junction between the free portion of the penis and the prepuce. This method also is helpful when collecting semen by electroejaculation. The penis is generally easier to extend when the animal is being held up on his rump than when he is in lateral recumbency.

Scrotal Circumference

The clinician should pull both of the ram's testicles ventrally into the scrotum and measure it at its largest circumference using a tape measure marked in centimeters. Care must be taken with breeds that have heavy scrotal wool because wool may falsely enlarge the measured circumference. Taking the average of several measurements can increase the accuracy of the SC measurements. The tape should be snug on the scrotum and barely indent the skin so that the tape does not slide on the scrotum (Figure 6-2). SC in the ram is highly heritable, and although controversy exists regarding its importance, it appears to be related to sperm output, age of puberty, and the propensity for multiple births in his female offspring.[1] During the selection of ram lambs the testicular diameter at 170 days provides a long-range prediction of postpubertal testicular size and sperm output.[9] SC is a major criterion in selecting replacement rams. Minimum accepted SCs of 30 cm for ram lambs weighing more

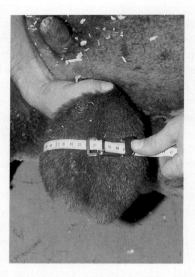

Figure 6-2 Measuring the scrotal circumference of a ram. The procedure is the same for bucks. The tape measure should slightly indent the skin, and the examiner should firmly push the testicles into the scrotum with the free hand. Care should be taken to read the measurement at the correct location on the measuring tape.

than 150 lb, 33 cm for 12- to 18-month-old rams, and 36 cm for rams weighing more than 250 lb have been suggested.[1] Based strictly on age, rams from 8 to 14 months should have 28 to 36 cm of SC to be classified as satisfactory and more than 36 cm to be classified as exceptional (Table 6-1). Rams older than 14 months should have 32 to 40 cm of SC to be classified as satisfactory and more than 40 cm to be classified as exceptional.[10] Scrotal size is usually greatest from August to October. Smaller testicular measurements (0.5 to 1.5 cm smaller) are to be expected when rams are tested outside of the normal breeding season (February to April) or during periods of extreme sexual activity.[1]

Semen Evaluation

The penis is extended as described previously. The ram is then placed in lateral recumbency to collect semen by electroejaculation. The same electroejaculators (EEs) described for use in bucks are used for rams (Figure 6-3). The clinician inserts the tip of the ram's penis and the urethral process into the warmed glass or plastic tube. Some rams ejaculate at this point of the examination. The rectum is cleared of feces and a lubricated electric rectal probe is carefully inserted. The clinician massages the accessory sex glands by moving the probe back and forth in a cranial to caudal direction 8 to 10 times while gently forcing the tip of the probe ventrally. Mild electrical stimulation is then applied for 5 seconds. The ram typically vocalizes during this procedure and attempts to escape. After the ram relaxes, the massage and electrical stimulation are repeated until the ram ejaculates into the tube. The spiraled urethral process straightens during the ejaculatory process. The collected semen is evaluated for motility, morphology, and the presence of inflammatory cells.

Motility. A drop of raw semen is first examined under low power (100×) to estimate the concentration and motility. A drop of warmed saline is placed on the slide.

The clinician then dips the corner of a coverslip into the drop of raw semen and mixes it with the drop of warmed saline. The resultant mixture should allow the examiner to watch the motion of individual spermatozoa. If the semen mixture is too concentrated to allow identification of individual spermatozoa, a new preparation should be made with less semen. With experience the observer will be able to determine the amount of semen to place on the coverslip to make an adequate slide. The examiner should visually estimate the number of progressively motile sperm. A common error is to overestimate the percentage of progressively motile sperm. The observer can minimize errors by mentally "freezing" the microscopic image before making the motility estimate. One technique to

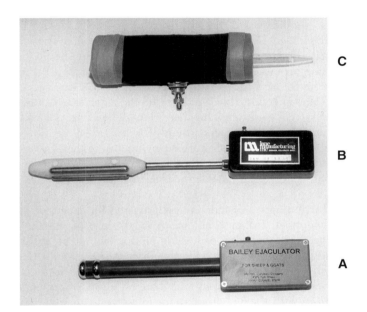

Figure 6-3 The two electroejaculators shown here are the Bailey **(A)** and Lane **(B)** electroejaculators. Both contain batteries and require no external power source. Other models are available. An artificial vagina also is shown **(C)**.

TABLE 6-1

SCROTAL CIRCUMFERENCE AND BREEDING SOUNDNESS EVALUATION BY AVERAGING THREE MEASUREMENTS FOR RAMS

8 to 14 Months		Older Than 14 Months	
SIZE*	RATING	SIZE*	RATING
Smaller than 28 cm	Questionable	Smaller than 32 cm	Questionable
28 to 36 cm	Satisfactory	32 to 40 cm	Satisfactory
Larger than 36 cm	Exceptional	Larger than 40 cm	Exceptional

From Yarney TA, Sanford LM: Pubertal development of ram lambs: physical and endocrinological traits in combination as indices of postpubertal reproductive function, *Therio* 40(4):735, 1993.
*Testicles may be 2 to 3 cm smaller in the off season.

TABLE 6-2

MOTILITY AND MORPHOLOGY PERCENTAGES REQUIRED TO PLACE RAMS INTO DIFFERENT CATEGORIES

	EXCEPTIONAL	SATISFACTORY	UNSATISFACTORY
Motility	Greater than 70%	Greater than 30%	Less than 30%
Morphology	Greater than 90%	Greater than 50%	Less than 50% normal

From Yarney TA, Sanford LM: Pubertal development of ram lambs: physical and endocrinological traits in combination as indices of postpubertal reproductive function, *Therio* 40(4):735, 1993.

make the estimate easier is to determine whether more or less than 50% of the spermatozoa are motile. After making that determination, the observer can try to arrive at the nearest 25%, then the nearest 10%. The observer also should record the number of round cells present in each image. If more than two round cells are seen in each medium power field, a smear of the semen should be made for cytologic evaluation (e.g., Wright's stain). The presence of white blood cells indicates inflammation and/or infection. The presence of early nucleated round germ cells indicates an aberration of spermatogenesis. Rams should have more than 30% progressively motile cells to obtain a satisfactory rating and more than 70% to have an exceptional rating[11] (Table 6-2). Motility is usually depressed outside the breeding season.

Morphology. A slide is next prepared for examination of spermatozoa morphology. A small drop of semen is placed on the edge of a slide, and a ribbon of eosin-nigrosin stain is placed slightly closer to the center of the slide. The corner of a second slide is dipped into the semen drop and the resultant "hanging drop" of semen is mixed with the ribbon of stain. The second slide is then pulled across the first slide in a manner similar to creating a blood smear. The amount of semen placed on the edge of the second slide is determined by experience. The resultant smear should have an even distribution of cells. Spermatozoa should be spaced so that individual cells are easily distinguished but each field should have approximately 10 cells. The slide is allowed to dry and then examined at 1000× with an oil-immersion lens. The observer should count at least 100 cells and determine a percentage of normal spermatozoa. Abnormalities are usually recorded as either primary or secondary. Primary abnormalities involve the head and midpiece of the spermatozoa, whereas secondary abnormalities involve the tail (Figure 6-4). The type of abnormality can be used to estimate the severity of problems in rams with an excessive number of abnormal cells. Abnormalities of the head and the acrosome are associated with severe testicular aberrations. Tail abnormalities are often associated with less severe problems or diseases of the epididymis. Round droplets of cytoplasm on the tail are usually seen in young rams and are associated with overuse, immaturity, or mild

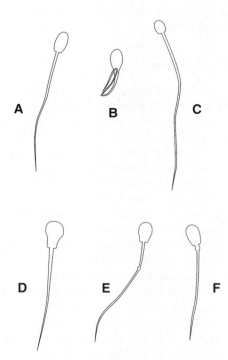

Figure 6-4 **A,** A normal spermatozoon; **B,** a spermatozoon with a primary abnormality—tightly coiled tail and midpiece; **C,** a spermatozoon with a primary abnormality—microcephalia, or small head; **D,** a pear-shaped head, which is a primary abnormality; **E,** a spermatozoon with a distal cytoplasmic droplet, which is a secondary abnormality; **F,** a spermatozoon with a proximal cytoplasmic droplet.

testicular degeneration. Droplets also can occur in samples taken from rams out of season. At least 50% to 70% of the observed spermatozoa should be morphologically normal for the ram to be considered a satisfactory breeder; more than 80% to 90% is considered exceptional[11] (see Table 6-2).

Breeding Soundness Prediction

The SC, progressive motility, and percentage of normal spermatozoa can be combined to classify rams into categories to help predict their usefulness in a breeding flock. Rams that are classified as satisfactory in all categories can be expected to impregnate about 50 ewes in a 60-day breeding season. Rams that receive exceptional ratings

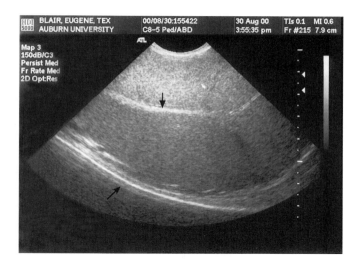

Figure 6-5 Ultrasonography of the ovine testicle (sagittal or longitudinal plane). The hyperechoic mediastinum is seen here as a distinct line on the image *(large arrow)*. The vaginal tunic can be best visualized in the field opposite the transducer *(small arrow)*.

can be expected to impregnate 100 ewes during a 60-day breeding season. Any ram that does not receive at least a satisfactory rating in all categories should either be culled or retested in 60 days. The decision to cull or retest should be based on the severity of observed lesions and the economic value of the individual animal.[9,10]

Ancillary Tests

Ultrasonography can be used to evaluate the testicles of rams (or bucks). Changes from the normal homogeneous testicular parenchyma such as hyperechoic and hypoechoic areas are indicative of fibrotic changes or cystic structures. The examiner should not confuse the normal hyperechoic mediastinum that is found in the center of the testicle for a fibrotic lesion. The mediastinum appears as a distinct round area in the center of transverse images of the testicle and as a hyperechoic line on longitudinal images (Figure 6-5). The epididymis and spermatic cord also can be examined for fibrosis and cystic structures. Areas of fibrosis or degeneration and testicular abscesses can usually be visualized.

Testicular biopsies using a 14-gauge biopsy needle can allow a direct examination of the testicular architecture. Testicular biopsies are useful in determining atrophy, degeneration, and hypoplasia. This technique is usually relegated to use in valuable animals. The clinician aseptically prepares the testicle and anesthetizes an area of skin. He or she then inserts the biopsy needle into the dorsum of the testicle, avoiding the epididymis and taking care not to penetrate the mediastinum. Tissue can be fixed in either Bouin's solution or 10% formalin for routine histopathologic analysis.[13]

Serologic screening for *B. ovis* should be performed on all rams at the time of the BSE.[12]

BREEDING SOUNDNESS EXAMINATION IN THE BUCK

All breeding bucks need to be evaluated for breeding soundness 3 to 4 weeks before mating season. As in the ram, the examination of the buck should include a physical examination, reproductive examination, measurement of SC, and semen collection and evaluation. BSEs are only able to evaluate the physical soundness and semen quality of the buck. A satisfactory finding cannot guarantee the buck's ability to produce live offspring.[14] Attempts to assess libido in the buck greatly aid in a complete reproductive evaluation. The libido measurement described for the ram can be adapted for the buck.

Physical Examination

Physical examination of the buck must include a general examination for health, with particular attention to assessment of body condition and musculoskeletal condition (feet and legs). To be a satisfactory breeder, a buck should be in good body condition. Thin or excessively fat animals should be avoided (see Chapter 2).[14,15] The buck should be free of known genetic defects such as hernias, jaw malformation, cryptorchidism, supernumerary teats, and intersex condition. Bucks should not be phenotypically polled.

Examination of the Reproductive Tract

Reproductive evaluation includes examination of the testes, epididymis, spermatic cord, and penis. Testis should be examined for size, symmetry, and consistency. A buck should have two large, oval testes of equal size; they are firm during the breeding season and slightly softer during the non-breeding season. If only one testicle is present, the male should be disqualified as a potential breeder. Ultrasonography may be useful in aiding detection or confirmation of abnormalities.[14-16] Gross changes in the epididymis are fairly rare in goats. The clinician should examine the penis for abnormalities when collecting a semen sample. The penis must be manually extended from the sheath so that a careful examination can be made. The urethra extends beyond the tip of the penis for about 2 to 3 cm, forming the urethral process. When bucks have a history of urinary calculi, the urethral process is usually removed during treatment because it is a common area of obstruction. The loss or removal of the urethral process appears to have no detrimental effect on the buck's fertility.[15] Because of its high correlation of testicular size and capacity for sperm production, SC is important in the buck. However, its use in the evaluation of breeding soundness is not well defined. SC is measured in the buck as described in the ram. SC in 45-kg dairy goats has been reported to be 25 to 28 cm, with larger bucks having SCs of 34 to 36 cm.[14,15] No age and breed standards exist for SC in meat goats. In 1999, during the Georgia and Southeast Meat Goat Buck Performance Test, SCs in 45-kg, 7-month-old Kiko and Boer bucks averaged 26 to 29 cm.[16]

Semen Collection

Semen may be collected with an artificial vagina (AV) in a trained buck or by electroejaculation.[13] The Bailey Ejaculator (Western Instrument Company, Denver, CO) and Lane Ejaculator (Lane Manufacturing Inc., Denver, CO) are the two most commonly used EEs (Figure 6-4). EEs should be 25 to 30 cm long and 2 to 3 cm in diameter. An AV can be built from a polyvinyl chloride (PVC) pipe or radiator hose with an inner liner made of a cut section of bicycle inner tube. An AV also can be purchased. The length of the AV should be 18 to 22 cm, and its outside diameter should be 6 cm. It should be filled with warm water to maintain proper turgor and warmth (38° to 40° C). A semen collection cone should be placed at one end. A nonspermicidal lubricant is placed in the open end. For electroejaculation bucks are restrained in chutes or held against the wall. The rectum is cleaned of feces and a well-lubricated probe is inserted. The prostate is massaged five to six times, electrical current is applied through the probe for 4 to 6 seconds, and then the probe turned off for 3 to 4 seconds. This pattern is maintained until ejaculation occurs (usually four to five cycles). Libido cannot be assessed when collecting semen by an EE. During and after collection, semen should be protected from direct sunlight and temperature shock, and sperm motility should be evaluated within 10 minutes.

Semen Evaluation

The volume of normal buck ejaculate is 0.5 to 1.5 ml (with an average of 1 ml). Semen is evaluated for color, gross and progressive mortality, morphology, and concentration.[15] Both semen quality and quantity may vary with age, season, temperature, breed, and even between individuals within the same breed. Normal semen values in the buck are as follows[15]:

Volume—1 ml (with a range of 0.5 to 1.5 ml)
Motility—80% (with a range of 70% to 90%)
Concentration—4 billion (with a range of 2 to 5 billion) per ml
Normal morphology—80% (with a range of 70% to 90%)

Minimally acceptable values are shown in Box 6-1.
Volume is measured directly from the graduated collection vial. Volume is of some value in evaluating semen collected using an AV, but of limited value when EEs are used. The color of semen depends on the number of sper-

---

BOX 6-1

MINIMAL ACCEPTABLE LEVELS FOR A SATISFACTORY POTENTIAL BREEDER BUCK

Volume—0.5 ml
Motile sperm—70%
Concentration—2 billion
Morphology—80% normal

Adapted from Memon MA, Mickelsen WD, Goyal HO: . In Youngquist RS, editor: *Current therapy in large animal theriogenology,* Philadelphia, 1997, WB Saunders.

---

matozoa per milliliter; it can vary from "whey-like" to "milky" to "creamy." Gross motility is measured as described for the ram. Even though concentration is not routinely assessed in field conditions, it is advisable to include it in the evaluation. Two of the authors (Drs. Mobini and Pugh) have evaluated meat bucks with very low sperm concentrations but with other satisfactory examination parameters.[16] Concentration can be easily assessed using a hemocytometer and a commercial Unopette system for white blood cell count.[15] Morphology can be determined by examination. An eosin-nigrosin–stained smear is evaluated using a 1000× objective; the examiner measures primary or secondary abnormalities in 100 to 200 spermatozoa per slide, as described for the ram (see Figure 6-4). Normal values for a buck to be classified as a satisfactory potential breeder are shown in Box 6-1. A questionable potential breeder may require reevaluation after 8 weeks or need to be culled. The classification of unsatisfactory potential breeder may be given for reasons other than semen quality (e.g., cryptorchid, lameness) Bucks showing depressed libido, slightly decreased SC, and increased sperm abnormalities should be identified and culled.[14,15]

REFERENCES

1. Burfening PJ, Rossi D: Serving capacity and scrotal circumference of ram lambs as affected by selection for reproductive rate, *Small Rumin Res* 9:61, 1992.
2. Groteluschen DM, Doster AR: Reproductive problems in rams, *NebGuide (http://www.ianr.unl.edu),* Lincoln, NE, 2000, Cooperative Extension, University of Nebraska.
3. Fitzgerald J: Applied reproductive physiology of the ram. In Youngquist RS, editor: *Current therapy in large animal theriogenology,* Philadelphia, 1997, WB Saunders.
4. Katz LS: Sexual performance tests in sexually inexperienced rams. In Dziuk PJ, Wheeler M, editors: *Handbook of methods for study of reproductive physiology in domestic animals,* Urbana, IL, 1991, University of Illinois.
5. Fitzgerald J, Perkins A: Serving capacity tests for rams. In Dziuk PJ, Wheeler M, editors: *Handbook of methods for study of reproductive physiology in domestic animals,* Urbana, IL, 1991, University of Illinois.

6. Perkins A, Fitzgerald JA, Price EO: Sexual performance of rams in serving capacity tests predicts success in pen breeding, *J Anim Sci* 70(9):2722, 1992.

7. Fitzgerald JA, Perkins A: Ram sexual performance: a relationship with dam productivity, *Sheep Res J* 7(1):7, 1991.

8. Fitzgerald JA, Perkins A, Hemenway K: Relationship of sex and number of siblings in utero with sexual behavior of mature rams, *Appl Anim Behav Sci* 38:283, 1993.

9. Yarney TA, Sanford LM: Pubertal development of ram lambs: physical and endocrinological traits in combination as indices of postpubertal reproductive function, *Therio* 40(4):735, 1993.

10. Kimberling CV, Marsh DJ: Breeding soundness evaluation and surgical sterilization of the ram. In Youngquist RS, editor: *Current therapy in large animal theriogenology*, Philadelphia, 1997, WB Saunders.

11. Bulgin MS: Ram breeding soundness examination and SFT form, Nashville, *Proceedings of the Society for Theriogenology*, 1992, Nashville, TN.

12. Pugh DG: Examination of the ram for breeding soundness, *Proc Hudson-Walker Therio Conf* 7:19, 1996.

13. Carson RL et al: Examination and special procedures of the scrotum and testes. In Wolfe D, Moll HD, editors: *Large animal urogenital surgery*, Baltimore, 1997, Williams & Wilkins.

14. Pugh DG: Breeding soundness examination in male goats, *Proc Hudson-Walker Therio Conf* 7:29, 1996.

15. Memon MA, Mickelsen WD, Goyal HO: Examination of the reproductive tract and evaluation of potential breeding soundness in the buck. In Youngquist RS, editor: *Current therapy in large animal theriogenology*, Philadelphia, 1997, WB Saunders.

16. Mobini S: Reproductive management in goats, *Proceedings of the North American Veterinary Conference*, vol 14, 2000, Orlando, FL.

DISEASES OF THE MALE

Varicoceles

A varicocele is defined as a localized dilatation and thrombosis of the internal spermatic vein and is recognized as a fluctuant to hard swelling in the spermatic cord. Varicoceles are more common in rams than in bucks. This condition is often manifested as rear limb lameness and awkward posture as the ram tries to relieve pressure on the swollen cords. Affected animals may become weak and susceptible to other diseases as a result of debilitation brought on by an unwillingness to walk to obtain food and water. Varicoceles can be diagnosed by palpation and diagnostic ultrasound. Abnormalities such as decreased total sperm count, reduced sperm motility, and morphologic abnormalities of the sperm are often associated with varicoceles. The exact etiology of the condition is not known but a genetic predisposition is suspected. No easy treatment is available, and affected rams or bucks should be culled.[1]

Epididymitis in Older Males

Epididymitis is a rare condition in the buck but a clinically important disease in rams. Epididymitis in rams should be considered to be caused by *B. ovis* until proven otherwise. This is especially true of older rams that have been actively breeding in multiple sire units. However, one case report involving an outbreak of *B. ovis* in a group of virgin ram lambs suggests that the disease may be spread in utero or neonatally, before any known sexual activity.[2] The primary means of spread is thought to be through contact with mucous membranes, which results in bacteremia. The organism localizes in the epididymis and secondary sex glands. Contact can occur among rams and from recently infected ewes; venereal and oral-nasal transmission also are possible.[3] Swelling of the epididymis is the primary presenting sign, occurring about 3 weeks after the initial exposure. Grossly, there is localized inflammation followed by hyperplasia and obstruction of the epididymal ducts. This obstruction causes a backup of spermatozoa, the development of sperm granulomas, and pressure necrosis. The seminal vesicles also are commonly affected, which may account for the large number of infected rams that show no palpable signs of epididymitis.[3] Semen collected from infected rams usually contains a large number of polymorphonuclear neutrophils that can be seen on the motility preparations or on Wright's stained specimens. Serology for *B. ovis* should be considered a routine part of a BSE. Both enzyme-linked immunospecific assay (ELISA) and complement fixation (CF) tests are available. Herd infections with *B. ovis* can result in a 15% to 30% reduction in lambing rate depending on the chronicity of the herd problem. This decrease in reproductive efficiency results from lowered fertility in the rams, failure of the ewes to conceive, reabsorption of embryos, abortions, stillbirths, and weak lambs.[5]

Recommendations outlined by Bulgin[4] include the following:

- Buying virgin rams that have been serologically tested for brucellosis
- Keeping newly purchased rams separate until all rams are tested free from *Brucella*
- Performing palpation and culling all rams with epididymitis before the breeding season
- Culling all *B. ovis*–positive rams
- Retesting all rams in the flock 60 days after any rams are found positive
- Performing BSEs yearly on all rams

If a large number of serologically positive rams is found after a year of adherence to these guidelines, efforts should be made to determine whether a serologically negative carrier ram is present in the flock by culturing semen from all rams.

Epididymitis in Young Males

In younger rams, and less commonly in bucks, epididymitis can be caused by a number of organisms such as *Histophilus*, *Actinobacillus*, and *Haemophilus* species, as well as *Corynebacterium pseudotuberculosis*. Lamb epididymitis can be spread from ram to ram by the oral or nasal route. The organisms responsible for lamb epididymitis can frequently be cultured from the preputial cavity of rams younger than 2 years of age and are commonly found in the mucous membranes of the prepuce, penis, mouth, and nasal cavity.[5] Colonization and subsequent disease of the reproductive tract may depend on the hormonal changes that occur during maturation and puberty, along with other unknown differentiating factors that allow most animals to eliminate the bacteria spontaneously while causing others to develop clinical signs.[6] Diagnosis of lamb epididymitis is made by palpation of the enlarged epididymis and by ruling out *B. ovis* infection. Semen from infected lambs is characterized by a large number of neutrophils and by the morphologically abnormal spermatozoa typical of epididymal disease. Although the signs of most cases of lamb epididymitis are restricted to the reproductive tract, occasionally an associated fever and hind limb lameness also occur. Lamb epididymitis can be treated with long-acting oxytetracycline (20 mg/kg intramuscularly [IM] or subcutaneously [SC]) injections for three treatments at 3-day intervals.[6,7] Inclusion of tetracycline (20 mg/kg by mouth [PO] daily) products in the ration may be appropriate in herds experiencing a high incidence of lamb epididymitis. Treatment should be reserved for valuable lambs and cases diagnosed in the early stages because most lambs develop scar tissue in the epididymis that prevents functional recovery.

Orchitis

Orchitis is a common occurrence in the ram and is occasionally seen in the buck.[8-10] Scrotal abscesses may be caused by trauma or may be an extension of epididymitis. Whenever testicular trauma or infection is encountered, it should be considered a medical emergency in breeding animals. Excessive heat from one testicle can result in possibly irreversible thermal injury to the germinal epithelium of the contralateral testicle. All the organisms discussed in the section on epididymitis can cause orchitis. The signs include a hot, swollen scrotum (usually unilaterally); inability to move the affected testicle freely in the scrotum; and pain on manipulation of the affected testicle and the scrotum. Some animals may show signs of systemic disease, pain on walking, and decrease in libido.[10] In cases affecting valuable animals, hemicastration in the acute phase may prevent permanent infertility.

Sperm Granulomas

Although testicular tumors are rare in rams and bucks, granulomatous swellings are occasionally encountered. Sperm granulomas are more common in goats than in sheep, and unlike abscesses or other forms of orchitis, they usually occur bilaterally. Sperm granulomas are often caused by a partial or complete blockage of the efferent ducts draining into the epididymis.[10] As pressure builds,

the ducts become distended and may rupture, resulting in a severe inflammation. As fluid accumulates, pressure continues to build and testicular degeneration may occur. Some animals are initially fertile but lose fertility after the efferent ducts become completely occluded. Granulomas are firm swellings found in the head of the epididymis. On palpation the testicles may be initially edematous, but they eventually become hard. The testicles may eventually become small and atrophic. Ultrasonographic evaluation may reveal mineralization of the testicles or the granuloma itself. No treatment is available for sperm granulomas, and the clinician should be cognizant of the potential association with the intersex condition.

Testicular Hypoplasia and Degeneration

Testicular hypoplasia and degeneration are difficult to differentiate during an initial examination.[8,10] In rams and bucks out of season, testicular size and palpation characteristics may be difficult to differentiate from subtle cases of testicular atrophy. More extreme differences are encountered in rams than in goats, but in general the testicle in the non-breeding season is smaller and lacks normal resiliency.[8] True hypoplasia can be associated with the intersex condition in bucks and a specific chromosomal abnormality in rams[8,10] (Figure 6-6).

Other causes of testicular atrophy include zinc deficiency, hypothyroidism (iodine deficiency, ingestion of goitrogenous plants), starvation diets, systemic disease, and heat and cold stress. Iodine-induced hypothyroidism has been associated with decreased testicular weight, depressed spermatogenesis, and decreased libido. Atrophic or degenerated testicles become elongated, small, and either softer or harder. Normal testicles usually have a homogenous echogenicity on ultrasound. Atrophic or degenerative testicles tend to have a heterogenous pattern and more hyperechoic areas. Testicular biopsy can be of value in diagnosis. Many cases of atrophy and degeneration are not treatable; the exceptions are cases caused by diet or certain diseases. In treating diet-related atrophy,

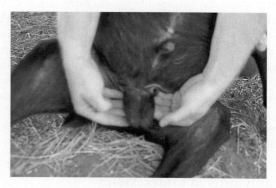

Figure 6-6 These small, thin, hard, hypoplastic testicles are from a polled yearling buck.

ensuring adequate protein-energy intake and free access to a good-quality trace mineral supplement is essential. If zinc deficiency is suspected, reducing the legume content of the diet and adding a chelated form of zinc (zinc methionine) to the diet or trace mineral mixture is useful. If iodine-induced hypothyroidism is diagnosed, the inclusion of iodine in a trace mineral mixture and the removal of goitrogenous plants from the diet should be undertaken; males should be kept off pastures with goitrogenous plants before and during breeding.

Intersex

Caprine intersexes are referred to as *male pseudohermaphrodites* because a majority of them have testes. True hermaphrodites have testicular and ovarian structures and generally constitute a much smaller proportion of intersexes.[11] Intersex is more prevalent in polled dairy goats (Saanen, Toggenburg, alpine, and Damascus breeds). The polled intersex condition is rare or not reported in some breeds (Nubian and Angora).[12] Cytogenetic evaluations of caprine intersexes clearly show that most polled intersexes are karyotypically female (XX), and the breeding histories of the parents indicate that intersexes are homozygous for the polled trait.[10]

Affected animals are genetically female but may exhibit male, female, or mixed external characteristics.[12] Generally they are female-appearing at birth, but as they reach sexual maturity they become larger than normal females, with masculine heads and erect hair on their necks.[10] An enlarged clitoris in a doe-like animal or a decreased anogenital distance in a more masculine individual is typical of intersex[12] (Figure 6-7). Intersexes may start to smell and may act aggressively toward other goats and people during the breeding season. Some dribble urine or stretch out with a concave back and urinate forward between the legs.[11] Whenever bilateral cryptorchidism is encountered, intersex should be suspected. The testes are generally intraabdominal (in the normal location of the

ovaries) but they may be partially or totally descended. Partially descended testes may be mistaken for udders, especially when they begin to enlarge during puberty.[11] Hypospadias (opening of the urethral orifice on the ventral aspect of the penis), sperm granulomas, and hypoplastic testicles should all be considered part of the intersex complex.[10]

The principal hormone produced by the gonads in caprine intersexes is testosterone, which accounts for masculine behavior. Intersex goats can be used as teaser animals because they do not produce sperm.[12] Gonadectomy is generally required if the animal is to be used as a pet. Identifying intersex animals with normal or nearly normal external genitalia is difficult. Failure to exhibit estrus, development of male behavior during the breeding season, a shortened vagina on speculum examination, and smaller than normal teats may be the first signs of the intersex condition.[12] The breeding of phenotypically polled bucks should be avoided.

Penile Abnormalities

Several penile abnormalities may occur, albeit rarely in sheep and goats. Both hypospadias and short penile length are associated with intersex in goats. Such animals should be culled. Careful examination of the penis in the fully extended state may reveal existing abnormalities. Occasionally urethral rupture (as a sequela to urethral stones), balanoposthitis (see Chapter 10), injuries to the villiform appendage, hair rings, and other abnormalities are identified.

Both phimosis (inability to extend the penis) and paraphimosis (inability to withdraw the penis into the prepuce) are occasionally seen in rams and bucks; both conditions can cause significant loss of libido and fertility. If they are not quickly diagnosed and treated, affected animals may be rendered infertile. These two conditions may be associated with hair ring, trauma, and balanoposthitis. In cases associated with a hair ring on the glans of the penis, inspecting the penis allows the clinician to identify the problem and remove the "ring" of hair. Shearing the wool or mohair just anterior to the sheath can minimize the incidence of this problem.[8,10] Phimosis also may occur as a sequela to trauma, balanoposthitis, and congenital abnormalities. In cases of trauma an adhesion may form in the sheath or in the sigmoid region, resulting in an inability to extend the penis. As a general rule these cases may be difficult to treat. In cases in which inflammation and scarring result in posthitis, the treatment is the same as that described for balanoposthitis. The clinician can attempt to "break down" the adhesions manually. The use of nonsteroidal antiinflammatory drugs (NSAIDs; flunixin meglumine 1 to 2 mg/kg twice a day [BID]) or antibiotics (procaine penicillin 22,000 IU/kg BID) and lavage of the sheath with mild antiseptics may be of value (see Chapter 10). In cases of

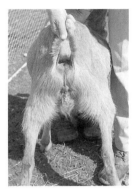

Figure 6-7 This intersex goat had two ovo-testes in the inguinal region. The vulva is positioned very ventrally and joins to an enlarged clitoris at its termination.

phimosis most animals experience a loss of libido and should be culled because the prognosis is poor.[10]

Paraphimosis also is associated with trauma, infection, and balanoposthitis. It is slightly more common in bucks than in rams, but it is rare in both. In cases of paraphimosis, applying antibiotic cream with or without corticosteroids, replacing the penis, and placing a purse-string suture into the preputial orifice may be of value. The inclusion of a tube in the sheath, exiting through the orifice, allows urine drainage. The clinician should take care to ensure proper urine flow. Flushing the sheath and penis with a mild antiseptic solution, providing penile hydrotherapy, and covering the penis with medicated ointments are valuable treatments for this condition. The penis should be extended at least every third day so the keeper or clinician can monitor healing. Sexual rest should be enforced throughout recovery. However, the prognosis in these cases is poor, particularly if the condition is more than 2 weeks old and the animal makes no attempt to retract the penis.[10]

REFERENCES

1. Kimberling CV: Disease of rams. In Kimberling CV, editor: *Diseases of sheep*, ed 3, Philadelphia, 1988, Lea and Febiger.
2. Bulgin MS: *Brucella ovis* epizootic in virgin ram lambs, *J Am Vet Med Assoc* 196(7):1120, 1990.
3. Kimberling CV: Sheep flock fertility, *Proceedings of the Society for Theriogenology*, 1990, Nashville, TN.
4. Bulgin MS: Epididymitis caused by *B. ovis, Proceedings of the Society for Theriogenology*, 1991, Nashville, TN.
5. Walker RL, Leamaster BR: Prevalence of *Histophilus ovis* and *Actinobacillus seminis* in the genital tract of sheep, *Am J Vet Res* 47:1928, 1986.
6. Bulgin MS: Ram lamb epididymitis, *Proceedings of the Society for Theriogenology*, 1991, Nashville, TN.
7. Ley WB: Ram epididymitis, *Agri-Pract* 14(5):34, 1993.
8. Bruer AN: Examination of the ram for breeding soundness. In Morrow DA, editor: *Current therapy in theriogenology*, ed 2, Philadelphia, 1986, WB Saunders.
9. Pugh DG: Breeding soundness evaluation in male goats, *Proc Hudson-Walker Therio Conf* 7:29, 1996.
10. Mickelsen WD, Memon MA: Infertility and diseases of the reproductive organs of bucks. In Youngquist RS, editor: *Current therapy in large animal theriogenology*, Philadelphia, 1997, WB Saunders.
11. Basrur PK, Yusoff RBH: Sex anomalies in goats. In Youngquist RS, editor: *Current therapy in large animal theriogenology*, Philadelphia, 1997, WB Saunders.
12. Smith MC, Sherman DM: *Goat medicine*, Philadelphia, 1994, Lea and Febiger.

SPECIAL PROCEDURES

Castration

Castration is the most common surgical procedure performed in small ruminant practice. Some of the complications that can occur include excessive hemorrhage, evisceration, infection, rupture or tearing of the ureter, and tetanus. The clinician should administer tetanus toxoids or antitoxins when castrating animals. Lambs and kids should receive 150 to 250 units of tetanus antitoxin; adults of unknown vaccination history should receive 500 to 750 units of antitoxin. Previously vaccinated adults should receive a tetanus toxoid booster. In some instances antibiotics may be of value. Evisceration may occur at any age but appears more common in young goats; some breed predisposition (pygmy, Spanish meat) is possible. Routine castration of lambs and kids is usually done during the first week of life. However, if the lamb or kid is to be a long-term pet, it is advisable to wait until the animal is at least 5 to 6 months old to allow for growth of the penis and urethra and detachment of penile adhesions.

Surgical castration. Surgical removal of the testes is superior to all other forms of castration. During the surgical removal of the scrotum and testicles, animals may be lightly sedated, anesthetized, or held by a helper or technician. Young lambs or kids 2 to 4 days old are often castrated by this method without anesthesia. However, sedation can be beneficial because of their vocalization and their greater tendency to develop hypotensive shock. Anesthesia can be achieved by local infiltration of lidocaine hydrochloride in smaller animals. A 1% solution is recommended to prevent lidocaine toxicity (see Chapter 16). Large bucks and rams should be sedated with xylazine hydrochloride (0.05 to 0.3 mg/kg IM) because they are susceptible to shock associated with the stress and pain of castration. In young kids or lambs the lower third of the scrotum is removed by a scalpel blade to expose both testicles. In weanlings and adult bucks or rams, the surgeon makes an incision over each testis or removes the distal third of the scrotum. The scrotal fascia is then stripped away from the testicles. The surgeon pulls the testicles ventrally by steady traction while breaking the cremaster muscle and the scrotal fascia away from the remaining spermatic cord. The spermatic cord should be torn in such a manner that it breaks dorsal to the pampiniform plexus.

When castrating rams or bucks older than 4 months of age and when castrating during the breeding season, the clinician may need to use an emasculator or place a transfixation ligature cranial to the pampiniform plexus to prevent or control hemorrhage. In cases in which hemorrhage appears to be clinically significant, the bleeding vessels should be located, cleaned, and ligated. If the bleeding vessel cannot be identified, the clinician should pack the scrotum with sterile gauze, antiseptic-soaked gauze (iodine), or epinephrine-soaked gauze and then suture the scrotum closed. If gauze is not available and the bleeding vessels cannot be located, the surgeon can close the scrotum with a purse-string suture or a through-and-through suture pattern to obliterate any "dead space." The scrotum should be reopened and the gauze removed

12 to 18 hours after the surgery. These animals may benefit from antibiotic therapy (penicillin 20,000 IU/kg) for 1 to 4 days. On rare occasions, when the testicles are pulled to allow the cord to rupture above the pampiniform plexus, the testicular artery may be avulsed from the aorta, resulting in fatal or near-fatal hemorrhage. Excessive tension can occasionally tear the ureter from the urinary bladder.[1]

Complications are rare with this method. It is easy to perform, and if done quickly, it appears to be associated with limited stress. Animals need exercise after castration to reduce postoperative swelling.

Elastrator. Elastrator castration is the simplest and most common technique used by producers. Lambs and kids younger than 1 to 3 weeks of age are the most suitable candidates for this technique. A very heavy rubber ring is placed around the neck of the scrotum with a special applicator. Care must be taken to ensure that the entire scrotum is included within the band. The penis should be palpated to ensure that it is not trapped within the band. Placing the band over the testicular cord and not directly against the abdominal wall helps prevent the trapping of any portion of the penis (sigmoid flexure). The rubber band method may initially appear to be less traumatic and stressful, but it is considered inhumane by some if it is performed on animals older than 3 weeks of age.[1] The scrotal sac and the trapped testicles become ischemic, die, and drop off within 2 weeks. No hemorrhaging occurs because no open wound is formed, but the risk of tetanus is increased compared with other techniques.[1] Occasionally the blood supply to one or both testicles does not become occluded, and the testicles continue to elaborate testosterone.[1]

Burdizzo emasculatome. A third method that may be used in older sheep and goats is castration by emasculatome. The main advantage of this technique is the absence of an open wound and the decreased risk of tetanus (compared with elastrator bands). Anesthesia is usually not required or used. A Burdizzo emasculatome crushes the spermatic cord and its blood vessels above each testis. The operator holds each cord tightly against the lateral aspect of the scrotum with one hand while applying the instrument twice on each side to crush the cord. The crushes are made 2 cm apart, ensuring that the midline of the scrotum is not crossed. The testicular cords may be clamped together or separately as previously described. When employing an emasculatome, the operator should ensure that both testicular cords are completely clamped. The complications of this method include testicular survival, scrotal sloughing, extreme scrotal swelling, tetanus, and undue suffering. One author of this chapter (Dr. Pugh) considers this the most inhumane method of castration. As with the banding method, the devitalized tissue is allowed to slough.

Hemicastration

A decision may be made to remove a diseased testicle to prevent the spread of disease or heat-induced testicular degeneration (such as that caused by inflammation) to the healthy testicle. The ram or buck should not eat for 48 hours and not drink for 24 hours before being put under general anesthesia; the clinician should administer a broad-spectrum antibiotic 2 to 4 hours before surgery. The animal should be anesthetized (see Chapter 16), placed in right lateral recumbency, and have the entire scrotum and surrounding areas clipped and prepared aseptically. The surgeon makes an elliptical skin incision on the lateral surface of the scrotum, starting near the base of the affected testicle and extending to near the apex. This incision should include the tunica dartos muscle. The surgeon should take care not to extend the incision into the normal hemiscrotum. This elliptical incision should be wide enough to remove any excess skin after the testicle is removed; however, the surgeon should be careful to leave enough skin to close the wound. The testicle and its associated tunics are bluntly dissected away from the scrotum. The vaginal tunics should be excised to expose the testicle and spermatic cord. The spermatic artery and vein should be ligated with a transfixation suture (0 gut) at a level above the pampiniform plexus. The cremaster muscle should also be ligated at a point proximal to the vascular ligature. A separate ligature should be placed around the entire spermatic cord. A clamp or suture is placed around the cord approximately 5 to 6 cm distal to the vascular suture, and the cord is transected. The remaining vaginal tunic is transected far enough distally to allow the tunics to be closed over the remaining cord. An inverting suture pattern (Connell or Parker-Kerr) is used with an absorbable material (0 gut). The tunica dartos muscle is closed over the wound with a simple continuous pattern. The longitudinal skin incision should be closed, and if excess skin is present it should be trimmed so that no dead space remains. The scrotum can be bandaged immediately after surgery if bleeding is expected. This bandage should be left in place no longer than 12 hours to avoid thermal damage to the remaining testicle. Routine presurgical antibiotics (penicillin or tetracycline) should be continued postsurgically as needed. NSAIDs may be indicated for control of pain, swelling, and other signs of inflammation.

Teaser Preparation

Teaser rams and bucks greatly facilitate estrus detection for artificial insemination (AI) and embryo transfer programs, particularly if they are used in conjunction with marking harnesses. In goats, one of the simplest teasers to attain is an intersex animal. Temporary teasers can be created hormonally. A wether, doe, or ewe that is not to be used for breeding can be given testosterone propionate (100 mg every third day or 150 mg weekly), beginning 3 weeks before intended use and continuing through the season.[2] A male used for estrus detection should be healthy and have good libido. A young postpuberal male is best, particularly if he is not so large that he injures females during mounting. The male should be incapable of intromission to minimize the spread of venereal disease. Moreover, in AI programs the introduction of bacterial pathogens into the anterior vagina before breeding should be avoided, which is another reason why males incapable of intromission are preferred teasers. The estrus-detecting male should not be able to ejaculate but should maintain a good libido.

Vasectomy

A properly performed vasectomy renders the male incapable of ejaculation but does not prevent intromission. The authors prefer mild sedation (xylazine 0.05 mg/kg IM) and local infiltrative anesthesia with lidocaine. The skin around the area proximal to the scrotum and the skin on the proximal scrotum is prepared for surgery. The surgeon identifies the vas deferens by palpation with one hand and cuts through the skin over the vas deferens. A combination of blunt and sharp dissection is used to isolate the vas deferens from the other structures of the spermatic cord (Figure 6-8). Two ligatures are placed 4 cm apart, and a 2-cm section of the vas deferens is removed. The skin is closed with sutures, staples, or by a subcuticular closure.[3] The procedure is then repeated on the other testicle. A surgeon can perform a bilateral vasectomy through a single, very "cranial" incision over the spermatic cord. The ram or buck should be rested for 30 days before use.

Epididymectomy

An alternative approach is to remove the entire tail of the epididymis. This technique, similar to vasectomy, does not prevent intromission but does result in infertility. Bilateral caudal epididymectomy is the simplest surgical procedure for teaser buck or ram preparation.[4] Although it is a "field procedure," the surgery should be performed under aseptic conditions. The clinician clips the scrotal wool, cleans the scrotum, aseptically prepares the area, and infiltrates a local anesthetic in the skin over the tail of the epididymis. He or she then grabs the testis and forces it to the distal segment of the scrotum. The tail of the epididymis bulges out on the ventral side of the scrotum. The clinician makes a 3-cm skin incision directly over the tail of the epididymis and continues it through the common vaginal tunic until the tail of the epididymis has extruded. He or she grasps the tail of the epididymis with a pair of towel forceps and, using a combination of blunt and sharp dissection, separates it from the testicle (Figure 6-9). Enough of the epididymis should be isolated so that sutures can be placed proximally on the body of the epididymis and distally on the tail of the epididymis. Alternatively, a pair of forceps can be clamped across the loop of epididymis that has been created and crushed. The loop of epididymis is now removed. If sutures were placed on the epididymis, and the procedure was performed under aseptic conditions, the skin may be closed. In less sterile conditions the skin wound may be left open to granulate. Advantages of epididymectomy over vasectomy include its technical ease and the fact that it can performed under less than ideal conditions. A minimum of 30 days of sexual rest should be enforced before the animal is used in a teaser program.[4]

Penile Translocation

One method of preventing intromission is to "free" the penis and move it over to the left flank. This method is useful in some teaser systems. The surgery prevents intromission, but not ejaculation. Therefore if penile transloca-

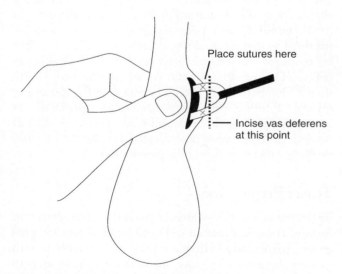

Figure 6-8   Isolation of the vas deferens away from rest of the testicular cord in preparation for vasectomy. As the vas deferens is lifted out of the incision, sutures are applied (at the *X*s) and the vas deferens is cut.

Place sutures here

Incise vas deferens at this point

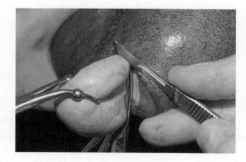

Figure 6-9   The tail of the epididymis is pulled away from the testicle. The scalpel is being held where the tail of the epididymis is to be cut. A hemostat can be placed proximal to the testicle and the epididymis cut distal to it.

tion is attempted, a vasectomy (epididymectomy) also should be performed. The clinician should give the buck or ram a systemic antimicrobial agent 2 or more hours before surgery. With the animal standing, the clinician marks an area 1 cm cranial to the flank fold.[1] The buck or ram is then heavily sedated, anesthetized with injectable anesthetics, intubated and maintained on gas anesthesia, or administered a lumbosacral epidural (see Chapter 16).[1,5] The animal is placed in right lateral recumbency, the ventral abdomen and left flank are clipped, and the surgical site is aseptically prepared.[1,5] The clinician excises a 4- to 7-cm circle of skin and cutaneous trunci muscle above the fold in the left flank. The lower edge of the circular incision should be 1 cm above the flank fold, just cranial to the mark made on the left flank. Hemostasis is achieved and the area is covered with saline-moistened gauze. The clinician then makes a circumferential incision 1 to 2 cm caudal to the preputial orifice through the skin around the sheath and extends the incision longitudinally along the ventral penile shaft, two thirds of the way to the scrotum.[9] The penis is left inside the prepuce, and the two structures are freed of all subcutaneous tissue by blunt dissection, avoiding large vessels. A single "reference" suture is placed in the skin at the most cranial aspect of the preputial orifice and a sterile glove is placed over the orifice.[1] From the circular incision in the flank to the most caudal aspect of the longitudinal incision, the clinician creates a tunnel using scissors and blunt dissection. The penis (along with the sterile glove covering the preputial orifice to maintain asepsis) is pulled through the tunnel.

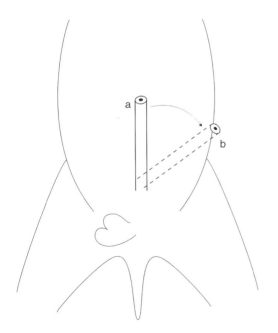

Figure 6-10 This view of the ventral abdomen shows the original site of the penis (a) and the translocated site (b) to the left flank. With this procedure the penis is moved 45° to one side to prevent intromission.

The penis should now be at a 45° angle to the long axis of the body[1] (Figure 6-10). The penis should not be restricted at any point through the tunnel, and the penis and prepuce should not be torsed. The reference suture should be used to align the cranial aspect of the preputial orifice to the dorsal portion of the circular flank incision.[1,5]

The circumferential incision should be sutured with a simple interrupted pattern using absorbable material. The subcutaneous tissue of the transposed prepuce should be sutured to the cutaneous trunci and followed with closure of the skin. The clinician then closes the longitudinal incision, attempting to diminish all open dead space with absorbable material. The authors prefer either a single interrupted or horizontal mattress type suture pattern. The skin over the longitudinal incision is closed by a simple interrupted pattern in all areas except the most cranial aspect of the original preputial incision. To allow for ventral drainage, this area is not sutured.[1,5] Fly control should be maintained, and tetanus prophylaxis should be provided (using tetanus toxoid or antitoxin). The clinician then performs a bilateral epididymectomy, continues administering antibiotics for 5 to 7 days (procaine penicillin 22,000 IU/kg BID), and removes the sutures in 14 days. The male is ready for use in 1 month.

SEMEN COLLECTION AND STORAGE

Rams

Semen from rams may be collected and used fresh or frozen for future use. Typically the rams are trained to service an AV (described in the section on buck evaluation) in the presence of females in estrus or treated ovariectomized females (i.e., females that have been given 1 mg estradiol benzoate per week or prepared as described in the section on libido testing). The semen is collected into a warm (39° C) AV and handled carefully to avoid exposure to any contaminants or ultraviolet rays. Temperature control is of utmost importance in the successful freezing of semen. The semen should be placed in an incubator or water bath (30° C).[6] Semen intended for freezing should have a concentration of more than 3×10^9/ml and a motility of more than 70% of the ejaculate. Semen should be extended in a warmed extender (30° C).[7] This extender can be as simple as whole milk or Dulbecco's phosphate-buffered saline (PBS) with 10% fetal calf serum. Other homemade or commercially prepared extenders containing antibiotics, tris, fructose, and egg yolk may be used. Many methods of semen freezing are used. Only a few are described here.

Straws. The ejaculate is normally diluted to a ratio between 1:1 and 1:4, with extenders added slowly by constant slow mixing.[6,7] The diluent is usually hypertonic; therefore rapid mixing may cause osmotic shock in

TABLE 6-3

EXAMPLES OF EGG YOLK–BASED SEMEN EXTENDERS

INGREDIENT	EXTENDER*	FREEZE BUFFER†
Tris (hydroxy methyl) amino methane (g)	3.634	24.2
Fructose (g)	0.50	10.0
Citric acid (monohydrate) (g)	1.99	13.6
Egg yolk (ml)	14	200
Distilled water (ml)	100	1000

From Evans G, Maxwell WMC: *Salmon's artificial insemination of sheep and goats,* Sydney, 1987, Butterworth Publishing.
*Used for both fresh, cooled semen and the initial extender in freezing.
†pH at 6.8.

spermatozoa.[6] The extended semen is slowly cooled to around freezing (4° to 5° C) over a 1.5- to 2-hour period. The cooled, extended semen should be diluted (usually at a ratio of 1:1) with an additional freeze buffer containing an energy source, a protein, an antibiotic, and a cryoprotectant (glycerol) before being placed into labeled serum straws. The extended semen is then rapidly chilled to between −80° and −100° C by placing the filled straws in liquid nitrogen vapors 4 cm over the surface of liquid nitrogen for 10 minutes. The semen is then rapidly cooled to its final storage temperature of −196° C by submersing the straws in liquid nitrogen. Formulas for mixing extenders and freeze buffers may be obtained by consulting the references. Some extenders are available commercially. An example of an extender with and without the cryoprotectant is shown in Table 6-3.

Pellets. Semen also may be frozen into pellets by dropping cooled semen into depressions drilled or scratched into dry ice. This is a convenient method for freezing, but semen treated this way is more difficult to thaw and use. In this method collected semen can be diluted by volume to contain 4% glycerol and 12% egg yolk in a slightly hypertonic, buffered solution.[6,7] Evans[6] described an example of 1 volume of semen to 4 volumes of diluent, with a diluent of 3.63 g tris (hydroxy methyl) amino methane, 0.50 g glucose, 1.99 g citric acid (monohydrate), 15 ml egg yolk, and 5 ml glycerol extended to 100 ml with distilled and deionized water. In a cooled, ventilated room the examiner makes several small circular cuts (0.5 to 0.8 cm diameter) on a flat piece of solid carbon dioxide (dry ice). Cooled pipettes (4° C) are used to drop 0.1 to 0.3 ml into the cut surface of the dry ice. The semen is allowed to dry for 2 to 3 minutes before the frozen pellets are transferred to the liquid nitrogen.[6]

Cooled Semen

Ram semen also may be collected and chilled for same or next day AI. This provides producers with the opportunity to use semen shipped from other farms.[8,9]

Bucks. No established health requirements exist for AI sires in goats. The health of the individual buck and the herd of origin should be evaluated. Two common semen collection methods are used in the buck: AV and EE. Dairy bucks are handled more often and are more easily trained to use an AV. Semen from meat bucks is more commonly collected by EE. The AV method is preferred because it is quicker, not stressful to the male, and results in the collection of better-quality semen.[7] Semen collected by EE is generally of larger volume but lower concentration than that collected by AV. The frequency at which semen may be collected depends on the age, condition, and temperament of the animal. Bucks can be collected two to three times daily on alternate days. Intervals of 30 minutes to 1 hour are advisable between daily collections to obtain good-quality semen.[7] Labeled ejaculates are placed in a water bath at 35° C until they can be evaluated. An immediate 1:1 extension with a diluent provides energy and buffer. The semen is evaluated for volume, motility, concentration, and morphology as described previously. Accurate determination of the concentration of the semen is important; the dilution ratio depends on it. Semen can be processed to be used fresh or frozen in straws in a similar fashion as described for rams.

COOLED OR FRESH SEMEN: The diluents commonly used to dilute buck semen contain either tris or citrate as the buffer, glucose or fructose as the energy source, and egg yolk to protect the spermatozoal cell membranes against cold shock. The concentration of egg yolk should be reduced to 2% to avoid it reacting with the coagulating enzyme present in the seminal plasma.[7] This enzyme occurs in greater concentrations when semen is collected by EE. To overcome any problems with the coagulating enzyme, a low-concentration egg yolk diluent or skim milk can be used or the seminal plasma can be removed by centrifugation immediately after collection.[7,10] Under field conditions the most readily available semen diluent is skim milk. The ultra–heat-treated milk is sterile and may be used directly as a diluent without any further treatment.[7] When does are inseminated with fresh spermatozoa by laparoscopic technique, PBS with the addition of 1000 IU of sodium penicillin and 1 mg of streptomycin per ml can be used as an extender.[7] The extended semen can be inserted by pipette into 0.5-ml straws and cooled gradually over 1 to 2 hours from 30° C to the storage temperature of 5° C. This semen should be used within 6 to 8 hours.[7] The semen should be cooled gradually over 1 to 2 hours.

FROZEN SEMEN: Many of the same principles described for the storage of frozen ram semen are applicable to goats. Buck semen can be placed in plastic straws and frozen in liquid nitrogen vapor by either slow or fast methods. Diluents for freezing buck semen should have similar properties to diluents used to extend fresh semen. In addition, they should contain an agent to protect the cell membrane during cooling (usually egg yolk) and a cryoprotective agent (usually glycerol) to protect the spermatozoa against membrane damage during freezing.[7,10] Dilution of semen can be performed in two ways. The two-step dilution method is similar to that used for bull semen. The semen is diluted at 30° C shortly after collection to half of the final diluted volume with a diluent containing no glycerol.[7] After cooling at 5° C for 1.5 to 2 hours, the semen is extended to the final volume with a diluent containing glycerol.[7] For one-step dilution the semen is gradually diluted to the final pre-freezing volume at 5° C in 1.5 to 2 hours in a refrigerator or cold room. The two-step dilution method has no advantage over the one-step method for buck semen. Therefore the one-step method is preferred because it simplifies diluent preparation and reduces the handling of semen before freezing.

After dilution the semen is loaded in 0.5-ml labeled plastic straws and sealed for freezing. The straws are placed horizontally on a cold rack (5° C) and lowered into liquid nitrogen vapor 3 to 4 cm above the surface of the liquid nitrogen in a Styrofoam or other suitable container. After 7 to 8 minutes the frozen straws are immersed in liquid nitrogen, carefully packaged into goblets of appropriate size, and transferred into liquid nitrogen storage tanks.[7]

FROZEN SEMEN HANDLING

Frozen semen for bucks and rams is stored in liquid nitrogen (−196° C). Any changes in this storage temperature can seriously alter semen quality.[11] Semen is most commonly packaged in 0.25- or 0.5-ml straws. The straw is placed in a holding goblet, with two goblets attached to a cane. Multiple canes are set inside a canister, which is immersed and maintained in a liquid nitrogen tank. The liquid nitrogen tank lid should be kept closed and the liquid nitrogen level checked and maintained at an adequate level. A schedule of tank maintenance should be set up and followed. A record of where particular semen is stored (goblet, cane, canister) helps expedite semen transfer and retrieval.[12] The tank should be kept in a cool, well-ventilated room. Straws should not be removed from the tank unless they are to be used; they should not be transferred from tank to tank unless the procedure takes less than 2 seconds.

To thaw the straws, the clinician should identify the canister holding the cane. The canister is raised until the cane tops can be seen (5 to 7 cm below the mouth of the tank). Straws should be maintained below the frost line in the neck of the tank at all times. Using a light source to identify the correct cane, the clinician removes

the straw to be thawed with tweezers or forceps. The cane is immediately dropped back into the canister, and the canister is immersed in the liquid nitrogen.[11,12] Straws should not be touched by the handler's hands.[11] The clinician should shake the straw (to remove any liquid nitrogen), quickly identify whether it is the correct straw, and then immerse it in a water bath (33° to 35° C). Straws should be thawed based on manufacturers' recommendations, but generally thawing requires only 40 seconds for 0.5-ml straws and 20 seconds for 0.25-ml straws.[11] Only as many straws as can be used in 10 to 15 minutes should be thawed at one time. If possible, the clinician should thaw no more than three straws at one time to avoid lowering the thaw water temperature.[11]

As goblets are emptied, they should be discarded to expedite the retrieval of straws in the lower goblets. However, if straws are to be retrieved from lower goblets, the cane is raised until the straws are even with the other cane tops, and then the straw to be used is removed.[11,12]

If pellets are used, the clinician removes the pellets from liquid nitrogen storage and places two or three directly in a dry, sterile tube. The tube is kept in a warm water bath (37° C). The thawed semen should be pulled into a pipette and used for AI immediately.[6] Alternatively, some processing techniques may require the addition of a warm diluent to the frozen pellets.

REFERENCES

1. Hooper RN: General surgical techniques for small ruminants: small ruminants for the mixed animal practitioner, *Proceedings of the Western Veterinary Conference*, 1998, Las Vegas, NV.
2. Smith MC, Sherman DM: *Goat medicine*, Philadelphia, Lea & Febiger, 1994; pp 411-463.
3. Kimberling CV, Marsh DJ: Breeding soundness evaluation and surgical sterilization of the ram. In Youngquist RS, editor: *Current therapy in large animal theriogenology*, Philadelphia, 1997, WB Saunders.
4. Wolfe DF, Baird AN: Urogenital surgery in goats. In Youngquist RS, editor: *Current therapy in large animal theriogenology*, Philadelphia, 1997, WB Saunders.
5. Riddell MG: Prevention of intromission by estrus-detector males. In Wolfe DF, Moll HD, editors: *Large animal urogenital surgery*, Baltimore, 1999, Williams & Wilkins.
6. Evans G: Freezing sheep semen. In Dziuk PJ, Wheeler M, editors: *Handbook of methods for study of reproductive physiology in domestic animals*, Urbana, IL, 1991, University of Illinois Press.
7. Evans G, Maxwell WMC: *Salmon's artificial insemination of sheep and goats*, Sydney, 1987, Butterworth Publishing.
8. Buckrell BC et al: Reproductive technologies in commercial use for sheep, goats, and farmed deer, *Proceedings of the Society for Theriogenology*, 1997, Nashville, TN.
9. Mylne MJA, Hunton JR, Buckrell BC: Artificial insemination of sheep. In Youngquist RS, editor: *Current therapy in large animal theriogenology*, Philadelphia, 1997, WB Saunders.
10. Cehmineau P et al: *Training manual on artificial insemination in sheep and goats*, Rome, 1991, FAO of the United Nations.
11. Buckrell BC: *Guelph system for transcervical AI (user manual)*, Georgetown, Ontario, Canada, Small Ruminant Genetics.

12. Marshall CE: Handling of frozen semen straws. In Dziuk PJ, Wheeler M, editors: *Handbook of methods for study of reproductive physiology in domestic animals*, Urbana, IL, 1991, University of Illinois Press.

FEMALE REPRODUCTION

Ewe

Anatomy. The reproductive tract of the ewe and doe is similar to that of other domestic animals. It is composed of the external genitalia (vulva, clitoris), vagina, cervix, uterus, oviducts, and ovaries. The vulva has two labia, which are composed of adipose tissue and portions of constrictor vulvae muscle covered with skin. The labia are marked by dorsal and ventral commissures. On parting the vulvar lips, the inner surface is easily visualized. The clitoris is homologous to the penis and has some erectile tissue. The vestibule is located cranial to the clitoris. It is lined with stratified squamous epithelium, rich in mucous glands. The vestibule of the ewe contains paramedian glands that exist along the urethral orifice; the doe lacks these glands.

The tubular portion of the tract (vagina, cervix, uterus, oviducts) is composed of an outer serosal surface, a double layer of muscular tissue, submucosa, and a mucosal layer. The vagina is located cranial to the vestibule. In the normal position the vaginal walls are collapsed into folds. The vaginal lumen is composed of stratified squamous epithelium. The cervix is located at the most cranial portion of the vagina and is found in a subtle depression near the vaginal floor. The canal of the cervix has 5 to 6 and 5 to 8 irregular overlapping rings in the ewe and doe, respectively. This tortuous, narrow, cervical lumen causes great difficulty in transcervical AI, particularly in the ewe. The cervix of the ewe and doe, unlike the vagina, is not easily dilatable. The cervix opens cranially into the uterine body. The bicornate uterus is composed of a short body and two horns that, in the nongravid state, are slightly coiled and lie in the pelvic canal. The serosal surface of the uterus is slung in the abdominal cavity by the highly vascular broad ligament. The endometrium is a pink-gray structure with folds that have convex caruncles. Melanin pigmentation is found in these caruncular regions in some breeds of sheep (Hampshire). This pigment is rare in goats.

The two oviducts attach the uterine horns to the ovarian bursa. The small (1.5 by 1 to 2 cm) oval ovaries are partially covered by the ovarian bursa. The ovarian surface is usually rough. During the breeding season or during gestation, the ovary can have two or more progesterone-secreting corpus lutea.

Physiology. Age, nutritional status, and season of the year all play roles in the development of sexual maturity in the sheep.[1-4] The approach of the breeding season or artificial manipulation of light to mimic shorter days hastens the onset of estrus in ewe lambs. Melatonin implants can cause a similar effect.[5,6] Differing reports about the effect of light manipulation and melatonin implants can be found in the literature.[7-9] The sex of siblings in multiple-birth lambings does not seem to affect the age of puberty in the ewe[10]; however, exposure to intact rams can decrease the time required for the ewe lamb to achieve her first estrus.[4] The attainment of puberty depends on the interaction of the juvenile hypothalamus, the anterior pituitary, and the ovary. Estradiol secreted by developing follicles has a negative feedback on LH secretion. As puberty approaches this inhibitory influence becomes less important and GnRH pulses from the hypothalamus and subsequent pituitary pulses of LH become more frequent. This stimulates further follicular development. As the follicle develops, it produces more estradiol until a threshold is reached, causing a positive feedback on LH secretion.[11] The resultant LH surge induces the luteinization of the follicle and usually ovulation. The life span of the resultant corpus luteum (CL) is usually shorter than that of subsequent cycles. This first ovulation in the sheep is not associated with behavioral estrus. The second and subsequent cycles of follicular growth, LH secretion, and CL development appear more normal and result in behavioral estrus. Follicle-stimulating hormone (FSH) also is released from the anterior pituitary gland in response to GnRH.[12]

Sheep are considered short-day breeders because their breeding season is regulated by the length of the day or, more specifically, by the increased duration of night.[13] Light duration and timing affect not only the induction of estrus, but short daylight regimens also can affect the length of the breeding season.[14] Seasonality is controlled by the visual perception of light that is transmitted by the superior cervical ganglion to the pineal gland. The pineal gland produces melatonin and secretes it during the night. Alteration in melatonin secretion provides cues to the hypothalamus in its pulse generations of GnRH.[12] The hypothalamus also changes in its sensitivity from a strictly negative feedback response to estrogen (from the developing follicles) to a positive feedback from increasing concentrations of estrogen.[15] The increased pulses of GnRH appear responsible for the induction of estrus during the breeding season.[16] In seasonally breeding animals a similar scenario occurs during puberty as is observed in the yearly transition from anestrus to the seasonal cycle. However, much variation occurs among breeds with respect to the occurrence and length of the breeding season. Dorset, Merino, Rambouillet, and Finnish-Landrace sheep tend to have longer breeding seasons, whereas the Southdown, Shropshire, and Hampshire breeds respond to day length and adhere to the short-day breeding season. Sheep living near the equator (or breeds that originated there such as the Barbados) are usually less sensitive to the effects of the seasons.

Estrus cycle. Estrus in the ewe lasts between 15 and 45 hours (with an average of 30 hours), and the interval between estrous activity is between 14 and 19 days (with an average of 17 days)—3 to 5 days of metestrus, 7 to 10 days of diestrus, and 2 days of proestrus). Ewe lambs, ewes cycling outside of the normal breeding season, and transitional ewes tend to have shorter estrus periods. As estrus approaches, the larger follicles of the FSH-induced follicular wave begin to produce more estradiol. This signals the hypothalamus to secrete GnRH, which results in the release of LH by the anterior pituitary gland. This LH surge typically occurs about 9 hours after the onset of estrus. The high estradiol concentration is partially responsible for the ewe showing signs of estrus. However, the sheep also must have been recently exposed to progesterone. Sheep ovulate toward the final third of estrus or occasionally after the end of behavioral estrus.[17] Ovulation typically occurs 14 to 26 hours after the LH surge. This coincides with about 21 to 45 hours after the beginning of estrus. The length of estrus may vary depending on the breed, with wool breeds generally having a longer estrus than meat breeds. Signs of estrus include vulvar swelling and anorexia in the ewe. The ewe may secrete small amounts of mucus, much less than that secreted by the cow.

After ovulation the follicle becomes luteinized and begins producing progesterone. The progesterone concentration remains elevated for about 12 to 13 days. In the absence of a conceptus the ovaries produce oxytocin and the uterine endometrium begins to secrete prostaglandin $F_{2\alpha}$ ($PGF_{2\alpha}$). The $PGF_{2\alpha}$ is transported away from the uterus by the uterine veins and is transferred directly to the ovarian arteries that run adjacent to the veins. The increased concentration of $PGF_{2\alpha}$ in the ovarian arteries leads to the regression of the luteal tissue and diminished progesterone secretion. The cycle begins again with a decrease in serum progesterone, concurrent development of the follicle, and a subsequent increase in serum estrogen concentrations. Ovum transport to the uterus takes 2 to 4 days in ewes. Approximately 12 days after conception, signals are sent to the endometrium and ovaries to prevent lysis of the luteal tissue and to maintain the pregnancy. The substance that inhibits uterine production of estrogen receptors is interferon-τ; the decrease in estrogen receptors in turn inhibits oxytocin receptors. This breaks a link in the production of luteolytic amounts of $PGF_{2\alpha}$.[18] Attachment of the embryo to the uterine endometrium is a slow process, beginning around day 18.

Gestation. The normal gestation length of the ewe is 145 to 150 days. Sheep have a cotyledonary, epitheliochorial placenta. The placental cotyledon and the maternal caruncle together form a placentome. In the pregnant ewe, 90 to 100 cotyledons are dispersed over the chorionic membrane. Around day 16 the chorion begins attaching to the uterine caruncles. This type of placenta

limits antibodies moving from the maternal to the fetal circulation, necessitating the ingestion of colostrum by the neonate for antibody transfer. After day 75 the concentration of progestin in the peripheral blood markedly increases. This increase results from the placental production of progestin and is of major clinical significance because luteolytic agents cannot guarantee abortion after day 75 of gestation. Parturition occurs as a result of a complex set of interactions involving the uterine musculature and fetus. As the fetal hypothalamus matures, it begins producing increasing amounts of corticotropin-releasing hormone, which stimulates the pituitary gland to produce and release corticotropin. This in turn stimulates the fetal adrenal glands to produce and release cortisol. Endogenous cortisol results in an increase in the estradiol, $PGF_{2\alpha}$, and prostaglandin-E2 (PGE2) concentrations. This in turn decreases progesterone production and relaxes the cervix. Uterine responsiveness to oxytocin also increases because of the estrogen-induced recruitment of oxytocin receptors. Normal parturition occurs over a period of 3 to 8 hours. The first stage of parturition (initiation of organized contractions) lasts from 1 to 4 hours. The second stage (active labor and delivery of the fetus) lasts as long as 2 hours. The final phase of parturition is the delivery of the placenta and should occur within 8 hours after the fetus is delivered.[12]

Doe

Physiology. From a pure physiologic standpoint, sheep and goats have great similarities. Nevertheless, they are dissimilar in length of the estrus cycle and maintenance of pregnancy. Goats in a temperate region are polyestrous and breed efficiently when day lengths are short (August to March), with a peak breeding season of October through December.[19] The transitional periods are approximately 2 months before and after breeding season, with deepest anestrus in April and May.[20,21] In tropical areas near the equator, native breeds show less seasonality and breed year-round (as do sheep). Variation in seasonality occurs among and within breeds, which allows for selection of out-of-season breeders.[20,22] For example, pygmy and Tennessee stiff-legged meat goat breeds tend to cycle year-round in North America, whereas Nubian, Spanish, Boer, and Kiko goats show more seasonality.[21] Producers can use this seasonality to their advantage in a synchronization program by introducing bucks during the summer transitional period to induce estrus in does. This "buck effect" is lessened when males live year-round with does.

Puberty. Does reach sexual maturity and begin to cycle at 6 to 8 months.[19] In pygmy goats, puberty may occur as early as 3 months. Generally a single-born doe has her first ovulation in the fall after her birth. Breeding should be delayed until a doe has attained 60% to 70% of her predicted adult weight (or 60 to 70 lb in meat goats and 70 to 90 lb in dairy breeds).[21]

Estrus cycle. The length of the estrus cycle in the doe is 21 days (with a range of 18 to 22 days). Although variations exist, estrus tends to be longer in does than in ewes. Short cycles of 5 to 7 days are more common at the beginning and end of the breeding season in does.[19] After midsummer, the decreasing day length causes increased melatonin release from the pineal gland, and the sequence of hormonal events is similar to that seen in the ewe. During estrus and seasonal anestrus, plasma progesterone concentrations are less than 1 ng/ml, whereas progesterone levels during the luteal phase are 4 to 8 ng/ml[19,20] (Figure 6-11).

Estrus varies from 24 to 72 hours, with most does exhibiting estrus for 36 hours. Does in estrus are restless, wag their tails, vocalize, and have swollen vulvas with clear mucous discharge that changes to cloudy toward the end of estrus. These behaviors may be pronounced in the presence of a buck. Milk production and appetite may decrease during estrus in dairy goats. Well-fed, healthy, mature does average two to three ovulations per cycle, which results in a high proportion of multiple births.

Gestation. Twins or triplets are more common than single kids. Oviductal transfer of the embryo(s) requires 3 to 4 days in goats. The average duration of gestation is 5 months, with a range of 147 to 155 days.[19] Similar to ewes, does have epitheliochorial, cotyledonary placentae. Pregnancy is maintained by progesterone, which is produced entirely by the CL of pregnant does and not by the placenta. This is different from ewes, which maintain sufficient progestogen output from their uteroplacental units. The plasma concentration of progesterone remains high until about 4 days before parturition.

REFERENCES

1. Mukasa-Mugerwa E, Kasali OB, Said AN: Effect of nutrition and endoparasitic treatment on growth, onset of puberty and reproductive activity in Menz ewe lambs, *Therio* 36:319, 1991.
2. Forcada F, Abecia JA, Zarazaga L: A note on attainment of puberty of September-born early-maturing lambs in relation to level of nutrition, *Anim Prod* 53:407, 1991.
3. McCann MA et al: Effect of rapid weight gain to puberty on reproduction, mammary development and lactation in ewe lambs, *Therio* 32:55, 1989.
4. Kassem R, Owen JB, Fadel I: The effect of pre-mating nutrition and exposure to the presence of rams on the onset of puberty in Awassi ewe lambs under semi-arid condition, *Anim Prod* 48:393, 1989.
5. Rajkumar RR, Argo CM, Rodway RG: Effect of melatonin on pulsatilla release of luteinizing hormone in female lambs, *Horm Metab Res* 24:229, 1992.
6. Fitzgerald JA, Butler WR: Sexual maturation of ewes raised without ram exposure in a controlled lighting environment, *Therio* 29:811, 1988.
7. Kennaway DJ et al: Pituitary response to LHRH, LH pulsability and plasma melatonin and prolactin changes in ewe lambs treated with melatonin implants to delay puberty, *J Repro Fert* 78:137, 1986.
8. Nowak R, Rodway RG: Effect of intravaginal implants of melatonin on the onset of ovarian activity in adult prepuberal ewes, *J Repro Fert* 74:287, 1985.
9. Sunderland SJ et al: Effect of photoperiod before and after birth on puberty in ewe lambs, *Bio Repro* 53:1178, 1995.
10. Meridith S, Kiesling DO: Age of puberty in ewes which developed prenatally with either a ram or a ewe fetus, *Small Rumin Res* 20:137, 1996.
11. Kinder JE et al: Endocrine basis for puberty in heifers and ewes, *J Repro Fert-Suppl* 49:393, 1995.
12. Stellflug JN, Weems YS, Weems CW: Clinical reproductive physiology in ewes. In Youngquist RS, editor: *Current therapy in large animal theriogenology*, Philadelphia, 1997, WB Saunders.
13. Sweeny T, O'Callaghan D: Physiology of seasonal reproductive transitions in the ewe—regulation by photo period and other environmental cues, *Repro Domestic Anim* 30:178, 1995.

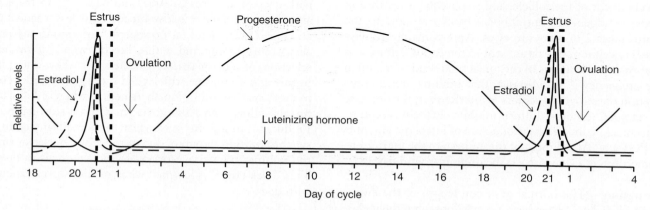

Figure 6-11 A schematic diagram of the caprine estrus cycle showing a follicular stage of the cycle. Plasma progesterone levels decline, removing the negative feedback from the pituitary and permitting the increased release of LH, which in turn acts on the follicle to subtly increase estrogen production and ovulation. Note that the LH and estradiol levels are highest when progesterone levels are lowest. The ewe's cycle is very similar, with one major exception: it is 3 to 4 days shorter.

14. O'Callaghan D et al: Role of short days in timing of onset and duration of reproductive activity in ewes under artificial photoperiods, *Bio Repro* 44:23, 1991.

15. Karsch FJ et al: Seasonal changes in gonadotropin-releasing hormone secretion in the ewe: alteration in response to the negative feedback action of estradiol, *Bio Repro* 49:1377, 1993.

16. Barrel GK et al: Seasonal changes of gonadotropin-releasing hormone secretion in ewe, *Bio Repro* 46:1130, 1992.

17. Keisler DH: Endocrine control of reproduction in the ewe and ram: a review. Small ruminant short course, *Proceedings of the Society for Theriogenology,* p 2, 1994, Nashville, TN.

18. Spencer TE, Becker WC, George P: Ovine interferon-tau regulates expression of endometrial receptors for estrogen and oxytocin but not progesterone, *Bio Repro* 53:732, 1995.

19. Smith MC: Clinical reproductive anatomy and physiology of the doe. In Youngquist RS, editor: *Current therapy in large animal theriogenology,* Philadelphia, 1997, WB Saunders.

20. Hill J: Goat reproductive management, *Proceedings of the Symposium on Health and Disease of Small Ruminants, American Association of Small Ruminant Practice,* p 114, 1996, Nashville, TN.

21. Mobini S: Reproductive management in goats, *Proceedings of the North American Veterinary Conference,* vol 14, p 219, 2000, Orlando, FL.

22. Wilddeus S: Reproductive management for meat goat production, *Proceedings of the Southeast Region Meat Goat Production Symposium,* Tallahassee, FL, 1996, Florida A & M University.

BREEDING SOUNDNESS EXAMINATION OF THE FEMALE

History is an essential component of a BSE of a doe or ewe because of the inaccessibility of the majority of the reproductive tract to palpation or visual inspection. Historical information of significance includes duration of heat, interestrous intervals, reaction to the male, and breeding and kidding history. A general physical examination emphasizing body condition, femininity, conformation of the mammary glands, and determination of whether the female is polled or horned is important in the evaluation of breeding soundness.

External genital examination should include evaluation of the anogenital distance and whether the clitoris is visible without parting the lips of the vulva. The vulva should be examined for abnormalities. A clear AI speculum or an endoscope can be used to evaluate the vagina and cervix. The clinician should note any discharges from the cervix or vagina. A normal, clear mucous vaginal discharge in early standing estrus that turns into a cloudy or creamy mucous discharge late in standing estrus is common, particularly in does. Transabdominal ultrasonography can be used to examine the uterus for pregnancy and pseudopregnancy. Pseudopregnancy is a more common problem in does than in ewes. Transrectal probes often allow visualization of the non-pregnant uterus and ovaries and early pregnancy.

BREEDING MANAGEMENT

Ewe

To maximize reproductive potential, keepers should maintain ewes in a healthy and disease-free state with a body condition score between 2.5 and 3.5 at the initiation of the breeding season. Ewe lambs should be bred so that they go through parturition earlier in the season than older ewes. Ewes require at least one cycle of increasing day length before the decreasing day length that signals the breeding season in order to cycle. Replacement lambs should be chosen from a pool of lambs born early in the previous lambing season. Ewe lambs should weigh approximately 70% of their projected mature weight at the time of breeding.

Doe

Replacement doe kids should be selected at weaning (4 to 5 months). Selection of meat does should emphasize traits such as reproduction and soundness. Milking does are selected based on production traits such as soundness of the udder and teats, adequate body size, and good body condition. Female goats that were born as twins or triplets, those born early in the season, and those whose dams gave birth more than once each year are preferable replacement does. All females of breeding age should be maintained in a single group. Breeding should be delayed until a doe has attained 60% to 70% of its adult weight at a body condition score of 3 to 3.5. Does that do not kid by the time they are 2 years old should be culled. Breeding does should not be allowed to become too thin or too fat. Thin does may fail to conceive, have low twinning rates, and produce kids with low weaning rates. Obese does can suffer from pregnancy toxemia and/or decreased milk production if they are allowed to become fat before the onset of puberty.

Control of the Estrus Cycle

With the increasing use of AI and the desire of producers to concentrate their efforts around lambing, control of the estrus cycle of the female is necessary. Estrus synchronization programs useful in goats and sheep are shown in Box 6-2. Producers often request estrus synchronization during the fall breeding season and to induce estrus during the winter anestrous period (nonbreeding season) and summer transitional period. To maintain a continuous milk supply from dairy goats and sheep, the flock should be divided into four equal breeding groups. This necessitates some form of estrus synchronization. In the Northern Hemisphere, these groups should be assigned to breedings in late August, mid-October, mid-November, and late December. Adequate nutrition, estrus detection, and adequate sire or insemination capabilities are essential components of a

BOX 6-2

Methods of Estrus Cycle Manipulation Used in Sheep and Goats in the United States

EWE

BREEDING SEASON
- Prostaglandins (single or double injections 9 to 11 days apart)
- Progesterone implants for 14 days used alone or in conjunction with PG 600*
- Oral melengestrol acetate (MGA, 0.125 mg/ewe/day BID for 14 days)

TRANSITIONAL SEASON
- Ram effect
- Progestin (MGA, implants, or pessary) for 8 to 14 days plus PG 600 up to 48 hours before progestin removal

OUT OF BREEDING SEASON
- Selection of breeds and individuals that cycle out of season or early in breeding season
- Progestin (MGA, implants, or pessary) for 8 to 14 days plus PG 600 up to 48 hours before progestin removal
- Ram effect
- Light manipulation
- Melatonin administration

DOE

BREEDING SEASON
- Prostaglandins (single or double dose)
- Progestins (PO or SC) for 14 days
- Progestins for 14 days plus 4 ml of PG 600 24 to 48 hours before or at the time of implant removal

TRANSITIONAL SEASON
- Buck effect
- Progestin for 14 days plus 5 ml of PG 600 48 hours before progestin removal

OUT OF BREEDING SEASON
- Progestin for 14 days plus 5 ml of PG 600 48 hours before progestin removal
- Lighting programs

*PG 600 (400 IU eCG and 200 IU hCG/5 ml vial), Intervet, Millsboro, NC.

synchronization program. Because any form of stress can affect the efficacy of a synchronization program, stress should be minimized as much as possible.

Ram or buck effect. Introducing a buck or ram into a group of transitional period does or ewes is a powerful tool to induce estrus.[5-7] Introducing a ram into a ewe herd induces estrus in most ewes within 6 days. The females should have no contact with the males for 3 to 4 weeks before their introduction. Suddenly placing the male with females induces an LH surge and ovulation within a few days. Similarly, fence line contact by males can be used to achieve a ram or buck effect for hand mating. The use of high-performing rams, as defined by serving capacity tests, has been shown to be more effective in inducing early ovulation than the use of low-fertility rams.[6] The response to male stimulation can be quite variable and is influenced by breed, previous isolation, depth of anestrus, nutrition, and length of time since parturition. This technique can be used in combination with pharmacologic out-of-season breeding programs and appears to enhance their efficacy. Males should be isolated from females for 30 to 60 days before introduction. When using the ram or buck effect in out-of-season breeding, producers should expose the male to a cycling female or an ovariectomized female treated

with estradiol cypionate (2 mg IM) for 2 weeks before using him to breed. Males that have undergone vasectomy or epididymectomy and castrated males treated with testosterone (100 mg weekly for 3 weeks) may be used. Regardless of the type of teaser male used, he should be introduced to the females for 2 to 3 weeks to bring them into heat before the desired breeding male is brought in. The first estrus after introduction of the male is usually silent.

Prostaglandins. $PGF_{2\alpha}$ can be used to lyse the CL and bring diestral females into heat. Goats and sheep are generally susceptible to prostaglandin-induced luteolysis after days 5 to 6 of the estrus cycle. This method of estrus synchronization should be used if the producer is sure that a significant number of ewes and does are actively cycling; it is most effective during the middle to late fall (October and November in North America). One shot of $PGF_{2\alpha}$ can be expected to result in 60% to 70% of the females in the flock exhibiting estrus within 30 to 60 hours. Ewes or does that do not show estrus after a properly administered prostaglandin injection have either been in estrus recently or are anestrous. A two-treatment method involving a second injection 9 to 11 days after the first results in tighter synchrony within the flock. An alternative is to observe the flock actively for 4 days, breed all females that come into estrus during this time, administer $PGF_{2\alpha}$ on the fourth day, and breed all females that come into estrus during the next 3 days. This should result in most females being bred within a 7-day period. Both $PGF_{2\alpha}$ (10 to 20 mg) and cloprostenol (75 µg per 45 kg of body weight) are used for estrus synchronization.[1] Producers should ensure that none of the ewes or does are pregnant at the time of administration of prostaglandins because abortion may be induced.

Progestins. Progestins are used to synchronize estrus by delaying its onset. Exogenous progestin can be used during the breeding season to control the length of the luteal phase artificially. The use of progestins is the most common method of estrus synchronization in goats for AI or embryo transfer. The most common route of application of progestin is transvaginal. After the progestin products are removed, estrus should occur within a few days. Placing sponges that contain progesterone into the vagina (controlled intravaginal drug-releasing devices, or CIDRs) is becoming a popular method of estrus control in some countries.[2] Several progesterone concentrations are available in CIDRs. However, devices containing 366 mg appear to yield the most reproducible responses in the experience of one of the authors (Dr. Pugh). Occasionally CIDRs may be difficult to remove if the string is not visible from the vulvar lips or the sponge has adhered to the vaginal wall. In both cases the examiner should restrain the female, introduce a gloved finger into the vaginal vault, identify the CIDR, and carefully remove it after separating it from the vaginal wall. The use of norgestomet implants ($^1/_2$ to 1 implant, or 3 to 6 mg) inserted between the skin and cartilage of the dorsal aspect of the ears' pinnae also are commonly used. Synchronization rates after feeding melengestrol acetate are similar to those encountered with norgestomet implants.[4] The feeding of oral melengestrol acetate (0.22 mg/ewe or doe for 14 days, or 0.125 mg/ewe or doe twice daily for 14 days) also is of value in controlling estrus. However, it is generally recommended that breeding be delayed until the second heat after the melengestrol acetate feeding is discontinued.[1] Also, if progesterone is added to the feed, a continuous adequate intake is imperative. This may be a problem in goats and some sheep, particularly if inadequate feeder or bunk space is available. All of these methods require the removal of the progestin after 9 to 14 days in the ewe, and 12 to 14 days in the doe. The removal of the progestin source can be used to synchronize the entire flock at one time. The flock can be divided, and the progesterone source removed daily, so that one ram can be used for breeding or the AI program can be spread out. Estrus can be expected about 24 to 48 hours and 24 to 36 hours after the removal of the progesterone sources in ewes and does, respectively.

Introducing a teaser male 24 hours after progestin removal enhances synchrony. Administering equine chorionic gonadotropin (eCG, 250 IU) or a combination of eCG and human chorionic gonadotropin (hCG) while removing the progestin can help tighten synchrony in the herd.[1] Administering prostaglandins 24 hours before progestin removal, followed by eCG 24 to 48 hours before or at the time of progestin removal may further tighten estrus synchrony. The use and removal of these progestin products also may hasten estrus in the non-breeding season.[3]

Seasonal manipulation. Seasonal manipulation of the female cycle can be used to hasten the onset of estrus to obtain more than one breeding per year. Seasonal manipulation also can change the time of lambing and kidding and lactation to better match forage availability. Dairy goats should be more than 120 days into the lactation period before the producer attempts an out-of-season breeding program.[8] All animals should be examined with real-time ultrasonography equipment to determine whether any reproductive abnormalities exist that may preclude the effectiveness of an out-of-season breeding program (e.g., pregnancy, hydrometra).[8] Artificial lighting, either by itself or in conjunction with exogenous melatonin can be used for effective manipulation of the breeding season. The sudden introduction of the male maximizes the efficacy of light-melatonin programs. Artificial lighting is mostly employed to mimic a long day. During the Northern Hemisphere winter, long days (approximately 20 hours of light) can be simulated for 2 months (in a barn) and then stopped on March 1. Animals are then exposed to natural daily sunlight. After 6 weeks of natural daylight exposure, males are introduced and a fertile estrus occurs within 10 to 20 days. Does undergoing this type of estrus manipulation have a short breeding season of around 60 days. Bucks and rams also may benefit from this type of treatment to increase libido and quality of semen. Light manipulation, although effective, is rarely practical (see Box 6-2).

Some producers combine hormones and lighting for out-of-season breeding. Lighting manipulation is used successfully in many dairy goat operations. Exogenous melatonin can be administered to supplement the endogenous release and thereby mimic the short days associated with the onset of breeding season. Exogenous melatonin can be given as a slow-release implant, repeatedly as an injection, or orally over 30 to 60 days to accelerate the onset of breeding. After the cessation of melatonin administration, females begin to cycle in 40 to 70 days. The lack of availability of this drug limits its use. Exogenous melatonin should be combined with the introduction of the male. Melatonin works most efficiently in dairy goats when combined with artificial lighting for out-of-season breeding.

The most commonly used program for out-of-season breeding is a combination of progestin (delivered as an implant in the ear [norgestomet] or vaginally [CIDR]) and pregnant mare serum gonadotropin (PMSG) or eCG. The progestin should be injected, fed, or implanted for 14 days. A gonadotropin, either FSH or PMSG, is administered 48 hours before progestin removal. PMSG (400 IU) is most commonly used because it requires only one injection. In areas where PMSG is not available for use, a product containing both hCG and PMSG can be substituted. Variable results have been reported with the use of these products depending on the timing and dosage of administration. The introduction of a buck or ram enhances the synchronization of these programs.

Increasing Twinning Rates

Most successful sheep-rearing enterprises depend on the number of lambs raised and sold per ewe per year. Genetic selection for prolific ewes can be slow because of the low heritability of the trait (10%), but some breeds tend to have this predisposition (Finnish-Landrace sheep). However, large variation occurs among flocks with regard to this trait. This variation allows for the selection of superior animals with a good potential for genetic progress.[9] A review of several studies suggests that an annual improvement of 1.3 lambs per 100 ewes can be obtained. Although this number may seem small, when results are compiled over several years, a sizable influence on flock revenues is apparent. The ability to select prolific females depends highly on accurate records. The more information that is collected on each individual ewe or doe, the more accurate the selection becomes. Replacement females should be selected from lambs or kids born to females that consistently produce a larger than average number of young per year. The management practice of providing supplemental feeding to ewes 2 to 3 weeks before breeding (commonly known as *flushing*) can result in increased ovulation rates (see Chapter 2). The most demonstrative response to supplemental feeding is seen in flocks that are experiencing a low lambing rate and whose nutritional status is not adequate. Flushing has little benefit if the ewes are already in good body condition. Ewes can be flushed by feeding 1 lb of a high-energy supplement (e.g., corn, oats, barley, or a combination) per day. An increase in numbers of twins and triplets requires a concomitant increase in the ovulation rate; the embryos also must be in an acceptable environment for survival. Stressors that may be associated with decreased embryonic survival include the female's age, body temperature of both the male and the female, lactation status during breeding, and overall nutritional status.[9] Females bred outside of the normal breeding season may not be as prolific as those bred during it.

ALTERNATIVE BREEDING PROGRAMS

Certain sheep breeds (Rambouillet, Dorset, Finnish-Landrace) and goat breeds (pygmy, Tennessee stiff-legged) can be encouraged to breed outside of the traditional breeding season. This may be done to match forage sources, decrease some parasite burdens, and improve lamb or kid supplies for some seasonal markets. Ewes and does can be selected to begin a fall lambing or kidding flock.[9] Selected females should be highly prolific and should have given birth early in the traditional lambing or kidding season. If they are normal, ewe lambs or doe kids from these reproductively efficient females should be saved as replacements. The producer should plan on retaining 30% to 40% more lambs or kids than are needed to select for out-of-season breeding potential.[9] This process should be repeated over several years to identify animals that will serve well in off-season breeding programs. Producers who do not have record systems to identify superior females should expose the flock to superior rams or bucks in the spring and retain any females that become pregnant to create a fall lambing flock. Females that do not lamb or kid can be exposed to males in the fall to follow traditional breeding programs. Males should be selected using a similar approach. Males born to the more prolific females should be selected as replacement males and older rams or bucks that have a proven history of superior fertility should be used. Good record-keeping systems and individual identification of females are essential in any selection program. Females born early in the lambing season as twins should be selected as replacements. With respect to growth traits, twins should be compared with other sets of twins because early selection based on size alone may discriminate against them compared with singletons. Ewe lambs of most meat breeds should weigh about 100 lb by the time they are 7 months old. Selected lambs should be bred at about 10 months so they will lamb at 15 months early in the spring. Ewes that bear twins early during lambing should be selected for the accelerated fall lambing flock.[10-12]

Sheep

A similar program for sheep, termed the *STAR management program,* has been developed at Cornell University. The STAR program's unique feature is that it allows for an almost continuous supply of market lambs. This is a good fit with the year-round niche market that many producers have developed. A chart of the calendar year is made using a 5-pointed star. The time lag between each point on the star is 73 days, which is also approximately half of the normal gestation length of the ewe. Therefore an individual ewe exposed to the ram at the time corresponding to one point on the star will lamb at the time corresponding to the third point on the star (146 days later). She can then be exposed to the ram at the fourth point on the star (216 days after the first breeding). This spreads lambing throughout the year, and provides five lambings in 3 years. The use of this system is contingent on the selection of highly prolific ewes that have the ability to cycle and conceive out of season. Accelerated breeding programs place demands on the producer to improve management of the flock's nutritional program and ensure that rams have excellent potential reproductive ability. These complex breeding schemes also demand the accurate identification of individual animals so that ewes capable of out-of-season breeding can be identified and replacement animals can be chosen from these females.[12]

Goats

In a controlled accelerated kidding program in which three kid crops every 2 years is desired, out-of-season breeding is necessary. This requires intense management, early weaning, and hormonal manipulation of does for induction and synchronization of estrus. Seasonal effects on reproductive characteristics also have been documented in bucks. Buck libido and ejaculate quality and quantity appear highest in late summer and fall, which coincides with the seasonal breeding patterns of the does. Distinct behavior changes and odors also occur in the males in the fall to trigger the buck effect in bringing the female into heat. Bucks can be used successfully for out-of-season breeding without any additional treatment.[13] However, they will benefit from winter light treatment to increase libido and quality of semen. Producers also can accomplish this by administering 50-mg GnRH injections three times daily for 4 days to boost testosterone production.[3]

References

1. Rowe JD: Reproductive management of sheep and goats, *Proceedings of the Annual Meeting of the American Veterinary Medicine Association,* p 616, 1998, Schaumburg, IL.
2. Wheaton JE et al: CIDR: a new progesterone releasing intravaginal device for induction of estrous and cycle control in sheep and goats, *Anim Repro Sci* 33:127, 1993.
3. Bulgin MS: Increasing reproductive performance of the ewe flock, *Proceedings of the Society for Theriogenology,* p 244, 1990, Nashville, TN.
4. Quispe T et al: Estrous synchronization with melengestrol acetate in cyclic ewes. Insemination with fresh or frozen semen during the first or second estrous post treatment, *Therio* 41:1385, 1994.
5. Cushwa WT et al: Ram influence on ovarian and sexual activity in anestrous ewes: effect of isolation of ewes from rams before joining and date of ram introduction, *J Anim Sci* 70:1195, 1992.
6. Perkins A, Fitzgerald JA: The behavioral component of the ram effect: the influence of ram sexual behavior on the induction of estrus in anovulatory ewes, *J Anim Sci* 72:51, 1994.
7. Haresign W: Manipulation of reproduction in sheep, *J Repro Fert* 45(suppl.):127, 1992.
8. Rowe JD, East NE: Reproductive management—estrous cycles, synchronization, artificial insemination, pregnancy diagnosis: small ruminants for the mixed practitioner, *Proceedings of the Western Veterinary Conference,* p 137, 1998, Las Vegas, NV.
9. Thomas DL: Improving reproductive performance of sheep through selection, *Proceedings of the Society for Theriogenology,* p 178, 1996, Nashville, TN.
10. Robinson JJ: Embryo survival in the sheep, *Proceedings of the Society for Theriogenology,* p 270, 1995, Nashville, TN.
11. Fitch GQ: *A breeding program for fall lambing,* OSU extension facts, no 3801, Stillwater, OK, 2000, Cooperative Extension Service, Oklahoma State University.
12. Keisler DH, Buckrell BC: Breeding strategies. In Youngquist RS, editor: *Current therapy in large animal theriogenology,* Philadelphia, 1997, WB Saunders.
13. Karatzas G et al: Fertility of fresh and frozen-thawed goat semen during the non-breeding season, *Therio* 48:1049, 1997.

NATURAL BREEDING SYSTEMS

Natural breeding is more commonly used in meat and fiber sheep or goat production systems, whereas AI or hand mating is the most common means of breeding in dairy goats or sheep and the method most commonly used by purebred breeders. In a meat production system, productivity is largely a function of the number of offspring born and weaned and the frequency with which they are produced. The desired date of parturition in a given farm dictates the breeding date and the management of the breeding male. Females are usually bred in the fall for spring kidding or lambing. Bucks should be kept separate from the does until they are to be used for breeding. After establishing a mating time, the producer should leave the bucks with the does for 32 days 1½ reproductive cycles) and the rams with the ewes for 27 days. This ensures that all kids or lambs are born within about 1 month of one another, reducing the amount of supervision required at kidding time. The male-to-female mating ratio depends on the age and SC of the male, the size of the mating area, and whether one or more rams or bucks are to be used. Meat goat production systems should have 1 buck per 30 does. A buck may breed 50 to 200 does in a single breeding season, but 3 to 4 bucks should be put with 100 does.[1] Most sheep producers should keep 3 to 5.5 adult rams per 100 ewes. A marking harness should be used on the males to identify which females have been bred. In commercial flocks, males should be changed at least every 2 years to prevent inbreeding. Bucks or rams of high libido and good semen quality can be used in a staggered breeding program in which seven or eight synchronized ewes or does exhibiting estrus at the same time are placed with the male for breeding. Hand mating of males can be used as a modification of staggered breeding, with the same female ratio of 7:1 to 8:1. Table 6-4 outlines a proposed male-to-female ratio.

ARTIFICIAL INSEMINATION

The goat and sheep industry has used AI commercially in North America for many years. The cervix of the doe is less of an obstacle to insemination than the cervix of the ewe. As a result, commercial AI programs using fresh or frozen semen have been developed and are used most commonly in goats. Advantages of AI include the following[2]:

- Maximal use of outstanding sires
- Elimination of the need for rams and bucks on the farm

TABLE 6-4

RECOMMENDED MALE-TO-FEMALE RATIOS FOR RAMS AND BUCKS

ANIMAL	COMMENT	MALE-TO-FEMALE RATIO
1-year-old	In a paddock or confined pasture	1:20 to 1:25
Adult	In a paddock or confined pasture	1:40 to 1:50
Adult	Range	1:25 to 1:30
Adult	Synchronized females in season	1:15 to 1:25
Adult	Synchronized females out of season	1:5 to 1:10

Adapted from Menzies PI: Reproductive health management. In Youngquist RS, editor: *Current therapy in large animal theriogenology,* Philadelphia, 1997, WB Saunders; Pugh DG: Breeding soundness evaluation in male goats, *Proc Hudson Walker Therio Conf* 7:29, 1996.

- Relatively inexpensive semen cost
- Decreased potential for venereally transmitted diseases
- Improved herd management

Disadvantages of AI include the following[2]:

- Cost for AI equipment and liquid nitrogen
- Increased labor for estrus detection and insemination
- Lack of standardization procedures for packing and quality control for goat semen
- Lack of suitable sire proofs for production traits
- Potential for spread of less desirable traits

The success of an AI program depends on many factors (fresh versus frozen semen, number and time of inseminations, insemination method, quality and quantity of semen, semen handling practices, and the management of the animals to be inseminated).

Females selected for AI should be in good health, have a body condition score of 2.5 to 3, and be put on an improved nutrition plan for 2 to 5 weeks before breeding. They also should be free of disease and have a history of giving birth to live, healthy young and raising those kids or lambs to weaning. Preference should be given to females that conceive early in the breeding season, those that lambed or kidded during poor weather conditions, and those that gave birth to and raised multiple young.

AI is usually performed in conjunction with estrus synchronization. Progestin implants or intravaginal devices are favored over prostaglandin regimens because of their tighter synchrony of estrus and ovulation. The producer may inject eCG (200 to 500 IU) when removing the progestin.

Because no uniform standards are available for freezing goat or sheep semen, any frozen semen to be used should be evaluated before an AI program is begun. Optimal timing of insemination is an important factor in the success of AI programs. Females do not ovulate until late estrus or shortly after the end of standing estrus. Therefore recognizing the signs of standing heat is important. However, the optimal timing of insemination is best determined by changes in cervical mucus. As the doe progresses through estrus, the mucus turns from clear and thin at the beginning of standing heat to cloudy and stringy at middle to late heat. Insemination should be performed in does before or at the time the mucus turns cloudy, usually 12 to 15 hours after the onset of estrus.[3] If the doe continues to exhibit heat after insemination, she should be inseminated again after 12 hours, particularly if the program uses cooled or frozen semen.

Timed insemination of synchronized meat goats and ewes tends to work well. Fixed-time insemination using fresh semen 50 to 55 hours after removal of the progesterone source is an excellent labor-saving technique. If a laparoscopic AI is to be performed, sheep and goats should be inseminated 55 to 60 hours and 52 to 60 hours after progesterone removal for frozen and thawed or fresh semen, respectively.[4] Australian workers suggest that observation for estrus before breeding has no advantage over timed insemination (laparoscopy) in the ewe.[5] In dairy goats, does should be observed for heat using a teaser animals and inseminated accordingly, whereas meat animals are usually synchronized in groups. Techniques that place the semen into the uterus should be used for frozen semen.

Vaginal Insemination

The vulva is wiped clean with dry cotton or paper towels. The practitioner carefully advances a pipette into the cranial vagina by sliding it along the dorsal vaginal roof to avoid entering the urethral orifice. A cleaned, lubricated speculum may afford better visualization for pipette placement. The equipment needed is shown in Figure 6-12. Insemination with 4×10^9 and 3×10^9 progressively motile, fresh, spermatozoa close to the cervix maximizes fertility with vaginal insemination in ewes and does, respectively.[2,6-9] The conception rate with this method ranges from 15% to 30%; experienced technicians may achieve better rates.

Cervical Insemination

Cervical insemination is more time consuming and requires greater skill than vaginal insemination. In this method the ewe's or doe's hindquarters (not its abdomen) are elevated and its legs are held over a table or more commonly a bale of hay. The operator gently introduces a lubricated vaginal speculum approximately 12 cm through the cleaned vulva and into the vagina. With the help of a good light source such as a transilluminator the cervix is visualized through the speculum. At this point the operator introduces an insemination pipette through the speculum and attempts to atraumatically pass the pipette as far into the cervix as possible. The long (7 to 8 cm) cervix and the 6 to 8 rear-directed cervical rings make completely traversing the cervix difficult in the ewe. Therefore semen is usually deposited into the caudal cervix. A 12-gauge tube attached to the semen delivery system allows deeper penetration of the cervix. The doe's cervix has a smaller luminal size but is slightly easier to pass. Approximately 1×10^9 sperm cells from fresh semen are needed to ensure good lambing and kidding rates using this method.[2,6-9] If cooled or frozen and thawed semen is used, these numbers may need to be expanded by a factor of 1.5 and 2, respectively.[2,6-9] The conception rate with this method ranges from 35% to 50% (and occasionally higher).

Transcervical insemination. The more invasive methods of insemination are designed to place semen directly into the uterus. With these methods a much smaller number of progressively motile sperm are needed. Transcervical insemination of dairy and meat goats is a relatively common procedure and one that can be easily mastered with some practice. The necessary speculum, light source, and insemination equipment are readily available through goat supply companies (Figure 6-13). All items that come into contact with the internal reproductive tract of the doe should be sterile. Dairy goats are usually restrained on a milking stand. Meat goats are not usually cooperative on stands and should be restrained by an assistant lifting the hindquarters and holding both hindlegs.

SHEEP: The most commonly used technique in sheep is known as the Guelph system for transcervical AI,[7] but variations of this technique also are available. The ewe is restrained on her back with the hind limbs pulled forward. Special cradles designed for foot trimming or a V-shaped wooden trough can be used. A specially designed Plexiglas vaginal speculum that has a 1-cm opening running along its entire length is introduced into the vagina and the cervix is identified. A wand-type light source that can be partially introduced into the speculum with a retaining clip can be used to provide a light for this procedure (Figure 6-13). The clinician inserts a pair of 25-cm Bozeman forceps into the speculum and grasps tissue near the cervical os. Any mucus preventing visualization of the cervical os can be aspirated with a syringe infusion pipette. The slit-like opening in the speculum allows the introduction of the forceps; after grasping the cervical tissue the operator can retract the cervix caudally and slide the forceps partially through the slit to allow better visualization of the cervix. Holding the speculum and forceps with one hand, the clinician next introduces a special bent-tipped insemination rod into the cervical os and attempts to traverse the cervical rings. Manipulating the AI rod and the cervix with the grasping forceps facilitates the placement of semen directly into the uterus. The tip of the insemination gun can be used to locate the cervical canal. By turning the gun, most of the cervical rings can be traversed (Figure 6-14).

Proper attachment of the forceps to the cervical os is crucial for maximal cervical penetration. If the AI pipette tip can be moved without resistance, it is in the cervical lumen or uterine body. The closer to the uterine body the semen is deposited, the higher the conception rate. This procedure requires 50 to 100 million progressively motile

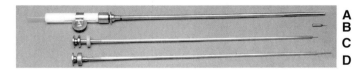

Figure 6-12 Equipment for intravaginal insemination and laparoscopic semination in sheep and goats. **A,** Laparoscopic insemination gun; **B,** needle to be attached to a syringe for laparoscopic insemination. Both can be successfully used in laparoscopic procedures. The needle **(B)** is useful when fresh semen is to be inseminated laparoscopically. **C** and **D,** Equipment used for intravaginal and intracervical insemination of goats. Cassou guns are designed to use semen frozen in straws. **C** is a standard Cassou gun, whereas **D** has a longer plunger and is better adapted for intracervical or transcervical insemination.

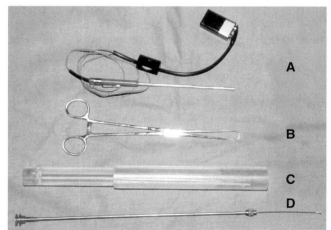

Figure 6-13 Equipment used for transcervical AI in sheep. **A,** Wand-type light source with retaining clip; **B,** Bozeman forceps; **C,** speculum; **D,** insemination pipette with special adaptor that allows movement into the cervix. This equipment is part of the Guelph AI system.

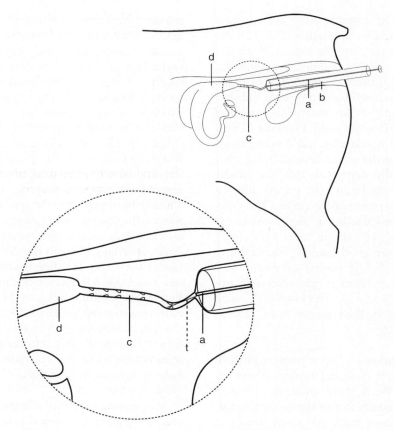

Figure 6-14 Cervical or transcervical insemination. The practitioner inserts an AI pipette *(a)* through a speculum *(b)* and into the ewe's cervix *(c)* and uterus *(d)*. *Inset,* The tip of the pipette *(t)* is moved slowly through the cervix, traversing the cervical rings. The cervix of the ewe is tortuous, with five or six cervical rings. These anatomic barriers make insemination difficult.

sperm cells. It also requires much experience and the reported results (40% to 70% lambing rates) are variable. Operators report a higher pregnancy rate when they can enter the uterus with the insemination pipette instead of depositing the semen into the cervix. Pregnancy rates may be similar to those achieved in laparoscopic methods when the semen is placed into the uterus.[10]

GOATS: For AI of goats, the perineal area is washed with soapy water, rinsed, and dried with a paper towel. A lubricated clear AI speculum is inserted into the doe's vagina and directed dorsally first and then slightly ventrally to pass over the ischial arch. The AI light is inserted into the speculum and the cervix is visualized. After locating the cervical opening, the clinician places pressure on the speculum to lock the cervix into the lumen of the speculum. An assistant should hold the speculum in the vagina while the inseminator prepares the semen. The frozen semen straw is placed in water based on the processor's recommendation (usually 30 to 60 seconds in 35° C water). The clinician dries the straw with a paper towel, cuts it, and places it in the AI gun. The insemination gun is manipulated through the cervical opening by gentle rota-

tion and forward movement, slowly depositing the semen in the interior cervix or uterine body. After insemination the doe is allowed to stand and relax for a few minutes. Conception rates between 50% and 85% have been reported, depending on the skill of the operator and the quality of the semen used. Fresh extended semen produces better fertility than frozen semen.[2,8,9] In the doe the desired number of motile sperm per insemination for fresh liquid semen is 150 million; 200 million sperm are required in frozen semen.[8,9] Both fresh and frozen semen should be evaluated for quality before insemination.

Laparoscopic Insemination

The use of a laparoscope (0°) allows visualization of the uterus so that semen can be placed directly into the lumen. The ewe and doe should be held off feed and water for 24 hours before surgery. The animals are sedated and positioned in dorsal recumbency, with the head tilted down at a 45° angle or more to allow the urinary bladder to fall away from the uterus as the procedure proceeds. The abdomen should be clipped and prepared for aseptic surgery. Local anesthetics are infiltrated

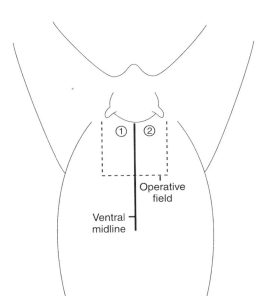

Figure 6-15 Sites for placement of trocars for laparoscopic insemination. The trocar and cannula for the optic instruments are placed at *1*, and the trocar and cannula for the insemination instruments are placed at *2*.

at two sites, both of which are 5 cm cranial to the udder and 4 cm to either side of the midline. A trocar or cannula is placed at the site of local anesthetic infiltration on one side of the midline and the abdominal cavity is distended with 1 to 2 L of carbon dioxide. A second cannula is placed opposite the first (Figure 6-15). The laparoscope (6.5 to 10 mm diameter, 0° telescope) is inserted into the first cannula, and the uterus is visualized. The clinician inserts the insemination pipette into the second cannula and inseminates each horn using a special needle on the end of the pipette. Alternatively, an insemination gun fitted with a brass injection tip (see Figure 6-12) or an aseptic needle (0.5 to 0.7 cm) is inserted through the other cannula into the abdominal cavity. An avascular area at the anterior uterine horn is identified and the needle is inserted into the uterine lumen at a right angle to the uterine wall. The clinician should place the needle in the center of the horn, taking care to ensure that the needle is in the lumen of the uterus. The authors prefer to make a quick, controlled thrust into the uterine lumen. The semen should easily flow through the insemination device and into the uterus. If it does not, the needle is likely in the wall of the uterus and should be redirected. After insemination the laparoscope and cannula are removed and the puncture sites are sutured, stapled, or covered with an antibiotic ointment. Ewes and does should be moved to a recovery area and left undisturbed for 1 to 2 hours. The desired number of motile sperm for laparoscopic AI using fresh or frozen semen is 20 million (both horns) for does and 50 million for sheep.[7,8,11,12] Conception rates of 20% to 90% have been

reported in sheep and goats. The success of insemination depends largely on the quantity and motility of spermatozoa being inseminated.[11] An experienced operator requires only 3 to 8 minutes to perform this procedure, and the females should recover uneventfully. Ewes and does may be laparoscopically inseminated many times throughout their lives.

EMBRYO TRANSFER

Traditional cross-breeding programs using AI focus on the male to produce offspring. Breeding programs using multiple ovulation and embryo transfer (ET) use genetically superior females to contribute to this genetic diversity. The limited economic value of most sheep and goats precludes the widespread use of ET for the average production unit. Also, the invasive procedure required makes ET less practical in goats than in cattle. Nevertheless, ET is an efficient method for moving genetics between flocks, across countries, and among continents. ET is less practical in ewes than in cows because surgical collection and transfer are usually required. A successful ET program requires advanced planning and lots of attention to detail in donor and recipient selection, superovulation, synchronization of donor and recipient, and successful recovery and transfer of high-quality embryos. ET can be carried out in or out of season, but the best response is attained during the breeding season when donors and recipients are cycling normally.[13-17]

Donor and Recipient Management

Donor and recipient selection and management are crucial to the success of an ET program. Recipient and donor ewes must be synchronized to cycle together. Donors respond most successfully to estrus synchronization and superovulation when they are young, healthy, and cycling normally. Does and ewes 2 to 5 years of age respond best to synchronization and superovulation programs. Unfortunately, does and ewes presented as potential donors may often be older animals, and therefore past their peak reproduction performance. Donors should be in good body condition (with a body condition score of 3 to 3.5) and good general health. They should be vaccinated against any infectious diseases prevalent in the area and kept in separate groups for 2 to 4 months before the beginning of the ET program. This helps acclimatize the donors and prevents stress.[15] Any changes in environment, feeding, and handling should occur well in advance of the initiation of an ET program. Premature luteal regression, a syndrome common in some breeds (Boer), appears to be caused by stress.

Recipients should be healthy animals with proven reproductive ability that are in good body condition (with a body condition score of 3 to 3.5) and cycling normally. Does 2 to 4 years of age with good mothering characteristics and adequate potential for milk production are preferred. Recipients also should be current on their vaccinations against diseases prevalent in the area.

Synchronization

Most ET programs rely on exogenous hormones to induce and synchronize estrus in donors and recipients as described in the section on control of estrus cycle. Synchronization is commonly achieved using progestin sponges, CIDR, or half of a norgestomet ear implant. Accurate detection of estrus can be achieved using a teaser buck or ram. The method of estrus synchronization should be the same for both donor and recipient, with the exception that superior results are obtained if progestin sources are removed from recipients 12 hours before they are removed from donors.

Superovulation

Superovulation of the donor is accomplished by injecting PMSG and pituitary extracts of FSH. PMSG has a longer half-life (about 72 hours). It is associated with overstimulation of the ovaries, resulting in the release of large numbers of eggs; an increased proportion of unfertilized embryos; and poorer-quality embryos. PMSG (1000 to 1500 IU) is administered in a single dose 48 hours before the progesterone source is removed. The donor also can be superovulated using an FSH product alone or in combination with eCG 2 days before the end of the artificially created luteal phase.[17] FSH has a half-life of about 6 hours and requires twice-daily injections beginning 48 hours before progestin removal. FSH is superior to PMSG in ovulation and fertilization rates and production of good-quality embryos. Does and ewes generally exhibit estrus 24 to 36 hours after progestin removal. Frequent observation of does for estrus with the aid of a teaser animal is needed to ensure accurate recording of the time of estrus. Donors can be hand mated 12 to 24 hours after estrus detection. Laparoscopic deposition of frozen and thawed semen into the uterine horns 24 hours after the animal is first seen in estrus yields adequate results. If donors are to be naturally bred, one buck or ram should be kept with one or two superovulated does or ewes.[16]

Embryo Recovery

Embryos are usually recovered from the donor's uterus on day 5 or 6 after breeding. In most instances, surgical collection may be employed. However, alternative techniques such as laparoscopic and nonsurgical embryo collection have been developed.[13-16]

Surgical. For surgical collection of embryos, does or ewes are taken off feed and water 36 hours before surgery.

The clinician or a helper anesthetizes the female, clips and prepares the abdominal area cranial to the udder for aseptic surgery, and positions the animal in dorsal recumbency. The uterus and ovaries are exposed through a small caudal ventral midline laparotomy beginning in front of the mammary gland. The clinician should examine the ovaries to determine the response to superovulation. This can also be accomplished with a laparoscope before laparotomy to minimize ovarian handling. The uterus is elevated out of the laparotomy incision. The clinician uses a 20-gauge, blunt needle to pierce the uterine wall near the uterotubal junction; he or she then inserts a "tom cat" catheter into the uterine horn. The tip of a small artery forceps is used to cut a small hole through the uterine wall for insertion of a 8- to 10-inch Foley catheter at the base of the uterine horn. The cuff is inflated with 5 cc of saline, and 20 ml of flushing media (Dubecco's PBS solution containing 100 IU/ml penicillin and 100 mg/ml streptomycin supplemented with 2% heat-activated goat serum) is infused through the catheter to lavage the uterus. The fluid should drain through the Foley catheter and into a collection bowl or Petri dish. The procedure is repeated on the opposite uterine horn. The uterine puncture sites are left unsutured. $PGF_{2\alpha}$ should be administered postoperatively to lyse all luteal tissue. If embryos are to be collected before the fourth day after breeding, oviductal flushing (through a cannulated oviduct near the fimbria) is necessary. The collection media is flushed in a retrograde direction through the oviduct using a catheter placed at the uterotubular junction.

Nonsurgical. Nonsurgical or transcervical embryo collection techniques avoid the risk of postsurgical adhesions and maintain the value of genetically superior donors after multiple embryo collections. Several reports of successful nonsurgical collection in sheep and goats have been published.[18] However, no practical technique is available yet that can be recommended for field use. In a recent report,[19] embryos were collected transcervically from 38 standing unanesthetized Boer goats. In this study the clinician inserted a duck-billed speculum into the vagina and grasped the external os of the cervix with Allis tissue forceps. The speculum was removed and the external os was carefully pulled caudally until it almost reached the vulvar opening in a similar fashion as that used for transcervical AI in sheep. A 3.2-mm outside diameter, #10 Rusch flushing catheter was passed through the cervix and directed into the left or right uterine horn with a finger in the vaginal fornix. The clinician performed 24 flushings, with a 2-hour pause between the first and last 12 flushings. The embryo recovery rate appears to be comparable to that achieved with surgical collection.[19]

Laparoscopic. Laparoscopic-assisted collection can be performed to exteriorize the tip of the uterine horn, with the flushing being performed in the same manner described for surgical collection. This method reduces the severity of adhesions that result from the handling required in a laparotomy approach.[14] Laparoscopy also can be used to collect the embryos within the abdomen without performing laparotomy. This technique requires considerable skill and is not practical for routine field use. A laparoscope-assisted procedure can be used to enhance this technique and decrease the risk of adhesion formation.[8] The laparoscopic method allows the operator to visualize the ovary, locate the CL, and more easily exteriorize the uterine horn. Advantages include reduced surgical time and a smaller abdominal incision.[8]

Embryo Handling

The flush medium is searched under a dissecting microscope, and the embryos are retrieved and placed in a holding dish after washing. Before freezing or transfer, they are carefully assessed for quality and stage of development. Morula and blastocyst stages are expected when embryos are collected at day 5 or 6. Embryos should be held in Dubecco's PBS with 5% to 20% fetal calf serum. The International Embryo Transfer Society (IETS) has defined handling procedures to reduce the risk of disease transmission during ET.

Embryos are pulled into the tip of a small-bore intravenous (IV) catheter attached to a 1-ml syringe for immediate transfer into recipients.[7] Alternatively, the embryos may be processed for freezing.

Embryo Transfer

Most transfers are done surgically. Recipients are selected for transfer based on the greatest synchrony of estrus to the donor doe. This synchrony is one of the most important factors in the success of ET programs. The recipient is prepared as for surgical embryo collection, and a small ventral midline incision is made in front of the mammary gland. The ovaries are examined for a CL, and the uterine horn ipsilateral to the CL is exteriorized. Embryos are transferred to the oviducts via the fimbria using a tom cat catheter or Pasteur pipette if the embryos are in an early stage of development (earlier than day 4). Older embryos (those collected after day 4) are transferred to the uterine horns through a small stab incision made with a rounded 20-gauge needle or with the "eye" of a suture needle. Before closing the abdominal incision, the clinician should examine the catheter used to make the transfer microscopically to ensure that no embryos are retained in it.

Recipient animals undergoing laparoscope-assisted transfer are prepared and placed on a surgical table or cradle as described for laparoscopic AI. Two cannulas are placed in the abdominal cavity, each 2 to 3 cm from the midline and approximately 10 cm cranial to the udder. The ovaries are examined through the laparoscope to identify the horn suitable for the ET. The tip of the uterus is grasped with forceps and gently elevated through the incision to the exterior. The tip of the uterus is punctured with a blunted needle and the embryos are introduced as previously described. The small incision in the midline is sutured.

Although the laparoscopic collection of embryos requires considerable expertise, laparoscopic transfer of embryos is relatively easy and recommended for large ET programs. However, laparoscopic-assisted transfer and surgical transfer are the techniques used most often for ET in goats.

For laparoscopic transfer the recipient animals are prepared as described for laparoscopic-assisted ET. The clinician examines the ovaries through the laparoscope and identifies the horn ipsilateral to the CL for transfer of the embryos. The embryos are loaded in a 0.5-ml straw and inserted into an AI insemination gun fitted with a brass injection tip. The Cassou gun is inserted into the abdominal cavity through the cannula, an avascular area at the tip of the uterine horn is identified, and the needle is inserted into the uterine lumen at a right angle to the uterine wall. The clinician depresses the plunger of the AI gun gently to expel the embryos.

Many factors can affect the success of an ET program. An average of 8 to 10 transferable embryos can be expected per flush, with expected pregnancy rates of 60% to 80% for the transfer of two fresh embryos per recipient.[20] Pregnancy rates from the transfer of frozen embryos are much lower.

IN VITRO FERTILIZATION

In vitro fertilization (IVF) and culture technology offer the advantage of producing embryos from animals when other techniques for producing embryos might be more difficult or impossible. In addition, efficient IVF procedure is important for the development of biotechnologies such as embryo sexing, nuclear transfer (cloning), and gene transfer. Recent progress in embryo biotechnologies has resulted in increased efforts in practical and commercial applications of IVF for the ET industry. Sheep and goat oocytes can be successfully matured during the breeding and non-breeding seasons.[21,22]

Oocytes for in vitro maturation (IVM) and IVF are usually obtained from superovulated does or ewes by aspirating follicles on the ovaries using midline laparotomy or laparoscopy. Ovariectomized ovaries or ovaries collected at slaughter also may be used. Oocytes can be aspirated from 2- to 6-mm follicles with a 20-gauge needle attached to a 5-ml syringe. The immature oocyte with surrounding cumulus cells is then washed in Dubecco's PBS in a Petri dish and incubated for 27 hours in tissue culture medium 199 (TCM-199) supplemented with 20% goat serum, 100 μg FSH/ml, and 1 μg estradiol 17B/ml. The in vitro matured oocytes are incubated in

100 μl droplets of medium under paraffin oil in a humidified 5% CO_2, 5% O_2, and 90% N_2 atmosphere at 38.5° C.[21] IVF is commonly performed with frozen and thawed spermatozoa after a process of sperm swim-up in Tyrode's albumin lactate pyruvate (TALP) medium with added heparin.[23] This procedure aids in both sperm selection and capacitation. Oocytes are incubated with sperm for 24 hours as described for IVM. Fertilized ova are then cultured in TCM-199 and 10% goat serum and monitored for development every 24 hours. Embryos reach the 4- to 8-cell stage at 48 to 72 hours and the morula to blastocyst stage at around 120 hours.[21,22] The reader interested in pursuing IVF and other advanced reproductive technologies should read and study as much of the current scientific literature on the subject as possible.

References

1. Alford A, Strickland J: *Meat goat production in Georgia*, Athens, GA, 1998, UGA Extension Bulletin.
2. Nuti L: Techniques for artificial insemination of goats. In Youngquist RS, editor: *Current therapy in large animal theriogenology*, Philadelphia, 1997, WB Saunders.
3. Mobini S: Reproductive management in goats, *Proceedings of the North American Veterinary Conference*, vol 14, p 219, 2000, Orlando, FL.
4. Karatzas G, Karagiannidia A, Varsakeli K: Fertility of fresh and frozen-thawed goat semen during the non breeding season, *Therio* 48:1049, 1997.
5. Moses D et al: A large-scale program in laparoscopic intrauterine insemination with frozen-thawed semen in Australian Merino sheep in Argentine Patagonia, *Therio* 48:651, 1997.
6. Mylne MJA, Hunton JR, Buckrell BC: Artificial insemination of sheep. In Youngquist RS, editor: *Current therapy in large animal theriogenology*, Philadelphia, 1997, WB Saunders.
7. Buckrell B et al: Reproductive technologies in commercial use for sheep, goats, and farmed deer, *Proceedings of the Society for Theriogenology*, p 185, 1997, Nashville, TN.
8. Evans G, Maxwell WMC: *Salmon's artificial insemination of sheep and goats*, Sydney, 1987, Butterworth Publishers.
9. Chemineau P et al: *Training manual on artificial insemination in sheep and goats*, Rome, 1991, FAO of the United Nations.
10. Halbert GW, Walton JS, Buckrell BC: Evaluation of a technique for transcervical artificial insemination of sheep, *Proceedings of the Society for Theriogenology*, p 293, 1990, Nashville, TN.
11. Rodriquez F et al: Cervical versus intrauterine insemination of ewes using fresh or frozen semen diluted with aloe vera gel, *Therio* 30:843, 1988.
12. Eppleston J, Maxwell WMC: Sources of variation in the reproductive performance of ewes inseminated with frozen-thawed ram semen by laparoscopy, *Therio* 43:777, 1995.
13. Buckrell BC, Pollard J: Embryo transfer in sheep. In Youngquist RS, editor: *Current therapy in large animal theriogenology*, Philadelphia, 1997, WB Saunders.
14. Scudamore CL et al: Laparoscopy for intrauterine insemination and embryo recovery in super ovulated ewes at a commercial embryo transfer unit, *Therio* 35:329, 1991.
15. Ishwa AK, Memon MA: Embryo transfer in sheep and goats: a review, *Small Rumin Res* 19:35, 1996.
16. Hill J: Maximizing the results of goat embryo transfer programs, *Proceedings of the American Association of Small Ruminant Practitioners, Research Symposium on Health and Disease*, p 120, 1996, Nashville, TN.
17. Husein MQ et al: Effect of eCG on the pregnancy rate of ewes transcervically inseminated with frozen-thawed semen outside the breeding season, *Therio* 49:997, 1998.
18. Flores-Foxworth G: Reproductive biotechnologies in the goat. In Youngquist RS, editor: *Current therapy in large animal theriogenology*, Philadelphia, 1997, WB Saunders.
19. Pereira RJTA, Shohenery B, Hollz W: Nonsurgical embryo collection in goats treated with prostaglandin F2a and oxytocin, *J Anim Sci* 76:360, 1998.
20. Rowe JD: Reproductive management in sheep and goats, *Proceedings of the American Association of Small Ruminant Practitioners, Research Symposium on Health and Disease*, p 39, 1998, Nashville, TN.
21. Keskintepe L et al: Term development of caprine embryos derived from immature oocytes in vitro, *Therio* 42:527, 1994.
22. Samake S et al: In vitro fertilization of goat oocyte during the non-breeding season, *Small Rumin Res* 35:49, 2000.
23. Keskintepe L, Simplicio AA, Brackett BG: Caprine blastocyst development after in vitro fertilization with spermatozoa frozen in different extenders, *Therio* 49:1265, 1998.

PREGNANCY DETERMINATION

Early pregnancy diagnosis and determination of the number of fetuses are of considerable value in goat and sheep reproductive herd health management. Goat owners frequently use clinical signs such as failure to return to estrus after breeding, enlarging abdomen, and developing mammary glands to make a presumptive diagnosis of pregnancy. However, pathologic conditions of the uterus and ovaries, physiologic anestrus late in the breeding season, and out-of-season breeding may cause post-breeding anestrus in non-pregnant does.[1,3] Many does and some ewes exhibit estrous behavior during pregnancy. Ultrasonography, hormonal assays, and radiography are the most useful methods of pregnancy diagnosis. Abdominal palpation or ballottement and rectal-abdominal palpation with a rod have limited use or have been abandoned.

The value of pregnancy determination lies in the identification of nonproductive females and ewes bearing multiple fetuses; early identification allows appropriate nutritional and management programs to be implemented. The ability to divide the flock into groups of animals based on pregnancy status and fetal numbers not only improves the health care of these animals by reducing the incidence of some disease, but also decreases production costs.

Ultrasonographic techniques for pregnancy determination include amplitude modulation (A-mode), Doppler, and real-time (B-mode) imaging.[2] A-mode ultrasonography can be used to detect pregnancy between 60 and 100 days' gestation. Detection of a fluid density is interpreted as pregnancy. Because of this hydrometra or a large bladder may give a false positive result. Therefore A-mode ultrasound is an unreliable method for diagnosing pregnancy. Doppler ultrasonography can be used to detect movement that may indicate pregnancy (blood flow in the middle uterine artery or umbilical arteries, fetal heart beat, and fetal movements). The external Doppler technique has an accuracy of 100% during the second half of gestation but is not as effective at 50 to 75 days or earlier.[2] The intrarectal technique for Doppler ltrasound may be attempted as early as 25 to 30 days after breeding, but waiting until day 35 to 40 produces better results.[2,3] False-negative and false-positive results are common, and determining fetal numbers is difficult.

Pregnancy detection in the ewe is now performed almost entirely with real-time ultrasonography. Linear array real-time ultrasound transducers can be used transrectally to diagnose pregnancy as early as 18 days and as late as 60 days. A homemade plastic extension can easily be fashioned from PVC pipe to allow easy introduction of the transducer into the rectum. A 5- or a 7.5-MHz transducer is recommended for rectal scans. After 60 days the gravid uterus is pulled down into the abdomen and may be difficult to visualize transrectally. Table 6-5 shows age of gestation and associated ultrasonographic findings for pregnant sheep and goats.

Transabdominal ultrasonography with a 3.5- or 5-MHz linear or sector scanner is used after 30 days of gestation. The transducer is placed on a fiberless area of the abdomen high in the inguinal region, preferably in the right flank.[1] A bland fluid (e.g., vegetable oil, methylcellulose) should be used to couple the ultrasound transducer to the skin. The clinician aims the transducer's beam toward the pelvis and scans the abdomen by slowly "sweeping" the transducer cranially. In goats, shearing the inguinal region increases the accuracy and speed of examination. Identification of the bladder (typically triangular in appearance) provides an excellent landmark. The uterus is normally located dorsal or cranial to the bladder. Pregnancy at this point can be diagnosed on the basis of

finding a fetus, placentomes, or, less reliably, numerous fluid-filled uterine luminal sections. The placentomes appear as round "doughnuts" or C-shaped structures (Figure 6-16). Transabdominal ultrasonography can be used as early as 30 days and as late as 120 days. After day 90 to 120 reliable identification of the number of fetuses becomes difficult because their individual size fills the screens; one fetus may be mistaken for two, or two different fetuses may be mistaken for one.

Twin pregnancies can often be determined between 45 and 90 days of gestation. Sector scanning units provide a wider visual angle or view of the abdomen.[1] This allows more of the uterus to be seen in the visual field, improving the accurate identification of multiple fetuses. The clinician should shear the belly wool just cranial to the udder and scan the abdomen slowly to make a mental image of all abdominal contents. Generally, the C-shaped placentomes can be seen "pointing" their concave portions toward the fetus. The fetal bones form "shadows," and the fetal ribs produce a characteristic striated appearance. Careful attention to a complete and thorough examination helps minimize errors, but viewing a single fetus too long can result in a false diagnosis of twins. After 120 days the fetal bones can produce a very distorted image, but a diagnosis can be made with some effort. To maximize the usefulness of ultrasound, ewes should be scanned between 45 and 60 days so producers can implement any management changes indicated by pregnancy status or number of fetuses. Clinicians also can

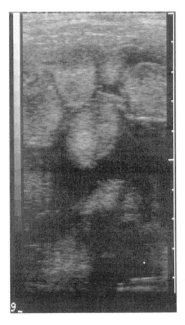

Figure 6-16 Real-time, linear array ultrasound using a 5-MHz transducer reveals positive signs of pregnancy (placentomes) at the top of the image. The hypoechoic area at the bottom of the picture is amnionic fluid, and the hyperechoic region at the bottom of the image is a fetus.

TABLE 6-5

ULTRASONOGRAPHIC FINDINGS WITH PREGNANCY

DAYS	COMMENTS
17 to 25	Transrectal; embryo visible after 24 days
26 to 35	Transabdominal; hypoechoic amnion and hyperechoic fetus
30 to 75	Transabdominal; doughnut-shaped to C-shaped placentomes
45 to 90	Best time for twin detection; mid-abdomen in front of udder
90 to term	Determination of number of fetuses is less accurate close to term

use ultrasonography to stage pregnancies by measuring the biparietal diameter of the fetus.[2-4]

Abnormal ultrasonographic findings include hydrometra, pyometra, fetal mummy, and macerated fetus. Hydrometra appears as an anechoic, fluid-filled uterus, often with membranous strands visualized in the lumen of the uterus. The uterus also does not have the typical placentomes characteristic of pregnancy. Hydrometra is often seen in does with apparently normal reproductive histories.[2,3] Pyometra also is manifested as a fluid-filled uterus with more hyperechoic densities and a swirling appearance.

Assessment of fetal viability may be crucial in cases such as pregnancy toxemia.[1] Fetal mummification may be identified as hyperechoic areas without any identifiable body parts within a relatively fluid-free placentome-less uterus. The fetal heartbeat can be easily recognized by 30 to 35 days after breeding.[2] Early fetal death may be recognized by finding free-floating fetal masses along with ribbon-like placental membranes.[4] These ribbon-like membranes may be found contralateral to a normally developing fetus. Lack of fetal movement, amniotic fluid, heartbeat, and blood coursing through the umbilicus can easily differentiate a dead lamb fetus from a living one with real-time ultrasonography. Soon after fetal death the placentomes lose their "crisp" margins.[1]

Hormone Assays

Measurement of hormones in blood, milk, or urine provides an alternative method of pregnancy diagnosis when ultrasound equipment is not available. The estrone sulfate test, pregnancy-specific protein B (PSPB), and progesterone measurement are examples.

Estrone Sulfate

Estrone sulfate is a pregnancy-specific hormone produced by the fetal placental unit. It can be detected in the urine, serum, or milk after day 50 of pregnancy. When performed any time after day 50 after breeding, this test has been characterized as almost 100% accurate in the detection of pregnancy. A positive test indicates a viable fetus. False positive results may occur if hemolyzed serum samples are assayed. False negative results may occur if samples are collected before day 50 of gestation. Commercial laboratories offering this test are limited and expensive.[1]

Pregnancy-Specific Protein B

PSPB is produced by binucleate giant cells of the placenta throughout gestation. It can be used in sheep and goats to detect pregnancy any time after day 25 after breeding. Both false positive and false negative results are possible,

and commercial laboratories offering the test are limited.[2] Multiple fetuses result in higher levels of PSPB.[1]

Progesterone

Progesterone analysis is not a test for pregnancy, and it more accurately detects non-pregnant rather than pregnant females. Goats depend on progesterone from the CL to maintain pregnancy throughout gestation. Plasma or serum progesterone concentrations below 1 to 2 ng/ml 21 days and 18 to 19 days after breeding in the doe and ewe, respectively, indicate non-pregnancy based on the absence of a functional CL. An elevated progesterone concentration may indicate pregnancy, hydrometra, pyometra, early embryonic death, fetal mummification, or irregular estrus cycle.[2] The accuracy of blood progesterone level analysis is reported as 80% to 100% for non-pregnancy and 67% to 100% for pregnancy. In some management scenarios, particularly in dairy goats, serum or milk progesterone is collected on day 19 to 22 after breeding. Serum or plasma progesterone concentrations more accurately reflect the true endocrine status of the doe and are more accurate than milk progesterone analysis. Commercial on-farm cattle progesterone test kits can be used in goats with good accuracy.[1,2]

Radiography

Abdominal radiography is useful for detecting pregnancy and fetal numbers in the individual pet goat brought to a clinic. It also provides an accurate alternative when ultrasound equipment is not available. This procedure is applicable but rarely used in ewes. Radiography is not practical for examining large numbers of animals. The fetal skeleton may be seen as early as 58 days after breeding and may be radiopaque after day 65. Radiography is probably best performed 90 days or later after breeding in goats to avoid false negative results.[2]

GENERAL FEMALE MANAGEMENT

Pregnant ewe and doe flocks should be intensely managed to control disease and lessen the chance of reproductive failure. A review of records provides the veterinarian the opportunity to look at the reproductive performance of the flock over the past several years. This can help in the implementation of management changes to enhance productivity. Particular attention should be paid to lambing percentages and dystocia rates to determine whether more aggressive monitoring and intervention may be necessary around the time of birthing. Some basic guidelines should be followed with respect to control of infectious disease. Producers should attempt to keep flocks closed during gestation and should be vigilant for potential fomite transmission among flocks. Biosecurity should be extended to include pest and stray cat control.

Pregnant Female Care

Females should be maintained at a body condition score of 2.5 to 3 and should be allowed free access to an acceptable mineral salt mixture (see Chapter 2) and clean water. All causes of stress should be avoided. Deworming, hoof trimming, shearing, vaccination, moving, and other stressful procedures should be minimized for 1 month before the ewes and does give birth.[1] Producers should determine the animals' pregnancy status and number of fetuses and sort and feed them accordingly. Females should be monitored and assessed for body condition score every 2 to 3 weeks throughout gestation. Basic feeding programs and herd health recommendations are covered elsewhere in this text (see Chapters 2 and 17).

References

1. Rowe JD, East NE: Reproductive management—Part I: estrous cycles, synchronization, artificial insemination, pregnancy diagnosis, *Small Ruminants for the Mixed Animal Practitioner Western Veterinary Conference*, p 137, 1998, Las Vegas, NV.
2. Buckrell BC: *Guelph system for transcervical AI (user manual)*, Georgetown, Ontario, Canada, 1999, Small Ruminant Genetics.
3. Mastas D: Pregnancy diagnosis in the goat. In Youngquist RS, editor: *Current therapy in large animal theriogenology*, Philadelphia, 1997, WB Saunders.
4. Haibel GK: Use of ultrasonography in reproductive management of sheep and goat herd, *Vet Clin North Am: Food Anim Pract* 6:597, 1990.

PARTURITION

Normal parturition requires the functional maturation of the fetal adrenal cortex. Parturition is triggered by activation of the fetal pituitary-adrenal axis. Adrenocorticotropic hormone (ACTH) is released by the fetal pituitary gland, stimulating the release of corticosteroids by the fetal adrenal glands. An increase in fetal corticosteroids stimulates placental estrogen biosynthesis, which in turn stimulates the synthesis and release of $PGF_{2\alpha}$ from the placenta and endometrium. $PGF_{2\alpha}$ causes luteolysis, which results in a decrease in progesterone. An increase in estrogen and decrease in progesterone stimulates myometrial activity, stimulating oxytocin release.[1]

Birth is much more likely to occur during the daylight hours than at night; it is most frequent around midday. When the female is close to birthing, the udder fills up rapidly, the pelvic ligaments relax, and the vulva enlarges and shows small amounts of colorless mucous discharge. The cervical plug is often shed just before parturition, but it may be lost as much as 1 week prepartum. Parturition can be divided into three stages. The first stage is initia-

tion of myometrial contraction, which lasts from 2 to 12 hours. In the first stage the female may leave the flock and act uncomfortable. The female is restless, lies down and gets up, and urinates frequently. During the first stage the cervix relaxes and releases the cervical seal. The second stage is delivery of the fetus, which is fairly quick, lasting about 1 to 2 hours. Does and ewes may prefer lateral recumbency during this stage, but some older, more experienced females may remain standing for delivery. Initially the amnion protrudes from the vulva, which should be followed shortly by the forefeet and the head. The lamb or kid should be in a position such that the dorsum of the lamb or kid is aimed toward the sacrum of the ewe or doe. NOTE: Any female that fails to continue progressing through parturition should be examined.

Some lambs and kids are born in posterior presentation, which is normal if both legs are extended and delivery occurs rapidly after the feet are delivered. In the case of multiple kids or lambs, the female may rest between deliveries or the deliveries may occur in quick succession. If a female strains without producing any kid or ewe for longer than an hour, intervention is indicated.

The third stage is characterized by delivery of the placenta within 6 hours and involution of the uterus. In the absence of septicemic or toxic signs, failure to deliver the placenta should be of no cause for concern until 12 to 18 hours. Involution of the uterus is complete by day 28 after birth. Lochia (a nonodorous, reddish-brown discharge) is normally discharged for as long as 3 weeks.

INDUCTION OF PARTURITION AND PREGNANCY TERMINATION

Termination of pregnancy in the doe can be achieved at any time because she depends on progesterone from the CL to maintain pregnancy throughout gestation. Therefore intentional or accidental administration of prostaglandins induces abortion or parturition at any stage of gestation. The typical reason for a client's request for early termination of pregnancy is mismating. The drug of choice to induce abortion or parturition in the doe is $PGF_{2\alpha}$ (5 to 10 mg) or cloprostenol (75 to 100 μg/45 kg). The ewe is similar to the cow in that $PGF_{2\alpha}$ may not induce abortion throughout gestation. To allow the CL to mature and become receptive to the effect of prostaglandin, the doe or ewe should not be treated earlier than 5 to 7 days after breeding. Successfully aborted does typically show estrus in 3 to 5 days.[1]

Ewe

Farm personnel can use induction of lambing as a management technique to ensure proper attention to the delivery process. Lambing can be reliably induced in ewes after day 137 of gestation with dexamethasone (15 to 20 mg IM), but better lamb survival rates may be expected if induction is initiated within 1 week of the expected due date.[2,3] Lambing can be expected within 36 to 48 hours after the injection.

Doe

The gestation age of a kid should be at least 144 days at induced parturition for the animal to be viable. Therefore accurate breeding records are very important. Females with enlarged udders filled with milk are the best candidates for induction. A doe induced in the morning at the correct stage of gestation can be expected to kid by the next afternoon. Prostaglandins may be given all at once (5 to 10 mg of $PGF_{2\alpha}$ or 75 to 100 μg/45 kg of cloprostenol) or in a step-wise fashion (100 μg cloprostenol followed in 10 hours by 50 μg). This allows owners to plan the time and day of kidding so that assistance is available. Unlike cows, does seldom retain placentas after induced parturition. If does are to be induced because of pregnancy toxemia, administering a glucocorticosteroid (10 to 20 mg dexamethasone IM) 6 to 12 hours before induction may enhance fetal maturation and improve postinduction survivability.[4]

DYSTOCIA MANAGEMENT

Dystocia can be a major cause of economic loss in sheep and goat flocks. The most common cause of dystocia is fetal postural abnormalities. Other causes include incomplete cervical dilation, simultaneous presentation of lambs or kids, cervicovaginal prolapse, uterine inertia, and occasionally fetal-maternal size disproportion. Cases of fetal-maternal size disproportion are usually associated with singleton births and overly finished ewes or does.[5] Most birthing problems are handled by owners, and only the more difficult cases are submitted for veterinary assistance. Most kids or lambs are born in cranial, longitudinal presentation. All manipulative procedures should follow general principles of veterinary obstetrics such as cleanliness, lubrication, and gentleness. Practitioners with small hands tend to have an advantage.

When a ewe or doe is presented for dystocia management, the clinician should first assess her overall condition and rule out the presence of concurrent disease. The 3-30 rule is employed by many practitioners. That is, the ewe or doe should be examined 30 minutes after contractions begin or after the breaking of the chorioallantoic membrane. If the female is normal and parturition is progressing normally, the clinician should wait at least 30 minutes before beginning any treatments or manipulations. Females should be examined 30 minutes after delivery to determine whether another fetus is still in the uterus or birth canal. Some females with dystocia may have a complicating uterine inertia because they have become fatigued; signs of pain and panting may occur. Hypocalcemia (both primary or secondary to respiratory alkalosis) contributes to poor uterine contractility. Administration of a caudal epidural analgesic facilitates corrections in fetal alignment and helps decrease the associated straining and pain. The area over the first two caudal vertebrae should be clipped and aseptically prepared. A 18- to 21-gauge, 4-cm needle is directed ventrally into the junction between the first two caudal vertebrae perpendicular to the slope of the tail head. In small goats a 25- to 27-gauge needle may be required. After penetrating the skin the clinician should fill the hub of the needle with 2% lidocaine (0.5 ml/45 kg body weight) and advance the needle slowly in a ventral direction. When the needle is in the proper position the lidocaine should flow into the space because of the negative pressure in the epidural space. Location of the site can be enhanced by moving the tail up and down. Epidural administration provides approximately 1 hour of analgesia. Ideally, the area around the vulva should be clipped of wool and thoroughly cleansed before any obstetric maneuvers. The clinician should next attempt to palpate the fetus and determine the cause of the dystocia. The use of copious amounts of lubricant should be encouraged when performing obstetric maneuvers in the ewe. Disposable gloves should be worn by all people participating in the birth process because of the potential for zoonotic disease transmission. Common causes of dystocia include deviations from normal presentation, position, or posture; flexion of the neck, carpus, and shoulder; fetal-maternal disproportion; and more than one fetus attempting to exit the vaginal canal at the same time.[5] However, not all cases of abnormal fetal presentation, position, or posture result in dystocia. Some does and ewes may give birth normally if only one forelimb is presented with the head. In dystocia caused by a relatively large head or fetus blocking the vaginal canal, one of the forelimbs may be repositioned into shoulder flexion, allowing room to pass the head and remaining forelimb; the kid can then be delivered by traction. In cases in which just the head is presented and both shoulders are in a flexed position, traction of the head with a snare may be sufficient for delivery if the vaginal canal has been well lubricated.

Carpal and shoulder flexions are corrected digitally by hooking a figure around the forelimbs below the flexed carpus and straightening the limb.

BREECH PRESENTATION

A true breech presentation implies that the fetus is in posterior presentation in a dorso-sacral position with both back limbs retained beneath the fetal body. Breech fetuses are handled similar to those with carpal flexion by straightening each flexed hindlimb. In these cases the rear quarters of the fetus and the tail are felt on vaginal examination. If the veterinarian's hands are small enough he or she may be able to correct this dystocia. The fetus should be pushed cranially and to one side. Raising the female's hindquarters can make this maneuver much easier. The clinician next should try to pull a hock back into the pelvic canal. After one hock is in the pelvis, it should be rotated laterally in relation to the long axis of the fetus while the foot is pulled ventrally and medially out through the vulva. The veterinarian should take care not to injure the ewe's vagina with the fetal hooves. The same procedure is then repeated on the contralateral limb, and the fetus is extracted from the ewe.

HEAD MALPOSITION OR LATERAL DEVIATION OF THE HEAD

Repulsion should be attempted to gain enough room to pull the head back around in normal position. If this cannot be accomplished the clinician can place a snare-type device over the laterally retained head and legs to keep the head of the fetus as tight against its body as possible and then extract the fetus by pulling on the forelimbs.

FRONT LEG MALPOSITION

One or both front legs can be retained. If both front legs are retained the head is usually in the pelvis or can be found protruding from the vulva. If the fetus is still viable it should be repulsed into the pelvic canal to create the room necessary to extract both legs one at the time. Lambs can be delivered with only one foot forward if repeated efforts to extend the second leg are unsuccessful. Care should be taken to ensure that the legs pulled into the pelvic canal are from the same fetus as the head. If no response is elicited from the fetus by pinching or pulling on the tongue and if the veterinarian is confident the fetus is dead, he or she can remove the head with a guarded wire saw or a fetotomy knife. This may allow for easier correction of the retained legs. The same basic procedure can be done if only one leg is retained. When both legs and the head present at the same time (i.e., the legs do not present before the head), the elbows often lodge against the inner entrance of the pelvic canal, creating an elbow lock. This can often be corrected by mild repulsion of the head followed by traction on one limb at a time.

RINGWOMB

Failure of the cervix to dilate properly is a relatively common occurrence in the ewe that also has been re-ported in goats. This condition is referred to as *ringwomb* and is considered to be a heritable condition. A similar clinical condition occurs when the natural birth process is disrupted and the cervix is not properly stimulated for normal dilation to occur. If the veterinarian's hand can fit into the pelvis, he or she can attempt manual dilation of the cervix. Oxytocin can be administered to induce uterine contractions; pushing against the closed cervix may aid in the dilation process. However, a Cesarean section is usually required. A fetotomy knife can be used to open the cervix if the animal's value does not warrant surgery and the fetuses are still viable. Euthanasia should be considered after this procedure depending on the condition of the cervix and uterus.

CESAREAN SECTION

Because of the small size of ewes and does relative to other farm animals, the veterinarian often cannot effectively perform vaginal manipulation of fetuses. Therefore Cesarean section is recommended if vaginal delivery is not possible and the animal's value does not preclude the cost of this procedure. Mild sedation with acepromazine in conjunction with leg restraints and local anesthetic infiltration is usually sufficient for most sheep. If deeper sedation is needed, Telazol (6.6 mg/kg IV) and ketamine (6.6 mg/kg IV) may be used (see Chapter 16). An inverted-L type block with 10 to 20 ml of 2% lidocaine provides good regional anesthesia (Figure 6-17). Although other approaches are possible, a simple recumbent, left flank approach has the advantage of easy restraint, and it is a familiar approach for most large animal practitioners. The ewe or doe can be placed in right lateral recumbency with the front and rear legs restrained in extension with soft cotton ropes. The owner or an assistant can hold the head to minimize stress. A rolled towel can be placed under the spine to tilt the ewe to a 30° angle to the surgeon. The paralumbar fossa is clipped and prepared for aseptic surgery. The clinician makes a

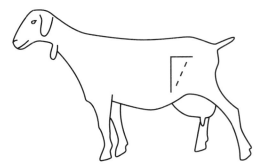

Figure 6-17   Cesarean section. The *solid lines* indicate the location for a local anesthetic block. The clinician injects 10 to 20 ml of 2% lidocaine both superficially and deep into the muscle along the *solid lines*.

15- to 25-cm skin incision near the center of the left paralumbar fossa. Depending on the size of the ewe the incision should start 5 cm ventral to the lateral processes of the lumbar vertebrae and continue in a slight ventrocranial direction to compensate for the bulging rumen and uterus. The external and internal abdominal oblique muscles are cut in the same plane as the skin incision. Alternatively the oblique muscles may be cut in the direction of their fibers to provide a grid-type entry. The clinician must be careful because the distended abdominal walls of sheep and goats are fairly thin compared with cows. A small nick incision can be made through the transverse abdominal muscle and peritoneum. This entry can be extended by inserting fingers into the incision and pulling dorsally and ventrally to separate the muscle along the direction of its fibers.

The uterus is located and exteriorized. The clinician should be aware that the ovine uterus is more fragile than that of the doe or cow. Sterile towels or laparotomy pads can be packed around the exposed uterus to decrease the chance of abdominal contamination. The uterus should be incised in a longitudinal plane over the greater curvature of the horn in a relatively avascular area. The incision should be made long enough to guarantee easy removal of the fetus without risking uterine tears. Separate incisions may be needed in the case of multiple fetuses. The incision should be closed with an inverting incision pattern (e.g., Utrecht pattern). In general a one-layer closure of the uterus is sufficient; however, the incision should be checked closely to ensure that a good seal has been obtained. If not, the entire incision can be oversewn in a second inverting pattern. The clinician generally closes the transverse abdominal wall and peritoneum with a simple continuous pattern using #1 absorbable suture. The internal and external abdominal oblique muscles may be closed together, after which the skin is closed. The authors prefer an interrupted suture pattern (cruciate) for skin closure. Antibiotics are generally not necessary unless abdominal contamination is suspected. However, in field conditions many clinicians administer a broad-spectrum antibiotic before the surgery. NSAIDs (flunixin meglumine) may be used for postoperative pain management.

FETOTOMY

A complete fetotomy, such as that performed in cows, is rarely practiced in either goats or does. Before performing a fetotomy the clinician should clean the animal's perineal area and lubricate the entire reproductive tract well; he or she should exercise extreme caution to avoid uterine rupture and cervical or vaginal damage. Partial fetotomy of the head in most cases is sufficient to allow enough room in the vagina for further manipulation or passage of the remaining fetal parts. In both sheep and goats, percutaneous fetotomy to remove the front legs may help reduce size so the fetus may be manipulated through the

pelvic canal. If two fetuses are wedged into the pelvic canal and repulsion of one or both is not possible, partial fetotomy may be beneficial. Partial fetotomy is warranted when the fetus has been dead for some time and the female's uterus is very friable. In such cases pretreatment with NSAIDs (flunixin meglumine) and antibiotics (penicillin) may be indicated.

PREPARTURIENT DISEASE

A variety of periparturient conditions such as pregnancy toxemia, vaginal prolapse, milk fever, and uterine inertia may interfere with normal parturition or adversely affect the health and fertility of the ewe or doe after parturition. With the exception of pregnancy toxemia, these conditions are more frequently encountered in sheep than in goats.

Fetal Hydrops

Consumption of legumes with high concentrations of estrogenic compounds, hypothyroidism secondary to iodine deficiency, and ingestion of goitrogens are all associated with hydrops uteri. Hydrops also may result from placental or uterine disease. Retention of large quantities of fluid may result in rupture of the prepubic tendon. Induction of parturition should be considered in cases of fetal hydrops.

Rupture of the Prepubic Tendon

Rupture of the prepubic tendon is occasionally seen in sheep and goats pregnant with multiple fetuses, pregnant females with fetal hydrops, and pregnant females that have experienced abdominal trauma. If the owner chooses to keep the female until parturition, applying a homemade canvas girdle (for added abdominal support), reducing rumen fill (increasing concentrate and decreasing forage intake), and reducing salt or trace mineral intake may all be effective treatments. Surgical correction is usually cost-prohibitive and may be unsuccessful. If an accurate breeding date exists, the clinician may consider performing an elective Cesarean section or inducing parturition. If parturition is induced, the clinician should closely observe the female in case she requires help to deliver. Preventing stress and trauma (e.g., deworming, shearing) in late-term females and selecting for animals that do not give birth to quadruplets may help prevent rupture of the prepubic tendon. Females that survive parturition should be culled.

Vaginal Prolapse

Vaginal prolapse is a relatively common problem in the ewe. It typically occurs during the last 3 weeks of gestation in multiparous ewes. Vaginal prolapse is relatively uncommon in goats but is occasionally encountered in dairy breeds. The ventral vaginal floor is usually the area that protrudes from the vulva lips. Many different theories have been advanced regarding the etiology of vaginal prolapse. The consumption of low-quality forage results in increased abdominal filling, which may lead to the vagina being forced out of the vulva. The estrogen content of some legumes also has been incriminated. Other nutrition-related problems include over- and under-conditioning and poor bunk management resulting in overcrowding. Other physical factors that have been implicated include obesity, persistent cough causing repeated episodes of high intraabdominal pressure, and improper or close tail docking in sheep. The tails of sheep should be docked beyond the sixth coccygeal vertebrae or left just long enough to cover the anus when pulled ventrally (see Chapter 9). Unfortunately show animals are often docked closer than this to improve the look of the rump area in the show ring.

Because of a possible genetic component the offspring of ewes or does that have experienced vaginal prolapse should not be kept as breeding stock.[7] An epidural (2% lidocaine 0.5 ml/45 kg) helps prevent straining. Alternatively, a combination of xylazine (0.07 mg/kg) and lidocaine (0.5 mg/kg) can be used to provide as much as 24 hours of relief from straining, although they may cause some pelvic limb ataxia.[8] The prolapsed vagina should be cleaned with a mild soapy solution before replacement. Occasionally the urinary bladder is found inside the prolapsed tissue. Real-time ultrasonography is beneficial in determining the location of the urinary bladder. If the bladder is within the prolapsed tissue, it can usually be drained by locating the urethral orifice beneath the prolapsed tissue (caudal to the vulvar commissures), inserting a finger into the orifice, and lifting the prolapse. A 12 French catheter can be inserted through the urethra and into the bladder if draining is required. The prolapsed tissue should be well lubricated with a water-soluble lubricant (methylcellulose), gently massaged, and carefully forced cranially to its natural position. Picking up the ewe by her hindlegs can facilitate the replacement of the prolapse. In the event that the prolapse has swollen and replacement is difficult to impossible, either a hydroscopic agent (e.g., Epsom salts, sugar) or steady pressure can be applied to the prolapse to decrease edema and reduce size.

A popular method of retaining the prolapsed tissue is through the use of a specially designed plastic prolapse retainer. This retainer has a broad spoon-shaped end that pushes down on the replaced vaginal floor and two retention arms that are tied into the wool or sutured to the skin on either side of the rump. These can be successfully used in some goats.

Various types of purse-string and mattress-type sutures also have been used. Making a shoelace pattern across the vulva with soft rolled gauze, using small loops

of umbilical tape placed lateral to each side of vulva, works well. The owner can loosen the lacing and check on the progress of parturition. If the female is 1 month from parturition, a Buhner suture can be used, with the clinician substituting a standard cadaver needle for a Buhner needle. The Buhner method results in a suture that may last longer and will rarely tear out.

A retention harness also has been described. A rope or stout cord is placed over the back so that half of the rope is on either side of the body. The rope is then crossed under the front legs and then brought back dorsally to be crossed over the back legs. The rope is then passed ventrally and under the rear limbs on either side of the udder and crossed again as it is brought dorsally over the perineal area. The two ends are now tied to the rope that is crossed over the back. This configuration discourages straining and secures the perineum.

Uterine Prolapse

Uterine prolapse generally occurs within 12 to 18 hours after lambing or kidding and may be associated with any condition that weakens the ewe or causes difficult delivery. Hypocalcemia may contribute to the flaccidity that predisposes to uterine prolapse. The prolapsed uterus is usually atonic and is slowly expelled from the vulva lips rather than being forcefully expelled by straining. The prolapsed tissue should be gently washed and well lubricated before replacement into the abdomen. The administration of a caudal epidural (lidocaine 2%, 0.05 ml/45 kg) before replacement decreases straining by the ewe or doe. The replacement procedure can be aided by raising the hindquarters off the ground. This allows the abdominal contents to fall away from the pelvic canal and promotes correct intraabdominal replacement of the prolapsed uterus.

Closure of the vulvar opening is accomplished using a Buhner or shoelace suture as described for vaginal prolapse. If hypocalcemia is suspected, the female should be given a calcium solution. Oxytocin is indicated to aid uterine contraction. The prognosis is normally good. Lacerated and severely soiled prolapses may be complicated by infection.

Retained Fetal Membranes

The placenta should be expelled by 6 hours after parturition. In the absence of toxemia, septicemia, or abnormal vaginal discharge, the clinician should take no action to remove the placenta until 12 to 18 hours postpartum. Retained fetal membranes (RFMs) may be caused by deficiency in selenium or vitamin A, infectious abortions (e.g., toxoplasmosis, chlamydiosis, listeriosis), obesity of the dam, hypocalcemia, dystocia, and possibly other factors.[9,10] RFMs are uncommon in goats but appear to be a problem in some sheep flocks. A higher incidence of

RFM has been reported in dairy goats and in does or ewes whose young have died or been removed. A retained placenta with no other concurrent clinical signs is of little significance, except that the RFM may be associated with certain diseases or deficiencies. Occasionally a vaginal examination can reveal the placenta if it is not visible externally.

Treatment. If the ewe or doe appears clinically normal, treatment should entail only the removal of the placenta. Manual removal should not be attempted. Instead, the doe or ewe can be given oxytocin (5 to 10 IU two to six times a day) or prostaglandins (PGF$_{2\alpha}$, 5 to 10 mg; cloprostenol, 75 µg/45 kg body weight). One of the authors (Dr. Pugh) prefers PGF$_{2\alpha}$ or its analogues and avoids using oxytocin in females with nursing young.

Metritis and Endometritis

Metritis is uncommon in sheep and goats but is encountered in dairy goat breeds and in association with RFM; dystocia; retained dead lambs or kids; abortion caused by toxoplasmosis, chlamydiosis, and listeriosis; and possibly other diseases.[9,10] A retained placenta may serve as a "wick" between the environment and the uterus.

Clinical signs and diagnosis. Clinical signs include a thin, watery, brown to red, possibly purulent, malodorous vaginal discharge. Infected females may be relatively normal or extremely ill and toxic. They may be febrile and exhibit decreased rumen motility, dehydration, increased scleral injection, and possibly depression. In severe cases animals can become infected with *Clostridium tetani*, other *Clostridium* species, or other toxin-producing bacteria. Peritonitis may develop as a result of severe uterine infection or postpartum uterine tears or ruptures. Uterine tears are more common after dystocia, but they also may occur spontaneously.[11] As expected, a CBC indicates toxemia or septicemia. Abdominocentesis may reveal increased protein, increased number of leukocytes, and possibly toxic leukocytes. Ultrasonographic examination usually reveals an enlarged fluid-filled uterus containing hyperechoic fluid. Both goats and ewes normally have a thick, nonodorous, brown to reddish brown vaginal discharge (lochia) for as long as 4 weeks after birth. This normal lochia requires no treatment. New, relatively inexperienced sheep or goat owners, particularly those with pet animals, may interpret this normal discharge as a sign of illness (e.g., metritis).

Treatment. Any underlying disease that is resulting in metritis should be treated. Affected ewes or does should be given broad-spectrum antibiotics (oxytetracycline 10 to 20 mg/kg once a day [SID] to BID) or antibiotics with good efficacy against anaerobic bacteria (penicillin 20,000 IU/kg BID). If a vaginal speculum examination reveals an open cervix, broad-spectrum antibiotics can be infused through the cervix and into the uterus. Uterine infusion is controversial, and clinicians performing it should take care not to damage the cervix, puncture the uterus, and cause greater uterine scarring or damage. A 12 to 14 Fr Foley catheter can be passed carefully through the cervix for uterine lavage and infusion. Uterine evacuation with prostaglandins (PGF$_{2\alpha}$, 5 to 10 mg; cloprostenol, 75 to 100 µg/45 kg body weight) or oxytocin (5 to 10 IU), rehydration as needed, and NSAIDs (e.g., flunixin meglumine 1 mg/kg) should be included in the therapeutic plan. If the placenta is retained, it should be removed, but not manually. Because of the potential for clostridial infections, particularly in animals with dystocia-induced uterine trauma, macerated fetuses, or uterine bacterial contamination, clostridial disease prophylaxis should be undertaken. Previously vaccinated females can be given a booster that includes *C. tetani*. In animals with no history of clostridial prophylaxis, antitoxin is indicated.[9,10]

Pyometra

Pyometra can occur as a sequela to cases of metritis in which the cervix has been damaged; it also occurs in females that cycle after parturition during the anestrous season (Nubians, dwarf goats). The late cycle can result in an ovulation and retention of the resultant CL for a prolonged period. Pyometra is a very uncommon disorder. Signs include anestrus, occasionally sustained elevated serum progesterone, ultrasonographic evidence of varying amounts of echogenic intrauterine fluid, and occasionally a purulent vaginal discharge.

Treatment. Treatment should include prostaglandins (PGF$_{2\alpha}$, 5 to 10 mg; cloprostenol, 75 to 100 µg/45 kg body weight) and/or oxytocin (5 to 10 IU BID).[9,10]

Pregnancy Toxemia

Pregnancy toxemia typically occurs during the final trimester of gestation in ewes and does. The condition is usually seen in females carrying multiple fetuses and may result from their inability to consume enough energy. Conditions that increase energy demands or decrease energy intake also can predispose to this disease. Ewes and does carrying multiple fetuses have a decreased dry matter intake compared with ewes carrying a single fetus. This decreased dry matter intake results from a decrease in rumen volume because of the enlarging uterus, an increase in heat production from the fetuses, and changes in free fatty acid concentrations.[12] Obese or extremely thin females may be more prone to developing the condition. Gestating ewes carrying twins require 180% more energy than those carrying singletons, and those carrying triplets require 240% more than ewes carrying singletons. Ewes and does may not be capable of consuming enough to meet these demands, resulting in a negative energy balance. Ewes and does perform little net glucose absorption from the gastrointestinal tract, but instead synthesize it in the liver.[4,12] A negative energy balance in late gestation results in changes in the insulin-glucagon ratio and activates lipases that mobilize fatty acids and glycerol from body energy reserves. The liver uses these fatty acids and glycerol as energy for fetal growth. If the energy demands are greater than the supply, the liver cannot produce enough glucose and may become overwhelmed with free fatty acids, resulting in the production of ketones.

Clinical signs and diagnosis. Pregnancy toxemia is characterized by depression and recumbency progressing to tremors, stargazing, incoordination, circling, and grinding of the teeth. Ketones and low glucose concentrations result in the observed clinical signs.[13] The diagnosis is confirmed by detecting an increase in urine and blood ketone concentrations. Urine concentrations are more sensitive and specific than blood concentrations. Other findings may include decreased serum calcium and potassium, increased blood urea nitrogen, elevated free fatty acid concentrations (more than 500 μg/ml), and elevated beta-hydroxybutyrate concentrations (more than 1 mmol/L).[13] Necropsy findings include a pale, swollen liver.

Treatment. Treatment of pregnancy toxemia must be immediate and aggressive. The fetuses must be removed as soon as possible. In critical cases a Cesarean section should be performed. If the animal is not critically ill or if its value does not warrant surgery, parturition should be induced. Glucose should be given to control the increased ketone production by the liver. A single injection of 50% (100 to 250 ml IV) dextrose may be effective, depending on the size of the ewe or doe. More frequent administration may result in a rebound hypoglycemia. If the animal's value warrants the expense, a slow drip of 5% dextrose can be used after the initial bolus. B vitamins can be given to stimulate the appetite and provide some of the necessary precursors for the liver to produce glucose. If hypocalcemia is suspected, the slow administration of 50 ml of calcium borogluconate (20 mg calcium/ml) is warranted. If the animal has been anorexic for several days, transfaunation with the rumen liquor from a healthy ruminant can produce a more favorable rumen environment. Propylene glycol can be given (15 cc BID) to treat the hypoglycemia.[14]

Prevention. Prevention of pregnancy toxemia entails providing a good nutrition plan and decreasing any stressors such as increased workloads and parasitism. The addition of niacin and ionophores may provide an additional means of combating this disease (see Chapter 4).[12] Shearing of pregnant sheep also is beneficial because it increases dry matter intake.[12,13,15] The weight of the fleece coat increases the workload for the ewe. Ewes in late pregnancy carrying multiple fetuses also tend to be larger and more awkward than their flock mates. Management must ensure that these animals are being allowed to eat and that adequate bunk space is available for them. Serum beta-hydroxybutyrate concentrations have been used as indicators of the nutritional status of ewes within a herd. Values greater than 0.7 mmol/L indicate that the herd is in a negative energy balance; the producer should take immediate steps to prevent pregnancy toxemia and not wait for clinical cases to appear. Ultrasonography is used to separate ewes that are carrying twins so that owners or caretakers can meet their additional nutritional needs.

Hypocalcemia

Hypocalcemia is typically seen during the last 2 weeks of gestation. Twin-bearing ewes require as much as 8 g of calcium and 4 g of phosphorus per day.

Clinical signs and diagnosis. The clinical signs can overlap the signs seen with pregnancy toxemia because the two diseases are often seen concurrently. Hypocalcemic ewes are initially ataxic and hyperactive but soon become recumbent. Other clinical signs include bloat and failure of pupillary light responses. The initial hyperactivity results from a lack of membrane stabilization by calcium. The subsequent paralysis occurs because little to no calcium is available to release acetylcholine at the neuromuscular junction and influence muscle contractility. Calcium concentrations can be measured to confirm hypocalcemia. The serum calcium concentration is less than 7 mg/dl in clinical cases.

Treatment. Clinical cases are treated with 1 g of calcium per 45 kg body weight, and the response is dramatic. Ewes should have a good supply of calcium in their diets during the final 6 weeks of gestation. Alfalfa hay provides a good source of calcium, as does a mineral mix containing calcium.[9]

NEONATAL CARE

Lambing Management

Ewes should be managed to ensure they have a body condition score of 3 to 3.5 at lambing. Producers should monitor body condition throughout gestation so that the ewes are not forced to try to create body reserves during the final few weeks of gestation. A good herd health program should be planned and implemented to decrease the incidence of disease in the prepartum ewe. Monitoring of blood calcium, phosphorus, magnesium, and selenium concentrations is warranted if a history of deficiencies has occurred in the geographic region. The ewe's energy balance also can be monitored by measuring beta-hydroxybutyrate concentrations in serum. A clean, dry lambing area that is protected from severe cold and wind should be provided for the ewe. She should be sheared before lambing and have her mammary glands examined to ensure that the lambs will be physically able to nurse and that no severe teat and udder lesions are present.[16] After lambing the ewes and lambs should be placed together in claiming pens for at least 24 hours. This allows the manager to observe the nursing behavior of the lamb and thereby enhances the opportunity to intervene. Newborn lambs should attempt to stand and nurse within 30 minutes of birth. Dipping the navel with an iodine solution (7% tincture), a weak iodine solution, or a chlorhexidine solution is recommended. The chlorhexidine solution appears to have a more residual antibacterial effect, and the strong iodine solutions may be associated with umbilical abscesses or patent urachus. Still, the "test of time" suggests that all of these solutions are safe and useful if used judiciously. Neonatal lambs are especially prone to hypoglycemia and hypothermia, so careful observation of newborns is mandatory. The newborn lamb should be up and nursing within the first 2 hours of life. If the lamb does not seem satiated after nursing or if the ewe has udder pathology with a potential for inadequate milk production, colostrum should be supplemented. Table 6-6 shows how to make and use a sodium sulfate solution that can be used to assess the success or failure of passive transfer of colostral antibodies. Recommendations for the supplementation of colostrum are 50 ml/kg in the first 2 hours after birth, and a total of 200 ml/kg in the first day. Lambs can be supplemented with ovine or caprine colostrum. Fresh or frozen colostrum from animal sources is generally considered superior to commercial supplements. If possible the colostrum donor should be from the same general location as the dam and be vaccinated against the clostridial diseases.[6]

PERIPARTURIENT CARE OF THE DOE

Prepartum care of does prevents most postpartum problems. Does should be examined with ultrasonography to confirm pregnancy status and the stage of gestation. The clinician or producer should determine their body condition scores. Dairy does should be "dried off" 60 days before the expected due date. During the final 4 weeks of the dry period, does should be supplemented with concentrates or good-quality pasture. They should be watched closely for signs of ketosis, hypocalcemia, hypomagnesemia, or abortion diseases.[16] Where possible, females should receive their annual vaccinations and be dewormed during the final month of pregnancy. Vaccination of females for enterotoxemia, tetanus, and other endemic diseases optimizes the presence of immunoglobulins in the colostrum. Dairy does should be brought into a kidding pen, and the hair around their udders, tails, and perineal areas should be clipped. Meat does should have access to a clean shelter for kidding and should be observed regularly.

At birth, kids should be observed for abnormal respiration and other evidence of fetal distress such as meconium staining. Mucus and fluids should be removed from the nose and mouth immediately. Normal kids attempt to stand within a few minutes of birth and nurse vigorously within the first few hours. The kid's respiration is stimulated by the doe licking it or the owner vigorously rubbing it with a towel. The umbilicus should be in-

---

TABLE 6-6

A METHOD OF ASSESSING THE SUCCESS OR FAILURE OF PASSIVE TRANSFER IN THE NEONATAL LAMB OR KID

Sodium Sulfate Test for Passive Transfer

- Place 14, 16, and 18 g of powdered sodium sulfate into labeled containers filled with 100 ml of distilled water.
- Place 1.9 ml of each of these solutions (14%, 16%, 18%) into three separate sterile tubes.
- Add 0.1 ml of serum to each container, then mix thoroughly.
- Allow the mixture to stand undisturbed at room temperature for 1 hour to permit maximal precipitation. Assess the tubes for clarity. A cloudy appearance (manifested by the inability to read newsprint through the tube) is associated with immunoglobulin precipitation.

IMMUNOGLOBULIN	14%	16%	18%	COMMENT CONCENTRATION (MG/DL)
More than 1500	Cloudy	Cloudy	Cloudy	Successful passive transfer
More than 1000	Clear	Cloudy	Cloudy	Successful to partially successful passive transfer
500	Clear	Clear	Cloudy	Partial failure of passive transfer
Less than 500	Clear	Clear	Clear	Failure of passive transfer

spected for hemorrhage or herniation, and the umbilical stump should be disinfected with 7% tincture of iodine or another suitable iodine or chlorhexidine solution. The way kids are raised and handled after birth depends on the type of goat and owner's preference. Meat and fiber goats raise their kids on pasture, whereas dairy kids are removed before they have a chance to nurse. Kids need to receive adequate colostrum within the first 4 hours of birth. Dairy kids are bottle fed heat-treated goat colostrum (at 56° C for 1 hour) to prevent caprine arthritis-encephalitis virus (CAEV) transmission. Weak kids should receive colostrum by an oral stomach tube or a lamb feeder. Kids should be fed 10% of their body weight in colostrum the first day, divided into three or four feedings. Colostrum substitutes are not suitable for kids and do not increase their immunoglobulin levels. Delayed colostrum intake, inadequate colostrum ingestion, and ingestion of poor-quality colostrum are common reasons for failure of passive transfer[16] (see Table 6-6). In meat and fiber production herds, adequate colostrum intake can be assessed by observing kids nursing and palpating their abdomens. Serum immunoglobulin levels can be assessed using a sodium sulfate test, zinc sulfate turbidity test, or other commercially available screening test. Levels higher than 1600 mg/dl are desirable; levels below 600 mg/dl may indicate failure or partial failure of passive transfer.[12] IV transfusion of 20 to 40 ml/kg of caprine plasma from the dam or another adult goat in the herd may be indicated for a valuable neonate exhibiting failure of passive transfer. Kids born in selenium-deficient areas should be injected with selenium at birth. Finally, kids are at greatest risk of hypothermia and hypoglycemia during the first few days of life. They should be protected from rain and cold weather and treated for hypoglycemia with glucose solution.

References

1. Thomas JO: Survey of causes of dystocia in sheep, *Vet Rec* 127:574, 1990.
2. Peters AR, Dent CN: Induction of parturition in sheep using dexamethasone, *Vet Rec* 131:128, 1992.
3. Owens JL et al: A note on the effects of dexamethasone-induced parturition on ewe behavior and lamb survival in prolific Booroola Merino ewes, *Anim Prod* 41:417, 1985.
4. Rowe JD: Reproductive management of sheep and goats. *Proceedings of the American Association of Small Ruminant Practitioners, Research Symposium on Health and Disease*, p 39, 1998, Nashville, TN.
5. Brawn W: Parturition and dystocia in the goat. In Youngquist RS, editor: *Current therapy in large animal theriogenology*, Philadelphia, 1997, WB Saunders.
6. Majeed AF, Taha MB: Preliminary study on treatment of ringwomb in Iraqi goats, *Anim Repro Soc* 18:1999, 1989.
7. Menzies PI, Bailey D: Diseases of the periparturient ewe. In Youngquist RS, editor: *Current therapy in large animal theriogenology*, Philadelphia, 1997, WB Saunders.
8. Scott PR et al: The use of combined xylazine and lidocaine epidural injection in ewes with vaginal or uterine prolapse, *Therio* 43:1175, 1995.
9. Rowe JD: Reproductive management—Part III. Small ruminants for the mixed animal practitioner, *Small Ruminants for the Mixed Animal Practitioner Western Veterinary Conference*, p 147, 1998, Las Vegas, NV.
10. Braun W: Periparturient infection and structural abnormality. In Youngquist RS, editor: *Current therapy in large animal theriogenology*, Philadelphia, 1997, WB Saunders.
11. Pugh DG, Hardin DK: Ovine uterine rupture, *Agri-Pract* 7:15, 1986.
12. Gessert ME: The use of niacin and other energy modifiers of energy metabolism for the prevention of pregnancy toxemia in ewes, *Proceedings of the Society for Theriogenology*, p 296, 1995, Nashville, TN.
13. Scott PR et al: Cerebrospinal fluid and plasma glucose concentration of ovine pregnancy toxemia cases in apparent ewes, *Br Vet J* 151:39, 1995.
14. Marteniuk JV, Herdt TH: Pregnancy toxemia and ketosis of ewes and does, *Vet Clin North Am: Food Anim Pract* 4:307, 1988.
15. Austin AR, Young NE: The effect of shearing pregnant ewes on lamb birth weights, *Vet Rec* 100:527, 1977.
16. Menzies PI, Bailey D: Lambing management and neonatal care. In Youngquist RS, editor: *Current therapy in large animal theriogenology*, Philadelphia, 1997, WB Saunders.

REPRODUCTIVE DYSFUNCTION

Reproductive Failure

During an investigation of reproductive failure in ruminants, the infectious causes always seem to garner the most attention. However, noninfectious causes can often be more problematic to diagnose but easier to treat. Deficiencies in iodine, copper, and other nutrients can result in reproductive failure in sheep and goats. These and other nutritional problems are covered in more detail in Chapter 2.

Plant Toxicity

Veratrum californicum.   Members of the *Veratrum* genus are associated with numerous congenital abnormalities in lambs. *V. californicum*, commonly known as *false hellebore*, contains a teratogenic alkaloid (cyclopamine) that is responsible for a number of congenital defects in lambs depending on the stage of gestation when they are consumed. Exposure to *V. californicum* during the first 10 days of gestation is associated with early embryonic death. The classic, demonstrable conditions associated with *V. californicum* ingestion—severe facial abnormalities such as a cyclops-like appearance, anophthalmos, and cleft palate—occur when exposure takes place between day 12 and 14. Exposure between day 25 and 36 results in hypoplasia of the metacarpals and metatarsals. Exposure has also been reported to cause inadequate development

TABLE 6-7

PLANTS THAT AFFECT REPRODUCTION

PLANT	COMMENT
Fusarium	• Found in moldy corn and wheat • Produces the estrogenic substance zearlenone • Signs include a decreased lambing and kidding percentage
Clovers (subterranean, crimson, red, white, alsike)	• Produce estrogen-like substances • Signs include cystic hyperplasia of the cervix and hydrops uteri • White clover also has cyanogenic ergotalkaloids • Alsike also can cause photosensitization, liver disease, and stomatitis
Ponderosa pine	• Signs include stillbirths, last-trimester abortions, renal tubular necrosis, pulmonary congestion, weak uterine contractions, and poor cervical dilation
Cottonseed	• Toxic substance is gossypol • Signs include testicle and spermatozoa abnormalities • Signs occur most often in young preruminants
Broomweed, Monterey cypress, jumpweed	
Veratrum californicum	• All parts of plant are toxic • Signs include salivation, diuresis, muscular weakness, incoordination, • Preventive measures include delaying grazing until after the first frost and breeding ewes 5 weeks before putting on range containing *Veratrum*

DAYS OF GESTATION	EFFECT
0 to 10	Failure to implant
12 to 14	Cyclopia
12 to 34	Motor nerve paralysis
22 to 30	Cleft palate
25 to 36	Hypoplasia of metacarpals and tarsals

PLANT	COMMENT
Tobacco	• Toxic effects are more common in swine
Poison hemlock	• Toxic effects are more common in cattle
Lupine	• Can cause arthrogryposis
Locoweed	• Can cause arthrogryposis
Sudan grass	• Can cause arthrogryposis and contracted tendons

of the fetal pituitary glands. This can result in prolonged gestations, abnormally large fetuses, and an increased incidence of dystocia. *V. californicum* is an erect herb with an unbranched stem. Large, wide, alternate, clasping leaves with prominent spiraling parallel veins are characteristic[1,2] (Table 6-7).

Locoweeds. Members of the genera *Astragalus* and *Oxytropis* are commonly referred to as *locoweeds;* they have been implicated as causing abortions, small weak lambs, and bent legs in newborns. The incidence of abortion and small weak lambs has been reported to be as high as 75% in exposed ewes. The toxin affects the fetal-placental unit, causing delayed placentation, decreased placental vascularization, fetal edema, and altered development of the cotyledons. It also is associated with decreased spermatogenesis in the ram.[3]

Broomweed. Broomweed *(Gutierrezia microcephala, Xanthocephalum lucidum)* ingestion can cause abortions and small, weak, premature lambs because of the toxic effects of an ecbolic toxin in these plants (triterpenoid saponin). Other clinical signs include gastrointestinal upset, hematuria, and death. Broomweed is a shrub found in arid regions of the western United States.[4]

Ergot alkaloids and ergot. The consumption of fescue *(Festuca arundinacea)* infected with the fungus *Netyphodium coenophialum* is associated with decreased reproductive efficiency.[4] The ergot alkaloids produced by the fungus have been shown to affect prolactin production in ewes and increase the interval from introduction of the ram until conception.[5] Ergot concentrations greater than 0.1% to 0.7% of the diet can reduce the number of live births in sheep.[6]

Estrogen-producing plants. Sheep appear to be sensitive to the effects of phytoestrogens from plants such as subterranean clover *(Trifolium subterraneum)*, white clover *(T. repens)*, and alfalfa *(Medicago sativa)*. Clinical signs associated with phytoestrogen consumption include infertility, irregular and prolonged heat cycles, lowered conception rates, and early embryonic death.[7] Physical changes that may be seen in ewes include vaginal prolapse, cystic glandular hyperplasia of the cervix and uterus, enlarged teats, and inappropriate lactation. Dystocia and uterine inertia also are observed.[6] Plants associated with depressed reproduction are shown in Table 6-7.

Nutritional Abnormalities

Poor body condition, depressed energy intake, and decreased mineral and vitamin intake all suppress reproductive activity in ewes and does. Lower overall nutritional intake results in poor or weak signs of estrus, depressed ovulation, abnormal estrus cycle length, and delayed puberty. Deficiencies in energy, protein, vitamins A and E, phosphorus, and many trace minerals are most commonly seen. Deficiencies in vitamin A, copper, manganese, and iodine are associated with irregular estrus cycles.

Heat Stress

Heat stress depresses reproductive ability and causes fetal wastage. Causes of heat stress include decreased water intake, obesity, exercise, and fatigue during hot weather. Both very young and very old animals are susceptible to heat stress. High ambient temperatures and high humidity result in poor or compromised cooling. As the ambient temperature approaches body temperature, skin vasodilation no longer aids in heat dissipation. In sheep the respiratory passages are important in cooling, so animals will pant when they are hot. Unsheared Angora goats and heavily wooled sheep, particularly young sheep, are especially susceptible to heat stress.

Clinical signs. Common clinical signs include decreased fertility and depressed signs of estrus in females as well as an increased number of abnormal spermatozoa and depressed libido in males. Angora goats experience high embryonic mortality if the heat stress occurs during the first 3 to 6 weeks of pregnancy. However, all breeds and both species can experience high embryonic losses. Other clinical signs include dullness, depression, rapid respiration, open-mouth breathing, congested conjunctiva, dilated pupils (early), constricted pupils (late), decreased feed intake, increased heart rate, weak rapid pulse, hyperthermia, acid-base alterations, dehydration, excessive loss of potassium and sodium from sweat, and increased packed cell volume (greater than 60% red blood

cells). Angora goats have a decreased ability to respond to heat stress compared with other breeds of goats. Sheep can tolerate external temperatures higher than 110° F if the humidity is less than 65%, but they will pant if the rectal temperature is higher than 106° F. Secondary bloat and acidosis can occur if high-energy feed is made available at night or if a break in the weather occurs because animals may engorge themselves.

Diagnosis. Diagnosis is based on the clinical signs. Necropsy findings include cerebral edema, rapid putrefaction, and large, distended veins. CBC results are unremarkable.

Treatment. Treatment should include lowering the body temperature with cold water submersion, cold water enemas, ice applications, or alcohol rubs. Affected animals should be sheared. Non-pregnant animals can be given glucocorticoids (dexamethasone 1 to 2 mg/kg IV). Normal hydration should be maintained. If animals are more than 10% dehydrated, IV fluids should be administered, but if animals are less than 10% dehydrated, fluids can be administered orally. Keepers should place affected animals in the shade and attempt to improve air circulation around them. Bucks and rams should undergo a BSE after periods of heat stress. If spermatic abnormalities are noted, the examination should be repeated in 49 to 60 days.

Prevention. Prevention is aimed at keeping animals cool. Woolly or hairy animals should be sheared before periods of hot weather. Long scrotal wool also should be shorn. Animals should be maintained at a good body condition score. Providing shade at feed bunks and spraying water on the animals' backs around the lounging areas are helpful in prevention. Spraying or misting at the feed bunks can increase feed intake. On hot, humid days, animals should only be worked or handled in the early morning. Trace mineral salt and cool water should be provided free choice. Animals should be fed in the early morning or late afternoon. Toxins and plants that decrease peripheral vasodilation should be avoided (fescue). Ventilation across the animals' backs and an open-ridge barn with a high ceiling help keep animals cool.

For dairy goats or sheep, sprinklers and good ventilation in holding pens helps minimize heat stress, but these measures may be contraindicated for the prevention of mastitis. Increasing the energy concentration of feed may improve production after a period of reduced intake. Feeding bypass protein (blood meal, fish meal, corn gluten meal, roasted soybeans, extruded soybeans) improves production, particularly if fat has been added to the feed. The addition of sodium bicarbonate (0.85% to 1%) may enhance milk production in hot weather. Less heat is generated from good-quality forage than from poor-quality forage. The acid-detergent fiber (ADF) content of the diet can be dropped to 21% of the dry matter intake for short periods. The addition of ionophores improves productivity and decreases intake for many animals, but may not benefit lactating females. The feeding of long-stem hay should be implemented. If green or wet feeds are fed, the bunks should be checked for spoilage on a routine basis on hot days.

Pseudopregnancy

Pseudopregnancy (mucometra, hydrometra, cloudburst) is caused by a prolonged luteal phase in goats. The incidence in dairy goats may be as high as 3% to 5% on some farms,[8] with the highest incidence occurring in November through December. It is much less common in fiber or meat breeds of goats and sheep. The cause of this condition is poorly understood, but possible modes of action that have been proposed include out-of-season breeding, sheep and goat hybrid pregnancy, and the overuse of hormonal manipulation of the reproductive cycle. Some cases probably occur as sequelae to abortion or early embryonic loss with a retained CL. Spontaneous CL retention outside of pregnancy, which may result from hormonal manipulation for superovulation or out-of-season breeding, also has been proposed as a cause of pseudopregnancy.[6,8] The condition may occur numerous times during the life of a doe, or it may occur only once.

Clinical signs and diagnosis. Some females may show signs of parturition, udder development, and a bloody vaginal discharge. Pseudopregnancy also is characterized by anestrus, occasionally increased abdominal size, and external and behavioral signs of pregnancy. Blood progesterone concentrations may be consistent with pregnancy and remain elevated for as long as 5 months. Real-time ultrasonography may reveal a uterus with varying amounts of fluid that is either clear, slightly cloudy, or clear with some flecks. The uterus usually appears thin-walled, and no placenta or fetus can be visualized. In females that undergo ultrasound examination before placentomes are visible (before day 30 of gestation), this condition may be falsely diagnosed as pregnancy. Therefore careful ultrasonographic examination with attention to the stage of pregnancy and positive signs of pregnancy (e.g., fetus, placenta, umbilicus) is imperative.

Treatment. The most common treatment for pseudopregnancy is the injection of $PGF_{2\alpha}$ (10 to 20 mg) or cloprostenol (75 to 100 μg/45 kg).

Vaginitis

Vaginitis has several causes (see Chapter 10). Whenever either nonparturient or parturient vaginitis is encountered, particularly in sheep, contagious ecthyma should be ruled out. Other causes of vaginitis include caprine herpes vulvovaginitis (edema and cloudy gray discharge), granular vulvovaginitis caused by *Mycoplasma* and *Acholeplasma*, and *Actinomyces pyogenes* and *Staphylococcus* infections.[6] Lavaging the vagina with mild antiseptic solutions (commercial chlorhexidine) may be all that is required. If animals are in a lot of pain, NSAIDs are useful.

Ectopic mammary tissue on the vulva is occasionally encountered. It appears as vulvar swelling before parturition. Because outflow tracts for milk are rare, this glandular tissue usually undergoes pressure atrophy. The glandular tissue can be surgically removed, but this form of therapy is rarely required.

Cystic Ovarian Disease

Cystic ovaries appear to be more common in goats than in sheep. In one study, 2.4% of more than 1000 female goats examined at slaughterhouses had ovarian cysts.[9] Owners often make the diagnosis based on short cycles or nymphomania,[8] so cystic ovarian disease is probably overdiagnosed. Graafian follicles larger than 12 mm may be considered cystic, but few studies have been performed to document a standard size.[8] The normal follicle diameter size of sheep (15 to 19 mm) is larger than that reported in the doe.[6] The use of some superovulation protocols (PMSG), possibly phosphorus deficiency, and the feeding of estrogenic compounds may be associated with the formation of cystic ovaries. Treatment with hCG (750 to 1000 IU) or GnRH (50 to 100 μg) may be effective.[8] Does that habitually develop cystic ovaries can be treated with hCG or GnRH, watched for signs of estrus, bred, and then retreated with hCG or GnRH 24 hours after breeding.

Ovarian Tumors

Ovarian tumors are rarely reported in sheep and goats.[6,10,11] A granulosa theca cell tumor is shown in Figure 7-5. This is the most common type of ovarian tumor occurring in ewes and does. Animals with these tumors may exhibit nymphomania, virilism, and inappropriate lactation syndrome. Ovarian ultrasonographic examination, either per rectum or transabdominal, usually reveals an enlarged ovary that is either solid or cystic. The contralateral ovary is devoid of structures and lacks a CL.

A tentative diagnosis can be based on elevated concentrations of testosterone or estradiol, diagnostic ultrasound findings, and clinical signs. The treatment is ovariectomy. The authors and others have suggested that does with granulosa cell tumors may have elevated concentrations of testosterone and estradiol.[10]

Ovariectomy

The animal should be heavily sedated and the flank blocked with a local anesthetic, or anesthetized (see

Chapter 16). Animals should be given antibiotics up to 4 hours preoperatively, and the clinician should adhere to aseptic technique. Either a flank or ventral midline approach is acceptable. For the removal of ovarian tumors, a flank approach made by positioning the animal with the affected ovary side up is preferred. For bilateral ovariectomy the authors prefer a ventral midline approach. Regardless of the approach selected, the abdomen should be entered as far caudally as possible. The technique to open and close the abdomen is the same as that described in the sections on Cesarean section and surgical ET. After locating the ovaries, the clinician should identify the pedicle and exteriorize the ovary and pedicle out of the incision. Slow tension usually enhances visualization of the ovary. A crushing hemostat is placed on the ovarian pedicle, and a transfixation ligature is placed through the pedicle on the side of the hemostat, opposite the ovary. The ovarian pedicle is transected next to the hemostat opposite the suture. The clinician then releases the hemostat and examines the pedicle for hemorrhage. If only one ovary is to be removed, the abdomen can then be closed. If the second ovary is to be removed, a hemostat may be placed around the pedicle of the removed ovary for easy retrieval in case of excessive bleeding. The second ovary is removed in the same manner as the first, after which the pedicles of both should be examined and the abdomen closed.[12] Bilateral ovariectomy is performed to produce females for semen collection and libido testing of males. These ovariectomized females should be given estradiol (100 mg) 24 to 48 hours before use.[13]

Others

Freemartins are rare in sheep and goats compared with cattle because both sheep and goats are adapted to multiple births.

References

1. Kampen KR, Ellis LC: Prolonged gestation in ewes ingesting *Veratrum californicum:* morphological changes and steroid biosynthesis in the endocrine organs of cyclopic lambs, *J Endocrin* 52:549, 1972.
2. James LF: Teratological research at the USDA-ARS poisonous plant research laboratory, *J Nat Toxins* 8:63, 1999.
3. James LF: Effect of locoweed feeding on fetal lamb development, *Can J Comp Med* 40:380, 1976.
4. Putman MR: Toxicologic problems in livestock affecting reproduction, *Vet Clin North Am: Food Anim Pract* 5:325, 1989.
5. Porter JK, Thompson FN: Effects of fescue toxicosis on reproduction in livestock, *J Anim Sci* 70:1594, 1992.
6. Roberts SJ: *Veterinary obstetrics and genital diseases (theriogenology),* North Pomfret, VT, 1986, David and Charles.
7. Adams NR: Organizational and activational effects of phytoestrogens on the reproductive tract of the ewe, *Proc Soc Exp Biol Med* 208:87, 1995.
8. Braun W: Noninfectious infertility in the doe. In Youngquist RS, editor: *Current therapy in large animal theriogenology,* Philadelphia, 1997, WB Saunders.
9. Lyngset O: Studies on reproduction in the goat. V. Pathological conditions and malformations of the genital tract of the goat, *Acta Vet Scand* 9:364, 1968.
10. DeWalque J: Tumeur ovarienne et masculinization chez une chamoisee de Alpas, *Annales de Med Vet,* p 322, 1963.
11. Lofstedt RM, Williams R: Granulosa cell tumor in a goat, *J Am Vet Med Assoc* 189:206, 1986.
12. Riddell MG: Ovariectomy. In Wolfe DF, Moll HD, editors: *Large animal urogenital surgery,* Baltimore, 1999, Williams & Wilkins.
13. Katz LS: Sexual performance tests in sexually inexperienced rams. In Dziuk PJ, Wheeler M, editors: *Handbook of methods for study of reproductive physiology in domestic animals,* Urbana, IL, 1991, University of Illinois Press.

ABORTION

Abortion (fetal loss or fetal wastage) is the loss of the conceptus anytime during gestation, but it is most commonly observed during the final 2 months. Fetal losses in early to middle gestation often go undetected. The ewe and doe are both normally very fertile animals but may have a high incidence of abortion compared with other farm animals.[1,2] Abortion rates of 5% for these two species are commonplace; rates less than 5% are considered good, and a less than 2% abortion rate is considered excellent.[3,4] Many infectious agents, stressors, pharmaceuticals, nutritional deficiencies, and toxic plants have all been indicated as causes of pregnancy loss.[2] Infectious causes are common and may be major sources of economic loss. During an abortion outbreak the safest approach is to assume that all causes of abortion are infectious in nature.[5,6] Several microbial agents have been incriminated as causes of abortion in sheep and goats, but the most common are *Chlamydia psittaci, Toxoplasma gondii,* and *Campylobacter* species.[3,7-9]

In a study of western North America sheep abortion and stillbirth specimens submitted during a 10-year period, *T. gondii, Campylobacter* species, and *C. psittaci* were diagnosed in approximately 25% of all cases.[9] Many of the organisms that cause abortion in sheep also are common causes of abortion in goats. Campylobacteriosis is the exception, as it appears to be rare in goats in North America.[10]

The most consistent finding in most cases of infectious abortion is placentitis (placental disease), which results in retarded fetal growth or death and occasional septicemia of the ewe or doe.[6] Regardless of the type of flock (commercial, hobby farm, pet), midterm and late abortions are of great concern to the owner from both an economic and emotional standpoint. When fetuses are lost, the unproductive females must be fed and cared for until the next breeding season or sold, both of which result in economic losses. In case of infectious abortion a prolonged period of uterine disease and infertility may follow.[10] Fetal

BOX 6-3

GENERIC ABORTION PREVENTION PROGRAM

- Institute a biosecurity program to quarantine all herd additions for as long as 30 days before introduction to the flock.
- Maintain good body condition scores and offer a complete, good-quality trace mineral–salt mixture free choice. Maintain a source of supplemental energy and protein for use during emergency situations.
- In endemic areas, vaccinate 4 and 2 months prepartum for *Chlamydia* and *Campylobacter* (and possibly other diseases) for animals not previously immunized; only one vaccination is required for those with a history of vaccination.
- Feed chlortetracycline (200 to 400 mg/head/day) and monensin (15 mg/head/day) or decoquinate (2 mg/kg body weight) during gestation. These can be included in a grain supplement or mineral mixture.
- Avoid exposure to cows or hogs
- Keep feed and water sources free of fecal-urine contamination
- Reduce numbers of rats, birds, and cats. Keep only spayed adult cats in barns.
- Do not place feed on the ground.
- Submit fetal samples (including placenta) to a diagnostic laboratory promptly.
- Keep first lambing and purchased ewes in separate areas from the rest of the flock.
- Keep postpartum and prepartum females in separate pastures.
- Respond aggressively to any abortions in a flock (diagnose, dispose of aborted tissue, separate aborting females, treat remaining animals).
- Maintain flock in a stress-free, sanitary, uncrowded environment.

mummification is not a common finding in sheep or goats. However, when fetal mummification occurs, toxoplasmosis, chlamydiosis, border disease, and *Coxiella* infection should be at the top of a differential list.[10]

Box 6-3 describes a generic abortion prevention program. Because of the zoonotic potential of many abortifacient conditions, pregnant women, persons with cancer, and those who are immunosuppressed should probably avoid handling aborted fetuses and placentas. In this discussion, causes of abortion or fetal wastage are discussed in terms of those that result in fetal deformities and those that do not.

ABORTION ASSOCIATED WITH DEFORMITIES

Bluetongue

Bluetongue is an infectious, noncontagious disease of ruminants, especially sheep, that is caused by an orbivirus. It is transmitted by a *Culicoides* gnat (or midge), and cattle may serve as reservoirs for infection.[3] Abortion associated with bluetongue occurs seasonally and is tied to the life cycle of the gnat.[3]

Clinical signs.　Infected ewes may become febrile; have a swollen tongue, ears, or face; exhibit an ulcerated mouth or nose; and become lame.[3] Ewes infected during pregnancy will abort or produce lambs with developmental defects (hydranencephaly). Goats are frequently infected in endemic regions as evidenced by serology, but clinical signs are rarely recorded. Bluetongue is an unlikely cause of abortions in goats.[7]

Diagnosis.　Bluetongue viruses can be isolated from the blood, semen, brain, and spleen of aborted fetuses. Viral isolation is enhanced if blood is collected during febrile periods (see Chapters 4 and 14).

Prevention.　Vaccination against bluetongue is of questionable value because of the large numbers of serovars. Housing sheep away from low-lying areas during gnat season, particularly at night, may help prevent the disease.

Akabane Virus Disease

Akabane viral abortion has been reported in sheep and goats.[2,10,11] Akabane virus is an arbovirus that is transmitted by gnats and mosquitoes.[5] It has been reported in Australia, Japan, South Africa, the Middle East, and Argentina, but it is rare in North America.[2,8,9]

Clinical signs.　Clinical disease has been observed in both sheep and goats. Infection of non-pregnant animals is subclinical. Pregnant animals may remain healthy but abort, deliver stillborn fetuses, or have mummified fetuses. Dystocia is common, particularly when arthrogryposis is present.[5]

Diagnosis.   The diagnosis of Akabane disease is made on the basis of arthrogryposis and/or hydranencephaly in the newborn. The identification of a positive antibody titer to this virus in live-born or aborted fetuses also is diagnostic.

Prevention.   Akabane viral infection is untreatable and prevention is difficult. However, effective vaccines have been developed and are used before breeding season in epizootic areas.[7]

Cache Valley Virus

Cache Valley virus is similar to Akabane virus and is an arthropod-borne disease. Mosquitoes are likely carriers of this virus. It is endemic in parts of the United States.

Clinical signs.   Clinical signs in sheep include aborted fetuses with arthrogryposis, brachygnathia, hydranencephaly, and microencephaly, as well as hypoplasia of the spinal cord in live-born lambs.[3,7] It appears to have a predilection for nervous tissues. The more severe the resultant lesion, the earlier in gestation the infection occurred. Early infection (between day 28 and 32 of gestation) may result in mummification or embryonic loss.[3] It is likely that goat fetuses also are susceptible to Cache Valley virus.

Diagnosis.   The diagnosis is aided by the detection of antibodies in fetal fluids or precolostral serum, concurrent with characteristic congenital abnormalities. Absence of titers from the dam also is significant, but absence from the lamb does not preclude diagnosis.[3]

Prevention.   In areas in which vaccines are available, their use 1 or 2 months before breeding may help prevent the disease.[3] Natural immunity derived from infection may be for life.[3] Reducing insect populations, fencing boggy low-lying areas with high insect populations, and using insect repellents are all potential preventative measures, but they are difficult to implement.

Border Disease

Border disease virus (BDV) infection, or hairy shaker disease, is closely related to bovine viral diarrhea. BDV causes abortion and congenital abnormalities of sheep in North America, Britain, Australia, New Zealand, and possibly other areas.[3,12] Goats appear fairly resistant to this disease.

Pathogenesis.   The ewe is infected by ingesting or inhaling the virus. Viremia ensues for 7 days. If a pregnant ewe is infected before day 85 of gestation, her fetuses are aborted, macerated, or mummified. Surviving lambs may have disturbances in the normal formation of the cerebellum and hair follicles. Some of these lambs may be born persistently infected. Lambs infected after 85 days of gestation may be born normal, weak, or stillborn; they may be negative for the virus or have viral antibody titers.[3]

Clinical signs and diagnosis.   Signs of infection include increased numbers of open females, mummified or macerated fetuses, stillbirths, and weak lambs with hairy fleece and tremors.[12] Fetal anomalies include cerebellar hypoplasia, hydranencephaly, and others. The hairy fleece of affected lambs is usually darkly pigmented and most prominent around the head and shoulder.[3] These "hairy shaker" lambs tend to grow poorly and may develop polyarthritis. Cotyledons are small or dysmature, with focal necrosis.[12] The virus can usually be isolated from fetal blood (buffy coat).[3]

Prevention.   All animals suspected of infection should be culled. Any replacement lambs should be screened (by BDV titers and/or viral isolation) before they are added to the flock.[3] Any flock additions should be quarantined for 30 days and tested for the presence of this and other diseases before being placed into the flock. Cattle and sheep should be separated, and the use of common water sources should be minimized. Modified live cattle vaccines should be avoided. The use of killed vaccines for BDV in cattle are of questionable efficacy but have been used.

Others

Teratogenic changes and abortion have been associated with several plant species, including *Gutierrezia* (broomweed), *Lupinus formosus* (arthrogryposis), *Conium maculatum, Nicotiana tabacum,* and *Veratrum californicum* (skunk cabbage). *Astragalus* (locoweed; causes arthrogryposis), *Lathyrus, Sophora,* and Sudan grass (ankylosis, contracted tendons) have been reported to cause congenital defects in sheep and goats similar to the malformations observed with Akabane virus and Cache Valley virus infections[7] (see Table 6-7).

Iodine deficiency may be a problem in certain locations around the world. Affected lambs are born with greatly enlarged thyroid glands, a condition commonly known as *goiter.* Late-term aborted fetuses with no wool and weak newborns are commonly seen. Flocks grazing on plants that are members of the *Brassica* family (e.g., rape, kale, turnips) and animals of certain breeds (polled Dorsets) are more susceptible to iodine deficiencies. Iodine should be supplied at a rate of 0.10 to 0.80 mg/kg of dry matter of feed intake. Supplementation with iodine in iodine-deficient areas has been associated with increased lambing rates and decreased lamb mortality.

Copper deficiency causes a condition in newborn lambs known as *enzootic swayback*. Lambs are typically normal at birth but develop rear-limb paresis or paralysis within a few weeks. The neurologic deficits are caused by a dystrophic demyelination of the white matter in the spinal cord. This lesion begins during gestation and cannot be corrected after diagnosis. Therefore the focus of attention should be on the gestating ewes and does. Pygmy goats appear to be the most susceptible of the goat breeds. Infertility problems also have been blamed on copper deficiencies. Copper supplementation in ewes should be done with caution because copper toxicity can result from oversupplementation and also may cause abortions and other systemic disease. Copper should be fed to ewes at a rate of 5 ppm (mg/kg) of the diet on a dry-matter basis. Copper is commonly supplemented in salt mixtures. These salt mixtures should contain between 0.0625% to 0.13% copper in the form of copper sulfate, which would be between 0.25% and 0.50% copper sulfate in the salt mix. Important interactions occur between copper and molybdenum and copper and sulfur. High concentrations of molybdenum (1 to 2 ppm) and sulfur (more than 2000 ppm) in feed and water sources can decrease copper availability.[2] Interaction with other minerals such as iron (more than 400 ppm), cadmium (more than 3 to 7 ppm), and zinc (more than 100 to 400 ppm) also can negatively affect copper absorption and metabolism.[2]

Manganese deficiency during gestation can result in abortion or weak, small, paralyzed, or deformed neonates.[2] As with other deficiencies, the addition of a palatable trace mineral salt mixture offered free choice, year-round, is usually preventative (see Chapter 2). Anthelmintics in the benzimidazole class (albendazole and cambendazole) given to pregnant females during the first trimester have been associated with fetal abnormalities and abortions.[7]

ABORTION NOT ASSOCIATED WITH DEFORMITIES, INFECTIONS

Campylobacter

Campylobacter (vibriosis) is the most significant cause of abortion in sheep in North America, particularly in western regions. However, it has rarely been documented in cases of goat abortion.[5,7,13,14] It also is an important cause of abortion in other areas of the world (Britain, New Zealand, Africa).[7,12]

Campylobacter jejuni and *C. fetus* (formerly *Vibrio fetus intestinalis*) have been identified as the causative species.[7,14] *C. jejuni* is the most common of the two in North America. These organisms are gram-negative, microaerophilic rods that live in the intestines of sheep, dogs, and some birds. The organisms can be shed by the intestinal tract and through the gallbladders of carrier sheep and occasionally guard dogs (that have ingested aborted fetuses). Infection occurs through ingestion of the organism by the pregnant female. After ingestion the organism enters the bloodstream through the intestinal lining, with a resultant bacteremia.

Clinical signs. Late-gestation abortions, stillbirths, and weak lambs are common. Aborted fetuses and placentas are expelled with little or no autolysis, but fetal retention may occur. Aborting does usually show no signs of systemic illness but may have diarrhea. A mucopurulent vaginal discharge is reported in most aborting does.[14] In South Africa, where *Campylobacter* abortion is common in goats, as many as 30% of aborted kids have grossly visible liver necrosis. The placenta is often edematous, with necrosis or swelling of the cotyledons.[7] The fetus may have some subcutaneous edema, pleuritis, hepatitis, and peritonitis. Necrotic areas on the livers of aborted lambs may occasionally look like "gray targets." Although abortion storms may occur in as much as 70% to 90% of a flock, they usually affect less than 20% of ewes in enzootically infected sheep flocks.[2] Ewes that become infected abort and then become immune. However, some become persistently infected and shed the organism in their feces. Ewes usually recover uneventfully but occasionally may die from retained dead fetuses, metritis, and possibly peritonitis.

Diagnosis. Definitive diagnosis of *Campylobacter* abortion is through isolation of the organism. Direct microscopic examination (dark field or contrast) and isolation of *Campylobacter* species from placenta, fetal abomasal contents, and maternal vaginal discharge is the preferred diagnostic procedure.[15] Stained cotyledonary impression smears are useful in identifying the organism.[3] A serologic test can be done at a few specialized laboratories. Whenever the organism is isolated, culture and antibiotic sensitivity patterns are useful for guiding possible flock treatment.

Treatment and prevention. The antibiotic regimen of penicillin or streptomycin injections or tetracycline in feed (300 mg/head/day) may be useful in the face of a disease outbreak.[13,14] Tetracycline in the feed (200 to 300 mg/head/day) before and during lambing or kidding season appears to decrease the incidence of abortion, as does the use of injectable long-acting oxytetracycline (20 mg/kg every 48 hours) during an outbreak. However, penicillin- and tetracycline-resistant strains have been identified.[3] In cases of apparent tetracycline resistance, sulfamethazine (110 mg/kg PO), or tylosin (30 mg/kg IM SID) may be given.

A combined killed bacterin of *C. fetus* and *C. jejuni* is available for use in sheep. In a confirmed outbreak, vaccination of all pregnant ewes and does with an ovine *Campylobacter* bacterin is advisable.[7] The vaccine is initially administered before breeding, with a booster in 2 to 3 months. Revaccination annually shortly before or just after breeding is recommended.[16] If an immunologic agent for *Escherichia coli* is combined with *C. fetus* or *C. jejuni,* it should be avoided in early gestation because it has been anecdotally associated with fetal wastage. On farms where *Campylobacter* is a confirmed cause of abortion, autogenous bacterins that are strain-specific are valuable. Because of the probable oral route of infection, maintaining sanitary conditions, avoiding fecal contamination of feedstuffs, and isolating aborting animals are recommended.[14] The placentas and aborted fetuses should be burned or buried and never fed to guard dogs. Occasionally *Flexispira rappini* is identified in suspected cases of vibriosis. Obviously, in these cases vaccination for *Campylobacter* is of no value.[3]

Zoonotic potential.   *C. jejuni* has been recognized as a cause of mild gastroenteritis and a possible cause of some neuromuscular disease in human beings. Domestic animals and unpasteurized milk are thought to be sources of *C. jejuni* infection in human beings. Aborted fetuses infected with *C. jejuni* should be handled carefully. Shepherds giving artificial resuscitation to infected lambs have reportedly acquired the disease.[14]

Chlamydia

C. psittaci is a gram-negative, intracellular organism that contains both ribonucleic acid (RNA) and deoxyribonucleic acid (DNA).[5] Chlamydial abortion is one of the most common causes of infectious abortion in sheep and goats in North America.[6,17,18] It also has been diagnosed in other areas (Britain, Europe).[19] Chlamydial infections also can produce pneumonia, keratoconjunctivitis, epididymitis, and polyarthritis in sheep and goats.[10,11,13,18] This organism was established as the causative agent of enzootic abortion of ewes (EAE) in the late 1950s.[20] The antigenic strains found in sheep and goats appear to be closely related. At least nine immunotypes and possible more have been identified.[3] Antigenic type 1 is implicated in abortions, stillbirths, weak kids and lambs, and neonatal chlamydial pneumonia. Type 2 isolates cause polyarthritis and conjunctivitis in adults.[21,22] However, serotype 2 has recently been reported as an abortion-inducing strain in ruminants as well.[18] Little or no cross-protection occurs between these two antigens.[21]

Pathogenesis.   Pigeons and sparrows may serve as reservoirs for the organism, and ticks or insects may play a role in the transmission of this disease.[22,23] *C. psittaci* can infect a non-pregnant female and remain dormant, eliciting little or no immune response. The organism can stay dormant, probably in the intestine, until it multiplies

at conception (cotyledon formation), resulting in both abortion and immune response. Inflammation and necrosis of the placenta caused by multiplication of the organism prevent normal transfer of nutrients across the placenta, resulting in fetal death and abortion.[7] Aborting females shed large numbers of the organism in the uterine discharge, fetus, and placenta, particularly during the first 3 weeks after abortion. After aborting the dam develops a good immune response, and elimination of *Chlamydia* from her uterus usually occurs within 3 months of the abortion.[24,25] However, some ewes that have aborted as a result of *C. psittaci* infection may shed the organism in vaginal secretions during estrus,[3] and susceptible females exposed for the first time in the last half of pregnancy may abort in the subsequent pregnancy.[18,20,26] These females may serve as sources of infection by shedding the organism from their vaginal secretions, feces, or expired air.[3,18,20] Regardless of the time of infection in the female, the organism does not proliferate and attack the placenta until about day 90 of gestation.[27] *Chlamydia* has been isolated from the semen of experimentally infected rams for as long as 29 days after inoculation.[22,23] Still, the primary modes of transmission are from vaginal or uterine secretions of aborting females and from females shedding the organism the following year.

During the subsequent breeding season the does show no signs of infertility, and the natural immunity after an abortion lasts about 3 years. Outbreaks of abortion among goats by dual infection with *Chlamydia* and *Coxiella burnetii* also have been reported.[28]

Clinical signs.   In newly infected flocks, 25% to 60% of ewes or does may abort.[17] In flocks in which the disease is epizootic, abortion rates tend to drop to between 1% to 15%, with abortions predominately occurring in flock additions.[3] Abortions often occur in the last month of gestation but may occur as early as day 100 of gestation.[6,10,24,25] Does and ewes may become anorexic and febrile and may show a bloody vaginal discharge 2 to 3 days before aborting. The fetus may be delivered in a fresh state, but if it is retained in the uterus for 1 or 2 days, it will be autolyzed. Some weak newborns may survive, and a few females may retain the placenta.[6,17] Occasionally, pneumonia may be seen in young animals during an abortion storm. Pathologic changes in the fetus are nonspecific. Regional to generalized placentitis involving the cotyledons and intercotyledonary space are usually noted.[6,17] The placenta may be thickened with white, gray, yellow, or red cotyledons.

Diagnosis.   Diagnosis is by history of abortion, clinical signs, and demonstration of the characteristic inclusion bodies in impression smears of placenta, fetal tissue or uterine discharge. Stained cotyledonary impression smears (Gimenez or modified Ziehl-Neelsen stain) and identification of elementary bodies also are good diagnostic indicators.[3] A definitive diagnosis is made by culturing the organism from the placenta or fetal tissue.[6,11,13,17] Serological testing also is a valuable aid in diagnosis. Ewes and does have significant increases in antibodies against chlamydial antigens after abortion.[29] Paired serum samples taken 2 to 3 weeks apart from the aborting female or the presence of antibodies in fetal serum can aid in diagnosis.[6,13,20] The tests of choice for *Chlamydia* are the enzyme-linked immunospecific assay (ELISA) and the indirect inclusion fluorescence antibody (IIFA) tests.[29] A four-fold increase in antibody titers between paired serum samples or titers in the range of 1:32 to 1:256 are highly suggestive of chlamydial infection, but not diagnostic. When chlamydiosis is suspected, the following samples should be submitted to a diagnostic laboratory:

1. Fresh placenta and fetus packed in ice
2. A vaginal swab taken within 3 days of abortion (if the placenta is not available)
3. Paired serum samples from both aborting and non-aborting females

Treatment. Success has been reported in controlling an outbreak by treating all females with tetracycline during the final 4 to 6 weeks of gestation.[6,13,17] Tetracycline (400 to 500 mg/head/day) mixed into the feed for 2 weeks can prevent the disease.[7,30] This is a reasonable approach for fiber-producing animals. However, in dairy herds it is customary to treat individual nonlactating does or ewes with injections of long-acting oxytetracycline (20 mg/kg IM or SC) every 10 to 14 days.[7] Others have given the drug twice a week during the final 4 to 6 weeks of gestation.[6,13,17] Considering the management difficulties and cost associated with this mode of prevention, the most effective protocol appears to be one injection of long-acting oxytetracycline 6 to 8 weeks before parturition, followed by a second injection 3 weeks after parturition.[22] The authors prefer to include tetracycline in the feed or energy-protein supplement when possible. Regardless of the route of administration, suppression of the organism with antibiotics may prevent additional placental damage and reduce shedding of *Chlamydia*. Tylosin (20 mg/kg IM SID or BID) also may be an effective treatment.

Prevention. Enzootic abortion is of such serious economic concern in some countries that compulsory vaccination programs have been implemented.[19] Killed vaccines for sheep are available in certain locales. These vaccines may be used in goats but have been associated with local and systemic reactions (marked soreness and stiffness).[8,16] Vaccines are usually available only in combination with *Campylobacter* bacterin or *Campylobacter* and *E. coli* bacterin.[8,16] Anecdotal evidence suggests that these three-way vaccines may result in fetal wastage if administered during the first month of pregnancy. If used,

the vaccine should be given IM or SC 8 weeks before breeding and followed in 4 weeks with a booster.[16] Even though trials in sheep have demonstrated that protection against abortion lasts for about 3 years, annual revaccination is recommended.[16,31] Vaccination helps prevent abortion but may not eliminate infection and should therefore not be considered 100% effective.[7]

Aborting females should be removed from the herd for at least 3 weeks, and fetuses and placentas should be burned or buried. Producers should take care to prevent the contamination of feed and water. No feedstuffs should be offered directly on the ground, and feeders should be designed to prevent animals from crawling into and contaminating feed.[19]

Zoonotic potential. *C. psittaci* is contagious to human beings. During lambing and kidding season, pregnant women assisting with parturitions may become infected and miscarry. An influenza-like syndrome also has been described in people assisting with lambing of infected animals.[7] Veterinarians and others assisting with normal parturition, dystocia, and abortion should wear masks and latex gloves and try to limit exposure to uterine fluids. The same precautions apply when collecting fetuses or placentas for disposal or diagnostic evaluation. Pregnant women should avoid contact with the flock during the kidding and lambing season.[7]

Q Fever

Query or Queensland fever (Q fever) is a zoonotic infection affecting a variety of animal species as well as human beings. It can cause abortion in sheep and goats[7,32] and has been reported in North America and many other countries.[6,7,10,32,33] Q fever is caused by *Coxiella burnetii*, an obligate, intracellular, rickettsial organism that can survive in a dried condition for extended periods.[3] Cattle, sheep, goats, and wildlife may carry the organism, which is shed in large numbers in placentas, uterine fluids, colostrum, and milk.[7,33] Cows may be a source of infection for sheep and goats when they share pastures, water, feed sources, and handling equipment. Animals and human beings can be infected by inhaling contaminated dust. Contact with aborted material, vaginal discharge, and mucous membranes of infected animals also are modes of contamination. This organism may be sexually transmitted. Grazing contaminated pastures and tick bites are other sources of infection.[7]

Clinical signs. The primary significance of this disease is its zoonotic potential. In livestock the disease is usually subclinical. However, occasional abortion outbreaks caused by *C. burnetii* have been reported in goats and, less commonly, in sheep.[8,34] Susceptible pregnant females develop placentitis, whereas non-pregnant females do not develop clinical signs.[3] Clinical signs are infrequent, but abortion and stillbirth may occur late in gestation as a result of severe damage to the placenta, necrosis of the cotyledons, and thickening of the intercotyledonary areas.[6,33,34] Some does abort without apparent clinical signs, whereas others show anorexia and depression 1 to 2 days before aborting. After the initial abortions or infections, animals become immune.

Diagnosis. Diagnosis is based on placental findings, serology, and isolation of the organism.[6,33] Although isolation of *C. burnetii* is the ideal means for diagnosis of the disease, it is usually not feasible because of the contagious and zoonotic potential of the organism. Some diagnostic laboratories are unwilling to handle such organisms because of strict biosafety procedures.[34] Ziehl-Neelsen staining of histologic sections of cotyledons or fetal abomasa may reveal the organism.[3] The fluorescent antibody test can be used to identify the organism in frozen placental sections. Even though a variety of serologic tests have been described, a diagnosis of Q fever abortion cannot be given solely on the basis of positive test results because symptomatic infections without abortions are possible.[35] Antibody titers of more than 1:20 indicate exposure to *C. burnetii*, although the organism may not necessarily be the cause of abortions. A four-fold increase in titers between acute and convalescent samples indicates recent infection.[34] A rapid presumptive diagnosis of infection with *C. burnetii* is possible by identifying a large number of characteristic organisms in the placental tissue and ruling out other causes of placentitis (*Brucella, Campylobacter,* and *Chlamydia*).[8,31]

Treatment and prevention. After the infection is established, the female can carry the organism indefinitely, shedding it in milk and at parturition. Producers should burn or bury placentas and aborted fetuses promptly.[33] In one outbreak of Q fever abortion in goats, abortions stopped after administration of chlortetracycline (200 mg anally every day) for 19 days.[33] The injection of long-acting oxytetracycline (20 mg/kg SC or IM) every 3 days or every 10 to 14 days has been recommended.[8] Prevention in sheep to be used in medical research is a major problem. No effective vaccine is currently available. However, using an autogenous produced vaccine and administering therapeutic levels of chlortetracycline may control the disease. Removing rodents, cats, and cattle that may serve as sources of infection also may aid in control efforts.[8]

Zoonotic potential. Q fever can be transmitted to human beings by ingesting milk from infected animals and having contact with placentas or feces. Disease in human beings is characterized by influenza-like symptoms, hepatitis, myalgia, and endocarditis.[3,11,33] The majority of human cases have a history of contact with infected sheep, goats, or cattle.[34] The organism is killed by pasteurization but is readily transmitted in nonpasteurized milk. All persons should wear masks and gloves when removing manure from the barn, assisting with lambing and kidding, and handling aborted fetuses.[7]

Brucellosis

Brucellosis is an infectious disease of goats characterized by abortion, weak kids, mastitis, and the formation of localized lesions in various tissue.[36] In sheep, brucellosis rarely causes abortion but it can cause epididymitis in rams. The incidence of brucellosis caused by *Brucella melitensis* in goats has historically been extremely low in North America, but recent sporadic outbreaks have been reported in goats in Texas and Colorado.[37] It is widespread in goats in the Middle East, India, Pakistan, Africa, Mexico, and parts of South America.[2,6,11] *B. ovis* is widespread in sheep throughout the western portions of North America.

Both *B. ovis* and *B. melitensis* are small, gram-negative coccobacillus organisms. Although considered goat-specific, *B. melitensis* may cause abortion in sheep.[3] It also is the cause of Malta fever in human beings.[2,6,11] Occasionally, *B. abortus* infection occurs in goats living in close contact with infected cattle or as a result of inadvertent vaccination of goats with live strains of the organism.[36]

Pathogenesis. As goats ingest contaminated feed or water, the organism enters through mucous membranes and becomes localized in the udder, uterus, testes, spleen, or lymph nodes.[2,36] In sheep the organism appears to be transmitted orally from ram to ram or ram to ewe, but not from ewe to ewe.[3] Infected rams, if they remain fertile, will pass the organism in their semen.[3] In pregnant animals, localization in the placenta leads to the development of placentitis with subsequent abortion. Goats excrete the organism in milk, urine, feces, and placenta and for 2 to 3 months in vaginal discharge. If ewes become infected and abort, they usually clear the organism within 2 to 4 weeks.[3] Non-aborting infected females often give birth to infected kids or lambs that are capable of shedding the organism.[2,7,30]

Clinical signs. Sheep and goats with brucellosis often abort during the final trimester.[36,38] Goat flocks may have an abortion storm after the disease is contracted. The initial flock abortions are followed by a period of resistance during which abortions are rare. Again, abortion appears to be more of a problem in goats than in sheep. In goats and rarely in sheep a systemic disease with fever, depression, weight loss, diarrhea, mastitis, lameness, hygroma, and orchitis in males can occur.[2,36] Infected ewes are rarely ill. On gross examination the placenta is normal in *B. melitensis* infection in goats, whereas *B. ovis* infection of sheep results in a thickened, necrotic placentitis.

Diagnosis. Identification of brucellosis as the cause of abortion is usually made by isolating the organism from the aborted fetus (abomasal contents), placenta (cotyledon), or vaginal discharge. Serologic testing alone may lead to a false diagnosis. Various agglutination, precipitation, and complement fixation tests are available to detect carrier animals.[7]

Treatment and prevention. No treatment is available for brucellosis in goats or sheep. In countries with a low prevalence of infection, slaughter of the entire flock is generally the control measure of choice.[2,7,38] In other situations a test and slaughter program may be more appropriate. In sheep, palpating the scrotum for epididymitis, serologic testing, and vaccinating ram-lambs may help control the disease.[3] Vaccination of goats is not permitted in the United States. In many countries in which caprine brucellosis is prevalent, the disease is controlled by an intensive vaccination program that is very effective. The killed vaccine occasionally used in sheep (*B. ovis*) appears to have poor efficacy. Where permitted, a live attenuated strain of *B. melitensis* can be given SC in kids and lambs 3 to 8 months of age.[7,38] This vaccine causes abortion in goats and should therefore be avoided in pregnant animals or those within 1 month of breeding. Immunity from a single vaccination for *B. melitensis* is considered to be lifelong.[7] All new animals should be serologically tested before introduction to the flock. Rams and bucks should be tested yearly before breeding season.[2] Placentas and aborted fetuses should be carefully burned or buried.

Zoonotic potential. Goats were the first species associated with transmission of brucellosis to human beings.[36] Malta fever is caused by *B. melitensis* and should be considered a serious human pathogen. Often the first indication of brucellosis is the occurrence of undulant fever in humans consuming unpasteurized goat milk or cheese.[2,7] Therefore a large percentage of human infections can be prevented by pasteurizing goat dairy products. *B. melitensis* and *B. abortus* infections in sheep and goats should be handled with precautions to minimize human exposure. *B. ovis* is not considered zoonotic, but the clinician should still exercise caution when handling suspected cases.

Leptospirosis

Sheep and goats appear to be less susceptible to leptospirosis than other domestic species. However, goats are more susceptible than sheep.[39] Several serovars of *Leptospira interrogans* (*icterohaemorrhagiae*, *grippotyphosa*, and *pomona*) have been reported as primary causes of abortion in goats.[33] The common serovars seen in sheep are *hardjo*, *bratislava*, *pomona*, and *icterohaemorrhagica*.[3]

Pathogenesis. Exposure to environments contaminated by urine from species other than sheep or goats appears to be the primary source of infection.[7] In a study

of goat abortion in Spain, 2.6% resulted from infection with *Leptospira*, with the serovar *pomona* being the most prevalent (75% of the abortions attributed to *Leptospira*), followed by the serovars *sejroe* (12.5%) and *icterohaemorrhagica* (12.5%).[39]

Clinical signs. Clinical signs include anorexia, fever, marked jaundice, hemoglobinuria, anemia, nervous manifestations, abortion, and occasionally, death.[7,39] Flaccid agalactia may occur in ewes.[3] Abortions have been reported during the final trimester of gestation in goats and to a lesser extent sheep.[39]

Diagnosis. Dark field microscopy, immunofluorescence testing, and silver stains on placenta, fetal tissue, and fluids are used to confirm the diagnosis.[7,39] The organism is difficult to isolate from contaminated specimens. Paired sera from aborted does and ewes showing a four-fold increase in titer is suggestive of leptospirosis.[7]

Treatment and prevention. Vaccination two to four times a year with multivalent cattle vaccines containing the serovar endemic to the area is indicated in regions where leptospirosis is prevalent. Other control measures include separating animal species, reducing the number of rodents, maintaining a clean water supply, and feeding tetracycline (300 to 500 mg/head/day) during middle to late gestation.[7]

Zoonotic potential. Producers or clinicians that suspect leptospirosis should exercise caution to minimize human contact with aborted tissues, the urine of affected animals, and potentially contaminated ponds and water sources. Human beings are susceptible, and infections can result in death.

Salmonellosis

Salmonella infection can cause abortion, metritis, and systemic illness in ewes and does.[30] The condition appears to be more of a clinical entity in stressful situations.[12] These include overcrowding, shipping, water or feed deprivation, and possibly the inappropriate use of antibiotics. *Salmonella abortus-ovis* was first implicated as a cause of abortion in pregnant females. Only sheep and goats are affected by *S. abortus-ovis*, which is uncommon in North America. *S. typhimurium*, *S. dublin*, *S. montevideo*, and *S. arizonae* also are associated with infections and abortion in persistently infected females.[3,7] Sources of infection include birds, cattle, and some wildlife species. Climatic changes, shipping, overcrowded conditions, and other diseases may all predispose to a flock abortion storm. The route of infection is by oral ingestion of the organism.

Clinical signs. Abortion storms affecting as many as 70% of the females may occur. Infected females may become febrile and depressed and have diarrhea. Metritis and retained placenta are common findings. A high mortality rate is seen in ewes after abortion. Abortion may occur throughout gestation but is more common during the final month.

Diagnosis.   A diagnosis can be made by culturing *Salmonella* from aborted fetuses, placentas, and uterine discharge. Specific agglutinins can be demonstrated in the sera of adults and aborted fetuses.

Treatment and prevention.   Prevention and control measures include treating pregnant females with appropriate antibiotics based on culture and antibiotic sensitivity. Administering two doses of an autogenous vaccine followed by an annual booster and cleaning the environment may help minimize this disease.[7]

Zoonotic potential.   *Salmonella* infections should be considered pathogenic to human beings. These organisms can cause abdominal pain, enteritis, and miscarriage in human beings. People who are being treated with oral antimicrobial therapy and those who are immunosuppressed should avoid handling affected sheep or goats.[3]

Toxoplasmosis

Toxoplasmosis has a worldwide distribution and is one of the most common parasitic infections in sheep and goats.[40-42] The protozoan *Toxoplasma gondii* is capable of causing abortion, fetal mummification, stillbirth, and the birth of weak lambs and kids.[7,40]

Pathogenesis.   Cats are vital in the transmission of *T. gondii*.[43] Cats become infected by ingesting infected rodents or birds and develop a transplacental infection. Kittens infected in utero can shed *T. gondii* oocytes after birth.[43] Unless they are immunosuppressed, cats apparently shed the disease only as kittens and rarely show signs of clinical illness. Cats defecate into and bury feces in hay and food bins. Ewes and does become infected by ingesting feed or water contaminated with oocytes found in the feces of infected cats. After ingestion the organism enters the blood and spreads to other tissues. In the pregnant ewe or doe, *Toxoplasma* can invade and multiply in the placenta, spread to the fetus, and cause fetal death, abortion, stillbirth, or the birth of weak lambs and kids; infected animals also may give birth to normal lambs or kids.[40] Abortion occurs as a result of necrosis of the placenta, particularly the cotyledons. Although *T. gondii* is found in goat semen, venereal transmission is an unlikely cause of abortion.[41]

Clinical signs.   Goats appear to be more susceptible to *Toxoplasma* infection than sheep.[44] Ewes and does infected before breeding usually do not abort. Those infected 30 to 90 days after breeding usually have fetal death with resorption or mummification. Most abortions

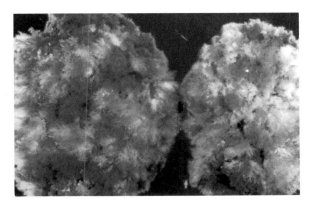

Figure 6-18   These cotyledons are from a goat that aborted as a result of toxoplasmosis. Cotyledons from such abortions typically have interspersed white foci, as shown here. These white foci are areas of coagulative necrosis that are mineralized in many cases. In *Toxoplasma* abortion the intercotyledonary space is usually normal. (Courtesy Dr. JP Dubey, Beltsville, MD.)

occur from infections during the latter half of gestation.[10] Does and ewes are often clinically normal at the time of abortion.[41] The incidence of abortion in a flock is usually low but can vary from 3% to 50%. Rarely, the pregnant female becomes febrile; if she is immunosuppressed, she may develop the neurologic form of the disease. The intercotyledonary areas of the aborted placenta are usually normal, with the cotyledons having gray-white to yellow, small focal areas of necrosis and calcification (1 to 3 mm in diameter). These lesions are clearly visible after the cotyledons are washed in saline[6,10,13,41,42] (Figure 6-18). However, *C. burnetii* and *Brucella* and *Chlamydia* species also can cause placentitis that includes the intercotyledonary region.[42] Fetal lesions include chalky-white necrotic brain lesions.

Diagnosis.   A presumptive diagnosis can be made from placental lesions alone. However, because of its rapid decomposition the placenta is often not available for examination.[44] The preferred diagnostic procedure is to identify *T. gondii* antibodies in fetal fluids or presuckling blood. Their presence indicates transplacental *Toxoplasma* infection.[45] The absence of *T. gondii* antibodies within 7 days of an abortion tends to rule out the possibility of infection. Serologic examination of neonates must occur before colostrum ingestion.[41] High antibody titers in doe or ewe serum is not diagnostic of recent infection because titers may remain elevated from one season to the next. However, the absence of antibodies is good evidence that toxoplasmosis was not the cause of abortion.[7,41] The modified agglutination test (MAT) can be used to detect antibodies in fetal and maternal serum and is more sensitive than other tests.[45] The ELISA and IFA tests also are useful in diagnosis.[41] Positive diagnosis of toxoplasmosis requires isolation of the organism from the placenta or the fetal brain, lung, or muscles.[45] Samples taken for isolation of the organism should be shipped to a diagnostic laboratory packed in ice, but not frozen.[41]

Treatment and prevention. Control of toxoplasmosis is based on preventing exposure of pregnant females to oocyte-contaminated pasture, food, water, and bedding. Fetal membranes and dead fetuses should be buried or incinerated so they do not serve as sources of infection for cats and other animals.[43] Cats should not be allowed near pregnant sheep and goats.[41,43] Spayed cats can be kept in the barn because this may help keep pregnant queens from nesting there. Attempts should be made to prevent cats from defecating in feeders, hay, and other feedstuffs. Cat litter boxes can be placed in strategic areas; if cats have access to hay, the top layers should be discarded or fed to non-pregnant animals. A vaccine containing tachyzoites that do not persist in sheep tissues is available in some areas of the world (Europe and New Zealand). Ewes vaccinated with the S48–strain vaccine remain immune for at least 18 months.[43] Goats that have been infected by *T. gondii* are likely to be resistant to reexposure in subsequent pregnancies.[46]

Feeding decoquinate (2 mg/kg body weight/day) or monensin (15 to 30 mg/head/day) throughout gestation may reduce the incidence of abortion. Anecdotal reports suggest that lasalocid is less effective than monensin in toxoplasmosis control.

Zoonotic potential. Aborted fetal membranes and fetuses should be handled with caution.[43] This organism can cause encephalitis or blindness in human fetuses infected in utero and in immunosuppressed adults. Toxoplasmosis has been reported in humans after drinking raw goat milk. Therefore goat and sheep milk should be pasteurized or boiled before human consumption. This is particularly true for goat and sheep milk fed to infants.[47]

Listeriosis

Listeriosis commonly causes meningoencephalitis, abortion, and septicemia in goats and sheep. *Listeria monocytogenes* and *L. ivanovii* are gram-positive, non–acid-fast facultative microaerophilic organisms. *L. monocytogenes* causes encephalitis, septicemia, and abortion in sheep and goats, whereas *L. ivanovii* causes abortion only in sheep.[3]

Pathogenesis. *L. monocytogenes* can be found in soil, water, plant litter, silage, and the digestive tracts of ruminants and human beings.[7] The organism can survive in soil and feces for extended periods and grows in poorly fermented silage (with pH levels higher than 5.5).[2,6,7,10] Abortion has been attributed to the feeding of contaminated silage. Abortions also have been reported in animals fed only hay or browse.[7,48-50] Of the cases observed by the authors, ingestion of contaminated silage is rarely a component, but grazing on boggy, high-pH soils is a consistent finding.

Clinical signs. Abortion results from infection early in gestation, whereas late gestational infection results in stillbirth or weak neonates. The abortifacient and encephalitic forms of listeriosis do not usually occur simultaneously in sheep, but may occur in goat flocks.[8] Abortion occurs in the final 2 months of pregnancy and is sometimes preceded by septicemia.[6,7] Signs of septicemia include fever, decreased appetite, and reduced milk production. Sheep and occasionally goats that abort may develop metritis. Kids grafted to the aborting female can contract listeriosis through the milk, develop septicemia, and die.[7]

Diagnosis. Culture of the organisms from the fetal abomasum or liver, placenta, or uterine discharge is diagnostic. Unfortunately, fetal autolysis can be so severe that culture may be difficult. In cases in which the liver can be examined, microabscesses are visible as white pinpoint spots. Identification of microabscesses of the liver and brain aids in diagnosis.[3,12]

Treatment and prevention. Feeding poor-quality or spoiled silage or grazing on contaminated pastures should be discouraged. The addition of chlortetracycline (300 mg/head/day) to a grain supplement has been reported to stop abortions during a listeriosis outbreak.[49] During outbreaks the administration of long-acting oxytetracycline (20 mg/kg of body weight every 48 to 72 hours) is also of value. Vaccination to produce cellular immunity has been investigated. Theoretically, live vaccines should be more effective than killed preparations. The administration of two doses of reduced-virulence live vaccine before breeding is reported to have provided significant protection against experimental challenge in pregnant does.[7]

Zoonotic potential. Persons should take care when handling aborted fetuses because *Listeria* can cause neurologic disease in human beings.

Mycoplasmosis

Mycoplasma species are significant pathogens of the goat, causing mastitis, arthritis, keratoconjunctivitis, and occasionally vulvovaginitis and abortion.[10,51,52] *M. mycoides* and *M. agalactia* have been reported as the species causing abortion in goats. Mycoplasmosis is uncommon in sheep, but a similar organism, *Ureaplasma*, has been isolated from ewes with a history of infertility and granular vulvitis.[10,52] *Ureaplasma* infection also may result in placentitis and low-birth-weight lambs.[3,10] Abortion is not the predominant clinical finding in an outbreak.

Abortion occurs in does (and rarely in ewes) in the final trimester of gestation. Females that abort generally shed the organism in their milk, amniotic fluids, and placenta. The organism also may be found in the cotyledons and in the liver and spleen of the fetus. Diagnosis of abortion caused by *Mycoplasma* species is by culture and serotyping of the isolate. Treatment with tetracyclines or tylosin may be of benefit, but identification and culling of all infected animals is the best course of prevention[51] (see Chapters 5 and 13).

Miscellaneous

Actinobacillus seminis has rarely been associated with abortion and metritis in ewes. It may be transmitted from carrier rams (see Chapter 14). This organism is rare in North America.

Several other organisms are associated with infectious abortion. Any diseases that result in debility (e.g., internal parasites, Johne's disease, caseous lymphadenitis) and infections with significant amounts of endotoxin production (gram-negative mastitis or septicemia) may result in fetal loss. Mycotic abortion, although rare, may occur in certain areas of the world.

NONINFECTIOUS CAUSES OF ABORTION

Noninfectious causes such as hereditary, stress, nutritional deficiencies, pharmaceutical effects, and toxic plant ingestion can result in pregnancy loss. Stress may trigger a higher percentage of abortions in goats than in sheep because of the goat's dependency on the CL for the maintenance of pregnancy. Predator attack, severe weather, or shearing may all trigger early regression of the CL in the doe, resulting in abortion. Angora goats experience some forms of abortion not typically seen in other breeds. Young Angora does are susceptible to stress abortions.[53] Some older Angora does experience habitual abortions as a result of adrenal dysfunction.[7,53] These does are heavier than average and have very fine mohair. This habitual, familial form of abortion usually starts when the doe is 4 or 5 years old. Abortions occur at approximately day 100 of gestation.[7] Mature Angora does that abort in this fashion should be removed from the breeding stock, and their offspring should be culled.[7] Heat stress also may result in early embryonic losses, abortions, stillbirths, or weak kids.[10]

Energy and protein deficiencies can result in embryonic loss, decreased fetal growth, depressed placental growth, fetal mummification, and the birth of weak young. Fetal wastage resulting from nutritional deficiencies often occurs between day 90 and 120 of gestation.[53] Deficiencies in a number of minerals and vitamins such as iodine, copper, magnesium, manganese, vitamin A, and selenium can cause abortion or the birth of weak kids and lambs.[7,53] Some heavy metal toxicities (lead) can cause fetal wastage in ewes.[10] High concentrations of dietary sulfur, particularly sulfate, may result in both selenium and copper deficiency.[10] Maintaining optimal body condition scores, ensuring adequate protein intake, and supplementing the diet with a good-quality, complete trace

mineral mixture offered free choice are usually protective (see Chapter 2).

Various pharmaceuticals have proven to be abortifacients, or at least their use has been reported to be followed by abortion. A number of anthelmintics such as phenothiazine and levamisole given in the final months of gestation may cause abortion.[7,52] Anecdotal reports of abortion following the use of other dewormers (ivermectin, fenbendazole) exist, but are largely unsubstantiated. Xylazine and high doses of acepromazine in the first half of pregnancy may cause abortion because of their adverse effects on uterine contraction and placental perfusion.[53] The administration of corticosteroids in late gestation and estrogen and prostaglandins throughout most of gestation may induce abortion.[53] Plants that accumulate nitrate such as sweet clover, Johnson grass, sorghum, lamb's quarter, Jimsonweed, sunflower, pigweed, and oat hay can cause abortion as a result of nitrate-nitrite toxicity.[53] If nitrate-nitrite toxicity is suspected, diluting the affected forage with other feedstuffs is a useful treatment. Cutting suspected forage 30 cm above the ground and avoiding the feeding of drought-stressed crops help decrease nitrate concentrations in feeds to less than 1000 ppm nitrate as nitrogen, or less than 0.44% nitrate. Concentrations higher than this should be avoided or diluted with other feeds. Feeds containing more than 3500 ppm of nitrate nitrogen, or more than 1.76% nitrate, should not be fed to pregnant animals.[54]

References

1. Smith MC: Some clinical aspects of caprine reproduction, *Cornell Vet* 68(suppl 7):200, 1978.
2. Smith MC: Causes and diagnosis of abortion in goats. In Morrow DA, editor: *Current therapy in theriogenology*, ed 2, Philadelphia, 1986, WB Saunders.
3. Menzies PI, Miller R: Abortion in sheep: diagnosis and control. In Youngquist RS, editor: *Current therapy in large animal theriogenology*, Philadelphia, 1999, WB Saunders.
4. Bulgin MS: Nutrition for the breeding flock, *Small Ruminants for the Mixed Animal Practitioner Western Veterinary Conference*, p 5, 1998, Las Vegas, NV.
5. Braun WF: Infectious caprine abortion, *Proceedings of the American Association of Sheep and Goat Practitioners*, 1983, Springfield, IL.
6. Braun WF: Manifestations and aberrations of caprine pregnancy, *Proceedings of the Society for Theriogenology*, 1986, Nashville, TN.
7. Smith MC, Sherman DM: Reproductive system. In Smith MC, Sherman DM, editors: *Goat medicine*, Philadelphia, 1994, Lea and Febiger.
8. Bretzlaff K: Problems of reproduction of goats, *Proceedings of the Small Ruminant Short Course, Society for Theriogenology*, 1994, Nashville, TN.
9. Kirkbride CA: Diagnosis in 1784 ovine abortions and stillbirths, *J Vet Diagn Invest* 5:398, 1993.
10. Roberts SJ: *Veterinary obstetrics and genital diseases (theriogenology)*, ed 3, Woodstock, VT, 1986, David and Charles.
11. Carter GR: *Veterinarian's guide to the laboratory diagnosis of infectious diseases*, Lenexa, KS, 1986, Veterinary Medicine Publishing.

12. Fielden ED: Infectious ovine abortion. In Morrow DA, editor: *Current therapy in theriogenology,* Philadelphia, 1986, WB Saunders.

13. Kimberling CV: Diseases of reproduction, *Proceedings of the First National Sheep Reproduction Symposium,* Fort Collins, CO, 1989, Colorado State University Press.

14. Anderson KL: Campylobacteriosis. In Morrow DA, editor: *Current therapy in theriogenology,* ed 2, Philadelphia, 1986, WB Saunders.

15. Dennis SM: *Campylobacter* abortion in sheep. In Kirkbride CA, editor: *Laboratory diagnosis of livestock abortion,* ed 3, Ames, IA, 1990, Iowa State University Press.

16. Council on Biologics and Therapeutics: Vaccination guidelines for small ruminants, *J Am Vet Med Assoc* 205:1539, 1994.

17. East NE: Chlamydiosis. In Morrow DA, editor: *Current therapy in theriogenology,* ed 2, Philadelphia, 1986, WB Saunders.

18. Sourian A et al: Differentiation of abortion-inducing and intestinal strains of *Chlamydia psittaci* isolated from ruminants by the microimmunofluorescence test, *Vet Rec* 132:217, 1993.

19. Mobini S: Infectious causes of abortion in the goat, *Proceedings of the International Goat Producers Symposium,* Tallahassee, FL, 1990, Florida A & M University Press.

20. Gatewood DM, Spire MF: *Chlamydial abortion in domestic ruminants,* theriogenology fact sheet B-5, Hastings, NE, 1990, Society for Theriogenology.

21. Schachter J et al: Serotyping of *Chlamydia* isolates of ovine origin, *Infect Immun* 9:92, 1974.

22. Timoney JF et al: Chlamydiaceae. In Timoney JF et al, editors: *Hogan and Bruner's microbiology and infectious diseases of domestic animals,* ed 8, Ithaca, NY, 1988, Comstock Publishing Associates.

23. Storz J: *Chlamydia*-induced diseases of sheep and goats. In Howard JL, editor: *Current veterinary therapy food animal practice,* ed 2, Philadelphia, 1986, WB Saunders.

24. Hall RF: Infectious abortions in ewes, *Comp Cont Ed Pract Vet* 4:S216, 1982.

25. Storz J: Chlamydia *and* Chlamydia *induced diseases,* Springfield, IL, 1971, Charles C Thomas.

26. Munro R, Hunter AR: Infection of lambs by orally administered ovine abortion strain of *Chlamydia psittaci, Vet Rec* 109:562, 1981.

27. Storz J: *Chlamydia*-induced diseases of sheep and goats, *Proceedings of the American Association of Small Ruminant Practitioners, WRCC Forty-Sixth Symposium of the Health and Disease of Small Ruminants,* Kerville, TX, 1991.

28. Schopf K, Khaschabi D, Dackau T: Outbreak of abortion among goats caused by dual infection with *Coxiella burnetii* and *Chlamydia psittaci, Tierarzll Prax* 19:630, 1991.

29. Storz J: Chlamydial absorption. In Kirkbride CA, editor: *Laboratory diagnosis of livestock abortion,* ed 3, Ames, IA, 1990, Iowa State University Press.

30. Hungerford TG: *Diseases of livestock,* ed 9, Sydney, 1990, McGraw-Hill.

31. Watson WA: The prevention and control of infectious ovine abortion, *Br Vet J* 129:309, 1973.

32. Behymer D, Riemann HP: *Coxiella burnetii* infection (Q fever), *J Am Vet Med Assoc* 194:764, 1989.

33. Miller RB, Palmer NC, Kierstad M: *Coxiella burnetii* infection in goats. In Morrow DA, editor: *Current therapy in theriogenology,* ed 2, Philadelphia, 1986, WB Saunders.

34. Moore JD et al: Pathology and diagnosis of *Coxiella burnetii* infection in a goat herd, *Vet Path* 28:81, 1991.

35. Zeman DH, Steen PL, Peacock MG: Ovine abortion caused by *Coxiella burnetii.* In Kirkbride CA, editor: *Laboratory diagnosis of livestock abortion,* ed 3, Ames, IA, 1990, Iowa State University Press.

36. Padmore CL: Infectious diseases of goats, *Proceedings of the International Goat Producers Symposium,* Tallahassee, FL, 1990, Florida A & M University Press.

37. Kahler SC: *Brucella melitensis* infection discovered in cattle for first time, goats also infected, *J Am Vet Med Assoc* 216:648, 2000.

38. Nicoletti P: Brucellosis. In Howard JL, editor: *Current veterinary therapy food animal practice,* ed 3, Philadelphia, 1993, WB Saunders.

39. Leon-Vizcaino L, Hermoso de Mendoza M, Garrido F: Incidence of abortions caused by leptospirosis in sheep and goats in Spain, *Comp Immun Microbiol Infect Dis* 10:149, 1987.

40. Dubey JP: Transplacental toxoplasmosis in goats. In Morrow DA, editor: *Current therapy in theriogenology,* ed 2, Philadelphia, 1986, WB Saunders.

41. Dubey JP: Toxoplasmosis in goats, *Agri-Pract* 8:43, 1987.

42. Dubey JP: Epizootic toxoplasmosis associated with abortion in dairy goats in Montana, *J Am Vet Med Assoc* 178:661, 1981.

43. Dubey JP: Toxoplasmosis, *J Am Vet Med Assoc* 205:1593, 1994.

44. Dubey JP et al: *Toxoplasma gondii*-induced abortion in dairy goats, *J Am Vet Med Assoc* 188:159, 1986.

45. Dubey JP: Diagnosis of livestock abortion due to *Toxoplasma gondii.* In Kirkbride CA, editor: *Laboratory diagnosis of livestock abortion,* ed 3, Ames, IA, 1990, Iowa State University Press.

46. Obendorf DL, Statham P, Munday BL: Resistance to *Toxoplasma* abortion in female goats previously exposed to *Toxoplasma* infection, *Aust Vet J* 67:233, 1990.

47. Dubey JP: Toxoplasmosis: zoonosis update, *J Am Vet Med Assoc* 196:123, 1990.

48. Antic S et al: Frequency of goat abortion and finding of *Listeria monocytogenes* as probable causative agent, *Vet Glas* 43:849, 1989.

49. Wiedmann M et al: Molecular investigation of a listeriosis outbreak in goats caused by an unusual strain of *Listeria monocytogenes, J Am Vet Med Assoc* 215:369, 1999.

50. Johnson GC et al: Epidemiologic evaluation of encephalitic listeriosis in goats, *J Am Vet Med Assoc* 208:1695, 1996.

51. East NE: Mycoplasmosis. In Morrow DA, editor: *Current therapy in theriogenology,* ed 2, Philadelphia, 1986, WB Saunders.

52. East NE: Common infectious conditions, *Small Ruminants for the Mixed Animal Practitioner Western Veterinary Conference,* 1998, Las Vegas, NV.

53. Braun WF: Pregnancy wastage in the goat, *American Association of Small Ruminant Practitioners, Proceedings of the Symposium on Health and Diseases of Small Ruminants,* 1997, Nashville, TN.

54. *Pioneer forage manual—a nutritional guide,* Des Moines, 1995, Pioneer Hi-Bred International.

Chapter 7

*D*iseases of the Endocrine System

DEBRA C. RUFFIN, UNDINE CHRISTMANN, AND D.G. PUGH

The endocrine system is rarely discussed as a separate entity in textbooks of sheep and goat medicine. This chapter presents current data, literary reviews, and available case reports regarding the endocrine systems of these two small ruminant species. It provides an overview of endocrine function and pathology to aid the clinician in treating some of the endocrinologic abnormalities of sheep and goats.

PITUITARY GLAND

Anterior Pituitary Gland

The anterior pituitary gland is located in the base of the skull in the sella turcica, which is the cavity of the sphenoid bone. It is composed of a variety of cell types: somatotrophs, which produce growth hormone (GH); mammotrophs, which produce prolactin (PRL); corticotrophs, which produce adrenocorticotropic hormone (ACTH); gonadotrophs, which produce luteinizing hormone (LH) and follicle-stimulating hormone (FSH); and thyrotrophs, which produce thyroid-stimulating hormone (TSH). Somatomammotrophs are unique cells that secrete both GH and PRL[1] in varying proportions depending on the action of other hormones such as cortisol and progesterone.[2] These cells have been identified in both sheep[3] and goats.[4] Hypothalamic hormones regulate (i.e., stimulate or inhibit) the release of hormones from the anterior pituitary cells (Table 7-1). Hormones from the hypothalamus are transported to the pituitary gland by the hypothalamic-pituitary portal circulation.

PRL is a hormone that stimulates udder development and subsequent lactation. Serum PRL levels fluctuate seasonally in photoperiodic seasonal breeders such as sheep and goats.[5,6] PRL levels are generally higher during the anestrous season of the year and lower during the breeding season.[6,7] In the Northern Hemisphere, PRL concentra-

tions are lowest from late October through late February (less than 39 ng/ml) and highest from May through September (200 to 350 ng/ml). Prolactin, unlike other pituitary hormones, is regulated primarily by hypothalamic inhibition.[7] Dopamine (prolactin-inhibitory hormone) inhibits the release of PRL from the anterior pituitary gland.[8]

GH is not only involved in the normal development of young animals but also influences milk and fiber production in adults. Administration of recombinant bovine somatotropin (rBST, a growth hormone) to lactating goats can increase milk yield,[9] as well as milk fat and lactose content.[10] Goats treated with rBST exhibit elevated serum levels of GH, insulin, thyroxine, and insulin-like growth factor-1. Studies have found that rBST significantly increases the secondary fiber growth rate and weight gain in goats.[11] However, in lactating does, no difference in fiber production was noted between animals treated with rBST and those that were not.[12] Still, the average daily gain of kids nursing from does given rBST was higher than the average daily gain of kids nursing from nontreated does.[12] This increased gain was seen only during the treatment period, and no posttreatment effect was reported. Sustained-release rBST has been shown to increase body weight gain by 22% in castrated male goats.[13]

Thyrotropin-releasing hormone (TRH), which is secreted by the hypothalamus, stimulates the thyrotrophs of the anterior pituitary to release TSH. TSH stimulates the production of triiodothyronine (T_3) and thyroxin from the thyroid gland. T_3 provides negative feedback to pituitary secretion of TSH. Therefore in the absence of adequate thyroid hormones, excessive TSH is released, resulting in enlargement in the thyroid gland (goiter).

Evaluation of anterior pituitary function. The literature contains very few reports of normal pituitary hor-

TABLE 7-1

HORMONES PRODUCED BY THE HYPOTHALMIC-PITUITARY AXIS

HYPOTHALMIC HORMONE	ACTION	PITUITARY CELL	PITUITARY HORMONE
Thyrotropin-releasing hormone (TRH)	Stimulatory	Thyrotroph Mammotroph	Thyroid-stimulating hormone (TSH) Prolactin (PRL)
Corticotropin-releasing hormone (CRH)	Stimulatory	Corticotroph	Adrenocorticotropic hormone (ACTH)
Growth hormone–releasing hormone (GHRH)	Stimulatory	Somatotroph Somatomammotroph	Growth hormone (GH)
Somatostatin	Inhibitory	Somatotroph Somatomammotroph	GH
Dopamine (prolactin-inhibiting hormone, PIH)	Inhibitory	Mammotroph Somatomammotroph	PRL
Prolactin-releasing hormone	Stimulatory	Mammotroph Somatomammotroph	PRL
Gonadotropin-releasing hormone (GnRH)	Stimulatory	Gonadotroph	Luteinizing hormone (LH) Follicle-stimulating hormone (FSH)

mone parameters in small ruminants. Lofstedt et al[14] performed an ACTH stimulation test in a normal and a lactating male. They found that within 10 minutes of the administration of porcine corticotropin hormone (80 IU intramuscularly [IM]), the blood cortisol rose to more than 120 nmol/L.[14] Blood cortisol levels in these two goats continued to rise throughout the 150-minute sampling period, reaching a maximum level of approximately 200 nmol/L and 280 nmol/L in the normal and lactating male goats, respectively.[14]

Little controlled research data are available regarding the use of the dexamethasone suppression test in sheep and goats. However, this test has been employed in the investigation of the endocrinologic status of a lactating male goat.[5] In one experiment dexamethasone (0.1 mg/kg IM) was administered and blood samples were then taken at hourly intervals for 10 hours. This dose suppressed cortisol to less than 30 nmol/L throughout the sampling period in both a normal male goat and a lactating male goat. The baseline cortisol level in the normal goat was reported to be between 40 and 70 nmol/L, whereas the baseline was 80 to 125 nmol/L in the lactating male goat with adrenal neoplasia. The authors of this chapter have administered the same dosage of dexamethasone in eight does and report suppressed cortisol output to very low levels (less than 14 nmol/L) for at least 8 hours. These eight does had baseline cortisol levels ranging from 36 to 257 nmol/L before the administration of the dexamethasone. Samples taken 12 to 13 hours after the dexamethasone injection tended to be erratic, but samples taken 24 hours after injection were significantly suppressed in seven of the eight does (Figure 7-1).

Posterior Pituitary Gland

The posterior pituitary gland (also known as the *neurohypophysis*) is an extension of the hypothalamus. Neuronal cell bodies within the supraoptic and paraventricular nuclei of the hypothalamus manufacture antidiuretic hormone (ADH) and oxytocin, which are transported along neurons to the posterior pituitary for storage and secretion.[7]

ADH regulates water and sodium balance in the body. Secretion of ADH in the dehydrated animal is stimulated by both the increased plasma osmolality and the decreased plasma volume. Either of these conditions alone also can stimulate ADH secretion. ADH is a vital component in effective recovery from hemorrhage-induced hypovolemia.[15,16] ADH increases plasma volume, enhances the permeability of the kidneys' collection ducts to water, and improves sodium chloride transport in Henle's loop. Without ADH, the animal cannot concentrate its urine and develops diabetes insipidus. An animal with this disease produces very dilute urine with no evidence of glucosuria. Naturally occurring diabetes insipidus is so rare in sheep and goats that the authors could find no reports in the scientific literature. However, the authors have noted many anecdotal reports of psychogenic polydipsia in sheep and goats. Polydipsia results in polyuria and could easily be confused with diabetes insipidus. Diabetes insipidus has been experimentally produced in goats by the creation of lesions in the median eminence of the hypothalamus.[16]

Oxytocin released from the posterior pituitary gland stimulates contraction of the myometrium myoepithelial cells of the mammary gland. Stimulation of the mammary

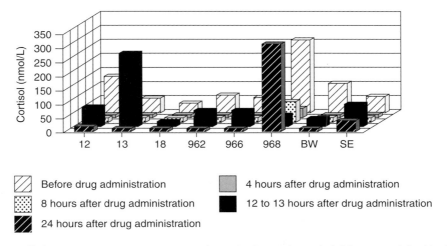

Figure 7-1   Dexamethasone suppression test (0.1 mg/kg dexamethasone) of eight apparently healthy does.

gland by the neonate or by milking causes afferent nerve impulses to be carried to the hypothalamus by the spinal cord. These impulses stimulate the supraoptic and paraventricular nuclei to release oxytocin from the posterior pituitary gland. Oxytocin is responsible for milk ejection or "letdown." The release of oxytocin from the pituitary each time the neonate nurses stimulates myometrial contractions that aid postpartal uterine involution. Exogenous oxytocin may be useful for the treatment of retained fetal membranes, metritis, and some other uterine diseases (see Chapter 6).

Pituitary Gland Tumors

Pituitary gland tumors are rare in sheep and goats. However, acidophilic adenomas of the anterior pituitary gland have been reported in both sheep and goats.[17,18] The pituitary lesions reported in does consist of distinct nodules of acidophil-type cells that compress adjacent pituitary tissue. Pituitary adenomas in ewes protrude dorsally into the optic chiasm and erode the sella turcica ventrally.[18] In most of these cases, animals have inappropriate lactation. Similar acidophilic adenomas have been reported in other species in association with abnormal mammary development.[19] Acidophil-type cells produce GH and PRL, both of which are lactogenic.[1] Anterior pituitary adenoma should be considered as a differential diagnosis for does with inappropriate lactation syndrome (ILS). However, no definitive antemortem diagnostic test is currently available for this condition. Several other pathologies have been reported in does with ILS. Two does with ILS described by Miller et al[17] also had concurrent pheochromocytoma and cystic endometrial hyperplasia. Furthermore, one of them had thyroid hyperplasia and follicular ovarian cysts.[17]

THYROID GLAND

The thyroid is a bilobed gland that lies just behind the larynx and lateral to the trachea. It is partially imbedded in the thymus in young animals. The lobes are connected by an isthmus. By iodinating tyrosine-containing compounds, the thyroid gland is responsible for manufacturing thyroxine (T_4) and T_3. These two hormones are produced by, stored in, and released by the thyroid gland in response to the anterior pituitary hormone TSH. Both T_3 and T_4 help moderate the animal's metabolic rate.

Thyroid Enlargement

Pathogenesis.   The most common causes of enlargement of the thyroid gland (goiter) are deficient iodine intake and the consumption of plants containing goitrogens.[20-22] Thyroid enlargement appears to be associated with increased TSH output by the anterior pituitary resulting from depressed blood T_4 and T_3 concentrations. Iodine deficiency–induced goiter is more common in neonates and has a worldwide distribution. Iodine-deficient soils result from rain-induced leaching. Iodine is absorbed in the small intestine, and any feedstuffs high in nitrates or other minerals decrease its absorption.[22] Because of the widespread use of iodine supplementation in trace mineral salt mixtures, the incidence of goiter caused by frank iodine deficiency is rare. Still, when treating animals that graze plants grown on sandy soils, iodine-deficient soils, or heavily fertilized soils, the clinician should be aware that iodine deficiency is a potential problem. Compared with other breeds polled Dorset sheep and Boer and Angora goats appear to be more susceptible to iodine deficiency–induced hypothyroidism.[20,21]

Neonatal hypothyroidism (cretinism) has been described in Angora goats.[23] Adequate levels of selenium are needed for proper functioning of thyroid hormones in peripheral tissue. Therefore if selenium is chronically deficient, decreased production ("ain't doing right") may ensue but not be the result of primary thyroid dysfunction. Goitrogenic compounds (e.g., thiourea, thiouracil) can decrease iodine uptake by the thyroid gland and decrease the iodination of tyrosine in the metabolic pathway for thyroxine production. Ruminants that ingest plants in the *Brassica* family may exhibit depressed iodine absorption and metabolism because of the thiocyanates in these plants. The most common plants that produce antithyroid compounds include the mustard family (e.g., kale, rape), the legume family (e.g., peanuts, soybeans, white clover), the prune family (e.g., cherries, apricots), and some grains (e.g., sorghum).

Hereditary, congenital goiter has been described in Merino sheep and in Dutch, pygmy, and Nubian goats.[24-28] The congenital thyroid goiters studied by Dutch researchers[27] originated from mixed strains of Saanen and dwarf goats. Goiter in Dutch goats was found to be inherited in an autosomal recessive manner. Early investigation of the disease indicated it was most likely caused by defective thyroglobulin synthesis,[28] which had previously been described in sheep.[25-27] Thyroglobulin is the iodoprotein necessary for thyroid hormone synthesis.

Clinical signs. Signs of hypothyroidism include goiter, poor quality and quantity of wool or hair, dry skin, tendon laxity or failure to form normal insertions in bone, and poor reproductive ability (depressed libido, poor semen quality, irregular estrus, depressed conception, abortion, and delivery of weak or dead fetuses; fetal hydrops, poor growth rates, and depressed milk production also may be seen). Kids born to dams with iodine-deficient diets or those that consume goitrogenic plants may be weak and woolless or hairless, have enlarged thyroid glands (swollen necks), and may show signs of respiratory difficulty. Lambs born to iodine-deficient ewes may exhibit an impaired development of wool-producing follicles. All animals can be affected, but signs of hypothyroidism are more common in young and growing lambs or kids, geriatric animals, and ewes and does in heavy production. In one study, eight Angora kids from 298 does showed signs of retarded growth, shortened heads, droopy eyelids, dullness, weight gain, and prognathism.[23] Bilateral goiter was easily palpable in all cases. These cases were thought to be caused by ingestion of thiocyanate precursors from highly fertilized forage.[23]

Goats with heritable, large, goitrous thyroid glands are born with a rough, sparse hair coat, thickened skin, retarded growth, and sluggish behavior[29]; they respond poorly or not at all to supplemental iodine. Gestation length in affected does may be increased to 153 days (with a range of 148 to 158 days).[30] Figure 7-2 shows a congenital goiter in a 1-week-old cross-bred goat. Heritable goiters are probably overdiagnosed because some

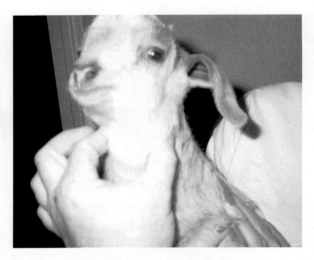

Figure 7-2 Congenital goiter in a 1-week-old cross-bred meat goat. The 4.5-cm swelling in the left thyroid gland was not associated with any signs of clinical disease. This goiter was noticed by the goat's owner at birth.

newborns have large thymus glands that can be mistaken for the thyroid.[31]

Diagnosis. Diagnosis of thyroid disease in sheep and goats is based on the following findings: a swollen thyroid gland, stunted growth, weight loss or obesity, subcutaneous edema, and rough and matted fleece. Blood analysis of affected animals may indicate decreased plasma protein-bound iodine and increased plasma protein, serum triglyceride, cholesterol, and phospholipid.[32] Iodine concentrations in serum, plasma, and milk and thyroxin concentrations in serum and plasma are usually depressed. Normal serum thyroxine levels for goats have been reported to be between 5.0 and 7.0 μg/dl[23] and between 6.1 and 8.3 μg/dl.[33] Normal serum iodine levels range from 2.1 to 9.3 μg/dl.[29,33] Smith[21] reported a doubling of serum thyroxine 4 hours after the administration of thyrotrophin (5 IU intravenously [IV]). The level and stage of production (meat, fiber, milk) affects blood thyroxine concentrations; thyroxine levels in does may drop by as much as 30% between the prepartal period and 1 week after birth.[34] Thyroid function in Angora goats has been shown to fluctuate with no apparent relation to the season.[35] Serum lipid concentration in goats is affected by thyroid status.[23,36] Triglyceride, phospholipid, and cholesterol levels steadily fall in a dose-dependent manner when animals are treated with T_3. Elevated serum cholesterol (higher than 7.0 mmol/L) has been reported in goats with congenital hypothyroidism.[23] A thyroid gland–to–body weight ratio greater than 0.46:1 has been associated with goiter caused by iodine deficiency.[37]

Treatment and prevention. Affected young can be treated with Lugol's iodine (3 to 5 drops) in the milk or can be given potassium iodine (20 mg) orally.[31]

Pregnant does and ewes in their final trimester should have free access to a trace mineral salt supplement containing iodine; this supplement should be the only source of salt. Iodized salt containing 0.007% to 0.01% iodine,[31] preferably in the iodate form, is usually protective against goiter. In deficient areas the form of iodine used in the mineral supplement is important. Iodine in the iodide form is less available than that in the iodate form.[22] Trace mineral salt intake may be depressed by many factors. Because the drive or desire to consume trace mineral salt is based on a craving for sodium, if other sources of dietary sodium are available (e.g., commercially prepared feeds, free choice sodium bicarbonate) or the "salt carrier" for the iodine has additives rendering it unpalatable (e.g., dicalcium phosphate, magnesium oxide), a less than optimal intake will occur. If this scenario is further complicated by the increased demands of pregnancy compelling ewes and does to consume more than normal amounts of nitrate-containing feeds or goitrogenic feeds (e.g., cabbage, kale, peanuts, rape, soybeans, sorghum, turnips), iodine deficiency–induced goiter and thyroid dysfunction may occur in their offspring. Therefore, when any or all of these situations occur, it is imperative to ensure adequate intake through individual iodine supplementation, painting adult animals with iodine (Lugol's iodine 2 ml weekly), or drenching with potassium iodine (200 to 300 mg by mouth [PO] once during late gestation).[31] Of course, iodine toxicity should be avoided. Culling, neutering, and removing parents should be considered to decrease the herd incidence of the heritable forms of goiter.

PARATHYROID GLAND

Parathyroid hormone (PTH) is a polypeptide hormone produced by the parathyroid glands and released in response to low serum ionized calcium. PTH interacts with osteoblasts, stimulating cytokine release, which in turn activates osteoclasts. Bone resorption by the osteoclasts releases calcium and phosphorus from bone into the blood. The number of functioning osteoclasts increases in response to PTH, which also acts on the distal renal tubules to increase calcium resorption and phosphorus excretion. Additionally, PTH increases the conversion of vitamin D to the active form, 1,25-dihydroxycholecalciferol, which increases calcium and phosphorus absorption from the intestine. PTH also has been shown to increase absorption of calcium and phosphorus from the forestomachs of sheep.[38]

Another closely related hormone is parathyroid hormone–related peptide (PTHrP). PTHrP acts similarly to PTH, with the exception that it decreases the serum level of 1,25-dihydroxycholecalciferol. It is produced by some neoplasms and is one of the causes of hypercalcemia (pseudohyperparathyroidism) associated with malignancy. PTHrP also is found in many normal adult and fetal tissues[39] and may act locally to influence the growth and development of some cells. It has been shown to increase placental calcium transport in sheep,[40] and it increases mammary blood flow in sheep[41] and goats.[42] High levels of the hormone are secreted into milk and have been detected in venous blood in the lactating goat, as well as in the hepatic portal venous plasma of suckling kids.[43] The more often the mammary gland is milked, the greater the concentration of this hormone in milk.[44] PTHrP may even play a role in ILS.

At least one study has demonstrated that diets rich in phosphorus (one to three times the daily requirement) have no adverse effect on bone mineralization in lambs as long as the minimum calcium requirement is met.[45] Low dietary phosphorus produces significant hypophosphatemia with corresponding hypercalcemia in both sheep and goats.[46,47] Still, the authors recommend a dietary calcium-to-phosphorus ratio of between 1:1 and 2:1. Primary hyperparathyroidism or hypoparathyroidism is rare, but nutritional secondary hyperparathyroidism is occasionally encountered.

Nutritional Secondary Hyperparathyroidism

Pathogenesis. Secondary nutritional hyperparathyroidism occurs when animals are fed a high-grain diet that is low in calcium and high in phosphorus. Such a diet decreases blood pH and increases blood concentrations of PTH. Hyperphosphatemia resulting from excessive phosphorus intake lowers blood calcium levels. This results in bone calcium mobilization. Chronic mobilization of calcium from bone leads to osteoporosis and replacement of reabsorbed calcium with fibrous connective tissue (osteodystrophia fibrosa). Excessive consumption of oxalate-containing plants (see Chapter 10) can decrease calcium absorption. Consumption of such a diet coupled with excessive cereal grain feeding can result in nutritional secondary hyperparathyroidism. Young and growing animals are more likely to succumb than adults.

Clinical signs. The disease is characterized by intermittent shifting leg lameness, loose teeth, pathologic fractures, and enlargement of the bones of the skull.

Diagnosis. The diagnosis is based on radiographic evidence of demineralization, increased urinary fractional excretion of phosphorus (see Chapter 10), and dietary mineral analysis. Early in the course of the disease hyperphosphatemia and hypocalcemia are seen. As the condition progresses, serum levels of calcium and phosphorus usually remain within normal limits. Serum alkaline phosphatase (SAP) may be normal, high normal, or high.

The effects of diet-induced changes in blood pH on mineral retention have been studied in lambs.[48] A diet supplemented with excessive ammonium chloride produces a mild metabolic acidosis and significantly higher plasma PTH levels than does a diet supplemented with sodium bicarbonate.[48] The amounts of calcium and phosphorus absorbed from the intestine were similar for each diet, but osteoclastic activity increased in animals consuming the acid diet. Although the plasma levels of the two minerals were not significantly altered by the diet, the retention of both calcium and phosphorus was lower in the animals consuming the acid diet because of increased urinary excretion of both minerals.[48] Ammonium chloride is rarely fed at a rate greater than 0.25% to 0.3% of the diet. However, demineralization of bone is a potential problem with long-term (years) feeding of ammonium chloride to pet goats. Although an acid diet is detrimental for growing animals, it can be helpful for animals at risk of periparturient hypocalcemia.

Treatment and prevention. Maintaining an adequate calcium-to-phosphorus ratio (1:1 to 2:1) is important in prevention, as is not feeding excessive amounts of cereal grains or oxalate-containing plants. Providing a mineral salt mixture for free choice consumption is always beneficial. Providing a mixture of equal parts trace mineral salt and dicalcium phosphate usually suffices for animals grazing grass pastures (see Chapters 2 and 9).

ADRENAL GLANDS

The adrenal glands are two small (2 to 4 cm × 1 to 2 cm) hormone-producing glands found near the kidneys. These glands function in sheep and goats as they do in other species. The cortex produces cortisol, aldosterone, and other steroid hormones, while the medulla secretes epinephrine, norepinephrine, and other vasoactive amines.

Necropsy of 2500 goats (80% of which were Angora) older than 5 years of age revealed that 314 of 2104 castrated males and 2 of 208 females had adrenal adenomas. No adrenal adenomas were diagnosed in the 188 intact males in this study.[49] The authors of the study theorized that testosterone inhibits the pituitary gonadotropins that mediate adrenal proliferation, as had been previously shown in laboratory rodents.[49] Adrenal cortical neoplasia has been described in a castrated male goat that was lactating.[14] Endocrine parameters in this goat consisted of elevated levels of estradiol 17β, GH, PRL, cortisol, and insulin-like growth factor-1. The elevation in the pituitary hormone levels was most likely caused by the lack of negative feedback by testosterone, whereas the elevation in cortisol levels occurred secondary to pituitary stimulation. The elevated estradiol 17β was thought be caused by the adrenal neoplasia.[14]

Pheochromocytomas have been reported in two does with aberrant or inappropriate lactation[17] and also from a family of does in Finland.[50] The association between ILS and pheochromocytoma has not yet been determined. The Finnish does examined at necropsy had histories of sudden nervous attacks. Gritz[50] reported that the pheochromocytomas in these does were histologically similar to those found in other species. Ultrastructural features corresponded with the classical descriptions of secretory granules in the adrenal medullas of other species. Both norepinephrine and epinephrine granules were found within the same cells.[50] Two of the does in this report had coincidental thyroid gland enlargement as previously described in association with pheochromocytoma in bulls[51] and does.[17]

Adrenal cortical hypertrophy and elevated plasma corticosteroids have been reported in animals that were maintained on a diet deficient in cobalt and vitamin B_{12}.[52] The animals in this study had plasma cortisol levels three to five times higher than normal (2 to 3 ng/ml). These investigators asserted that the effect of vitamin B_{12} deficiency was remarkably similar to the effects of chronic malnutrition in other species.[52]

A habitual abortion syndrome described in Angora goats appears to be associated with hypoadrenocorticism. Some Angora does have an impaired ability to respond to stress during gestation. This impairment grows worse as gestation progresses. The affected females may have small adrenal glands and decreased plasma cortisol levels.[53] This heritable hypoadrenocorticism most likely has genetic linkage to fine mohair production. Stress (e.g., nutritional, climatic, physical) may result in abortion.[54] Most abortions occur between day 90 and 110 of gestation. Because of the dam's inability to respond to stress, the fetus develops adrenal hyperplasia. This results in increased fetal cortisol output and thereby prematurely induces the parturition cascade. Aborted fetuses are typically dysmature and anemic and have adrenocortical hyperplasia.[53,54]

PANCREAS

The pancreas of sheep and goats functions similarly to that of other ruminant animals. This bilobed gland is located in the craniodorsal abdomen and attached to the descending duodenum. The pancreas has both exocrine functions (production and release of digestive enzymes) and endocrine functions (production and release of insulin and glucagon). Diabetes mellitus (DM) has been described as any condition in which there is a permanent elevation of blood glucose and glucosuria. Primary DM involves beta-cell damage (insulin-producing cells) followed by decreased insulin levels and hyperglycemia. Secondary DM results from a resistance to the effect of insulin even with normal or elevated plasma insulin levels. DM is rare in goats. Only one case report of spontaneous DM could be found in the scientific literature.[55] Other case reports describe the features of experimentally induced DM by administration of alloxan[56] or streptozocin.[57]

Clinical signs of diabetes in goats include weight loss, poor appetite, and lethargy.[56] Polyuria and polydipsia are invariable findings, with some animals exhibiting two to three times their normal water intake. A 90% decrease in milk production has been observed in lactating goats with experimentally induced DM. Insulin treatment has been tried in both spontaneous and experimental DM. In general a response to treatment is observed within 4 days and results in a partial relief of clinical signs and normalization of laboratory values.[55,56] However, improper insulin dosage can result in life-threatening hypoglycemia. Recurrence of clinical signs is observed with discontinuation of therapy.

ABERRANT LACTATION, GALACTORRHEA, PRECOCIOUS UDDER (INAPPROPRIATE LACTATION SYNDROME)

Although only a few cases of ILS in goats are described in the scientific literature, the anecdotal reports of this problem are seemingly endless. ILS has been reported in both castrated and intact males, as well as in female goats.[14,17,58,59] It is, however, more common in females than males. Rare in ewes, it appears to be more of a clinical concern in pet does. Does with ILS usually have an enlarged udder with no history of being bred. A thorough history, including assessment of possible exposure to a male and investigation regarding whether the doe is being nursed or milked, should be taken. Results of a routine physical examination are generally within normal limits. The udder may be slightly enlarged or so large that the animal has difficulty walking and is in danger of secondary orthopedic disease (Figure 7-3). The udder is usually soft, non-inflamed, and non-painful to palpation. The initial examination of these animals should rule out impending parturition through the use of ballottement, palpation, or real-time ultrasonography. After pregnancy and "milk removal" have been ruled out as causes of lactation, a more comprehensive examination should follow. Examination of mammary secretions usually reveals a substance that appears to be milk. However, a thinner, more translucent to clear fluid also may be found. The expression of milk is generally difficult during the initial examination because of plugged teat orifices. If the teats are plugged and milk is not easily expressed, the animal is probably not being nursed or milked. The mammary secretions from does with ILS may look like milk on the first milking but later change to a straw-colored fluid with continued or intermittent milking. However, continued milking of these animals may stimulate milk production in some does, and a normal lactation may ensue. The authors of this chapter have noted a mild familial association with ILS.

It is a common presumption that milk removal is necessary to sustain lactation. Without milk removal, intraudder pressure should develop and inhibit milk secre-

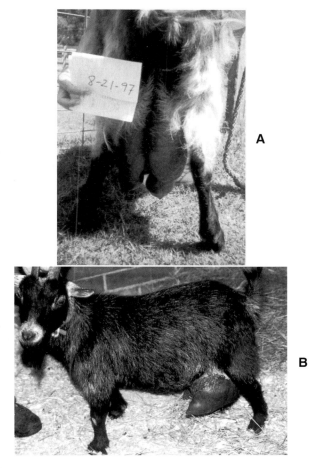

Figure 7-3   Udders of two does with inappropriate lactation. **A,** A 4-year-old Spanish crossed goat that had given birth to a single kid 3 years previously. **B,** An aged pygmy goat that had been displaying ILS for several years.

tion. Although many does are not being nursed, milk remains in the teat cistern. The teat cisterns of these does are often abnormally large ("bottle teats"), either as a result of prolonged filling or because the enlarged cistern prevents the needed back-pressure from occurring. Bruckmaier et al[60] described two different patterns of milk ejection during machine milking of goats: one with a sharp peak and the other with a prolonged plateau. Does with prolonged plateaus had larger teat cisterns than does producing sharp-peaked ejection patterns. The larger teat cisterns seem to have a permissive effect on lactation. Perhaps a bottle teat is so expandable that adequate back-pressure cannot be established. Another possibility is that abnormal apoptosis of mammary gland cells may occur in the udders of these does in response to back-pressure.

Pseudopregnancy is one possible cause of ILS (see Chapter 6). Most practitioners recommend treating these does with luteolytic hormones (prostaglandin $F_{2\alpha}$ [$PGF_{2\alpha}$] 10 mg IM) after pregnancy has been ruled out. Although this does not usually result in a cure, it can and should be used to rule out pseudopregnancy. The authors have not evaluated the fertility of females with ILS because most are older animals that are kept as pets. However, their fertility is most likely impaired by the vast array of endocrinologic and reproductive organ abnormalities (e.g., pituitary adenomas, adrenal pheochromocytomas, cystic ovaries, cystic endometrial hyperplasia) that have been reported in goats with ILS.[14,17]

A complete history of dietary intake should be performed in all cases of ILS. Possible grazing of estrogenic forage such as legumes (e.g., clover) or grains infected with _Fusarium roseum_ should be investigated. _F. roseum_ produces the mycotoxin zearalenone, which has the physiologic effect of estrogen. Evaluation of the diet also may be of value because adrenal hypertrophy and elevated plasma cortisol levels have been reported with malnutrition and certain B vitamin deficiencies. Parenteral vitamin B_{12} supplementation or the addition of cobalt to the diet may be beneficial if the diet is found to be inadequate or marginal.

Although most references to ILS in the literature suggest that PRL levels in these animals are elevated,[17,58] this may not always be the case. The authors have measured serum PRL in four does with ILS and found that all had low serum PRL. Two of these measurements were taken in the winter months, when PRL is ordinarily low (less than 39 ng/ml). LeProvost et al[61] described the presence of PRL mitochondrial ribonucleic acid (mRNA) in the mammary glands of lactating sheep and goats, thus demonstrating that de novo synthesis of PRL is the likely cause of elevated milk PRL levels during the periparturient period in normal ruminants. Local PRL production may play a role in the establishment of ILS in goats.

PTHrP also may be involved with this syndrome. Thompson et al[44] demonstrated that removing milk from one mammary gland of a normal doe in late gestation resulted in an increase in PTHrP from the milked gland. These researchers also demonstrated that the more often milk was removed from a single gland, the higher the milk concentration of PTHrP.[44] When milking was discontinued in the single gland, PTHrP levels declined,[44] indicating that PTHrP has a local (autocrine) lactogenic role in the goat. Goats with tumors may have elevated levels of PTHrP that could theoretically stimulate lactation. If this is the case, hypercalcemia of malignancy should also be expected.

Bromocriptine mesylate, a dopamine agonist, has been suggested as a treatment for does with inappropriate lactation. It should inhibit PRL release by the anterior pituitary gland. However, successful use of this drug to stop inappropriate lactation has not been reported. Failure of response to bromocriptine mesylate can be anticipated for a number of reasons:

1. Some of the does with inappropriate lactation may already have low serum PRL (especially if the condition occurs in winter, when PRL is normally low).[6]
2. Normal does treated with PRL for 4 days before and 4 days after parturition showed prolonged suppression of PRL but resumed lactation within 10 days and produced 32% higher milk yields than the previous year.[62]
3. Local production of PRL by the mammary gland could be maintaining the inappropriate lactation and would most likely be unaffected by bromocriptine therapy.[61]
4. Other hormones such as PTHrP may be playing a role.
5. A defect in normal mammary gland involution may be present in these animals.

Pituitary adenomas (which can be PRL-secreting tumors in other species) have been reported in two does with ILS.[17] The authors have examined the pituitary glands of normal does and a doe with ILS (Figure 7-4). The pituitary gland of the doe with inappropriate lactation (Figure 7-4, _B_) is larger and protrudes further dorsally than the pituitary gland in the normal doe (Figure 7-4, _A_).

Spontaneous lactation of does also has been reported in association with ovarian abnormalities. DeWalque[63] described a doe with a granulosa cell tumor that exhibited virilism concurrent with inappropriate lactation. Lofstedt

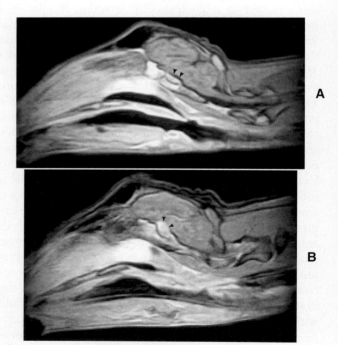

Figure 7-4 Midsagittal, T1-weighted, post-contrast magnetic resonance imaging (MRI) of the brain of a normal female goat **(A)** and a female with ILS **(B)**. The contrast-enhanced area shows that the pituitary gland _(arrows)_ of the female with ILS is enlarged compared with that of the normal doe, extending dorsally to the dorsal extent of the pituitary fossa. (Courtesy John Hathcock, Auburn, Alabama.)

and Williams have reported udder engorgement in a doe 6 days after removal of a granulosa cell tumor.[58] The authors of this chapter also have seen masculine behavior and granulosa cell tumors in a doe (Figure 7-5) with a history of ILS (1-year duration) and mastectomy (2.5 years before the onset of masculine behavior). In addition, one of the does with ILS described by Miller et al[17] had ovarian follicular cysts. Does with granulosa cell tumors have elevated serum levels of testosterone and estradiol and variable serum levels of progesterone. These does often exhibit virilism and abnormal estrus cycles.

The current treatment of choice for inappropriate lactation in pet goats is mastectomy (see Chapter 13). Although this obviously stops outward clinical signs, an underlying problem may remain. Therefore these does should be closely monitored throughout their lives for other conditions that have been reported to occur concurrent with inappropriate lactation. These include endometrial hyperplasia and uterine fluid retention (which could predispose these does to pyometra, endometritis, or acute septic metritis), pituitary adenomas, pheochromocytoma (which may present clinically as nervousness and abnormal behavior), and ovarian granulosa cell tumor (which may present as virilism). Although the fertility of many of these does is limited, they should nevertheless not be allowed any exposure to a buck after mastectomy. Not only is a lack of milk for the offspring a problem, but also the loss of mammary tissue in goats has been associated with an increased incidence of periparturient complications in goats, most likely because of the absence of hormones such as estradiol-17β that are normally produced by the mammary gland during the final few days of gestation. These reported complications include premature labor, prolonged onset of labor, lack of cervical dilatation, and maternal death at parturition.[64] The authors have observed prolonged labor and poor cervical dilatation in a female that had a mastectomy and was then inappropriately bred.

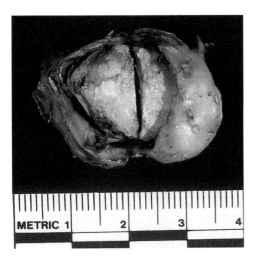

Figure 7-5 A granulosa cell tumor that was removed from an approximately 7-year-old Spanish crossed female goat. She had a history of ILS for 2 to 3 years before displaying virilism.

REFERENCES

1. Frawley LS, Boockfor FR: Mammosomatotropes: presence and functions in normal and neoplastic pituitary tissue, *Endocrine Rev* 12(4):337, 1991.
2. Kineman RD et al: Steroids can modulate transdifferentiation of prolactin and growth hormone cells in bovine pituitary cultures, *Endocrinol* 130(6):3289, 1992.
3. Thorpe JR, Ray KP, Wallis M: Occurrence of rare somatomammotrophs in ovine anterior pituitary tissue studied by immunogold labeling and electron microscopy, *J Endocrin* 124:67, 1990.
4. Sanchez J et al: Identification of somatomammotroph cells in lactating goats *(Capra hircus)* by fluorescence and immunogold techniques, *Acta Anatomica* 149(1):39, 1994.
5. Prandi A et al: Circannual rhythm of plasma prolactin concentration in the goat, *Anim Repro Sci* 17:85, 1988.
6. Walton JS et al: Changes in concentrations of follicle stimulating hormone, luteinizing hormone, prolactin and progesterone in the plasma of ewes during the transition from anestrus to breeding activity, *J Endocrin* 75:127, 1977.
7. Goodman HM: Hormonal control of reproduction in the female II. Pregnancy and lactation. In Ganong WF, editor: *Basic medical endocrinology,* ed 2, New York, 1994, Raven Press.
8. Thomsett MG et al: Hormone ontogeny in the ovine fetus VIII. The effect of thyrotrophin-releasing factor on prolactin and growth hormone release in the fetus and neonate, *Endocrinol* 106(4):1074, 1980.
9. Faulkner A: Changes in plasma and milk concentration of glucose and IGF-1 in response to exogenous growth hormone in lactating goats, *J Dairy Res* 66(2):207, 1999.
10. Chadio SE et al: Effects of recombinant bovine somatotropin administration to lactating goats, *Sm Rumin Res* 35(3):263, 2000.
11. Villar D et al: The effects of bovine somatotropin on hair follicle activity and cashmere fibre growth in goats, *Aust J Agri Res* 50(8):1365, 1999.
12. Davis J et al: The effect of bovine somatotropin treatment on production of lactating Angora does with kids, *J Anim Sci* 77(1):17, 1999.
13. Skarda J: Effect of bovine growth hormone on growth, organ weights, tissue composition and adipose tissue metabolism in young castrated male goats, *Livestock Prod Sci* 55(3):215, 1998.
14. Lofstedt RM, Laarveld B, Ihle SL: Adrenal neoplasia causing lactation in a castrated male goat, *J Vet Intern Med* 8(5):382, 1994.
15. Goodman HM: Pituitary gland. In Ganong WF, editor: *Basic medical endocrinology,* ed 2, New York, 1994, Raven Press.
16. Rundgren M et al: Effects of hemorrhage on vasopressin secretion and arterial blood pressure during experimental diabetes insipidus in goats, *Acta Physiol Scand* 116:57, 1982.
17. Miller CC et al: Lactation associated with acidophilic pituitary adenoma, pheochromocytoma, and cystic endometrial hyperplasia in two goats, *J Am Vet Med Assoc* 210(3):378, 1997.
18. Olson DP, Ohlson DL, Davis SL: Acidophil adenoma in the pituitary gland of a sheep, *Vet Path* 18:132, 1981.
19. Lipman NS et al: Prolactin-secreting pituitary adenomas with mammary dysplasia in New Zealand white rabbits, *Lab Anim Sci* 44(2):114, 1994.

20. Menzies PI, Miller R: Abortion in sheep: diagnosis and control. In Youngquist RS, editor: *Current therapy in large animal theriogenology,* Philadelphia, 1997, WB Saunders.

21. Smith MC, Sherman DM: *Goat medicine,* Philadelphia, 1994, Lea and Febiger.

22. Smart ME, Cymbaluk NF: Trace minerals. In Naylor JM, Ralston SL, editors: *Large animal clinical nutrition,* St Louis, 1991, Mosby.

23. Bath GF, Wentzel D, Van Tonder EM: Cretinism in angora goats, *J South African Vet Assoc* 5(4):237, 1979.

24. Falconer IR: Biochemical defect causing congenital goitre in sheep, *Nature* 205:978, 1965.

25. Falconer IR: Studies of the congenitally goitrous sheep. Composition and metabolism of goitrous thyroid tissue, *Biochem J* 100:197, 1966.

26. Rac R et al: Congenital goiter in Merino sheep due to an inherited defect in the biosynthesis of thyroid hormone, *Res Vet Sci* 9:209, 1968.

27. Dolling CE, Good BF: Congenital goitre in sheep: isolation of the iodoproteins which replace thyroglobulin, *J Endocrin* 71:179, 1976.

28. De Vijlder JJM et al: Hereditary congenital goiter with thyroglobulin deficiency in a breed of goats, *Endocrinol* 103:2105, 1978.

29. Rijnberk A et al: Congenital defect in iodothyronine synthesis. Clinical aspects of iodine metabolism in goats with congenital goitre and hypothyroidism, *Brit Vet J* 133(5):495, 1977.

30. Piosik PA et al: Effect of maternal thyroid status on thyroid hormones and growth in congenitally hypothyroid goat fetuses during the second half of gestation, *Endocrinol* 138(1):5, 1997.

31. Bretzlaff K, Haenlein G, Huston E: Common nutritional problems feeding the sick goat. In Naylor JM, Ralston SL, editors: *Large animal clinical nutrition,* St Louis, 1991, Mosby.

32. Sreekumaran T, Rajan A: Clinicopathological studies in experimental hypothyroidism in goats, *Vet Path* 15:549, 1978.

33. Reap M, Cass C, Hightower D: Thyroxine and triiodothyronine levels in 10 species of animals, *Southwestern Vet* 31:31, 1978.

34. Emre Z, Garmo G: Plasma thyroxine through parturition and early lactation in goats fed silage of grass and rape, *Acta Vet Scand* 26:417, 1985.

35. Wentzel D, Viljoen KS, Botha LJJ: Seasonal variation in adrenal and thyroid function of Angora goats, *Agroanimalia* 11:1, 1979.

36. Ibrahim RE et al: The effect of altered thyroid status on lipid metabolism in Nubian goats, *Compar Biochem Physiol* 77B(3):507, 1984.

37. Sargison ND, West DM, Clark RG: An investigation of the possible effects of subclinical iodine deficiency or ewe fertility and perinatal lamb mortality, *New Zealand Vet J* 5:208, 1997.

38. Dua K et al: Effects of parathyroid hormone and parathyroid hormone-related protein on the rates of absorption of magnesium, calcium, sodium, potassium and phosphate ions from the reticulo-rumen in sheep, *Exper Physiol* 79(3):401, 1994.

39. Ratcliffe WA: Parathyroid hormone-related protein: a polyhormonal enigma, *Equine Vet J* 29(3):174, 1997.

40. Care AD et al: Stimulation of ovine placental transport of calcium and magnesium by mid-molecule fragments of human parathyroid hormone-related protein, *Exper Physiol* 75:605, 1990.

41. Thompson GE: Parathyroid hormone-related protein and mammary blood flow in sheep, *Exper Physiol* 78(4):499, 1993.

42. Prosser CG, Farr VC, Davis SR: Increased mammary blood flow in the lactating goat induced by parathyroid hormone-related protein, *Exper Physiol* 79(4):565, 1994.

43. Ratcliffe WA et al: Production of parathyroid hormone-related protein by the mammary gland of the goat, *J Endocrin* 133:87, 1992.

44. Thompson GE et al: Local control of parathyroid hormone-related protein secretion by the mammary gland of the goat, *J Pharm Med* 4(1):485, 1994.

45. Wan Zahari M et al: The effect of high phosphorus intake on calcium and phosphorus retention and bone turnover in growing lambs, *Exper Physiol* 79(2):175, 1994.

46. Breves G, Ross R, Holler H: Dietary phosphorus depletion in sheep: effects on plasma inorganic phosphorus, calcium, 1,25(OH)$_2$-Vit-D$_3$ and alkaline phosphatase and on gastrointestinal P and Ca balances, *J Agri Sci* 105:623, 1985.

47. Schroder B et al: Binding properties of goat intestinal vitamin D receptors as affected by dietary calcium and/or phosphorus depletion, *J Vet Med* 42:411, 1995.

48. Damir HA et al: The effects of feeding diets containing either NaHCO$_3$ or NH$_4$Cl on indices of bone formation and resorption and on mineral balance in the lamb, *Exper Physiol* 76:725, 1991.

49. Altman NG, Streett CS, Terner JY: Castration and its relationship to tumors of the adrenal gland in the goat, *Am J Vet Res* 30(4):583, 1969.

50. Gritz BG: Hereditary caprine pheochromocytomas, *J Vet Med Assoc* 44:313, 1997.

51. Wilke BN, Krook L: Ultimobranchial tumor of the thyroid and pheochromocytoma in the bull, *Path Vet* 7:126, 1970.

52. Mgongo FOK, Gombe S, Ogaa JS: Influence of cobalt/vitamin B$_{12}$ deficiency as a stressor affecting adrenal cortex and ovarian activities in goats, *Repro Nutr and Develop* 24(6):845, 1984.

53. Roberts SJ: *Veterinary obstetrics and genital disease (theriogenology),* ed 3, Woodstock, VT, 1986, David and Charles.

54. Basrur PK, Koykul W, Yusoff RBH: Genetic disorders of the goat. In Youngquist RS, editor: *Current therapy in large animal theriogenology,* Philadelphia, 1997, WB Saunders.

55. Lutz TA et al: Secondary diabetes mellitus in a pygmy goat, *Vet Rec* 135:93, 1994.

56. Nowak J, Dzialoszynski L: Effect of experimental alloxan diabetes on the secretion and composition of goat milk, *Acta Physiol Polonica* 18(4):488, 1967.

57. Stangassinger M, Peruche T, Giesecke D: Diabetes Mellitus bei Zwergziegen: Modellversuche mit Streptozocin, *Zentralblatt fur Veterinaria Medicine A* 29:297, 1982.

58. Lofstedt RM, Williams R: Granulosa cell tumor in a goat, *J Am Vet Med Assoc* 189(2):206, 1986.

59. Jassim RA, Khamas W: Gynaecomastia and galactorrhea in a goat buck, *Aust Vet J* 75(9):669, 1997.

60. Bruckmaier RM et al: Machine milking of dairy goats during lactation: udder anatomy, milking characteristics and blood concentrators of oxytocin and prolactin, *J Dairy Res* 61:457, 1994.

61. LeProvost F et al: Prolactin gene expression in ovine and caprine mammary gland, *Neuroendocrin* 60:305, 1994.

62. Forsyth IA, Lee PD: Bromocriptine treatment of periparturient goats: long term suppression of prolactin and lack of effect on lactation, *J Dairy Res* 60:307, 1993.

63. DeWalque J: Tumeur ovarienne et masculinization chez une chevre chamoisee des alpas, *Annales de Med Vet* 107:322, 1963.

64. Diamond JM: Mammary gland as an endocrine organ: implications for mastectomy, *Nature* 295:191, 1982.

Chapter 8

Diseases of the Integumentary System

DAVID E. ANDERSON, D. MICHAEL RINGS, AND D.G. PUGH

Disease conditions affecting the skin and hair of sheep and goats are common. These diseases result in significant economic losses to livestock producers because of poor growth, weight loss, and loss of fiber and leather products. Veterinarians often are consulted for diagnosis and treatment of these diseases but may become frustrated because of economic limitations imposed by owners. Therefore history, clinical signs, and physical examination are important in developing an accurate differential diagnosis. This chapter discusses specific diseases of the skin and hair of sheep and goats with emphasis on diagnosis and treatment strategies.

ANATOMY

The skin functions as a protective barrier to the environment. It also aids in thermoregulation, acts as a sensory organ, and communicates through the secretion of chemicals.[1,2] The skin acts as a barrier to bacteria partly by its acidic surface pH. It is a layered structure made up of the epidermis, dermis and hair follicles, and subcutis. The epidermis is further stratified histologically into four regions. These regions are, from the superficial to the deep layers, the stratum corneum, stratum granulosum, stratum spinosum, and stratum basale. Areas exposed to frequent abrasion (e.g., muzzle, plenum, hoof margin) also have a stratum lucidum or clear layer, which is composed of a nuclear, homogenous material containing retractile droplets (eleidin).[3] The ability of the skin to heal depends on the severity of damage incurred by the cells of the stratum basale. Skin thickness varies with anatomic regions; it is thicker dorsally and thinner ventrally. Overall, skin thickness in sheep averages 2.6 mm; it is 2.9 mm in goats.[2] Specialized cells found in the skin include melanocytes, which give color to the hair and skin; Langerhans' cells, which process antigens; and Merkel cells, which function as mechanoreceptors.

The dermis lies immediately beneath the epidermis and is composed of collagen, elastin, neurovascular structures, arrector pili muscles, and a variety of cells and cellular products such as proteoglycans. The superficial dermis is a loosely arranged network of collagen and elastin fibers. The deep dermis is more structured with collagen fibers arranged parallel to the skin surface. Blood is supplied to the skin by intercommunicating vessels between the plexuses of the deep, middle, and superficial layers. The subcutis is a composite of bundles of collagen and elastin intermixed with adipose tissue.

In goats, wattles may be present—typically along the ventral neck caudal to the angle of the mandible. Although the function of wattles is unknown, they contain extensive neurovascular structures and cartilage. The presence of wattles is controlled by an autosomal dominant gene.

Sebaceous (holocrine) scent glands are located caudal and medial to the base of the horn tissues on the head of goats. In male goats these glands produce a pungent odor. Surgical procedures to remove the scent glands of goats (descenting) involve excising the sebaceous glands caudal and medial to the horn base. This procedure is easily done in young buck kids at the time of dehorning. In sheep, scent glands are present rostral and medial to the eye and may produce a pungent odor in rams. Sweat (apocrine) glands are present throughout the body in goats but are most pronounced around the eyelids, scrotum, udder, and perineal regions. These glands are not innervated, but respond to heat by producing sweat at a rate as high as 208 g sweat/m^2 skin/hour in males and 216 g sweat/m^2 skin/hour in females in response to temperatures in excess of 41° C (106° F).[3]

The hair coat of sheep (wool and hair) and goats (fiber) has variable economic potential based on the texture of the hair. Two types of hair follicles are found in the skin of goats: primary and secondary. Primary hairs are long and coarse and may occur singly or in groups of two or three. Primary hairs often are referred to as *guard hairs*, *outer coat*, or *kemp*. Secondary follicles produce fine, shorter hairs (undercoat and lanugo hairs in goats are nonmedullated hairs), creating an undercoat often referred to as *down*. Secondary hairs include larger, medullated hairs (undercoat) and smaller, nonmedullated hairs (lanugo). Some fiber breeds of goats are genetically selected for down production.[1] The ratio of secondary to primary hairs ranges from 3 : 1 to 25 : 1.[3] Primary hair follicles have associated sebaceous and apocrine sweat glands and arrector pili muscles. The number of primary hairs per square centimeter for goats ranges from 175 hairs/cm^2 for sexually intact males to 216 hairs/cm^2 for sexually intact females and 259 hairs/cm^2 for castrated males.[3] Secondary follicles also have associated sebaceous glands.

Livestock owners specifically interested in wool or fiber production are concerned about disease processes that damage the quality of the product. They may consult veterinarians about pathologies such as fungal dermatitis, lice, and skin mites that cause noticeable lesions in the coat. The hair follicle is composed of a bulb of tissue that produces the hair shaft, an arrector pilus muscle that changes the angle of the hair shaft to the surface of the skin, and various sebaceous and sudoriferous glands that excrete coatings onto the shaft. The growth of hair follicles is controlled by a variety of factors, including genetics.[4-6]

Active hair growth is referred to as the *anagen phase*. It occurs for variable time periods and is followed by a resting, or telogen, phase. The telogen phase disrupts the integrity of the hair shaft; when the anagen phase begins again the previous hair shaft breaks away and is shed. Goats may shed in the spring and fall, but sheep do not undergo a noticeable shedding period and continuously grow wool. Hair growth in goats can be influenced by ambient temperature, photoperiod, or both; hair growth is not affected by castration. One study found that wool growth intensity is greatest in autumn and winter and least in spring in sheep.[7] Also, sebaceous and sudoriferous gland volume was greatest in winter and spring and wool sulfur content was greater in autumn and winter, corresponding to larger diameter hair shafts.

APPROACH TO DIAGNOSIS

The diagnosis of skin disease is confirmed in the same way as that of diseases affecting other body systems: complete historical data, including environment and commingling risk assessment; detailed clinical signs; thorough physical examination; and diagnostic testing based on differential diagnosis lists. Often skin diseases in sheep and goats are diagnosed based on risk factors such as species, clinical signs, age, and exposure risk within the

herd without confirmatory testing. Specific diagnostic tests may be performed when diseases fail to respond to seemingly appropriate therapy or when animals are scheduled for sale or show activities.

Historical data should include the signalment of the animal: species, breed, age, gender, weight, and color. Some breeds have a higher likelihood of developing specific disease conditions (Table 8-1). Therefore breed information is useful to assess for susceptibility. The clinician should note details concerning the origin of and exposure risks to the animals. Origin of the animal includes whether the animal was born and raised on the farm, purchased by farm contracts, purchased through sale barns, or imported from another state or country. Exposure risks include transportation to another farm; commingling in sales, shows, or fairs; farm tours involving children or livestock owners; and diseases that are endemic to the particular farm. In the latter case the clinician should also note when the last outbreak occurred. Chronologic data are important in making a differential diagnosis. The date of the first observation of clinical signs should be determined, the duration of clinical signs should be evaluated, and details regarding the progression of the disease within the affected animals should be described. The region of the body affected and the spread of disease to other regions of the body also are important. Often the current state of disease is so severe that the

TABLE 8-1

BREED PREDILECTIONS FOR SKIN DISEASES IN SHEEP AND GOATS

BREED	DISEASE
Border Leicester-Southdown cross sheep	Cutaneous asthenia
Finnish crossbred sheep	
Merino sheep	
Norwegian Dala sheep	
Romney sheep	
Corriedale sheep	Congenitohereditary photosensitivity
Southdown sheep	
Dorset sheep	Viable hypotrichosis
Merino sheep	Hereditary goiter
Saanen dwarf cross goat	
Scottish blackface sheep	Epidermolysis bullosa
Southdown sheep	
Suffolk sheep	
Suffolk sheep	Scrapie

Adapted from Scott DW: *Large animal dermatology*, Philadelphia, 1988, WB Saunders.

point of origin cannot be determined by physical examination. Assessment of whether the disease has spread from one animal to another within the flock or herd is particularly important. Finally, the veterinarian may assemble a detailed chronology of any treatments applied, the dosage and route used for administration, and the duration of treatment.

Clinical signs are important in the development of a differential diagnosis. They can vary widely and depend on the tissues involved in the disease process. Differential diagnoses are most easily determined early in the course of disease, when the primary lesions are abundant (Table 8-2). As the disease progresses, secondary lesions such as infection, thickening, crusting, and hair loss may overwhelm the primary disease and make assessment of skin disease extremely difficult. Therefore animals with newly emerging disease should be selected for examination.

Erythema refers to reddening of the skin. It is not a disease-specific change but usually indicates the presence of inflammation.

Papules are solid masses, small in diameter (less than 1 cm), that are reddened, raised from the surface of the skin, and may be painful to palpation. They are consistent with infection, allergic reaction, and ectoparasites. When the papule is centered on a hair follicle, bacterial or fungal folliculitis and ectoparasites such as demodectic mange should be suspected. When papules occur independent from hair follicles, allergic skin reactions and ectoparasites such as scabies mites should be suspected.

Vesicles are similar in size and shape to papules, but these masses are filled with a serous fluid and are fluctuant. Vesicle formation may be preceded by a papule. Vesicles are most often associated with viral skin diseases such as poxvirus infections, contact allergies, and autoimmune diseases such as pemphigus.

Pustules are similar to vesicles but are purulent in nature. Purulent exudate is formed because of migration of neutrophils either in response to infection or because of an autoimmune disease. Vesicles and pustules are ruptured by abrasion or spontaneous disruption of the overlying membrane. The fluids accumulated on the skin surface form crusts, and the underlying skin becomes thickened in response to the injury.

Crusts are firm, adherent amalgamations of serum, pus, blood, cellular debris, and associated organisms. The presence of crusts indicates an exudative process but is not disease-specific. Microscopic examination of crusts may reveal infectious organisms such as fungi, bacteria, or cells. The term *scale* simply refers to desquamated stratum corneum and is not disease-specific.

Thickening of the skin (specifically, thickening of the stratum corneum) often is referred to as *hyperkeratosis*. The term *orthokeratosis* is used to describe hyperkeratosis without the presence of nuclei. Parakeratosis is hyperkeratosis with nuclei present in the keratinized skin. Unfor-

tunately, these findings are consistent with chronic dermatopathy and are not disease-specific. The distribution of lesions may be more important than the actual histologic description in this scenario.

Alopecia is hair loss. It may be associated with disease or other stressors, producing a stress-induced telogen phase. This "stress break" in the hair shaft may result in generalized hair loss. Stress alopecia usually is associated with normal skin and normally growing hair. Systemic disease causing prolonged pyrexia also can disrupt normal hair and fiber growth and result in easily epilated hair. In sheep this is referred to as *wool break*. Nutritional deficiencies in zinc, selenium, and vitamin E may cause hair loss. A congenital form of alopecia, termed *hypotrichosis*, is well described in cattle and is associated with a recessive genetic trait.[8]

Scratching associated with skin disease is termed *pruritus*. Assessment of the severity of pruritus can aid in the formulation of an accurate differential diagnosis. Severe pruritus typically is seen with ectoparasitism. Mild pruritus is more often associated with nutritional deficiency, allergic skin disease, bacterial or fungal skin disease, and autoimmune disease. It is a common clinical sign associated with scrapie that also is seen in pseudorabies virus and rabies virus infections.

Changes in skin and hair pigmentation are uncommon in most ruminant diseases. Exceptions to this include the hair pigment lightening seen in cattle with chronic copper deficiency and molybdenosis and the black wool pigment that develops in blackfaced sheep after skin injury (abrasions, laceration, chronic irritation). The development of dark pigmentation also has been observed in Saanen goats exposed to excessive sunlight.

Lesion location can be used to establish a differential diagnosis (see Table 8-2). Regions commonly affected in the early stages of skin disease include the face, ears, feet, udder, and perineal region. Fungal skin infections more commonly occur on the face, neck, and ears, whereas bacterial skin diseases also affect the feet, udder, and perineum. Nutritional deficiencies typically involve all regions to various degrees. Photosensitization is more severe in areas that receive little protection by the hair coat and areas with slight or no pigmentation. Ectoparasite lesions are most severe around the feet, face, and ears.

Diagnostic Tests

Although many skin diseases are diagnosed based on clinical signs and intuition, specific diagnosis requires confirmation by laboratory tests (Table 8-3).

Skin scraping.   Skin scraping and cytology are easily performed under field conditions and may be diagnostic of certain diseases. Observation of bacteria on cytology is not diagnostic because bacteria are ubiquitous on the

TABLE 8-2

TYPICAL DISTRIBUTION OF LESIONS ASSOCIATED WITH SELECTED DISEASES OF THE SKIN

AREA INVOLVED	DISEASE	PRIMARY LESION TYPE
Head and neck	Dermatophytosis	Papulocrustous
	Dermatophilosis	Pustolocrustous
	Demodicosis	Papulonodular
	Elaeophoriasis	Ulcerative
	Fly bites	Papulocrustous
	Actinobacillosis	Nodular
	Clostridiosis	Edematous
	Sarcoptic mange	Papulocrustous
	Contagious viral pustular dermatitis	Pustolocrustous
	Ovine viral ulcerative dermatitis	Ulcerative
	Goat pox	Pustolocrustous
	Sheep pox	Pustolocrustous
	Pemphigus foliaceous	Vesiculopustular, crusts
	Zinc deficiency	Crusts
	Contact dermatitis	Variable
	Viral papillomatosis	Papulonodular
	Squamous cell carcinoma	Nodular, ulcerative
Ears	Dermatophytosis	Papulocrustous
	Dermatophilosis	Pustolocrustous
	Sarcoptic mange	Papulocrustous
	Fly bites	Papulocrustous
	Pemphigus foliaceous	Vesiculopustular, crusts
	Ergotism	Necrotizing
	Fescue toxicosis	Necrotizing
	Frostbite	Necrotizing
	Photodermatitis	Edematous, necroulcerative
	Squamous cell carcinoma	Nodular, ulcerative
Mucocutaneous	Contagious viral pustular dermatitis	Pustolocrustous
	Goat pox	Pustolocrustous
	Sheep pox	Pustolocrustous
	Bluetongue	Erythema, edema
	Zinc deficiency	Crusts
	Bullous pemphigus	Vesiculoulcerative
	Pemphigus foliaceous	Vesiculopustular, crusts
	Dermatophytosis	Papulocrustous
	Dermatophilosis	Pustolocrustous
	Squamous cell carcinoma	Nodular, ulcerative
Dorsum	Dermatophilosis	Pustolocrustous
	Fly bites	Papulocrustous
	Psoroptic mange	Papulocrustous
	Contact dermatitis	Variable
Ventrum	Dermatophilosis	Pustolocrustous
	Fly bites	Papulocrustous
	Sarcoptic mange	Papulocrustous
	Contact dermatitis	Variable

Adapted from Scott DW: *Large animal dermatology,* Philadelphia, 1988, WB Saunders.

TABLE 8-2

TYPICAL DISTRIBUTION OF LESIONS ASSOCIATED WITH SELECTED DISEASES OF THE SKIN—cont'd

AREA INVOLVED	DISEASE	PRIMARY LESION TYPE
Ventrum—cont'd	Goat pox	Pustolocrustous
	Sheep pox	Pustolocrustous
	Contagious viral pustular dermatitis	Pustolocrustous
	Zinc deficiency	Crusts
	Corynebacterium pseudotuberculosis infection	Abscesses
Trunk	Dermatophytosis	Papulocrustous
	Dermatophilosis	Pustolocrustous
	Psoroptic mange	Papulocrustous
	Psorergatic mange	Alopecia, pruritus
	Keds	Alopecia, pruritus
	Ovine fleece rot	Moist dermatitis
	Pemphigus foliaceous	Vesiculopustular, crusts
	Demodicosis	Papulonodular
	Caprine viral dermatitis	Papulonodular
	Scrapie	Excoriation, pruritus
	Vitamin A deficiency	Hyperkeratosis
	Iodine deficiency	Alopecia, scaling
	Biotin, niacin, riboflavin, pantothenic acid deficiency	Alopecia, scaling, crusts
	Vitamin C–responsive dermatosis	Alopecia, erythema, purpurea
	Copper deficiency	Depigmentation
Hindquarters	Dermatophilosis	Pustolocrustous
	Chorioptic mange	Papulocrustous
Legs and feet	Dermatophytosis	Papulocrustous
	Dermatophilosis	Pustolocrustous
	Chorioptic mange	Papulocrustous
	Contact dermatitis	Variable
	Elaeophoriasis	Necroulcerative
	Clostridiosis	Edema
	Sarcoptic mange	Papulocrustous
	Zinc deficiency	Crusts
	Vitamin C–responsive dermatosis	Alopecia, erythema, purpurea
	Ovine viral ulcerative dermatitis	Ulcerative
	Pemphigus foliaceous	Vesiculopustular, crusts
Tail	Psoroptic mange	Scales, pruritus
	Selenosis	Alopecia
Coronary band	Pemphigus foliaceous	Vesiculopustular, crusts
	Bluetongue	Erythema
	Contagious viral pustular dermatitis	Pustolocrustous
	Ergotism	Edema
	Fescue toxicosis	Edema
	Dermatophilosis	Pustolocrustous
	Zinc deficiency	Crusts

TABLE 8-3

TESTS USED FOR DIAGNOSIS OF SKIN DISEASE

CAUSE OF SKIN DISEASE	TESTS USED
Parasites	Acetate tape
	Skin scraping
	Fecal flotation
Fungi	Potassium hydroxide
	Mineral oil mount
	Wood's lamp
	Fungal culture
	Cytology
Bacteria	Direct smear
	Bacterial culture
Viruses	Viral isolation
	Electron microscopy
	Serology
Allergy	Intradermal skin tests
Miscellaneous pathology	Histopathologic tests— biopsy sections, immunofluorescent tests, antinuclear antibody tests, special stains

Adapted from Scott DW: *Large animal dermatology*, Philadelphia, 1988, WB Saunders.

TABLE 8-4

NORMAL MICROBIAL INHABITANTS OF THE SKIN IN SHEEP AND GOATS

SPECIES	BACTERIA	FUNGI
Goat	*Staphylococcus aureus*	*Aspergillus*
	Coagulase-negative	*Mucor*
	Staphylococcus	
Sheep	*Bacillus*	
	Escherichia coli	
	Micrococcus	
	S. aureus	
	S. epidermidis	
	Streptococcus	

Adapted from Scott DW: *Large animal dermatology*, Philadelphia, 1988, WB Saunders.

surface of the skin. Bacteria observed in pustule fluid are more diagnostic. The contents of skin pustules or abscesses may be aspirated and cultured for identification. A direct smear should be done and a Gram's stain performed for immediate identification of infectious bacteria. The presence of phagocytized bacteria supports a diagnosis of bacterial infection. Bacteria in the absence of neutrophils or macrophages suggests that the bacteria are contaminants rather than causes of disease.

Description of the morphology of groups of bacteria may be helpful. For example, *Dermatophilus congolensis* is a gram-positive filamentous branching bacterial colony. Scales and crusts also can be examined under a microscope. Direct examination is usually not rewarding, but softening the material with sodium nitrate solution may allow for visualization of ectoparasites or fungal hyphae. These organisms often float to the top of the solution; a slide placed on top of the solution aids in identification because mites often are carried with the water adhesion onto the slide.

Skin scrapings can be frustrating to interpret. The scraping should be done firmly and deeply into the skin surface. The presence of blood at the site of scraping indicates that the depth is adequate to collect any infesting ectoparasites. Careful microscopic examination of the debris is useful to identify mites or their eggs. Potassium

hydroxide solution may be used to clear the sample for examination.

Microbial culture. Bacterial and fungal cultures can be used to determine the presence of pathogenic organisms. Culture results may be challenging to interpret because some cultured microbes may be part of the normal resident flora of the skin of sheep and goats (Table 8-4). Bacterial cultures may be obtained by aspirating pustules, abscesses, and other nodules. If a skin biopsy is to be performed, bacterial culture may be obtained from a sample of skin tissue. The clinician cleanses the desired sample area with alcohol and obtains a hair sample from the periphery of an active lesion. Cultures for dermatomycotic agents must be set up on special media. Fungal cultures may require weeks in a favorable environment before a positive or negative result can be reported.

Impression smear. Impression smears may be of some (albeit limited) value, particularly in the diagnosis of very exudative or very dry lesions. A moist lesion or an area from which a scab has just been removed is selected. A clean glass microscope slide is carefully pressed against the lesion and is allowed to air dry or is fixed. The slide is then suitably stained and the cytologic evaluation is performed.

Biopsy. Skin biopsy is most useful to identify lesions consistent with ectoparasites and allergic and autoimmune disease. Skin biopsy is indicated when a lesion is unusual, has failed to respond to treatment, is suspected to be neoplastic, or is persistently ulcerative or exudative. It also can be used to rule out various pathologies during differential diagnosis. Biopsy specimens should be obtained from primary lesions and ideally should include the junction of normal and abnormal skin. Commercial skin biopsy instruments (with internal diameters of 4 to 8 mm) provide the best quality samples for pathologists. Areas with minimal skin tension should be chosen. A needle and scalpel blade can be used to harvest a skin sample, or the entire lesion may be submitted if surgical excision is performed. Full-thickness skin biopsy is recommended to allow examination of all layers of the epidermis and dermis. Sedation or tranquilization of the patient may be required. The clinician may clip the hair surrounding the area of skin biopsy; however, hair emerging from the skin sample is desirable to enhance the pathologist's evaluation. Therefore only minimal clipping should be performed, and a razor blade should not be used. A small amount of lidocaine hydrochloride 2% is deposited in the subcutaneous tissue deep within the specimen. This should be done carefully and immediately before biopsy because the side effects of lidocaine include vascular dilatation and edema, both of which may confuse histologic evaluation. Many pathologists prefer that skin specimens be preserved attached to a wooden plank such as a piece of a tongue depressor. Fixatives for skin samples include 10% neutral buffered formalin for routine light microscopy and glutaraldehyde for electron microscopy. Skin biopsies may be fixed with Michel's fixative or fresh-frozen without fixative if immunohistochemistry or other such tests are desired. In one study shrinkage was similar for formalin-fixed and fresh-frozen specimens (approximately 20%).[9] Skin biopsy specimens should be submitted to a veterinary pathologist experienced in the interpretation of skin histology (dermatohistopathologist). Because skin histology varies dramatically among species, a pathologist experienced in evaluation of the skin of sheep and goats is preferable. If preferred by the clinician or owner the biopsy site can be closed (using a simple interrupted or cruciate pattern) with either absorbable or nonabsorbable material.

References

1. Scott DW: *Large animal dermatology,* Philadelphia, 1988, WB Saunders.
2. Smith MC, Sherman DM: Skin. In Smith MC, Sherman DM, editors: *Goat medicine,* Baltimore, 1994, Williams & Wilkins.
3. Scott DW, Smith MC, Manning TO: Caprine dermatology. Part I. Normal skin and bacterial and fungal disorders, *Comp Cont Ed Pract Vet* 6:S190, 1984.
4. Abouheif MA, Johnson CL, Botkin MP: Heritability estimates of wool follicle traits in sheep skin, *Anim Prod* 39:399, 1984.
5. Eythorsdottir E: Genetic variation in woolskin quality of Icelandic lambs, *Livestock Prod Sci* 57:113, 1999.
6. Henderson M, Sabine JR: Secondary follicle development in Australian cashmere goats, *Small Rumin Res* 4:349, 1991.
7. Dragnev Z, Nedelchev D, Vladov K: *Zhivotnovudni Nauki* 13:80, 1976.
8. Steffen DJ: Congenital skin abnormalities, *Vet Clin North Am* 9:105, 1993.
9. Steinhagen O, Bredenhann AEJ: The effect of histological processing on sheep skin samples, *S Afr J Anim Sci* 17:151, 1987.

VIRAL DISEASES

Contagious Ecthyma

Contagious ecthyma (contagious viral pustular dermatitis, orf, sore mouth, contagious pustular dermatitis, cutaneous pustular dermatitis, scabby mouth) affects sheep and goats and is caused by an epitheliotrophic *Parapoxvirus* (140 kilobase [kb] deoxyribonucleic acid [DNA]).[1-7] Lesions occur most severely on the mouth and face but also occur on the feet, teats, and genitalia. The poxvirus is present worldwide and can remain infective in scabs in the environment for months or years. Transmission occurs either by direct contact or indirectly from environmental contaminants. The poxvirus gains entry through abrasions; morbidity is highest among animals subjected to coarse feeds and pasture plants that cause injury to the oral mucosa. The virus remains in the local tissues and is shed with the scab. Infection of the respiratory and gastrointestinal systems is rare.[2] The incubation period can be as short as 4 days or as long as 2 weeks. Commingling sheep is a common risk factor and younger sheep, especially 3- to 6-month-old feeder lambs, are most susceptible. The infection is self-limiting, with most sheep developing protective immunity. However, reinfection is possible. If it occurs, the course of the disease is less severe and more rapidly cleared. Neonatal lambs may achieve only limited protection through passive transfer of maternal antibodies in colostrum, and maternal protection wanes near weaning age.

Clinical signs. Early clinical signs of contagious ecthyma include papules, vesicles, and pustules in affected skin. Thick, brown-to-black crusts form rapidly and are most evident at the commissures of the mouth. Lesions may spread to the oral cavity, feet, eyelids, and teats. Mastitis may develop because of compromise to the teat defense mechanisms. Lesions typically resolve in 14 to 21 days but may persist in immunocompromised patients. Nursing lambs may spread the infection to the udders of susceptible ewes. Oral lesions may be severe enough in lambs to cause anorexia, weight loss, and dehydration or malnutrition. Lesions involving the coronary band may cause lameness and udder lesions may result in mastitis in affected sheep. Rarely, the respiratory and gastrointestinal systems are involved. In these cases pneumonia and diarrhea, respectively, may occur. Secondary bacterial infection of the skin is common. Differential diagnoses include ulcerative dermatosis, sheep pox, and dermatophilosis.

Diagnosis. Observation of typical histopathologic lesions in skin biopsy specimens is supportive of a diagnosis of contagious ecthyma. These lesions include epithelial proliferation, ballooning degeneration, and eosinophilic intracytoplasmic inclusions. Viral particles may be observed in vesicular fluid, skin, and crusts with electron microscopy. Fluorescent antibody tests may be performed on cell cultures that have been inoculated with material from lesions.

Treatment. Treatment of individually affected animals is not provided unless lesions are severe. In these cases therapy is supportive and includes the administration of oral fluids and nutrients. Application of topical astringent agents may speed recovery.

Prevention. Control measures should be implemented immediately, and affected sheep should be isolated. However, these measures alone may not be effective in controlling contagious ecthyma because of the short incubation time and survivability of the agent in the environment. Commercial vaccines are available; they require application to the surface of scarified epithelium in the axilla, groin, inner thigh (not in lactating ewes), underside of the tail, or ear. These vaccines are not recommended for use in disease-free herds because the vaccine virus remains viable in the environment for a long period. Development of immunity occurs over a period of 3 weeks and may persist for as long as 2 years. Contagious ecthyma is highly zoonotic and may produce lesions on the hands or fingers of persons handling infected sheep or goats. Therefore hygiene is imperative during handling of infected herds. In endemic flocks vaccinating lambs and kids at 2 to 3 days of age may help reduce the severity of a flock outbreak. In lambs this may be coordinated with tail docking.

Malignant Contagious Ecthyma

A persistent form of contagious ecthyma known as *malignant contagious ecthyma* has been recognized in a limited number of sheep within infected flocks. Proliferative lesions develop, especially on the distal legs and feet and less commonly on the head. However, unlike ordinary contagious ecthyma, the lesions fail to regress and may continually enlarge (Figure 8-1). Secondary bacterial infections, fly strike, and hemorrhage are major complications. Although a poxvirus morphologically similar to the contagious ecthyma virus has been identified by electron microscopy in typical lesions, the disease has a different course. Affected sheep do not pass the infection to commingling animals. Preliminary studies of the cellular immune systems of affected sheep have failed to demonstrate any deviation from normal.

Ulcerative Dermatosis

Ulcerative dermatosis occurs most commonly in sheep in the western United States. It is caused by a similar but antigenically distinct virus from that causing contagious ecthyma.[3,4] Transmission occurs by direct or indirect

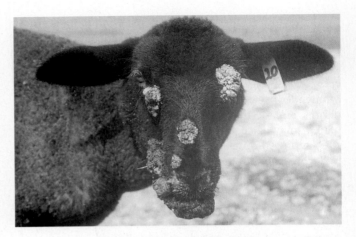

Figure 8-1 Malignant contagious ecthyma. Note the proliferative lesions around the face. In traditional contagious ecthyma, lesions last only 2 to 4 weeks. Lesions around the mouth make grazing painful and can result in weight loss. Lesions around the udder can result in the refusal of dams to allow nursing. Lesions may become infected with secondary bacteria, at which time topical antibiotics may be indicated.

contact. Infection is typically complicated by pathogenic bacteria such as *Fusobacterium necrophorum*. These viral and bacterial agents cause ulcers, necrosis, and scabs. Morbidity with ulcerative dermatosis is less than that seen in contagious ecthyma in a susceptible population, seldom exceeding 20% of the flock.

Clinical signs. During breeding season, ulcerative dermatosis appears clinically as vulvitis or balanoposthitis. Epithelial abrasions that occur during breeding allow transmission from one animal to the other. Infected tissues become red and swollen and develop a moist exudate. During winter or periods of high risk for feet and lip abrasions, ulcerations may develop on the feet and mouth. Lesions do not involve the oral mucosae. Lesions are present for 2 to 6 weeks and are self-limiting. When lesions are severe, scar tissue may cause phimosis or paraphimosis. When necrosis is severe, sepsis of the interphalangeal joint, urethral fistula, or sloughing of the urethral process may occur.

Diagnosis. Ulcerative dermatosis is differentiated clinically from contagious ecthyma because of the ulcerative nature of the disease, rather than the proliferation typical of contagious ecthyma. Histopathologic lesions observed in skin biopsy specimens confirm this differentiation.

Treatment. Treatment should include isolating affected animals, cleansing wounds and treating them with antiseptic or antimicrobial (triple antibiotic) ointments, and managing secondary infections. Control may include removing hair from the animals' genital areas to prevent abrasion of genital tissues.

Sheep Pox

Sheep pox is caused by an extremely virulent poxvirus. It produces marked pyrexia, anorexia, and apparent depression.[3,7] Sheep pox is found in Eastern Europe, North Africa, and Asia. Lesions rapidly transform from macules to papules and then to vesicles on skin with limited wool coverage (mouth, face, eyelids, perineum, udder, prepuce). Tissue necrosis and scab formation ensues. The epithelial tissues of the lungs and gastrointestinal system may become involved, with a mortality rate as high as 50% among affected sheep.

Goat Pox

Goat pox virus infection causes papules, vesicles, pustules, and scabs that can be difficult to distinguish from those of contagious ecthyma.[1,6,8] However, these lesions usually occur on the teats, udder, scrotum, and thighs but are uncommon on the face. Although not diagnosed in the United States, a virulent strain of goat pox has been documented to cause anorexia, pyrexia, rhinitis, and conjunctivitis in herds in Africa and the Middle East. Research into the nature of goat pox virus revealed the presence of numerous precipitinogens, some heat stable and some enzyme resistant.[1,7] Death may ensue, with pulmonary lesions found at necropsy.

Scrapie

A discussion of scrapie is beyond the scope of this chapter (see Chapter 11).[3,4] However, scrapie-infected sheep may demonstrate intense pruritus and body tremors. Wool may be missing or distorted because of the scratching, but the underlying skin is normal.

Bluetongue

A discussion of bluetongue is beyond the scope of this chapter (see Chapters 4 and 14).[2] However, bluetongue virus infection may cause ptyalism, lacrimation, conjunctivitis, oral ulceration, and swelling of the mouth, muzzle, and ears. Hyperemia and eczema may be noted in hairless areas. The coronary band may be inflamed and lameness may occur. Lesions can be severe enough to cause sloughing of the hooves.[1]

Vesicular Stomatitis

Vesicular stomatitis may cause vesicle formation on the commissures of the lips in goats.[1] Pseudorabies can cause intense pruritus in goats. Viral encephalitis and rapid death are typical of pseudorabies infection. Viral isolation and serology are recommended to differentiate the various viral diseases (see Chapter 14).

REFERENCES

1. Smith MC, Sherman DM: Skin. In Smith MC, Sherman DM, editors: *Goat medicine*, Baltimore, 1994, Williams & Wilkins.
2. Haig D et al: Cytokines and their inhibitors in orf virus infection, *Vet Immunol Immunopath* 54:261, 1996.
3. Lofstedt J: Dermatologic diseases of sheep, *Vet Clin North Am Large Anim Pract* 5:427, 1983.
4. Mullowney PC: Skin diseases of sheep, *Vet Clin North Am Large Anim Pract* 6(1):131, 1984.
5. Mullowney PC, Baldwin EW: Skin diseases of goats, *Vet Clin North Am Large Anim Pract* 6(1):143, 1984.
6. Scott DW, Smith MC, Manning TO: Caprine dermatology. Part II. Viral, nutritional, environmental, and congenitohereditary disorders, *Comp Cont Ed Pract Vet* 6:S473, 1984.
7. Kimberling CV: Diseases of the skin. In Kimberling CV, editor: *Jensen and Swift's diseases of sheep*, ed 3, Philadelphia, 1988, Lea & Febiger.
8. Smith MC: Dermatologic diseases of goats, *Vet Clin North Am Large Anim Pract* 5:449, 1983.

BACTERIAL DISEASES

Dermatophilosis (Streptothricosis, Lumpy Wool Disease, Rain Scald)

Dermatophilosis causes a severe suppurative inflammation of the skin.[1-4] *Dermatophilus congolensis* is the causative organism and is a gram-positive, filamentous, aerobic bacteria. This disease is associated with skin abrasion and moist conditions. Therefore the ears, muzzle, face, and tail are common sites for disease. In geographic areas with long periods of rainfall and high humidity, the disease also may affect the dorsum of the neck and back. The bacteria may be spread by mechanical vectors (shears, flies), by contaminated dipping solutions, and by direct contact. Animals debilitated by malnutrition, parasitism, or other disease are most susceptible to clinical infection.

Clinical signs. Clinical signs include the formation of thick crusts with a significant inflammatory response in the skin. Crusts contain infective zoospores of the bacterium that are released when the crust softens in moist conditions. These zoospores are stable in the environment within crusts for at least 4 months. Sheep may carry the infection subclinically and serve as carriers of the disease. Periods of prolonged moist skin allow penetration of the bacterium into the skin and establishment of infection. *Strawberry footrot* is another name for *D. congolensis* infection of the distal extremities and large crust formation around the carpus, tarsus, and coronary bands. Pastures contaminated with *D. congolensis* may produce widespread disease in a flock; clinical cases are most severe in young stock (less than 1 year old). Lesions heal by granulation, which is observed with forced removal of crusts (hence, the strawberry appearance).

Diagnosis. Cytologic examination of the deep layer of the crusts (adjacent to the granulation tissue) reveals coccoid bacteria branching into formations similar to "railroad tracks." Maceration of crusts may allow identification of motile zoospores. Diagnosis is confirmed by culture of a skin biopsy or crusts. Secondary mycotic dermatitis is common and confuses diagnostic efforts.

Treatment. Local and systemic treatment of dermatophilosis has been recommended. Empirical antibiotic therapy may include procaine penicillin G (dosage range 20,000 to 70,000 units/kg body weight) or oxytetracycline (20 mg/kg subcutaneously [SC] or intramuscularly [IM] every 72 hours). Topical treatment may include administration of copper sulfate (0.2%), zinc sulfate (0.2% to 0.5%), or potassium aluminum sulfate (1%). Clinicians should take precautions during treatment because *D. congolensis* is capable of infecting human beings. Improving the dietary protein, energy, and mineral intake and providing shelter from rain are all good methods of promoting skin healing and preventing the disease.

Fleece Rot

Excessive moisture trapped by the wool and held against the skin for a prolonged time can result in a bacterial dermatitis known as *fleece rot*.[2,5] Prolonged wetting of the skin causes hyperkeratosis, acanthosis, and edema. Economic losses are incurred because of discoloration of the wool by exudate or chromogenic bacteria. Although it is not the exclusive cause of fleece rot, *Pseudomonas aeruginosa* is commonly isolated from lesions.

Clinical signs. Infection with *P. aeruginosa* may cause a greenish discoloration of the wool, and infection with *P. indigofera* may cause a bluish discoloration. Lesions are most commonly found on the back and withers. The underlying skin is soft, macerated, and cyanotic. Sheep with dense hair follicles and a variety of hair shaft diameters are most susceptible to *Pseudomonas* infection. Fleece rot is distinguished from dermatophilosis in that no scab is associated with the infection.

Treatment. Marked improvement of lesions occurs after shearing and drying of lesions.

Malignant Edema (Swelled Head, Bighead)

Malignant edema is a rare condition most commonly affecting young rams.[1,3,5] The disease is caused by *Clostridium novyi*, *C. sordelli*, and *C. oedematiens* and is most commonly seen in summer and autumn. Rams 6 months to 2 years of age are most commonly affected. The bacterial spores gain entry to the skin through fighting wounds among pubertal rams.

Clinical signs. Characteristic lesions include head and neck edema, especially of the eyelids, that is not associated with hemorrhage or emphysema. Early in the course of disease, rams have marked pyrexia (41° to 43° C) that can progress to death within 72 hours.

Treatment. Treatment (penicillin, oxygen insufflation of affected tissues, antitoxins) is usually futile. Prevention is easily attained with multivalent clostridial vaccines at least 6 weeks before the onset of the first breeding season.

Actinobacillosis

Actinobacillus lignieresii, a non–spore-forming, gram-negative rod, causes a pyogranulomatous bacterial infection of the soft tissues of the head.[6] These bacteria usually are inoculated into the tissues by grass awns or stemmy forage. A local granulomatous reaction occurs, but these bacteria also may spread to regional lymph nodes or the bloodstream. They can produce chains of small nodules leading to the lymph nodes.

Clinical signs. Purulent material may be observed draining from lymph nodes. Severe enlargement of submaxillary or parotid lymph nodes may cause difficulty in breathing or eating; sheep may die from malnutrition. Nasal exudate may be noted if the infection drains into the nasopharynx.

Diagnosis. The diagnosis is made by performing cytology and a Gram's stain on the exudate. The gram-negative rods are filamentous and form sulfur granules in the pus that can be seen without the aid of a microscope.

Treatment. Therapy includes surgical drainage, antibiotics (procaine penicillin G, 22,000 to 66,000 units/kg body weight SC every 24 hours for 7 days), and iodine therapy. Sodium iodide can be administered (80 mg/kg body weight) intravenously (IV) and repeated once or twice at 7-day intervals. Alternatively, organic iodides can be added to the feed (7.5 to 15 g/head/day) for 14 to 21 days.

Staphylococcal Dermatitis

Staphylococcus aureus can cause a bacterial infection of the skin.[2,4,7] The bacteria become established when puncture wounds or other injuries allow entry into the skin.

Clinical signs. Affected animals have an exudative dermatitis that is most severe around the eyes, ears, base of the horns, and bridge of the nose. In goats, vesicles and pustules may be found on the teats and udder soon after parturition.

Diagnosis. The diagnosis is made by culture of hemolytic *S. aureus*. This disease must be differentiated from elaeophoriasis because of the distribution of lesions on the head.

Treatment. The application of topical antiseptics or antimicrobial ointments may be of benefit. If clinical signs are severe or the distribution of lesions is widespread on the body, systemic antibiotic therapy should be based on results of culture and sensitivity tests. Empirical antibiotic therapy may include penicillin (22,000 IU/kg once a day [SID] or twice a day [BID]), ampicillin (10 to 20 mg/kg IM or IV BID), or oxytetracycline (10 mg/kg IV BID or 20 mg/kg SC or IM every 48 to 72 hours). The causative bacterium is contagious and affected sheep should be isolated from the flock. Affected dairy goats should be removed from the milking line or milked last. Careful attention to hygiene is necessary to prevent staphylococcal mastitis and spread of these pathogenic bacteria to other lactating does.

Abscesses

Abscesses of the soft tissues are not uncommon in sheep and goats. Abscesses usually begin when wounds allow entry of surface bacteria through the epidermis. Therefore *Staphylococcus* species, *Corynebacterium* species, *Actinomyces* species, and streptococcal bacteria are expected on culture. Noncontagious abscesses may be treated by lancing after infiltration of local anesthesia. The interior capsule of the abscess is débrided and flushed with a dilute iodine solution (1%). Systemic antimicrobial agents are not indicated in most cases but may be administered if numerous abscesses or deeply seeded abscesses are present.

Caseous Lymphadenitis

Caseous lymphadenitis is caused by *Corynebacterium (Actinomyces) pseudotuberculosis*, formerly called *C. ovis. C. pseudotuberculosis* is a facultative, gram-positive, coccoid bacillus that is an intracellular parasite of macrophages and monocytes.[8,9] It may cause abscesses in the skin or subcutaneous lymph nodes that may break open to the skin surface (Figure 8-2).[8] Bacterial infection may spread rapidly through a sheep flock at the time of shearing because of skin abrasions and contamination of shears, tail docking equipment, and dip tanks. Experimental studies have described abscess formation as early as 41 days after inoculation.[10] In many animals the organism disseminates to the viscera, most commonly the mediastinal lymph nodes or lungs, resulting in dyspnea and tachypnea. Therefore some animals may present with a history of respiratory disease. This disease may be spread by the respiratory route, and lung abscesses may pose a potential source of flock contamination in high-density areas such as barns and dry lots. This organism can survive for extended periods in dark, damp areas, soil, and

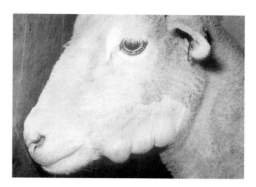

Figure 8-2 Caseous lymphadenitis abscesses in a young adult ewe.

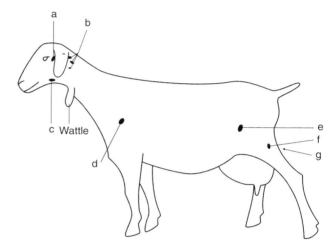

Figure 8-3 Locations of the most common palpable lymph nodes that can become enlarged in caseous lymphadenitis. The nodes are the parotid *(a)*, retropharyngeal *(b)*, mandibular *(c)*, prescapular *(d)*, prefemoral *(e)*, and popliteal *(f)*; the *arrow* points to the superficial inguinal lymph node *(g)*. This illustration also shows the most common location for wattles. However, wattles also can be found in other areas of the cervical region. (Adapted from Williams CSF: Routine sheep and goat procedures, *Vet Clin North Am Food Anim Pract* 6(3):753, 1990.)

manure. Some breeds (Merino, because of their wrinkled skin) and certain management practices (e.g., the use of dip tanks, improper shearing techniques, housing with nails or wire) predispose to this disease.[9] These lesions have thick, often caseated exudate. Spontaneous rupture of the abscess causes clumping of wool or hair with exudate. In an experimental study, draining abscesses continued to contaminate the environment for as long as 37 days after rupture.[9,10]

Clinical signs. Clinical signs include swelling of superficial lymph nodes (i.e., prescapular, prefemoral) (Figure 8-3), occasionally with draining tracts. In sheep these abscesses initially contain pale green material that eventually forms an "onion ring"–like structure and matures into a calcified mass. Abscesses in goats usually remain greenish-cream colored with a pasty texture.[9] These skin lumps may occur in chains or as solitary lesions. As abscessation of the viscera occurs, chronic weight loss may be encountered, more commonly in sheep than in goats. Poor fertility, decreased milk production, decreased lamb crop and weaning weights, and poor growth and wool production also are encountered. The organism can spread to the central nervous system or superficial inguinal lymph nodes and mammary glands, resulting in neurologic signs and mastitis, respectively.[9]

Diagnosis. Diagnosis is based on serologic testing of infected animals, culture of the organism (particularly from the peripheral portions of the necrotic area), and necropsy with consistent pathologic findings. *C. pseudotuberculosis* is a catalase-positive, urease-negative, phospholipase-D–positive, pyrazinamide-negative organism.[10,11] To culture the abscessed lymph node, the skin over the node is clipped and surgically scrubbed. The clinician inserts a sterile needle and aspirates the abscess. If no fluid can be withdrawn, sterile saline is injected and the node is re-aspirated. If the abscess is plated onto blood agar after 48 hours, the organism grows as a thin colony with slight hemolysis. Organisms should stain gram-positive, but occasionally they are variable in their staining characteristics. *C. pyogenes* may be a secondary invader and is not uncommonly cultured. The hemolysis synergistic inhibition test measures antibodies to exotoxins produced by the organism. Most infected animals produce antibodies to the exotoxins within a month of infection. A complete blood count (CBC) may reveal a leukocytosis with a normal lymphocyte-to-neutrophil ratio, anemia of chronic disease, and hypoproteinemia, although findings are usually nonspecific. Occasionally an increase in total serum protein and gamma globulin is seen before the onset of symptoms. Other diseases that cause chronic weight loss should be considered, including parasitism, ovine progressive pneumonia (OPP), caprine arthritis-encephalitis (CAE), *Actinobacillus* infection, tuberculosis, and Johne's disease.[9]

Treatment. *C. pseudotuberculosis* abscesses should not be opened within the vicinity of the flock. Affected animals should be isolated for treatment; however, antimicrobial treatment is usually unrewarding. When economically feasible, the authors of this chapter prefer to surgically remove the intact abscess, including the capsule. Complete removal of the abscess markedly reduces the likelihood of contamination of the environment. This procedure is best done under general anesthesia because these abscesses are often located in areas with vital neurovascular structures. If abscesses have already ruptured, the animal should be isolated, the abscessed area flushed with an antiseptic solution (3% iodine or 2% chlorhexidine), and the area packed with antiseptic-saturated gauze.[11] Bulgin[12] has described a treatment technique using a 60-ml syringe filled with 10 to 25 ml of formalin (10% solution) attached to a 14-gauge needle. The needle is inserted into an infected node and the caseous material is aspirated. The clinician leaves the needle in the node, detaches the syringe from the needle, caps it, and mixes its contents. If fluid easily runs out of the needle in sheep the etiologic agent is probably *C. pyogenes* (or others) and not *C. pseudotuberculosis*. Abscesses may be more commonly caused by *C. pyogenes* rather than *C. pseudotuberculosis* in pre-weaning and weaning-age lambs. If the aspirated material is very thick, after it is shaken into solution the syringe is uncapped, reattached to the needle, and injected back into the node.[12] Controversy exists regarding the use of such "autovaccines" in animals intended for food because of the potential for formalin to be introduced to the food chain. However, one of the authors (Dr. Pugh) has used this procedure for many years in pet goats and sheep with excellent clinical success. Culling such animals is still the best treatment.

Prevention. Identification of infected animals and removal from the flock is the most effective method of control. Housing should be maintained free of objects that can cause skin injury. Needles, surgical equipment, and tattoo pliers should be cleansed and disinfected after use. All animals with open draining lesions should be culled or quarantined. Both agglutination tests and hemolysis synergistic inhibition tests may aid in identification, but they are not accurate enough for clinicians to base decisions to cull animals that have early nonclinical infections. Special care should be taken to keep all shearing and hoof trimming equipment and dipping vats clean and free of contamination from infected draining wounds. Animals with poor body condition should be culled. Although controversial, the use of commercially produced or autogenous formalized vaccines may be beneficial. Vaccination is of value and can reduce the incidence of abscesses in a flock by more than 70% but will probably not result in disease eradication in a flock.[9] Box 8-1 presents a generic lymphadenitis control program.

FUNGAL DISEASES

Dermatophytosis (Ringworm, Lumpy Wool, Club Lamb Fungus)

Fungi are not major pathogens in sheep.[2,5,11] Fungi cultured from clinical lesions include *Trichophyton verrucosum, T. gypseum, T. mentagrophytes,* and *Microsporum canis.* Dermatophytosis is transmitted by direct contact or indirect contact with contaminated equipment or environmental vectors. These fungi invade keratinized tissues and hair fibers. Breaks in the hair and alopecia occur because of breakdown of the hair shaft. The close shearing and washing practices used on show lambs leave them susceptible. Crust formation occurs because of the accu-

A Generic Caseous Lymphadenitis Control Program

- Quarantine new flock additions
- Identify and cull suspects:
  Palpate lymph nodes
  Evaluate animals with a hemolysis synergistic inhibition test
- Isolate all affected animals:
  Cull or treat and cull
  Disinfect housing and equipment with which affected animals had contact
  Disinfect all equipment used on animals (e.g., shears, hoof nippers)
- Perform necropsies on all dead animals to assess for the presence of disease
- Perform slaughter checks to assess for the presence of disease
- Vaccinate to reduce disease incidence in endemic flocks (NOTE: Vaccines may only reduce abscesses in animals in number and possibly in severity)
- Vaccinate lambs at time of tail docking
- Vaccinate all replacement lambs and kids two or three times between 6 weeks and 6 months of age
- Vaccinate rams, bucks, ewes, and does 4 to 6 weeks before lambing

Adapted from Gessert ME: *Proceedings of the 1998 Symposium on Small Ruminants for the Mixed Animal Practitioner Western Veterinary Conference*, 1998, Las Vegas, NV.

mulation of fungal hyphae and epithelial debris on the skin surface.

Clinical signs. Some pruritus may be seen with infection with *Trichophyton* species. Typical circular lesions may be seen on the face, and involvement of the ears and neck is common. Young stock are most severely affected, and mild pruritus may be observed when significant scaling or crusting is present.

Diagnosis. Use of the Wood's lamp during clinical examination may help with differential diagnosis. However, *Trichophyton* species do not fluoresce. Diagnosis is confirmed by culture of skin and hair samples on Sabouraud's dextrose agar. A 20% potassium hydroxide solution can be used to prepare wet mounts of arthrospores on the hair shafts for microscopic examination. The course of disease is 4 to 5 weeks in animals with competent immune systems.

Treatment. Treatment can help limit spread of the disease to other herd members. Topical iodine compounds (2% to 5%), chlorhexidine (2%), lime sulfur (2% to 5%), and topical antifungal medications (3% captan) are useful for local treatment of lesions. Administration of systemic drugs such as griseofulvin produces variable results. Persons providing treatment should wear gloves because these diseases have zoonotic potential.

Prevention. Dermatophytosis is spread by clippers, blankets, and other equipment. Therefore proper cleaning of equipment after use with antiseptic solutions helps control the spread of this disease.

Mycetoma

Mycetomas may be formed by fungal or bacterial elements or a combination of both.[4] Lesions most often occur on the limbs and may be initiated by a wound. These lesions cause focal swelling and have an exudate that contains granules composed of microbial organisms coated with host immune elements (e.g., immunoglobulins, fibrin).[1] These granules may be red, yellow, or purple. *Actinomadura madurae* and *A. pelletierii* have been found in goats with mycetoma, as has *Nocardia brasiliensis*. Although success rates are unknown, treatment strategies include the use of antimicrobial drugs, surgical excision, and limb amputation depending on the severity of the disease.

Candidiasis

Yeast or *Candida* dermatitis has been diagnosed in goats.[1,4] *Candida albicans, C. tropicalis, C. pseudotropicalis, C. stellatoidea, C. parapsilosis, C. krusei, C. parakrusei, C. stellatoidea, C. guilliermondii*, and other yeasts may be isolated from lesions. If yeast dermatitis is diagnosed, a compromised immune system or malnutrition must be suspected. Chronic moist conditions resulting in maceration of the skin allow the yeast to become established.

Clinical signs. Clinical signs include alopecia, scales, crusts, a greasy layer to the skin, and lichenification of the skin.

Diagnosis. Diagnosis is made by observation of budding yeasts and pseudohyphae on skin cytology.

Others

Several other fungi have been isolated from chronic dermatopathy in goats. *Peyronella glomerata* is associated with hyperkeratotic lesions of the ears of goats in the United Kingdom.[1] *Aspergillus* species can cause clinical disease in animals with compromised immune systems. These fungi also may cause granulomatous lesions in the skin.

REFERENCES

1. Scott DW, Smith MC, Manning TO: Caprine dermatology. Part I. Normal skin and bacterial and fungal disorders, *Comp Cont Ed Pract Vet* 6:S190, 1984.
2. Lofstedt J: Dermatologic diseases of sheep, *Vet Clin North Am Large Anim Pract* 5:427, 1983.
3. Kimberling CV: Diseases of the skin. In Kimberling CV, editor: *Jensen and Swift's diseases of sheep*, ed 3, Philadelphia, 1988, Lea & Febiger.
4. Smith MC: Dermatologic diseases of goats, *Vet Clin North Am Large Anim Pract* 5:449, 1983.
5. Mullowney PC: Skin diseases of sheep, *Vet Clin North Am Large Anim Pract* 6(1):131, 1984.
6. Smith MC, Sherman DM: Skin. In Smith MC, Sherman DM, editors: *Goat medicine*, Baltimore, 1994, Williams & Wilkins.
7. Mullowney PC, Baldwin EW: Skin diseases of goats, *Vet Clin North Am Large Anim Pract* 6(1):143, 1984.
8. Fubini SL, Campbell SG: External lumps on sheep and goats, *Vet Clin North Am Large Anim Pract* 5:457, 1983.
9. Pugh DG: Caseous lymphadenitis in small ruminants, *Proc North Am Vet Conf* 11:983, 1997.
10. Lloyd S: Caseous lymphadenitis in sheep. In Melling M, Adler M, editors: *Sheep and goat practice*, ed 2, London, 1998, WB Saunders.
11. East NE: Common infectious conditions, *Proceedings of the 1998 Symposium on Small Ruminants for the Mixed Animal Practitioner Western Veterinary Conference*, 1998, Las Vegas, NV.
12. Bulgin MS: Central nervous disorders of sheep, *Proceedings of the 1998 Symposium on Small Ruminants for the Mixed Animal Practitioner Western Veterinary Conference*, 1998, Las Vegas, NV.

PARASITIC DISEASES

Parasitic diseases are presented here with respect to their importance in causing lesions in the skin and hair. A summary of common treatments for ectoparasites is provided in Table 8-5.

Lice (Pediculosis)

Lice infestation is most common during winter months, presumably because temperatures, crowding, and feeding management practices are optimal for spread and proliferation of these pests.[1-6] Infestations are more severe in debilitated animals such as those suffering malnutrition and intestinal parasitism. Lice can be divided into two forms: biting and sucking. The body louse, *Damalinia ovis*, is the biting louse of sheep, and *D. caprae* is the biting louse of goats. *D. crassiceps* and *D. limbata* also have been found to infest Angora goats and can cause significant damage to the fleece. *Linognathus ovillus* (sucking face lice) and *L. pedalis* (sucking foot louse) are the sucking lice of sheep. *Linognathus stenopis* is the sucking louse of goats. *L. ovillus* infests the wool around the face, and *L. pedalis* infests the tissues distal to the carpus or tarsus. Lice may be transmitted by direct contact or by contact with contaminated areas of the environment. *L.*

TABLE 8-5

REPORTED THERAPEUTIC STRATEGIES FOR TREATMENT OF EXTERNAL PARASITES

DRUG	TREATMENT	PARASITE EFFICACY
Amitraz	250 ppm dip	Mites
Chlorpyrifos	0.05% to 0.25% spray	Keds, lice, mites
Coumaphos	0.05% to 0.3% spray or dip 0.5% to 1% dust	Keds, lice, mites
Lime-sulfur	2% to 5% dip	Keds, lice, mites
Lindane	0.03% to 0.05% spray	Keds, lice, mites, ticks
Trichlorfon	0.2% spray or dip	Keds, lice, mites
Methoxychlor	0.5% spray or dip 5% dust	Keds, lice, mites, ticks

pedalis may survive in the environment away from the host for at least 2 weeks.

Clinical signs. The clinical signs associated with lice infestation include intense pruritus, wool loss, weight loss, and anemia, if infestation is severe. Lameness may be observed with infestation.

Treatment. Therapy is centered on the animal because the life cycles of lice depend on the host. Keepers and veterinarians must exercise caution in treating meat- and milk-producing animals to avoid volatile residues. Treatment of the environment is usually impractical. Treatment may include dips, sprays, or dusts of coumaphos (0.125% as spray or 0.5% as dust), malathion (0.5% as spray or 4% as dust), or permethrin. Injections of avermectin anthelmintics (ivermectin or doramectin; 0.2 mg/kg body weight) are useful in treating sucking lice but have limited efficacy against biting lice. Treatments should be repeated at 2-week intervals for at least two treatments to ensure that lice emerging from eggs are killed. Oral administration of these drugs is of very limited value. If used topically, cypermethrin can penetrate sheep skin at a rate of approximately 11 cm per hour.[7] The drug penetrates to the stratum compactum and then spreads laterally with some penetration of the dermis. The effect of deltamethrin on sheep skin has been evaluated.[8] This drug was found to cause irritation, edema, disruption of the lipid layer, and some degenerative changes in the epidermis. This reaction was determined to be caused by the solvent mixture of the formulation. A formulation of deltamethrin was found to spread from the back to the lower body within 24 hours, but peak concentrations in the wool did not occur for 4 to 5 days with a xylene-based formulation and 11 days with a water-based formulation.[9] A concentration of deltamethrin in the skin sufficient to kill lice was present for approximately 12 days, but remained high in the tips of wool fibers. However, insecticide in the fleece was insufficient to kill lice after 14 days, suggesting that inactivation occurred in vivo. Topical drugs should be carefully evaluated before they are applied to small ruminants.

Melophagus ovinus (Sheep Ked)

The sheep ked spends its entire 6-week life cycle on the host; therefore transmission is by direct contact with infested animals. These blood-sucking insects cause skin irritation and pruritus, stain the wool, and may cause discomfort. Although they may occur year-round, most of their damage occurs during the winter.

Treatment.   Treatment is similar to that for lice and should be repeated at 14- to 21-day intervals.

Mange Mites

Mange occurs rarely in sheep but more commonly in goats.[1-6,10] Mange mites known to infest sheep include *Psoroptes communis* var *ovis, Sarcoptes scabiei ovis, Psorergates ovis, Chorioptes bovis* var *ovis,* and *Demodex ovis.* Mange has been essentially eradicated from sheep in the United States, with the exception of demodectic mange. In goats, clinically important forms of mange include sarcoptic mange, demodectic mange *(D. caprae),* psoroptic mange *(P. cuniculi),* and chorioptic mange.

Treatment.   Treatment for mange is most easily performed after shearing. Various products have been used with variable success, including coumaphos (0.3% dip), toxaphene (0.5% dip), lime sulfur (2% dip), and phosmet (0.15% to 0.25% dip) (see Table 8-5).

Psoroptic Mange (*Psoroptes cuniculi,* Common Sheep Scab)

Psoroptic mange is a reportable disease in the United States.[1-5,10] These mites have elongated heads, are oval in shape, and their first pair of legs are jointed. These mites are transmitted by direct contact, are host-specific (no zoonoses), have a 2-week life cycle, and can live off the host for as long as 3 weeks. In sheep, clinical disease is most severe in the fall and winter. The saliva of the mite causes an intense inflammatory reaction in the skin, with severe pruritus resulting in self-trauma and alopecia. These lesions are primarily distributed along the trunk. In goats, *P. cuniculi* usually infests the ears and may cause alopecia, pruritus localized to the ears, and head shaking. Infestation of the ears may be seen in goats as young as 10

days old. In sheep these mites infest heavily wooled areas and cause papules, crusting, and matting of wool. These mites may be observed on the skin surface with a magnifying lens. Local administration of louse medications is curative.

Sarcoptic Mange

S. scabiei is rare in sheep and goats and is not known to be present in the United States.[1-6,10] Scabies is a reportable disease in the United States and is zoonotic. This mite prefers to infest the skin around the eyes and ears and causes intense pruritus. The mites are round in head and body and have long, nonjointed stalks for the first pair of legs. These mites burrow through the epidermis, and the female lays eggs in these tunnels. The life cycle of *Sarcoptes* ranges from 10 to 17 days. The mites are most commonly transmitted by direct contact but can survive in the environment for variable periods. Excoriations, alopecia, and crusting occur on the face and non-wooled areas but do not spread to the bodies of the affected sheep. Chronic infection causes hyperpigmentation and lichenification of the skin, and affected sheep and goats suffer weight loss and ill thrift because of the discomfort. In goats, sarcoptic mange may affect the entire body, causing alopecia, crusting, pruritus, and subsequent weight loss. Regional lymph nodes may become enlarged because of the severity of skin damage. Diagnosis requires deep skin scraping of the periphery of active lesions, but mites are difficult to find and diagnosis is often based on clinical signs and response to therapy. Numerous scrapings may be required to find these mites. An alternative to direct examination is to mix skin scrapings and crusts with sodium nitrate solution, a technique similar to fecal floatation. Treatment consists of ivermectin anthelmintic administration and dips such as 1% lime sulfur. Dips may be required weekly for 4 to 12 weeks before the condition resolves completely. Spontaneous resolution of sarcoptic mange can occur in goats.

Psorergates ovis (Sheep Itch Mite)

The smallest of the sheep mange mites, *Psorergates ovis,* has a rounded body with indentations between the attachments of the legs.[1-6,10] This mite has a 4- to 5-week life cycle and lives in the epidermis. Alopecia, crusts, and scales are primarily distributed along the trunk (withers and sides) of the body. Infested sheep demonstrate severe pruritus, including biting at affected regions. These mites may be observed on the skin surface with a magnifying lens.

Chorioptic Mange

The *Chorioptes* mite (*Chorioptes ovis, C. caprae)* has an oval body shape; the first pair of legs are short, unsegmented,

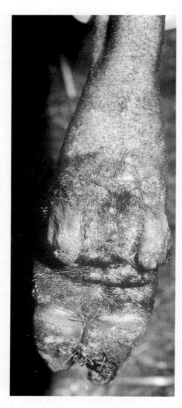

Figure 8-4 Chorioptic mange in a ewe that was associated with pruritus. Chorioptic mange mites cause wrinkling of the skin and pustules in the interdigital spaces, legs, scrotum, and brisket.

and have suckers attached to the ends.[1-6,10] *Chorioptes* is host-specific (no zoonoses), has a 2- to 3-week life cycle, and can only live off the host for a few days. These mites and their associated lesions are limited to the scrotum and distal rear limbs of sheep and the lower limbs, abdomen, and hindquarters of goats (Figure 8-4). Lesions include alopecia, erythema, excoriation, crusts, and pruritus. Infested sheep may be restless, stomp, and chew at their feet because of discomfort. Scrotal infestation may cause dermatitis and temporary infertility in rams. These mites may be observed on the skin surface with a magnifying lens. Lime sulfur dips are usually curative.

Demodectic Mange

Demodectic mange *(D. ovis, D. caprae)* affects the face, limbs, and back.[1-6,10] *D. ovis* mites infest hair follicles, causing severe folliculitis often complicated by secondary pyoderma (evidenced by the presence of pustules or abscesses). Diagnosis requires deep skin scraping and should include follicles bordering active lesions. *D. caprae* infestation may be the most common mange of goats. Disease is characterized by 2- to 12-mm diameter nodules in the skin along the neck, shoulders, and trunk.

These nodules exude a thick exudate. Cytology of this exudate reveals the presence of large numbers of cigar-shaped mites. These mites are readily spread among kids and may remain unnoticed for many months. Spread among adults is not common, therefore isolation of affected animals from kids is prudent but not necessary from adult herd members. Severe infestation suggests a compromised immune system. Therefore clinicians and keepers should pay close attention to the nutrition program and general health of affected goats. Treatment may include weekly dipping with 0.5% malathion, 0.2% trichlorfon, or 0.5% amitraz.

Fly Strike

Fly strike has been known to effect the skin of sheep. Screw-worm *(Cochliomyia hominivorax)* has been eradicated from the United States but continued surveillance for larvae of this fly is prudent. These larvae are 1 to 2 cm long, pink, and tapered. The adult fly is blue-green, with an orange head and three dark longitudinal stripes on the body. Cutaneous myiasis (black blowfly, *Phormia regina*) occurs in sheep in the United States and is most common among breeds that have excessive skin folds such as Merino sheep. In Australia the sheep blowfly, *Lucilia cuprina*, is the major ectoparasite of sheep, causing severe damage from myiasis and death from secondary infections.[11-13] However, a variety of fly larvae can infest wounds that have necrotic tissue present. Skin lesions cause staining of wool and alopecia.

Elaeophorosis (Sorehead)

Elaeophora schneideri is a filarial nematode that can cause dermatopathy. The filaria cause thrombosis of capillary beds and terminal arteries. Tissue ischemia resulting from vascular injury causes severe lesions that appear similar to those of photosensitization and ulcerative dermatitis (Figure 8-5). Horse flies *(Hybomitra, Tabanus)* are intermediate hosts that transmit infective larvae from one host to another. Infective larvae migrate and develop to young adults in the leptomeningeal arteries. If thrombosis occurs at this level, circling, opisthotonos, convulsions, and other neurologic signs or sudden death may occur. Alternatively, the young adults may migrate to the common carotid and maxillary arteries and develop into mature adults. These adults produce microfilaria that embolize the capillary beds of the face and may cause ischemia or an allergic reaction. Lesions primarily occur on the face but may develop on other areas of the body. They are focal and consistent with vascular compromise and may require months or years to heal completely. Elaeophorosis should be included in the differential diagnosis of any unilateral lesions of the head. Skin biopsy may reveal the microfilaria either by histo-

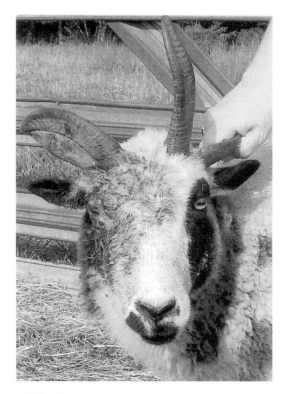

Figure 8-5   Suppurative dermatosis with lesion distribution typical of elaeophoriasis. Filarial showers result in thrombosis of the capillary beds of the face. (Courtesy Dr. Mike Pope, Paris, Kentucky.)

logic examination or by tissue maceration and harvest of larvae. Avermectin drugs (ivermectin 200 μg/kg SC) can kill the microfilaria, but repeated doses may be required. Adult nematodes can be killed by the administration of piperazine salts (50 mg/kg by mouth [PO]) or ivermectin.

Onchocerca Species Infestation

Onchocerca species can parasitize sheep and goats. Adult *Onchocerca* species can live in the connective tissues of sheep and goats, where they induce nodules. Adults produce microfilariae that migrate into the dermis of the ventral abdomen and thorax. Alopecia, erythema, and thickening of the skin develop because of the host's response to dying larvae.

Other nematodes diagnosed in cases of focal dermatitis include *Pelodera strongyloides*, *Strongyloides papillosus*, and *Parelaphostrongylus tenuis*. These nematodes have been associated with dermatitis, but their clinical significance is minimal. Strongyloidiasis is seen on dependent regions of the body; the localized dermatitis is caused by an immune reaction to migrating larvae. *P. tenuis* infestation of the central nervous system may cause focal regions of hyperesthesia. This may lead to self-trauma that the

keeper or clinician notes as excoriations or nonhealing ulcers.

REFERENCES

1. Smith MC, Sherman DM: Skin. In Smith MC, Sherman DM, editors: *Goat medicine*, Baltimore, 1994, Williams & Wilkins.
2. Lofstedt J: Dermatologic diseases of sheep, *Vet Clin North Am Large Anim Pract* 5:427, 1983.
3. Mullowney PC: Skin diseases of sheep, *Vet Clin North Am Large Anim Pract* 6(1):131, 1984.
4. Mullowney PC, Baldwin EW: Skin diseases of goats, *Vet Clin North Am Large Anim Pract* 6(1):143, 1984.
5. Smith MC: Dermatologic diseases of goats, *Vet Clin North Am Large Anim Pract* 5:449, 1983.
6. Manning TO, Scott DW, Smith MC: Caprine dermatology. Part III. Parasitic, allergic, hormonal, and neoplastic disorders, *Comp Cont Ed Pract Vet* 7:S437, 1985.
7. Jenkinson DM, Hutchinson G, McQueen DJL: Route of passage of cypermethrin across the surface of sheep skin, *Res Vet Sci* 41:237, 1986.
8. Britt AG et al: Effects of pour-on insecticidal formulation on sheep skin, *Aust Vet J* 61:329, 1984.
9. Johnson PW et al: Kinetic disposition of xylene-based or aqueous formulations of deltamethrin applied to the dorsal midline of sheep and their effect on lice, *Int J Parasitol* 25:471, 1995.
10. Fadok VA: Parasitic skin diseases of large animals, *Vet Clin North Am Large Anim Pract* 6(1):3, 1984.
11. Colditz IG, Eisemann CH: The effect of immune and inflammatory mediators on growth of *Lucilia cuprina* larvae in vitro, *Int J Parasitol* 24:401, 1994.
12. Sandeman RM et al: Hypersensitivity responses and repeated infections with *Lucilia cuprina*, the sheep blowfly, *Int J Parsitol* 22:1175, 1992.
13. Young AR, Meeusen EN, Bowles VM: Characterization of ES products involved in wound initiation by *Lucilia cuprina* larvae, *Int J Parasitol* 26:245, 1996.

AUTOIMMUNE DISEASES

Pemphigus Foliaceus

Pemphigus foliaceus is a rarely diagnosed autoimmune skin disease of goats characterized by widespread crusty, pruritic lesions.[1] It has been classified as a type II hypersensitivity reaction. Lesions are often first noted over the face or limbs but may be found on the abdomen, perineum, and scrotum as well (Figure 8-6). The proposed mechanism is the development of autoantibodies directed against the skin, specifically the glycocalyx of keratinocytes. Loss of intercellular cohesiveness results in blister formation and acantholysis.

Diagnosis.   A diagnosis of pemphigus foliaceus may be made from skin biopsy specimens obtained from characteristic skin lesions. Numerous biopsies should be taken from suspect goats to improve the accuracy of the diagno-

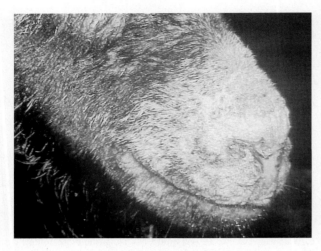

Figure 8-6 Pemphigus foliaceus in a pygmy goat. This autoimmune disease results in vesicles, pustules, and crusts over the body. Immunofluorescence of biopsied skin is a good diagnostic tool.

sis. The presence of acantholytic keratinocytes within vesicles is a diagnostic feature of pemphigus. Because acantholysis can be seen in other dermatologic conditions, biopsies should be evaluated by a veterinary pathologist with expertise in dermatopathies.

Treatment. Treatment of pemphigus is aimed at diminishing the body's immune response. Prednisolone (1 mg/kg every 24 hours for 7 days) in conjunction with aurothioglucose (1 mg/kg IM every 24 hours for 7 days) has been reported effective in controlling symptoms, followed by 1 mg/kg of prednisolone every 48 hours.

NUTRITIONAL DISEASES

Nutritional deficiencies and excesses are beyond the scope of this chapter and are discussed in other chapters (see Chapter 2). However, changes specific to the skin or hair are briefly discussed in the following paragraphs.

Fescue Toxicity

Fescue toxicosis is caused by ingestion of tall fescue grass *(Festuca arundinacea)* contaminated with an endophyte *(Acremonium [Neotyphodium] coenophialum)*. During winter months the toxins may cause a peripheral vasoconstriction leading to a gangrenous necrosis of the distal limbs and tail. Of the 35 to 40 million pasture acres in the United States, approximately 80% is infected. About 8 million acres of fescue grass are not infected with the endophytic fungus and therefore do not contain the ergovaline toxin. Sheep and goats appear to be less sensitive to the toxin than cows. Feeding noninfested fescue and diluting fescue by planting other species of grasses both help reduce the incidence of this condition.

Copper Deficiency

Copper deficiency or molybdenosis decreases wool quality and color. Wool quality suffers because of decreased crimp and a limp and steely texture. Dark wool loses color intensity until it is gray-white in color. This disease can result from absolute copper deficiency (pasture grass with less than 3 ppm dry matter copper) or excessive molybdenum (pasture grass with more than 10 ppm dry matter molybdenum), sulfur, or iron in the diet. Diagnosis can be made by assessing copper concentrations in the blood or liver. Copper deficiency is diagnosed if the blood copper concentration is less than 0.7 mg/dl or the liver concentration is less than 80 mg/kg dry weight (see Chapter 2).

Iodine Deficiency

Iodine deficiency (goiter) of newborn lambs manifests as alopecia, thick scaly skin, weakness, and enlarged thyroid glands.[2] Neonatal death, poor reproductive performance, and abortion may be seen in the flock or herd. Familial goiter occurs in Merino sheep, Dutch goats, and Nubian and Angora goats, among others. Iodine deficiency causes kids to be born hairless or with fine hair. The kids may be weak or stillborn and have goiters. Goiter also may be caused by congenital defects or ingestion of goitrogens in the diet. Dietary iodine deficiency is most common in geographic regions with sandy soil and heavy rainfall. Ingestion of large amounts of calcium, cyanogenic glycosides, and cruciferous plants also may induce iodine deficiency. Diagnosis of iodine deficiency can be made by identifying protein-bound iodine in serum (normal serum protein-bound iodine for adult ewes is 2.4 to 4 µg/dl serum). In herds known to be at risk for iodine deficiency, potassium iodide (250 mg) may be administered at 60 and again at 30 days before lambing (see Chapters 2 and 7). Providing a good-quality iodine-containing trace mineral supplement and removing pregnant animals from pastures containing goitrogenous plants decreases the occurrence of goiter.

Zinc Deficiency

Zinc deficiency is associated with parakeratosis and may cause reduced growth rate, wrinkled skin, swollen hocks, and salivation in sheep. Parakeratosis is most pronounced on the face, feet, and scrotum of affected animals. Rams fed a zinc-deficient diet develop abnormal testicles and experience impaired spermatogenesis. In goats the most prominent clinical signs include rough hair coat; hair loss on the head, limbs, and scrotum; overgrowth of the dental pad; small testicles; and fissures of the feet. The predominant histologic lesions are hyperkeratosis and parakeratosis.[3] Increased calcium and phosphorus intake decreases zinc absorption. Some goats may have a genetic predisposition to depressed zinc absorption. This is magnified in the face of high calcium (and other mineral) intake.[4] Diets rich in legumes (high calcium) or "homemade" high-phosphorus grain supplements (corn-soybean, corn-oats-barley) with no added minerals all predispose to zinc deficiency. A biopsy of the affected area indicating parakeratosis coupled with properly collected serum zinc concentrations of less than 0.8 ppm is diagnostic.[3] Blood drawn for zinc analysis should be collected in a special tube that does not have a butyl rubber stopper. Animals benefit from supplementation of a good-quality trace mineral salt offered free choice. Adding zinc to the feed or administering zinc sulfate (1 g/day PO) is usually effective.[3] If calcium makes up 1.5% of the diet, the zinc sulfate may not be effective and chelated zinc should be administered or added to a premixed salt supplement. Response to zinc supplementation should be rapid (within 14 days) (see Chapter 2). Removing legumes and cereal grains from the diet and feeding grass hay and commercially prepared concentrate feeds (with added zinc) is usually preventative.

Vitamin A Deficiency

Vitamin A deficiency may cause hair loss and night blindness, overgrown hooves, and corneal ulceration in adult goats.[2] Deficiency is rare if animals have access to green forage. If dry, brown forage is fed, inclusion of vitamin A in a supplement (mineral mixture) or use of a commercial injectable product helps prevent deficiency disease.

Photosensitization

Photosensitization is segregated into primary and secondary causes based on the pathophysiology of disease (Table 8-6). *Photosensitization* refers to conditions under which photodynamic chemicals accumulate in the skin and become stimulated by sunlight on exposed and unpigmented areas of the skin.[2,5-7] These substances damage the capillary beds and result in skin necrosis and sloughing. *Primary photosensitization* refers to ingested photodynamic substances that do not require alteration in the body to cause disease (Figure 8-7) (see Table 8-6). Primary photosensitization may occur after ingestion of St. John's wort, which contains hypericin; aphids containing an unknown photodynamic agent; or lush forage with accumulated phylloerythrin. This condition is most common in late summer and early autumn during periods of rapid pasture growth. Ingestion of alfalfa and other plants, including clover, lucerne, vetch, and oats, has been associated with photosensitization. The mechanism of pathology is not well understood. Secondary photosensitization occurs when liver damage results in the accumulation of photodynamic substances such as phylloerythrin in the bloodstream (Table 8-6). Liver damage may be

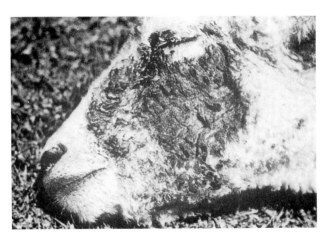

Figure 8-7   Phenothiazine photosensitization in a goat. Photosensitization is associated with edema, erythema, and pruritus. Lesions occur on unpigmented regions (e.g., back, ears, face). The primary form of the disease results from ingestion of a photodynamic chemical (in this case phenothiazine).

caused by the ingestion of plants containing pyrrolizidine alkaloids or carbon tetrachloride, *Pithomyces chartarum*–infected grasses, or blue-green algae *(Anacystis cyanea)*.

Clinical signs and diagnosis.   Clinical signs of photosensitization include head shaking, restlessness, erythema, and edema of eyelids, muzzle, ears, and tail. Skin lesions characteristically affect exposed, nonpigmented regions of the skin. Yellow serum may seep through the skin within 2 days and pruritus causes self-trauma. The transudate accumulates as a crust and superficial skin sloughing occurs. Secondary bacterial infection is common. Necropsy reveals subcutaneous edema and sloughing tissue. In cases of secondary photosensitization, liver disease may be obvious.

Treatment.   Treatment for photosensitization is symptomatic and includes the provision of shade, control of secondary infections, treatment of primary disease if liver damage is present, removal of animals from high-risk forage, allowance of grazing at night only, maintenance of hydration and access to electrolytes, and administration of nonsteroidal antiinflammatory drugs (NSAIDs) and antibiotics in severe cases. Photosensitization can be prevented by good pasture management and provision of adequate shade.

MYCOTOXINS

Pithomycotoxicosis

Pithomycotoxicosis (facial eczema) occurs in sheep and cattle of all ages in Australia, New Zealand, and South Africa. *Pithomyces chartarum* is a fungus that produces the

TABLE 8-6

CAUSES OF PHOTOSENSITIZATION IN SHEEP AND GOATS

SOURCE	TOXIN	SPECIES AFFECTED
PRIMARY PHOTOSENSITIZATION		
Plants		
St. John's wort	Hypericin	Any ruminant
Buckwheat	Fagopyrin, photofagopyrin	Any ruminant
Bishop's weed	Furocoumarins	Any ruminant
Dutchman's breeches	Furocoumarins	Any ruminant
Wild carrot	Furocoumarins	Any ruminant
Perennial ryegrass	Perloline	Any ruminant
Burr trefoil	Aphids	Any ruminant
Toxins		
Phenothiazine	Phenothiazine alkaloids	Any ruminant
Thiazides		Any ruminant
Methylene blue		Any ruminant
Sulfonamides		Any ruminant
Tetracyclines		Any ruminant
HEPATOGENOUS PHOTOSENSITIZATION		
Plants		
Rape, kale		Any ruminant
Kleingrass		Sheep
Caltrops	Saponins	Sheep
Lantana	Triterpene	Any ruminant
Ragworts, heliotrope	Pyrrolizidine alkaloids	Any ruminant
Mycotoxins		
Pithomyces chartarum (pasture grass, especially ryegrass)	Sporidesmin	Sheep, cattle
Anacystis (blue-green algae)	Alkaloid	Any ruminant
Periconia (Bermuda grass)		Any ruminant
Phomopsis leptostromiformis (lupin)	Acid-phenolic compounds	Any ruminant
Chemicals		
Copper		Any ruminant
Phosphorus		Any ruminant
Carbon tetrachloride		Any ruminant
Phenanthridium		Any ruminant
Bacterial hepatitis		
Viral hepatitis		
Parasitic hepatitis		
Hepatic neoplasia		

Adapted from Scott DW: *Large animal dermatology,* Philadelphia, 1988, WB Saunders.

mycotoxin sporidesmin; it is most often found in ryegrass. Sporidesmin is a hepatotoxin that causes hepatogenous photosensitization and phylloerythrin accumulation in the bloodstream. Morbidity is highest in summer and fall, especially when rains follow a period of drought.

Clinical signs. Clinical signs of pithomycotoxicosis include conjunctivitis, keratitis, restlessness, stomping of the feet, and lethargy. Edema of the eyelids and ears may be noted. Exudate accumulates on the skin, which then begins to slough. Sheep may suffer secondary infections and die in 2 weeks to 2 months.

Treatment. Feeding zinc sulfate (0.5 to 2 g/head/day) is protective for sheep grazing infected pastures. Applying thiabendazole (1 kg per acre) to the pasture has been reported to control the fungus.

Stachybotryotoxicosis

Stachybotryotoxicosis (poisoning by fungi of the genus *Stachybotrys*) has been reported in sheep. This fungal mycotoxin causes cutaneous necrosis, ulceration, petechiae, and ulceronecrotic areas, most pronounced in the mucocutaneous junctions. The toxin is a macrocyclic trichothecene that also causes bone marrow suppression, neutropenia, and thrombocytopenia.

ENVIRONMENTAL PATHOLOGIES

Intertrigo

Intertrigo occurs in areas of skin-to-skin contact; excessive motion results in moist dermatitis and inflammation because of friction. This most commonly occurs in ruminants between the udder and the inner aspect of the thigh. Treatment includes cleansing the region and applying an astringent ointment with the goal of drying the lesion. The disease is self-limiting in most animals, but pain may cause apparent lameness; moreover, the area may have a foul odor and secondary infection may increase the risk of mastitis.

Callus

A callus is formed on areas of the skin that receive chronic mild to moderate abrasion from objects in the environment. The most common location in sheep and goats is the dorsal aspect of the carpi and the sternum. Other locations include the cranial aspect of the stifle and the caudal aspect of the elbow. These lesions are normal unless they have associated exudate, swelling, or pain.

Hematoma

Blunt trauma can result in the formation of a hematoma. Hematomas may develop in exposed highly vascular tissues such as the ears or on the main body. Causes of trauma include injury from horned breeding males, fighting injury, attack by dogs or other predators, equipment-related injury, and entanglement with fences or other objects. Spontaneous bleeding under the skin is rare but may occur if ingestion of toxins causes coagulopathy.

Cutaneous Ulceration

Pressure sores (or cutaneous ulcerations) form when bony prominences are in prolonged contact with hard surfaces. They most commonly occur when sheep or goats rest in lateral recumbency because of musculoskeletal or neurologic disease. Pressure sores form because of prolonged ischemia and cellular injury (pressure necrosis). They can therefore be prevented or controlled by frequent movement of the animal. Contact with moist surfaces can accelerate this process because hydration of the skin weakens its resistance elasticity.

Foreign Bodies

Foreign bodies can become lodged in the skin by injury or surgery. In a study of skin reaction to suture materials in Borno white goats, researchers found that a prolonged inflammatory phase was associated with nylon and silk but not cotton or stainless steel suture material.[8] Stainless steel and nylon sutures produced a moderate amount of granulation tissue reaction, cotton suture produced a marked granulation response, and silk produced the smallest amount of granulation. Wounds sutured with cotton or stainless steel healed faster than those sutured with nylon or silk.

Subcutaneous Emphysema

Penetrating wounds or full-thickness lacerations that act as one-way valves can result in subcutaneous emphysema. In these cases air is allowed to enter but not freely exit from the subcutaneous tissues (bellows effect). Subcutaneous emphysema also occurs in sheep and goats with pneumonia, especially after parturition. The weakened lung parenchyma may rupture into the mediastinum if excessive intrathoracic pressure is applied against a closed glottis (as occurs during parturition). The air dissects along tissue planes and exits through the thoracic inlet to the subcutaneous spaces.

Clinical signs.   Subcutaneous emphysema typically is noted along the neck, dorsal to the shoulder; it may dissect along the back. The condition also may occur with clostridial infections. Often affected animals are found dead and subcutaneous emphysema is discovered during necropsy. However, emphysema may be noted on physical examination early in the infectious process. Clostridial disease should be considered in the differential diagnosis if the animal exhibits severe systemic disease in the presence of subcutaneous emphysema.

Burns

Skin burns are most commonly found on animals that have been trapped in building fires. Pour-on products containing alcohol are flammable but usually do not ignite the hair coat and do not continue to burn after the fluid volume is consumed. Burns may be classified by severity and extent of the body surface area involved. Sequelae of burn injuries include secondary infection, especially with *Pseudomonas*, and hypoproteinemia from protein exudation from the wounds. Severe or extensive burns are more likely to result in fatal infection or protein losses. Smoke inhalation and thermal damage to the lungs also can cause death. The clinician should perform a thorough evaluation of the thorax after the initial injury and follow up later because the onset of clinical disease may be delayed. Burns in sheep and goats are likely to occur as a result of inappropriate heat lamp placement in maternity pens. Lambs and kids stand under the lamps for warmth and may burn the dorsum as a result. Pour-on products or irritants such as creosote and strong iodine can cause chemical burns on areas of skin contact.

Clinical signs. Depending on its severity a burn may produce only superficial scabbing or it may result in serum exudation and suppuration with deeper skin layer involvement. Because wool is fire-retardant, the most severe burns on sheep exposed to barn or grass fires are likely to be found around the head and limbs, whereas goats are likely to have severe burns over their entire bodies.

Treatment. Evaluation of the patient's overall condition is essential in a fire because smoke inhalation and thermal damage to the respiratory tract may cause death. Treatment is aimed at preventing or controlling secondary infection. Pain management and administration of plasma (if needed to address hypoproteinemia caused by excessive serum exudation from the wounds) are common therapeutic elements.

Sunburn

Sunburn in animals, as in human beings, is caused by skin damage from ultraviolet light. Sunburn is different from photosensitization.[3,4] It is more commonly seen in white-faced sheep (especially on the face and ears), particularly those that have been recently shorn, and light-colored goats (especially on the udders, ears, and nose).[3] Prolonged sun exposure is associated with tumors (e.g., squamous cell carcinoma).

Clinical signs. Clinical signs of sunburn include erythema, swelling, crusting of skin, head shaking, and pruritus. If the udder is affected, animals will resent milking or being nursed.[9]

Treatment. Treatment includes the application of pigmented teat dips and the application of sunburn lotion on the udder (for dairy goats), the provision of adequate shelter, and gradual light exposure for light-pigmented animals. In cases of secondary bacterial infection the use of topical or systemic antimicrobial agents is warranted.[3,4]

Frostbite

Prolonged exposure to extremely cold temperatures may result in frostbite. Young stock are most prone to frostbite injury, and the extremities (ears, tail, feet) are most com-monly involved. Death from low body core temperature ensues if treatment is not initiated before vital organs are compromised. Frostbite may occur at a variety of temperatures depending on environmental conditions (sunlight, moisture, wind). The crucial temperature threshold for milk-fed neonates has been suggested to be 13° C (55° F).[7] Injury is caused by vasoconstriction, subsequent arterial thrombosis, and ischemic necrosis. After sloughing, damaged ears tend to be rounded with alopecic tips.[3] If the surface of the skin is wet, ice crystals can form, accelerating the process. Frostbite injuries occur in four phases.[10,11] Phase one (pre-freeze) is characterized by arteriolar constriction, venous dilatation, congestion, and serum transudation. Phase two (freeze-thaw) begins with extracellular ice crystal formation. Phase three (vascular stasis) is denoted by more severe and persistent venous dilatation and arterial spasm, which causes arteriovenous shunting and tissue hypoxia. Phase four (ischemia) is denoted by nervous tissue damage caused by prolonged local hypoxia.

Treatment. The therapy for frostbite may result in reperfusion injury. Nevertheless, it should be instituted immediately and continued for at least the first few days after injury. Warming in water of 104° to 106° F is recommended, as is the use of antibiotics and antiinflammatory drugs as needed to control tissue damage. Necrotic tissue should be débrided as needed to facilitate healing and limit secondary bacterial infection.

Prevention. An easily accessible shelter should be provided. For each degree drop in ambient temperature below 0° C, the keeper should offer a 0.5% to 1% increase in feed. Feeding ewes and does in barns keeps them and their lambs and kids out of the cold weather and in a warmer condition.

Wool Slip and Wool Break

Goats naturally shed their coats in spring. Sheep, however, continuously grow wool and should not shed it. Shorn sheep being housed for winter can, however, experience complete loss of wool (wool slip).[3,9] The affected skin is smooth, free of ectoparasites, and shows no signs of disease. No treatment is required and the wool does grow back.[3,9] Wool slip has been associated in some sheep with copper deficiency (low serum copper and cold stress).[9] Therefore possible deficiencies in dietary copper should be investigated.

Stressors such as parasitism and systemic disease can cause sheep to undergo a cessation in wool growth and can weaken the fiber (wool break). Wool can be lost within days of a systemic stress (anagen defluxion) or within 2 to 3 months after the stress (telogen defluxion). In both cases the wool does grow back over time. The practical application of this information is in educating the owners of pet sheep that survive a systemic illness—the clinician should warn the neophyte owner of the potential for fiber loss.

CONGENITAL PATHOLOGIES

Several forms of congenital skin disorders are of clinical interest. Because of good identification and culling practices, most are fairly rare.[12,13]

Hepatogenous Photosensitization

Southdown lambs have an autosomal recessive trait that can result in hepatogenous photosensitization.[13] The defect causes congenital hyperbilirubinemia and subsequent photosensitization. Corriedale lambs have an assumed inherited condition, similar to Dubin-Johnson syndrome in human beings, characterized by a failure to transfer phylloerythrin and conjugated bilirubin.

Epitheliogenesis Imperfecta

Epitheliogenesis imperfecta has been diagnosed in numerous breeds of sheep. It is an autosomal recessive genetic defect in cattle. Epithelial defects in the oral cavity (including the tongue and hard palate) are noted at birth. Hoof horn can easily be separated from the underlying laminae.

Collagen Tissue Dysplasia (Ehlers-Danlos Syndrome)

Collagen tissue dysplasia, or Ehlers-Danlos syndrome, appears to be a hereditary skin disease of Norwegian sheep. Skin wounds develop rapidly after birth because of collagen defects.[13] Affected lambs die soon after birth because of secondary infection. This genetic defect results in the failure of collagen bundles to form in a functional configuration.

Hypotrichosis Congenita

Hypotrichosis congenita is a viable hypotrichosis—that is, the disease is not immediately fatal to affected neonates. It is hereditary in polled Dorset sheep. Affected lambs have sparse hair fibers, most pronounced on the face and limbs.

Epidermolysis Bullosa

Epidermolysis bullosa is a recessive heritable defect of Weisses Alenschaf sheep and has been diagnosed in Suffolk and South Dorset Down breeds of sheep as well.[13,14] Affected animals are born without type VII collagen and develop wounds rapidly after epidermal abrasion.[13] Skin biopsy reveals separation of the dermal-epidermal junction in the absence of epidermolysis. The hooves may slough and ulcers of the gingiva, hard palate, tongue, and mouth form rapidly.[14]

Hairy Shaker Disease of Lambs

Border disease, or hairy shaker disease, is a congenital condition caused by a pestivirus that may be transmitted vertically from the ewe to the fetus in utero. Newborn lambs have domed heads, short limbs, and thick trunks. Viral infection of the fetus before day 80 of gestation may interfere with the development of primary hair follicles and result in the formation of "kempy" fibers and long halo fibers in the fleece. Affected lambs appear abnormally hairy and are called *hairy shaker* lambs because tonic-clonic contractions of their skeletal muscles cause them to shake. Diagnosis is confirmed by virus isolation or a necropsy finding of hypomyelinogenesis in the central nervous system (see Chapters 6 and 13).

NEOPLASIA

Neoplasia is occasionally diagnosed in sheep and goats. Some breed predilections have been described for various tumors (Table 8-7).

PAPILLOMAS (WARTS, FIBROPAPILLOMATOSIS)

Warts in sheep are caused by species-specific papovaviruses. These DNA viruses cause papillomas on the face and legs that vary in size but may be as large as 4 cm in diameter and 2 cm in height. These lesions are vascular and bleed when disrupted. Secondary bacterial infection may occur with repeated trauma to the lesion. A cellular immune response eventually clears the lesions, which may require months to regress. Failure of lesions to regress or excessive numbers of lesions suggests that the immune

---

TABLE 8-7

BREED PREDILECTIONS FOR SKIN TUMORS

BREED	TUMOR
Saanen goats	Udder papillomatosis
Angora goats	Squamous cell carcinoma
	Melanoma
Merino sheep	Squamous cell carcinoma
	Follicular cysts
Suffolk sheep	Melanoma
Nubian goats	Wattle cysts

Adapted from Scott DW: *Large animal dermatology*, Philadelphia, 1988, WB Saunders.

system is not competent. A viral cause has not been confirmed in goats. Papillomas on the udder of Saanen goats have been documented; they tend to persist without undergoing the regression typical of viral papillomas.

SQUAMOUS CELL CARCINOMAS

Squamous cell carcinomas are most commonly diagnosed in Merino sheep and are usually seen in sheep older than 4 years. The peak incidence (12%) was observed in 12-year-old sheep. Tumors occur on the face, ears, and vulva but most commonly involve the ears. As the tumor grows, the surface may become ulcerated because of tissue necrosis or self-trauma. Diagnosis is made by histopathologic examination of tissue specimens. Characteristic lesions exhibit acanthosis, pseudoepitheliomatous hyperplasia, and hyperkeratosis. Inflammation associated with ulceration or secondary bacterial infection is not uncommon. Ultraviolet radiation has been implicated in squamous cell carcinoma; photosensitive sheep are at greatest risk. Lesions in the ear, such as from ear tags, are more prone to mutate into squamous cell carcinoma. Treatment is by surgical excision with wide margins, but early culling is common.

MELANOMA

Melanoma has an unknown incidence in sheep and goats. One survey of the skins of 37,026 sheep and 23,429 goats found only two melanomas, both occurring on goats.[15] Another survey indicated an incidence of 0.03% cutaneous melanoma in goats.[12]

HEMANGIOMA

Hemangioma has been diagnosed in a sheep by one of the authors (Dr. Rings). The lesion affected the distal rear limb of a ewe (Figure 8-8). Diagnosis was confirmed by histology after surgical excision.

DRUG RESIDUE ISSUES

Preservation of a wholesome product, free of contaminants, is paramount to the sheep and goat industry.[16] Nearly all treatments for skin diseases are performed in an extra-label manner because relatively few drugs are approved for use in sheep and goats. Veterinarians must work diligently with industry personnel to ensure quality. In the United States keepers and clinicians should respect the treatment guidelines described in the Animal Medical Drug Use and Clarification Act (AMDUCA) to avoid residue contamination of meat and milk. Sheep and goats differ from cattle in both size of drug dosages and drug elimination times. Therefore whenever possible, drug withdrawal times should be established from research performed specifically on sheep and goats.

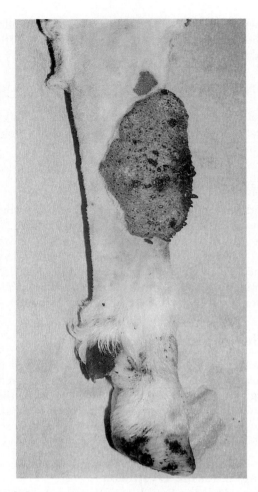

Figure 8-8 Hemangioma on the frontal surface of the rear leg of a ewe. Note the proliferative nature of the lesion. Such lesions can be surgically excised.

References

1. Scott DW: *Large animal dermatology*, Philadelphia, 1988, WB Saunders.
2. Scott DW, Smith MC, Manning TO: Caprine dermatology. Part II. Viral, nutritional, environmental, and congenitohereditary disorders, *Comp Cont Ed Pract Vet* 6:S473, 1984.
3. Smith MC: Small ruminant dermatology, *Proceedings of the 1998 Symposium on Small Ruminants for the Mixed Animal Practitioner Western Veterinary Conference*, 1998, Las Vegas, NV.
4. Linklater KA, Smith MC: *Color atlas of diseases and disorders of the sheep and goat*, Aylesbury, UK, 1993, Wolfe Publishing.
5. Smith MC, Sherman DM: Skin. In Smith MC, Sherman DM, editors: *Goat medicine*, Baltimore, 1994, Williams & Wilkins.
6. Kimberling CV: Diseases of the skin. In Kimberling CV, editor: *Jensen and Swift's diseases of sheep*, ed 3, Philadelphia, 1988, Lee & Febiger.
7. Smith MC: Dermatologic diseases of goats, *Vet Clin North Am Large Anim Pract* 5:449, 1983.
8. Mohammed A, Rabo JS, Ibrahim AA: Reaction to skin suture materials in Borno white goats, *Small Rumin Res* 16:191, 1995.
9. Mitchell GBB: Non-parasitic skin diseases in sheep. In Boden E, editor: *Sheep and goat practice*, London, 1991, Bailliere Tindall.

10. Gonzalez-Jimenez E, Blaxter KL: The metabolism and thermal regulation of calves in the first month of life, *Br J Nutr* 16:199, 1962.
11. Pelton JA et al: Frostbite in calves, *Comp Cont Ed Pract Vet* 22:S136, 2000.
12. Venkatesan RA et al: Survey of the incidence of various surface defects in goat and sheep skins in Madras, *Leather Sci* 24:255, 1977.
13. Basrur PK, Yadav BR: Genetic diseases of sheep and goats, *Vet Clin North Am Food Anim Pract* 6:779, 1990.
14. Steffen DJ: Congenital skin abnormalities, *Vet Clin North Am* 9:105, 1993.
15. Venkatesan RA, Nandy SC, Santappa M: A note on the incidence of melanoma on goat skin, *Ind J Anim Sci* 49:154, 1979.
16. Bretzlaff K: Special problems of hair goats, *Vet Clin North Am Food Anim Pract* 6:721, 1990.

REMOVAL OF WATTLES, SCENT GLANDS, AND HORNS, AND OTHER SKIN PROCEDURES

Wattles

Wattles are skin appendages that are found in the cervical regions of some goats (see Figure 8-3). Although they are usually encountered in the mid-neck, they also may be found on the face or ears.[1] They are composed of connective tissue, nerves, blood vessels, smooth muscles, and a cartilaginous core.[1] Cysts may be found in the bases of some wattles.[1] These cysts may be hereditary and either bilateral or unilateral. If swollen, the cysts will be filled with a clear fluid. Wattles may become injured (e.g., caught in feeders or fences), detract from the appearance of show animals, make clipping and grooming difficult, and may be chewed or nursed by other kids or adults.[1,2] For these reasons, some owners wish to have them removed. When animals are young (2 to 4 days), wattles can be removed at castration or dehorning. Slight tension can be placed on the wattle before its base is cut with scissors.[1,2] If excessive bleeding occurs, pressure should be applied. The skin should heal without further therapy.

Disbudding

Some management styles prefer that goats (and occasionally rams) have their horn buds removed during the first 2 weeks of life.[2] However, many meat, fiber, and pet goat owners prefer to keep horned animals. Disbudding is more common among dairy goat producers to reduce fighting-related injuries. Kids can be held or placed in a dehorning box. They can be sedated (xylazine 0.05 to 0.2 mg/kg), have a ring of tissue around the horn anesthetized (2% lidocaine SC), or be placed under general anesthesia. A dehorning box encloses all of the body except the head. The heat from a commercial electric de-

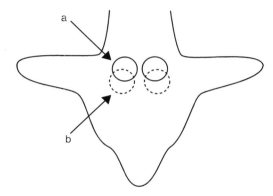

Figure 8-9 A view of the kid from the top of its head. The area for applying the cauterizing unit for descenting *(a)* and dehorning *(b)* is shown. The clinician should take care to avoid causing excessive thermal damage to the underlying bone and nervous tissue. (Adapted from Williams CSF: Routine sheep and goat procedures, *Vet Clin North Am Food Anim Pract* 6(3):753, 1990.)

horning iron (for cattle or goats) or an electric cautery unit may be used. Regardless of the method, clipping all hair around the area aids the process. If an electric dehorning iron is used for this purpose, Williams[2] has recommended allowing it to heat and then applying it to a pine board. If the iron makes a slightly depressed black ring on the board, the proper temperature has been achieved.[2] The dehorner should be applied in a rocking manner over the horn buds (Figure 8-9). The area should be burned until a copper color is attained. If the hot iron is correctly applied the horn "cap" should be easily removed. Williams[2] recommends burning the horn until the central core is removed. Common mistakes with this method are heat-induced meningitis and underheating of the germinal epithelium of the horn, resulting in the regrowth of abnormal horn tissue.[1,2] If the germinal horn tissue is not completely destroyed, the scar that regrows can be removed later. The calvarium of a kid is thin and the cornual sinus is small compared with those of calves. Heat-induced malacia of the underlying cerebrum can result in depression, blindness, abscess formation, and death.

Meat-induced meningitis and malacia is rarely reversible. Still, in such cases immediate treatment with glucocorticosteroids (dexamethasone sodium phosphate 1 to 2 mg/kg IV), mannitol (0.25 to 1 mg/kg IV over 5 minutes), and possibly NSAIDs are indicated.

An alternative to cauterization of the horn buds is surgical removal. This can best be accomplished in 2- to 4-day-old kids using a similar method as described for heat removal. Instead of using a dehorning iron or electric cautery, the clinician makes a circumferential incision through the anesthetized skin and removes the horn bud and germinal tissue. To control hemorrhage the area can be cauterized or firm digital pressure can be applied.

Caustic paste also is used to remove the horns of young kids. Clipping the hair around the horn buds aids in the application of the paste. If caustic paste is used, lanolin or petroleum jelly should be applied around the area, particularly around the eyes. The clinician should take care to prevent the caustic ointment from injuring the kids' eyes or other soft tissues. This method should be relegated to animals kept indoors (out of the rain), kids not nursing their dams, and those not able to rub the caustic ointment onto other kids.

Dehorning

Kids older than 2 to 3 weeks of age, those whose previous dehorning has resulted in the growth of an abnormal horn tissue (scur), and adult goats are all candidates for dehorning. The animal can be sedated or placed under general anesthesia; alternatively, a ring of skin around the horn or the cornual branches of the lacrimal and supratrochlear nerves can be anesthetized (see Figure 16-7).

In adults and particularly in males with large horns, general anesthesia is recommended. However, sedation (xylazine 0.05 to 0.2 mg/kg) and local anesthesia of the cornual branches of the lacrimal and infratrochlear nerves may be employed. The owner should be forewarned that this procedure is usually a "bloody mess." The wounds can take a long time to heal, result in secondary sinusitis, leave holes that never completely heal, or possibly result in brain abscesses. The skin around the horns should be clipped and surgically prepared. The clinician makes a circular incision through the skin 2 mm outside of the horn-skin junction.[3] The strip of skin between the two horns should be left to improve and shorten healing time. An obstetric wire is then "laid into" the incision. A helper-technician holds the head to prevent excessive motion, and the surgeon stands in front of the animal. The cut should be made in a rostral-ventral direction. Hemorrhage can be controlled by cautery or pressure. If the animal has a small horn base, the surrounding skin can be undermined and stretched over the opening created by the horn removal.[1] Pulling the skin over the surgical site allows for a more speedy recovery but is rarely possible in adult males. An antibiotic ointment (triple antibiotic) can be applied and a gauze pad or other absorbable material can be placed over each horn. The pads can be held in place by tape wrapped around the head or by a stocking with eye holes.[1] Animals can be given antibiotics (penicillin 20,000 IU/kg BID), NSAIDs, tetanus prophylaxis (tetanus antitoxin 150 to 300 IU), or tetanus toxoid. Fly control measures should be instituted. The bandage should be changed and the area examined every 2 to 4 days or as needed. An alternative is to use a small Barnes dehorner to cut or nip off the horn tissue. The cut should be made carefully to avoid injuring the thin skull. The area can then be cauterized to control bleeding and destroy all remaining germinal epithelium.

An alternative method is to cut the horn off at the tip, mid-horn, or as close to level with the skull as possible, depending on the desire of the owner and the animal's use. This should be done on a sedated or an anesthetized goat. The horn can be cut with obstetric wire or a dehorning saw. The animal should be monitored for sinusitis, and the horn will continue to grow.

Descenting

Because of the smell associated with bucks, some owners request the removal of these animals' sebaceous glands. Removal of these glands may improve the smell, but odor will probably not be completely prevented. In young buck kids the area behind the horns (see Figure 8-9) can be cauterized during dehorning. In the adult the glands are located in thickened, folded skin caudad-medial to the horn base. The gland opening is a hairless area at the base of a skin fold.[2] Washing the head helps the clinician visualize the scent glands. The buck should be anesthetized or heavily sedated, the hair clipped, and the area surgically prepared. The clinician then makes an incision through the skin 1.5 to 2 cm around the gland opening. The incision should be deepened to the periosteum, the area dissected, and the gland identified and removed.[2] The clinician should attempt to close the skin defect. However, this is most difficult in older males because of the skin hypertrophy in this area. If the skin is not easily sutured, an antibiotic ointment can be applied and the area allowed to granulate.

References

1. Smith MC, Sherman DM: *Goat medicine*, Philadelphia, 1994, Lee & Febiger.
2. Williams CSF: Routine sheep and goat procedures, *Vet Clin North Am Food Anim Pract* 6:737, 1990.
3. Hooper RN: General surgical techniques for small ruminants: Part I, *Proceedings of the 1998 Symposium on Small Ruminants for the Mixed Animal Practitioner Western Veterinary Conference*, 1998, Las Vegas, NV.

Chapter 9

Diseases of the Musculoskeletal System

LAURA K. REILLY, A.N. BAIRD, AND D.G. PUGH

EXAMINATION

Sheep and goats are naturally herd animals that prefer living and staying in a group. Therefore any examination of these animals on the farm should include initial observation of the entire group if possible. Flock observation is probably less important in the evaluation of traumatic musculoskeletal conditions than when animals are affected by infectious diseases, parasitism, nutritional disorders, and improper management. When the herd has a higher than expected incidence of fractures or injury, the practitioner should look for potential hazards around feeders and other objects. Veterinarians should look closely for animals that lay down or walk on their knees when their herdmates are moving around. Animals also should be observed for difficulty in rising, swollen or enlarged joints, lameness, and abnormal stance.

When examining an individual animal, the clinician should perform careful, meticulous palpation and close examination. Some animals may have obvious fractures and wounds. Those with more subtle problems require thorough examination. The clinician should first examine the feet for overgrown hooves, abscesses, interdigital lesions, exudate, and any foul smell. The coronary band should be examined for swelling, hyperemia, and proliferative lesions. All limb joints should be evaluated for swelling associated with trauma, septic arthritis, and infectious disease. The clinician should flex and extend the animal's joints through the entire range of motion to detect pain or laxity. In cases of hindlimb lameness, the clinician also should evaluate the patella for laxity, movement, and pain. Any asymmetry associated with swelling or muscle atrophy should be noted. Sciatic or peroneal nerve injury can occur after intramuscular injections and may produce lameness and muscle atrophy.

ANATOMY

Sheep and goats, like cattle, are members of the *Bovidae* family. They join several other even-toed animals in the order *Artiodactyla*. Animals in this order share three skeletal characteristics: the talus has distal and proximal trochleae; the calcaneus and fibula articulate with each other; and the limb axis divides the fused third and fourth metacarpal-metatarsal bones and the associated digits.[1] Sheep have short, blunt spinous processes of the cervical vertebra, whereas those of goats are longer, pointed, and have sharp edges. Small ruminants have 7 cervical vertebrae, 13 thoracic vertebrae, 6 or 7 lumbar vertebrae, 4 sacral vertebrae, and 16 to 18 caudal vertebrae. The presence of seven cervical vertebrae is a reliable trait in identification. However, variations are not unusual, such as 12 or 14 thoracic vertebrae or 5 lumbar vertebrae. Occasionally, an unusual transitional vertebra that is difficult to classify is found between the thoracic and lumbar vertebrae.[1] The authors describe a few of the musculoskeletal differences between sheep and goats within this chapter, as well as some of the variations from cattle. However, a thorough description of small ruminant anatomy is beyond the scope of this text.

REFERENCE

1. Getty R, Sisson S: *Sisson and Grossman's the anatomy of domestic animals*, ed 5, Philadelphia, 1975, WB Saunders.

GENERAL HOOF CARE

Most lameness in small ruminants is associated with pathology of the foot. Surveys have found that the incidence of foot disorders varies from approximately 10% to 19%.[1,2] Overgrown hooves are one of the most common foot disorders. Many foot disorders can be attributed to environmental, nutritional, and anatomic factors, but some can be prevented by proper trimming and management. With increased nutritional intake, and particularly with enhanced protein intake, hooves tend to grow more rapidly.

The hooves of small ruminants have fewer problems in a dry environment. The incidence of hoof disorders is higher in seasons of more precipitation and when housing is allowed to become humid, wet, or muddy. Fewer problems are seen when the animals can move about on hard, dry surfaces. Most sheep and goats require hoof trimming because of lack of adequate exercise on a hard, dry surface to wear down hoof material naturally; because of chronic laminitis; or because of fast hoof growth resulting from intensive feeding practices designed to increase production. Some herds may require foot trimming every 6 weeks to 2 months to minimize the incidence of foot disorders. Hooves can usually be trimmed adequately with shears, although a hoof knife also may be useful.[1]

During trimming some goats will stand, others need to be "set up" on their rumps, and others will stand in a stanchion. Some individuals prefer to trim the feet of sheep with them restrained in a tilt chute. The authors of this chapter prefer to trim the feet of sheep with them sitting on their rumps; foot trimming in goats is easier if the animals stand and the operator stands to the side. If an animal is allowed to stand, it should be tied. This allows the animal to be secured between the operator and a wall during foot trimming.[1] Regardless of the method, complete restraint is crucial to proper hoof care.

The clinician or keeper should shape the foot to match the angle of the coronary band while trimming the toe wall and sole (Figure 9-1). Dirt that has become packed into the toe should be cleaned out so the operator can de-

termine the amount of toe horn to be removed. After trimming, the hoof wall and the coronary band should be almost parallel. Trimming of the lateral wall corrects many hoof problems. After trimming the toe and lateral wall, the clinician or keeper should cut the inner wall shorter than the outer wall. The rubbery heel should be cut if it is excessively long or overgrown. The outer hoof wall should be slightly longer than any other hoof structure because it is a weight-bearing surface (Figure 9-2). If the hoof is improperly trimmed, the sheep or goat may walk on the toe or side of the foot or on the heel with the toe pointing up. A common cause of foot problems is an inward-turning outer wall that produces areas that accumulate debris and become infected. The inner wall may occasionally overgrow toward the interdigital cleft and predispose the animal to interdigital disease. The foot will be better balanced if the operator removes the toe curl by trimming the solar surface of the hoof and keeping it level rather than dubbing or shortening the toe. In sheep and goat flocks kept on soft pastures or paddocks, placing feeders on rough surfaces helps decrease the amount of trimming needed. Building or stacking rough material (cement or concrete blocks) for goats to play on also may help minimize the need for frequent trimming.

Feeding affects hoof condition and growth. Animals being overfed energy and protein and living on soft ground may be more prone to some abnormalities. As a general rule a well-balanced feeding program with a free choice mineral salt supplement consisting of calcium, phosphorus, and trace minerals is all that is required. However, some feeding programs may enhance hoof growth and health and are useful in special circumstances.

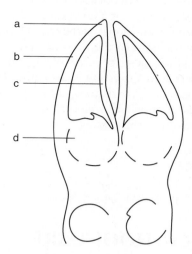

Figure 9-1 The bottom of the sheep or goat's foot. The toe *(a)* should be cleaned out, and the outer hoof wall *(b)* should be cut to remove all overgrowths, bring the wall down to the sole, and make the outer wall parallel with the coronary band. The inner hoof wall *(c)* is then cut, with more inside wall than outside wall being removed. The heel *(d)* should not be cut unless it is badly overgrown.

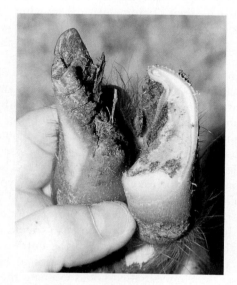

Figure 9-2 This hoof requires trimming. After cleaning the toe, the practitioner trims the toe and lateral walls. The inner wall is then trimmed, and the procedure is repeated on the other toe.

In other ruminants (cattle), diets that change normal rumen function by increasing the fermentation rate negatively affect the hoof health.[3] The ingestion of high-energy feeds coupled with inadequate fiber intake can result in suboptimal hoof health. In rations in which concentrates and roughage are fed separately, the concentrated portion of the diet should be divided into two or more equal feedings each day. This not only promotes overall health but also may help reduce the microflora changes that alter normal rumen fermentation and predispose animals to founder. Forage should always make up more than 30% to 50% of the dry matter content of the ration. Lush, young forage rarely provides enough effective fiber to optimize rumen fermentation. The feeding of buffers, particularly in high-concentrate diets, may help the rumen resist digestive upsets and thereby prevent subsequent hoof disease. Abnormal rapid hoof growth can occur when abnormal rumen fermentation is induced by the ingestion of lush, well-fertilized pastures.[3]

Hoof health also can be affected by certain vitamins and minerals. The addition of 20 mg of biotin improves short-term healing of hoof and claw lesions and decreases hoof disease in cattle.[3] Furthermore, diets that acidify the rumen decrease the microbial synthesis of biotin. One of the authors (Dr. Pugh) prefers to include biotin (3 to 4 mg/day) in sheep and goat rations for animals with a history of hoof disease. Other vitamins that play major roles in hoof health include vitamins A and E and the vitamin A precursor beta-carotene. Adequate dietary vitamin A and beta-carotene are needed for normal cell replication, epithelial repair, and immune function. Vitamin E maintains cellular integrity and normal immune function. Diets should be fortified with both of these nutrients if hoof problems occur and in cases in which production practices predispose to hoof disease (see Chapter 2).

Calcium is the largest mineral component of hooves and is required for normal hoof growth. Dietary calcium concentrations should range between 0.6% and 0.8% of the diet, with the calcium-to-phosphorus ratio being maintained between 1:1 and 2:1. Of the trace minerals that appear to affect hoof growth, zinc, copper, and, to a lesser extent, molybdenum and manganese, are most crucial.[3] Zinc is required for normal immunity, horn tissue production, vitamin A metabolism, epithelial repair, and hoof hardness. Studies in range, dairy, and feedlot cattle have all shown improved hoof health and decreased lameness when zinc is added to the diet, particularly in a chelated form (zinc methionine).[3] The use of such minerals also may be of value in improving overall hoof health. In sheep the administration of oral zinc sulfate (0.5 g daily) to prevent footrot has shown mixed results.[4-6] In cases of high legume intake (high calcium), zinc in the chelated form (zinc methionine) may be beneficial. Copper is needed for keratin synthesis and normal immune function and as a cofactor for many enzyme systems in the body. Copper deficiency in the body may be primary (inadequate copper in the diet) or conditioned by other dietary factors (excessive dietary molybdenum, sulfur, or iron). The dietary copper-to-molybdenum ratio should be maintained between 4:1 and 6:1 to maintain adequate copper availability.

Excessive nitrogen fertilization and liming of soils may depress copper and selenium uptake by plants. Heavily fertilized forage and roughage harvested after a drought may be sources of nitrates, which are reduced to nitrites by anaerobic microbial metabolism in the rumen. Nitrites can have a direct effect on hoof growth, resulting in abnormal horn tissue in cattle and possibly other ruminants.[3]

The key to maintaining healthy hoof tissue with respect to nutrition lies in minimizing rumen acidosis and fortifying the diet with certain nutrients (e.g., biotin, calcium, zinc).

DISEASES OF THE FOOT

Infectious Footrot

Infectious footrot is a severe, contagious disease of sheep, and to a lesser extent goats, that leads to significant economic losses as a result of weight loss, low fleece weight, labor and treatment costs, and premature culling. Many factors contribute to the disease, but the primary agent is the anaerobic bacterium *Dichelobacter nodosus (Bacteroides nodosus)*. Previous infection by *Fusobacterium necrophorum* contributes to the development of footrot. *Corynebacterium (Actinomyces) pyogenes* infection may increase the susceptibility of the hoof to the other two bacteria. Many strains of *D. nodosus* have been identified, and they can generally be classified as benign or virulent. Virulent strains have a greater keratolytic ability, which is associated with the production of a heat-stable protease.[1,2,7-9]

Footrot occurs worldwide wherever periods of warmth and prolonged wetness occur. In many regions the spring and fall are the times when transmission is most likely. If conditions are favorable, a significant portion of the flock can be affected. All ages are susceptible, but the severity of disease generally increases with age. Merino sheep are most susceptible to disease, and some breeds (Gulf Coast native) are more resistant. Some individuals do not become infected or have less severe signs, and a genetic basis for resistance is suspected.[8,9] Excessive hoof growth and, anecdotally, hoof color (white) may predispose to the condition.[4]

The source of *D. nodosus* is the feet of infected animals, which transfer the organism to the soil where it contacts the feet of other sheep.[8] The organism can survive only a few days to a few weeks in the environment but can persist for years in carrier sheep and goats. New infections usually are preceded by the introduction of new animals or exposure to ground that has recently been occupied by an infected flock. Management practices that allow the concentration of animals in small areas, irrigated pastures, long grass (which may abrade the interdigital skin), and wet or rainy conditions all predispose to infection.[4,8]

Pathogenesis. Wet conditions leading to maceration of tissue encourage infection with *F. necrophorum* (and occasionally *A. pyogenes*) which is thought to be necessary for infection by *D. nodosus* to occur.[4] *F. necrophorum* produces a mild clinical syndrome known as *interdigital dermatitis* in sheep that usually resolves when the ground becomes drier.[8] Interdigital dermatitis may produce severe lameness in goats.

When sheep or goats with interdigital dermatitis are exposed to a benign strain of *D. nodosus*, the soft horn becomes under-run but no further pathology occurs. This condition is known as *benign* (or *nonprogressive*) *footrot*. If sheep come into contact with a virulent strain of *D. nodosus*, a much more severe disease known as *virulent footrot* results.

Clinical signs. Footrot usually affects both claws in more than one foot. Benign footrot is characterized by inflammation and necrosis of the interdigital tissue. The soft horn is pale, pitted, and may be separated from the skin, but this separation does not involve the hard horn. With benign footrot, often only one or a few animals in a flock are affected. Virulent footrot, in contrast, is marked by severe lameness in numerous animals in the flock, with under-running of the hard horn beginning near the heel on the axial surface. In severe cases the entire horn may separate from the underlying tissue. Affected areas produce a malodorous exudate. Animals may carry the affected leg, graze on their knees, or remain recumbent. Some animals develop fever, anorexia, and weight loss. Secondary bacterial infection and flystrike may complicate footrot infection.

Footrot in goats is generally less severe than in sheep, although significant lameness may develop. Interdigital dermatitis is a more prominent sign, and under-running of the horn is a less prominent sign compared with sheep infected with the same virulent strain of *D. nodosus*.[7,10]

Diagnosis. The diagnosis of virulent footrot is usually based on the clinical presentation of interdigital dermatitis and lameness in numerous flock members (virulent footrot). A Gram's stain of the interdigital exudate may show the large, curved, gram-negative, barbell-shaped rods characteristic of *D. nodosus;* however, they may not always be isolated because of their special growth requirements.[11] Several tests may be performed to differentiate between benign and virulent strains.[8] Serologic tests are of limited utility but may aid in identifying carrier animals. Antibody levels are only elevated for a short time and are not always accurate. Vaccination may confound the interpretation of the antibody tests. Footrot is the most common cause of lameness in sheep. However,

other differential diagnoses include foot abscess, laminitis, bluetongue, and foot and mouth disease.

Treatment. The mainstay of therapy is proper hoof trimming. Trimming can increase short-term lameness, but appropriate trimming also can produce very high cure rates without other forms of therapy.[4] Applying antibacterial agents to the foot after trimming it further improves cure rates. Topical treatments include antibiotics (tetracycline) and antiseptics (copper sulfate, zinc sulfate, cetrimide, or 4% to 5% formalin). If only a few animals are affected, these agents may be applied with a spray applicator or brush; bandaging ensures contact of the medication with affected tissue.[8]

The use of foot baths is a more practical method to treat numerous animals. Typically, affected animals should be separated from unaffected animals. Both groups of animals are passed through a foot bath and then kept in a dry place for a few hours before being placed on separate clean pastures. If this procedure is repeated several times, the majority of the animals will be cured, and the rest should be culled. A prolonged soaking time (1 hour) may be more effective than brief passes through foot baths, even when they are performed every 10 days.[12] Copper sulfate (5%), zinc sulfate (10%), and formalin (5%) have been used in foot baths and seem to have similar efficacy. Zinc sulfate is preferred because it is less hazardous and causes less discomfort than formalin, does not stain the wool, and has a reduced risk of toxicity compared with copper sulfate. An anionic surfactant, sodium lauryl sulfate, appears to enhance penetration of the zinc sulfate solution.[8,12] Dry foot baths (85% powdered limestone, 15% zinc sulfate) also may be beneficial. The clinician should remember that sheep are capable of jumping long distances and goats can walk on the thin edge of a small plank. Therefore foot baths should have solid sides and be at least $2\frac{1}{2}$ to 3 m long. Regardless of the type of foot bath used, trimming the feet before the therapy greatly enhances its effectiveness.

Several systemic antibiotics have been shown to be effective in the treatment of footrot. Penicillin (20,000 to 30,000 IU/kg intramuscularly [IM] twice a day [BID]), long-acting oxytetracycline (20 mg/kg subcutaneously [SC] every 72 hours), erythromycin (3 to 5 mg/kg IM BID), lincomycin, spectinomycin, and florfenicol (20 mg/kg IM every 48 hours) have been used successfully, especially when conditions are dry. These treatments are not approved in all countries.[13,14]

Vaccination has been shown to shorten the course of disease in flocks. However, a significant number of injection reactions are reported.[8] The decision to vaccinate during an outbreak must be carefully considered.

Prevention. Eradication of virulent footrot is possible but often difficult, especially in areas that are wet most of

BOX 9-1

FOOTROT PREVENTION PROGRAM*

- Trim feet, separate infected animals, and disinfect trimming equipment between animals.
- Move all animals through a 15% zinc sulfate foot bath. Where possible, have them stand in the foot bath for 30 minutes. Foot baths should be repeated two to 4 times at weekly intervals.
- Put both affected and nonaffected sheep in a previously unused (clean) pasture or paddock.
- Cull all severely affected animals and those not responding to treatment.
- Vaccinate 8 to 12 weeks before the season when large numbers of footrot cases are anticipated (disease tends to occur at the same time each year).
- Selectively breed for animals that appear less susceptible.

*Some or all of these procedures can be employed. The main ingredient in any protocol for footrot prevention is vigilance.

the year.[8] Box 9-1 describes a footrot prevention program. Treating affected animals, culling chronic cases, and isolating new animals are the mainstays of an eradication program. New animals should be segregated through a wet season before they are placed with a footrot-free flock. Obviously, any animal showing signs of footrot during quarantine should be culled.

In flocks with endemic footrot, vaccination may be useful in reducing the number and severity of footrot cases, but aggressive hoof trimming, foot bathing, and culling should be continued for the best control. Several types of vaccines are available. Two doses given at least 6 weeks apart, followed by boosters a few weeks before the wet season may improve effectiveness.[4] The protection is not complete and only lasts for a short time (4 to 12 weeks). Knowledge of seasonal infection patterns and vaccination before the predicted increase in clinical cases improves vaccination effectiveness.[4] Some animals develop fairly severe local reactions to the vaccine that may reduce production and be undesirable in show or sale animals. Genetic selection for resistance to footrot should be a primary adjunct to disease control.

Laminitis

Laminitis (inflammation of the dermal and epidermal laminae) is fairly common in sheep and goats. The history often includes consumption of a highly concentrated or lush forage diet. Laminitis also may be associated with systemic illness such as pneumonia, mastitis, and metritis; it can occur after parturition.[15]

Clinical signs.   Clinical signs of laminitis include lameness and warm feet. Animals move with a stiff gait and prefer recumbency. In chronic cases, foot deformity, marked by "turning up" of the toes, occurs. Laminitis is often accompanied by signs of primary gastrointestinal illness such as bloat, diarrhea, and toxemia. Differential diagnoses include footrot, caprine arthritis-encephalitis (CAE), and nutritional conditions that produce lameness, stiff gait, and recumbency.

Treatment and prevention.   The mainstay of treatment is nonsteroidal antiinflammatory drugs (NSAIDs) such as phenylbutazone (10 mg/kg by mouth [PO] once a day [SID]), flunixin meglumine (1 mg/kg SID), and aspirin (100 mg/kg PO BID), as well as treatment of the primary disorder. If the inciting cause can be corrected, many animals recover.[16] The risk of laminitis can be reduced by *slowly* increasing the amount of grain being fed. Preventing accidental exposure to large amounts of concentrate, ensuring adequate forage intake, and adding rumen buffers to the diet all help decrease the incidence of laminitis.

Hairy Heel Wart

Cases of unusually severe footrot in sheep in the United Kingdom have been described in the past few years. Affected animals usually have only one digit involved but the severe undermining of the hoof wall causes pain that leaves the animal unable to bear weight. Examination with dark field microscopy of swabs taken from these animals revealed the presence of spirochetes. The spirochetes isolated were enzymatically and biochemically similar to those found in dermal dermatitis (hairy heel warts) cases in cattle.[17] This condition may become severe enough that amputation is the treatment of choice. However, topical therapy with tetracycline should be attempted before resorting to amputation. Tetracycline can be placed in a foot bath, injected, or painted onto the lesion.

Interdigital Fibromas

Interdigital fibromas occasionally occur in small ruminants but are much more common in cattle. This hyperplasia of the interdigital skin may not cause lameness until the lesion is quite large or infected. Some reports speculate that predisposing factors include obesity, footrot, and abnormal hoof conformation.[13] Complete surgical excision under general anesthesia or sedation and local anesthesia is the treatment of choice, although cryotherapy, cautery, and topical caustic agents also have been employed. After surgery the foot is bandaged. Healing may be enhanced by securing the toes with wire to prevent spreading and movement of the interdigital skin. Recurrence of interdigital fibromas is not uncommon. [13]

REFERENCES

1. Cottom DS, Pinsent PJ: Lameness in the goat, *Goat Vet Soc J* 9(1):14, 1988.
2. Chakrabarti A: Incidence of foot disorders in goats in Tripura, *Indian Vet J* 74:342, 1997.
3. Greenough PR, Schugel LM, Johnson AB: *Illustrated handbook on cattle lameness*, Eden Prairie, MN, 1996, ZinPro.
4. Morgan K: Footrot. In Boden E, editor: *Sheep and goat practice*, London, 1991, Bailliere Tindale.
5. Cross RF, Parker CF: Oral administration of zinc sulfate for control of ovine footrot, *J Am Vet Med Assoc* 178(7):704, 1981.
6. Cross RF, Parker CF: Zinc sulfate foot bath for control of ovine foot rot, *J Am Vet Med Assoc* 178(7):706, 1981.
7. Egerton JR: Footrot of cattle, goats, and deer. In Egerton JR, Yong WK, Riffkin GG, editors: *Footrot and foot abscess of ruminants*, Boca Raton, FL, 1989, CRC Press.
8. Stewart DJ: Footrot in sheep. In Egerton JR, Yong WK, Riffkin GG, editors: *Footrot and foot abscess of ruminants*, Boca Raton, FL, 1989, CRC Press.
9. Kimberling CV, Ellis RP: Advances in the control of foot rot in sheep, *Vet Clin North Am Food Anim Pract* 6:671, 1990.
10. Ghimire SC, Egerton JR, Dhyngyel OP: Transmission of virulent footrot between sheep and goats, *Aust Vet J* 77:450, 1999.
11. Rings DM: Ovine contagious foot rot. In Howard JL, Smith RA, editors: *Current veterinary therapy 4, food animal practice*, Philadelphia, 1999, WB Saunders.
12. Bulgin MS et al: Comparison of treatment methods for the control of contagious ovine foot rot, *J Am Vet Med Assoc* 189:194, 1986.
13. Radostits OM et al: *Veterinary medicine*, ed 9, Philadelphia, 2000, WB Saunders.
14. Vandyke S et al: Treatment of ovine foot rot: use of florfenicol versus oxytetracycline for treatment of ovine foot rot, *Sheep and Goat Res J* 15:54, 1999.
15. Guss SB: *Management and diseases of dairy goats*, Scottsdale, AZ, 1977, Dairy Goat Journal Publishing.
16. Bulgin MS: Diagnosis of lameness in sheep, *Compend Contin Educ Pract Vet* 8:F122, 1986.
17. Naylor RD, Martin PK, Jones JR: Isolation of a spirochete from a case of severe virulent ovine footrot, *Vet Rec* 25:690, 1998.

CONGENITAL CONDITIONS

Myotonia Congenita

Myotonia congenita is a heritable condition of goats in which the animal experiences tetanic muscle contraction when startled. Occasionally the contraction is severe enough that the goat collapses to the ground. This phenomenon has led to affected animals being referred to as *fainting goats*. This condition is caused by an autosomal dominant trait. [1] Some speculate that the variability in clinical signs and intensity of muscle contractions may be related to the animal being homozygous rather than heterozygous for the trait. [1] The condition closely resembles one form of myotonia congenita in human beings and has therefore been used as a research model for the human disease. The condition is related to a block of the normal conductance of chloride in the membrane of muscle fibers. [2] The primary abnormality is a delay of relaxation of contracted muscle that is most likely caused by repeated firing of action potentials. Histochemical and ultrastructural abnormalities are present in goats with myotonia congenita. [1,2]

Hereditary Chondrodysplasia (Spider Lamb Syndrome)

Spider lamb syndrome is an inherited musculoskeletal condition seen primarily in the Suffolk and Hampshire breeds. [3] Clinical signs may be present at birth or affected lambs may appear normal at birth, only to have the severe skeletal abnormalities develop by 6 weeks of age. [4] This latter group may have longer legs with angular deviations, shallower bodies, and narrower chests than normal lambs, [4] and these animals display the expected radiographic abnormalities associated with this condition at birth. Skeletal abnormalities exhibited by affected lambs vary in severity and type. Chondrodysplasia is evident in the skull, sternum, appendicular skeleton, and vertebrae.

Radiographically, the dorsal silhouette of the skull may be rounded, the occipital condyles may be elongated (occasionally with cartilage erosion), and thickening of the occipital bone between the condyles and the poll may be evident. The sternebrae may be of abnormal size and shape. The sternum is often misaligned, dorsally deviated, and not fused across the midline. The scapula and olecranon usually have more cartilage and less bone distally than normal. Animals with spider lamb syndrome have several islands of ossification near the anconeal process that can be seen on flexed lateral radiographs of the elbow. The distal physis of the radius is flared, and angular limb deformities are common. Generally the forelimbs are more severely affected than the hindlimbs. Erosion of articular cartilage is common if the lamb survives for a few months. The vertebrae commonly have abnormal and excessive cartilage. Vertebral body abnormalities may contribute to scoliosis or, less commonly, kyphosis. [4] Histologically, the typical osseous lesion is manifested as uneven growth cartilage.

Spider lamb syndrome is inherited as an autosomal recessive trait with complete penetrance but variable expression. The pathologic changes are found by the end of the second trimester of gestation. [4] The carriers of the recessive gene have a normal phenotype that makes elimination of the condition difficult. The locus that causes spider lamb syndrome has been localized to ovine chromosome 6, and deoxyribonucleic acid (DNA) tests may soon allow identification of carrier animals. [5]

Arthrogryposis

Arthrogryposis and hydranencephaly are congenital conditions that must be differentiated from spider lamb syndrome. The two conditions cause severe deformities in sheep. Arthrogryposis and hydranencephaly may result from infection with Akabane virus, Cache Valley virus, bluetongue virus, and possibly other organisms that affect the developing fetus. Affected animals have severely flexed forelimbs and overextended hindlimbs. A spiral deviation of the spine also is present. Neurologic conditions that may be seen with arthrogryposis and hydranencephaly include cerebellar hypoplasia, hydrocephalus, micromelia, and hydrocephaly.

Polydactyly

By definition, polydactyly is a congenital anomaly in which extra digits are present. It is seldom seen in sheep and goats. The condition is certainly heritable in cattle and probably heritable in pigs, where cleft palate may concurrently be seen. Polydactyly is suggested to be heritable in horses. One report of polydactyly in goats describes an affected female that was sired by a male with polydactyly.[6] Polydactyly usually has only cosmetic consequences for affected animals. However, polydactyly may cause serious gait abnormalities in some animals. The practitioner must thoroughly examine animals with gait abnormalities to determine whether the lameness is because of some other anomaly or clinically significant lesion. Radiographs are necessary to assess the anomaly fully and determine any treatment to be rendered.

Treatment. Treatment involves surgical removal of the extra digits and primary closure of the skin incision. Removal of some of the digits can be done by sharp excision; however, orthopedic instrumentation is sometimes required to disrupt osseous attachment. Appropriate postoperative care should be given after surgical excision.

Patella Luxation

Animals with congenital patella luxation are usually brought to veterinarians shortly after birth because they tend to crouch on the rear legs when attempting to stand. The patella luxation functionally disrupts the quadriceps apparatus, rendering the animal unable to hold the stifle in extension. The primary differential diagnosis that must be ruled out with this presentation is femoral nerve injury, which also causes failure of the quadriceps apparatus because of lack of strength in the quadriceps muscle, producing the same abnormal stance. Femoral nerve injury is more commonly seen in calves after dystocia than it is in small ruminants. A diagnosis of patella luxation is easily made by palpating the patella; a luxated patella easily dislocates either medially or laterally. In se-

verely affected animals the patella remains luxated and is difficult to reduce into its normal position. This manipulation is more easily accomplished with the stifle held in extension.

Standard radiographic views with the addition of a skyline image demonstrate the position of the patella, the depth of the trochlear groove, and other osseous abnormalities that may be present. The skyline view, which allows the best assessment of the trochlear groove, is taken with the stifle flexed and the x-ray beam directed proximally to distally perpendicular to the tibia. However, the ease of luxation on palpation of the patella is much more important diagnostically than is the location of the patella on a single craniocaudal radiograph. The affected patella is often in a normal position for a given radiograph if it is not purposely luxated by the examiner before the radiograph is taken.

Surgery is usually indicated for young animals with congenital patella luxation. Most young animals respond well to imbrication of the fibrous joint capsule and overlying fascia on the side opposite the direction of patella luxation. However, the veterinarian must fully evaluate the limb before surgery and assess the joint at surgery. Some severe cases may require trochleoplasty or tibial crest osteotomy and relocation. The reader should refer to small animal surgery texts for detailed descriptions of the more complex stifle surgeries.[7]

Affected animals should be thoroughly examined for other congenital abnormalities. Specifically, severely affected newborns may not be able to stand and suckle. Therefore failure of passive transfer and associated illness may become more significant to the health of these animals than even the primary patella luxation. Small ruminants may compensate for mild cases of patella luxation (especially if the condition is unilateral) and go undiagnosed until they are seen by veterinarians as adults with lameness caused by luxation or degenerative joint disease caused by intermittent luxation. Adult animals also may exhibit acute lameness as a result of traumatic patella luxation. Surgical treatment of these adults tends to be more involved in that orthopedic implants such as screws and wires may be required to secure the patella. The prognosis for a return to soundness is not good compared with the prognosis for treated neonates with congenital luxations.[8,9]

Spastic Paresis

Spastic paresis has been described in pygmy goats.[10] Affected goats suffer constant contraction of the gastrocnemius muscles in the hind legs. The contraction produces extension of the tibiotarsal joint and arching of the back. Clinical signs are not significantly different than those described in several breeds of cattle.[11-13] The condition is suspected to be inherited, but the exact mode of transmission is unknown. No lesions have been noted in the spinal cord, tibial or peroneal nerves, or gastrocnemius muscle. The clinical signs appear to be caused by a defect in the myotactic reflex that results in an overstimulation or relative lack of inhibition of the efferent motor neurons.[10]

REFERENCES

1. Bryant SH, Lipicky RJ, Herzog WH: Variability of myotonia signs in myotonic goats, *Am J Vet Res* 29(12):2371, 1968.
2. McKerrell RE: Myotonia in man and animals: confusing comparisons, *Equine Vet J* 19:266, 1987.
3. Rook JS et al: Diagnosis of hereditary chondrodysplasia (spider lamb syndrome) in sheep, *J Am Vet Med Assoc* 193(6):713, 1988.
4. Oberbauer AM et al: Developmental progression of the spider lamb syndrome, *Small Rumin Res* 18:179, 1995.
5. Cockett NE et al: Localization of the locus causing spider lamb syndrome to the distal end of ovine chromosome 6, *Mammal Genome* 10:35, 1999.
6. Al-Ani FK, Hailat NQ, Fathalla MA: Polydactyly in Shami breed goats in Jordan, *Small Rumin Res* 26:177, 1997.
7. Hulse DA, Shires PK: *Textbook of small animal surgery*, Philadelphia, 1985, WB Saunders.
8. Baron RJ: Laterally luxating patella in a goat, *J Am Vet Med Assoc* 191(11):1471, 1987.
9. Gahlot TK et al: Correction of patella luxation in goats, *Mod Vet Pract*, p 418, May 1983.
10. Baker J et al: Spastic paresis in pygmy goats, *J Vet Int Med* 3(2):113, 1989.
11. Leipold HW et al: Spastic paresis in beef shorthorn cattle, *J Am Vet Med Assoc* 151(5):598, 1967.
12. Thomason KJ, Beeman KB: Spastic paresis in Gelbvieh calves: an examination of two cases, *Vet Med* 82(5):548, 1987.
13. Harper PAW: Spastic paresis in Brahman crossbred cattle, *Aust Vet J* 70(12):456, 1993.

TRAUMATIC CONDITIONS

Predator Attack

Sheep and goats are of the stature and disposition to make them susceptible to predators. Small ruminants seldom survive attacks by wild carnivores. However, veterinarians are sometimes called to treat survivors of attacks by domestic animals or interrupted attacks by wild animals. These survivors often ultimately die because of either lethal injury to internal organs or physical exhaustion from the chase and the attack. A veterinarian treating animals that survive the initial trauma may face a significant challenge. Although skin wounds are quite obvious after the animal is thoroughly examined and clipped, injuries to deeper structures and serious myopathy are more difficult to assess.

Attacking predators tend to "go for the jugular," which leads to a concentration of wounds in the head and neck area. The associated injury to the great vessels is usually obvious and often fatal. Tracheal puncture can cause res-

piratory difficulties and subcutaneous emphysema. Subcutaneous emphysema also can result from the undermining skin wounds alone, making diagnosis of tracheal perforation difficult in some cases and adding to the difficulty of detecting a tracheal wound. Perforation of the esophagus is common. Esophageal injury may lead to abscess formation and tissue necrosis as a result of contamination of surrounding tissues by esophageal contents. Abscess formation may physically impinge on the airway and make swallowing difficult. Neurologic damage from the primary injury or damage caused by abscess formation may inhibit normal function of the soft palate.

Tetanus antitoxin should be administered to these animals, as well as broad-spectrum antibiotics (florfenicol 20 mg/kg every 48 hours) to combat wound infection and sepsis. Antibiotics with good efficacy against anaerobic bacteria (penicillin 20,000 IU/kg BID) should be considered in cases in which massive trauma has resulted in some tissue devitalization. All skin wounds must be thoroughly cleaned of organic debris and foreign material. Establishing drainage in undermined skin wounds also is important. Some of these wounds lend themselves to débridement and delayed primary closure, whereas others are best managed by allowing second intention healing. The veterinarian must be conscious of injury to muscle and joints deep beneath these skin wounds. Supportive care in the form of fluids and NSAIDs (flunixin meglumine 1 to 2 mg/kg intravenously [IV]) is important in treating any myopathy.

Fractures

The hallmark of long bone fracture in small ruminants is acute non–weight-bearing lameness. A thorough physical examination must be performed to rule out other causes of severe lameness, including septic arthritis, joint luxation, and severe footrot. The clinician should readily detect instability and crepitance on palpation of the fracture site. The exception is an incomplete or greenstick fracture that manifests itself as a less severe acute lameness that improves with time. The clinician should not overlook the possibility that an incomplete fracture may suffer a catastrophic breakdown and become unstable rather than heal. Because of economic constraints, radiographic examination may be impractical. However, whenever possible, radiographic evaluations before and after repair enhance the success of the procedure.

The most commonly treated fractures occur in the metacarpal and metatarsal bones.[1] These fractures are usually treated successfully with a cast. Fractures of the distal half of the metacarpal and metatarsal bones often respond well to lower limb casts that incorporate the foot and extend proximally to a point just distal to the carpus and tarsus. Proximal or comminuted metacarpal and metatarsal fractures may require full-limb casting with or without transfixation pins to stabilize the fracture properly and prevent collapse.

Many fractures of the carpus or tarsus also respond to treatment with a full-limb cast.[2] However, these injuries are often associated with contamination of the joint, and the incidence of septic arthritis is high. Septic arthritis requires more intensive antibiotic therapy, as well as local treatment through a window in the cast. One complication with using treatment windows in casts is the "window edema" that sometimes develops. The cast window should be cut out as one piece. Edema can be avoided by securing this piece in the window with tape between treatments. The management of carpal tarsal fractures with concomitant septic arthritis is difficult. Ankylosis of the joint often results even if successful fracture healing occurs.[2]

Radial fractures must be evaluated individually to determine the best mode of treatment. Fractures of the distal radius may respond to a full-limb cast. Proximal radius fractures may heal better with the use of an external fixator, a transfixation cast, or possibly a modified Thomas splint. Splints may be very applicable for neonates, and need only stay in place for 2 to 4 weeks in most instances.[3] Some radial fractures may require internal fixation with plates and screws. However, internal fixation is seldom required and often not economically feasible in small ruminants. If a splint is used for radial fractures, it should extend to the elbow and preferably above it.[3]

Treatment decisions for tibia fractures are very similar to those for radius fractures. Distal fractures heal well with full-limb casting.[4] The tibia is an area where one of the authors (Dr. Baird) often chooses to employ an external fixator or in larger goats a transfixation full-limb cast.

Fractures of the humerus and femur occur less frequently in small ruminants.[1] Humeral fractures often heal with stall rest alone. However, the distal limb frequently suffers carpal contracture, rendering the animal unsound regardless of fracture healing. Femoral fractures may heal if the limb is taped in a modified Ehmer sling (made of tape placed in figure eights around the limb) that is taped to the abdomen.[3] This method is less costly but is still an effective method in young or light-weight animals.[3] Fractures of the humerus and femur usually require internal fixation with plates and screws or intramedullary pins. The mode of internal fixation depends on the complexity of the fracture and the experience of the veterinarian. Financial considerations may dictate the use of intramedullary pins rather than plates and screws if possible.

Fractures in other areas such as the scapula and pelvis can be treated much as they are in the dog. Small ruminants are usually good orthopedic patients because of their relatively small size and ability to maneuver well on three limbs. Often pelvic or scapula fractures heal if the animal is confined for 3 to 6 weeks.[3] The veterinarian can form a plan for treating unusual orthopedic injuries in small ruminants by considering principles of small animal orthopedics and cost-benefit decision-making processes of food animal medicine.

Mandible fractures may occur in small ruminants that have been kicked by a large animal such as a horse or cow and those that have caught the rostral mandible in a fence or some other object. A kick injury may result in any number of fracture configurations; the veterinarian must refer to information on small animal fundamentals to determine whether plates, wires, or pins are the most appropriate surgical stabilizers. Occasionally external fixators can be used to treat mandibular fractures (Figure 9-3). Rostral fractures may involve mostly teeth and soft tissues but very little bone. They often cause loss of teeth but minimal instability. Therefore the veterinarian may wish to débride the area, institute antibiotic therapy, and modify the animal's diet. If the mandibular fracture occurs between the incisors and the cheek teeth, it may be stabilized by securing wires from the rostral mandible to the cheek teeth.[5,6] Animals with these types of fractures require nutritional support, either orally or parenterally (see Chapter 2). Many of these animals can be fed a moistened pelleted diet.

Occasionally digit or leg amputation is required to treat septic conditions, fractures, or luxations (Figure 9-4). Amputation can be done with the animal under general anesthesia or with the animal sedated and under local anesthesia (see Chapter 16). For digit amputation a tourniquet should be applied proximal to the fetlock after the surgical site is prepared in an aseptic manner. A circumferential skin incision is made just proximal to the coronary band. Many texts recommend two incisions per-

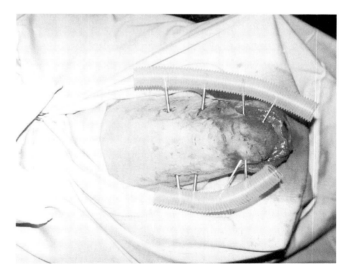

Figure 9-3 This intraoperative photograph shows the repair of a mandibular fracture with an external fixator. The pin ends are within the pieces of 2-inch plastic tubing, which will be filled with hoof acrylic to function as connecting rods.

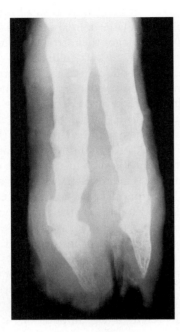

Figure 9-4 A dorsoplantar radiographic view of the phalanges of a sheep with lameness caused by a chronic wound of the medial digit. Note the pronounced soft tissue swelling with minimal osseous changes.

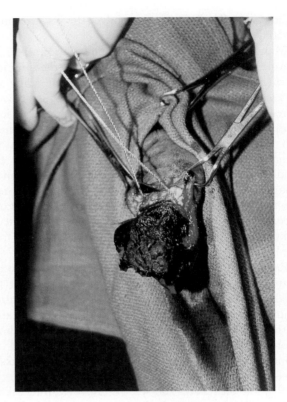

Figure 9-5 Intraoperative photograph of digit amputation showing the flaps of the inverted T incision being retracted with towel clamps and the Gigli wire being crossed as the amputation is performed.

pendicular to the circumferential incision (one dorsal and another palmar or plantar) to create a skin flap that is elevated to allow amputation with Gigli wire. The authors prefer to make one incision over the abaxial aspect of the affected digit perpendicular to the coronary band to create an inverted T incision. The two flaps of the inverted T can be undermined to allow the passage and crossing of the Gigli wire (Figure 9-5). The amputation should be completed on an angle at the distal aspect of the proximal phalanx, with the clinician removing all of the articular cartilage and synovial membrane of the proximal interphalangeal joint while leaving the interdigital ligaments intact to provide stability to the fetlock. The corners of the flaps of the inverted T can be trimmed to minimize dead space when the surgical site is closed. The site can be closed completely if the amputation is performed as a treatment for fracture or luxation. However, if infection is present in the form of septic arthritis or osteomyelitis, the clinician should consider the advantages of drainage facilitated by partial closure. With either closure, a bandage should be placed on the foot to aid in hemostasis before the tourniquet is removed. The bandage should be changed as needed until the incision site has healed. The use of broad-spectrum antibiotics (oxytetracycline 10 mg/kg IV or IM BID, or 20 mg/kg SC every 48 hours) and antiinflammatory drugs

should be considered. If all or part of a leg is to be amputated, as much of the limb as possible should be left in place. Similar techniques as those used in other small animals can be applied to limb removal in sheep and goats.

Cast. The previous description of fractures discussed casting as a primary treatment option for fixation of fractures. The clinician should prepare the limb for cast application by removing any organic debris to ensure the leg is clean. Cotton or gauze sponges should be placed in the interdigital space to prevent pinching of the interdigital skin within the cast by the hooves. Orthopedic felt or gauze sponges should be placed over the dewclaws to provide padding; however, holes should be cut to allow the dewclaws to protrude. Without this precaution, pressure from the cast over the dewclaws can cause skin ulcerations and may even result in dewclaw sloughing. The clinician then applies a double layer of stockinette to the limb and places a strip of orthopedic felt around the limb where the most proximal part of the cast will end. The authors prefer to put this proximal felt between two layers of stockinette so the felt is encased in the stockinette when it is rolled down over the felt during application of the cast. However, others place the felt beneath the stockinette. Other padding materials may be used according to preference, but the clinician should remember that the relatively small size of many sheep and goats demands that the cast not be overly heavy or bulky. The authors believe no padding beyond the previously mentioned interdigital cotton, orthopedic felt, and stockinette is necessary to prevent skin ulceration under a properly applied cast. If the wool of heavily wooled animals is not clipped, it may act as excellent padding.[3] The one exception in which more padding is useful is for very young animals, which are likely to experience significant growth while in the cast and tend to be more prone to cast sores than adults.

Fiberglass casting material has replaced plaster in most practices because of its increased strength, lighter weight, and faster drying time. The foot should be included in the cast. The clinician should be careful to apply the cast without wrinkles (which may cause cast sores) and in a timely manner so that all layers bond together as one rather than laminate in several layers. The cast is not as strong if it dries in laminated layers. The solar surface of the cast should be protected from wear in some manner. Methods of protecting this part of the cast include tape alone, a section of tire inner tube and tape, and a walking pad made of hoof acrylic. The particular method chosen is less important than achieving the desired result of preventing exposure of the hoof through a worn cast.

Any animal in a cast must be monitored closely to detect complications as soon as possible. The clinician should consider complications under the cast as the cause of any abnormal clinical signs such as fever, inappetence, increased lameness in the cast limb, and swelling proximal to the cast. The cast should be palpated daily to determine its fit and check for any areas of increased heat that may indicate the formation of cast sores. However, some areas of the cast (e.g., over wounds and bony protuberances) are normally warmer than other areas of the cast. Therefore, it is more important to recognize changes in relative warmth in the same area of the cast from day to day than differences in temperature between different areas of the cast. A fiberglass cast applied over stockinette is porous, and exudate from a wound or cast sore will penetrate the cast. If the environment makes fly control difficult, flies may be observed concentrating over these localized areas of the cast before exudate can be seen penetrating the cast. This part of the cast also may have an increased relative temperature before the exudate penetrates it.

Transfixation casts add stability in cases in which cast immobilization alone is not adequate.[1] Transfixation pins help immobilize proximal fractures in ways that casting alone does not. In some cases comminuted distal fractures collapse unless transfixation pins transfer the weight away from the distal limb to the transfixation pins.[7] Application of a transfixation cast often requires general anesthesia, although casting of hindlimbs can be done with sedation and spinal anesthesia. Pin diameter and placement depend on animal size, bone diameter, and fracture con-

BOX 9-2

Zipp Formula*

Zinc oxide—4 parts
Iodoform—4 parts
Mineral oil—4 parts

---

*Zipp formula can be applied under a cast and may have an antibacterial effect for as long as 2 weeks. If zinc oxide ointment is used, no mineral oil is required, and the ointment can be made of equal parts zinc oxide and iodoform (30 ml of each).

figuration. The transfixation pins are placed through stab incisions using aseptic technique. Intraoperative radiographs are helpful in the placement of the transfixation pins. However, this technique is usually successful even when pin placement is directed by palpation alone. Antimicrobial ointment ("Zipp" ointment or neomycin-polymyxin B-bacitracin) can be applied to the skin at the pin sites and covered with gauze sponges. The limb is then prepared as previously described for cast application. The formula for an ointment that can be applied under a cast and has an antibacterial effect for as long as 2 weeks is given in Box 9-2. The clinician should cut holes into the stockinette to accommodate the pins and cut the pins so that they protrude about 1 to 1.5 cm beyond the anticipated thickness of the cast. The cast material should be applied so that the bone pin ends perforate the cast material or the material placed around the pin. When the cast material has set or become hardened, the pin ends should be covered to prevent injury to the contralateral limb. Hoof acrylic or cotton and tape can be used to cover the pin ends (Figures 9-6 and 9-7). As the fracture heals, bone resorption occurs around the pins, causing them to loosen. Neither special instrumentation nor general anesthesia is required for pin removal (Figure 9-8).

External fixation. External fixators are preferable to simple casts or transfixation casts in some fractures of the radius and tibia. Either traditional fixators or modified fixators using cast material to support the transcortical pins work well in small ruminants. Traditional external fixation techniques described for small animals can be used for sheep and goats.[8] A modified fixator designed to treat calf tibia fractures is less technically demanding to apply than a traditional external fixator[9] but allows more flexibility in pin placement. The authors have found this technique to be most useful in tibia fractures but also of value for treatment of other fractures. The procedure is performed on a surgically prepared animal, under general anesthesia (see Chapter 16) and according to aseptic technique. At least two pins must be placed proximal and two pins distal to the fracture site. The pins can be placed

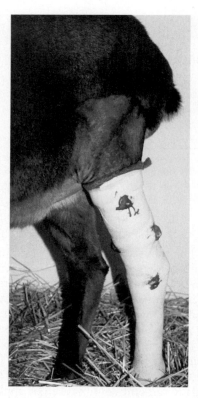

Figure 9-6   A transfixation cast used to treat an open fracture in a 175-pound goat. In this case the transfixation cast was chosen to give added stability to enhance healing of the open fracture. Note the hoof acrylic covering the pin ends. This cast also had a window on the medial side of the limb for wound management, which is not shown.

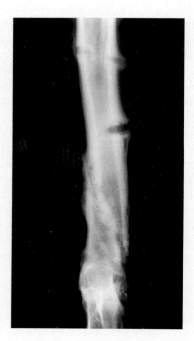

Figure 9-8   Craniocaudal radiograph of the goat in Figure 9-6 at the time of cast removal 6 weeks after the initial injury.

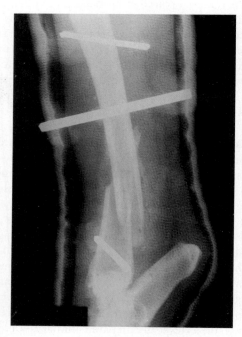

Figure 9-7   Lateral radiograph of the goat in Figure 9-6 at the time of transfixation cast application.

through stab incisions from lateral to medial (type II pins) through the skin on each side. One major advantage of this technique is that a single type I pin can be placed from the dorsal aspect. The type I pin passes through one skin surface and both cortices of the bone, but not through the caudal soft tissues and skin. A second type I pin is not required because the cast material itself connects and stabilizes the pins. This is a major advantage in fractures (either proximal or distal) in which the fragment size does not allow placement of two type II pins. The pins should be incorporated into a cast of the same length described previously for the transfixation cast and the limb treated with topical ointment. This technique incorporates more padding than that used with a standard cast. Cotton or some other padding should be wrapped around the entire length of the tibia. No stockinette or orthopedic felt is required. Fiberglass cast material should then be placed over the length of the tibia to incorporate the pins, as is done with the transfixation cast. After the cast hardens completely, the caudal quarter to third of the cast can be removed and the padding cut away from the caudal part of the limb. This modification allows unencumbered movement of the gastrocnemius. Occasionally the dorsal distal portion of the cast also must be trimmed to allow flexion of the hock. Some patients initially require a splint or bandage over the fetlock to ensure the

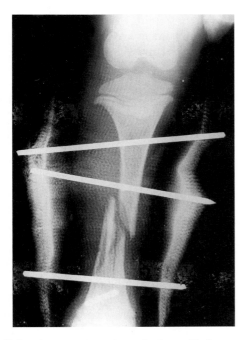

Figure 9-9   Craniocaudal radiograph of a modified external fixator in a 3-month-old lamb with a tibia fracture.

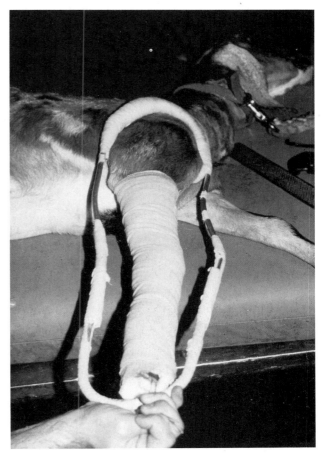

Figure 9-10   Application of a Schroeder-Thomas splint on the front limb of a goat. Note the wire in the hoof wall being used to secure the foot to the distal aspect of the splint. The splint is finished with adhesive tape to secure the entire limb within the splint.

animal bears weight on the solar surface of the foot. Most patients become fully ambulatory in 48 to 72 hours. Treatment of young animals should be tailored to prevent a compensatory tarsal varus of the contralateral limb (Figure 9-9). This procedure is technically less difficult because the practitioner is allowed more variation in pin placement than if traditional connecting bars are used. The pin ends should be covered as they are in transfixation casting.[9]

Splints.   Splints can be useful in treating some musculoskeletal conditions in small ruminants. However, the veterinarian should be selective in using them. Many practitioners are more comfortable using casts and external fixators than applying and monitoring splints. The majority of small ruminants referred to one of the authors (Dr. Baird) for malunion or delayed-union healing of fractures had been treated with splints before referral. For this reason alone, practitioners should consider using other techniques that achieve more stable fracture fixation. However, splints can be useful in selected cases if the practitioner is skilled at splint management. In emergency situations a splint can be made of cut polyvinyl chloride (PVC) pipe or other such material.[6]

A spoon splint, either commercially manufactured or fashioned from cast material, is probably best used to support greenstick fractures of the distal limb. When used in this way it helps prevent catastrophic breakdown of the fracture. However, a more important role may be in preventing the limb contracture that can occur if the carpus is allowed to remain flexed for a prolonged period in a non–weight-bearing animal. With this technique a padded bandage is placed on the limb and the splint is conformed to the bandage and secured with adhesive tape.

Another type of splint occasionally used in small ruminants is the traction splint, commonly referred to as the *Schroeder-Thomas splint* (Figure 9-10). This splint is usually made of aluminum rods and consists of a ring that fits in the axillary or inguinal region of the animal with bars on the dorsal and palmar or plantar aspect of the limb joined distally. The shape of the splint varies, as does the way particular parts of the limb are secured to the splint depending on the specific reason the splint is applied. Traction is applied by securing the foot to the distal splint with adhesive tape or by placing wires through the hoof wall. A soft bandage should be placed on the limb, after which the limb is secured strategically to the splint. Usually tape is placed over the entire limb and distal splint[10] (see Figure 9-10).

INFECTIOUS AND TRAUMATIC CONDITIONS

Septic Arthritis

Bacterial infections of the joints (septic arthritis) occur most commonly in neonates. However, older sheep and goats sporadically suffer from joint infection as a result of a penetrating injury or spread from adjacent infected tissues, as in the case of footrot. In neonates, septic arthritis is most often a sequela to septicemia and often a consequence of failure of passive transfer. The bacteria isolated from lambs include *Streptococcus, Escherichia coli, A. pyogenes, Erysipelothrix insidiosa (rhusiopathiae), Pasteurella haemolytica, Corynebacterium pseudotuberculosis,* and *Fusobacterium necrophorum. Staphylococcus aureus* arthritis is associated with tick pyemia, a disease seen in lambs 2 to 6 weeks old in areas infested with *Ixodes ricinus. Streptococcus dysgalactiae* has been reported as a cause of arthritis in dairy goats and was the most common pathogen isolated from arthritic lambs in England and Wales. Other isolates included *E. coli,* coagulase-positive *Staphylococcus, E. rhusiopathiae,* and *A. pyogenes.*[12] Coexisting omphalitis was found in 16% of arthritic lambs.

Erysipelothrix polyarthritis is a nonsuppurative condition usually seen in 2- to 6-month-old lambs, but it also can cause neonatal disease. Outbreaks may affect as many as 40% of the lambs in a flock. Hallmarks of this infection are fever and lameness, with minimal swelling of joints. This nonsuppurative polyarthritis will progress to chronic arthritis if not treated appropriately.[11]

Pathogenesis. Septicemia often contributes to hematogenous seeding of joints with bacteria that localize in the synovial membrane. The resulting synovitis causes the affected animal to exhibit joint pain, heat, swelling, and synovial effusion. Progression of the septic arthritis and associated synovitis causes damage to articular cartilage and subchondral bone. As bacteria proliferate, an influx of inflammatory cells produce hydrolytic enzymes that destroy bacteria and normal cartilage, resulting in cartilage erosion. In the chronic stages of infection animals develop thickening of the synovial tissue, fibrosis of the joint capsule, and signs of degenerative joint disease.

Clinical signs. The hallmarks of septic arthritis are lameness and warm swelling of the joints. The joints most commonly involved are the carpus, tarsus, and stifle. Any joint may be infected, including the hip, shoulder, or elbow; infection here may be more difficult to diagnose than in the more commonly affected joints. Several joints may be affected, and the practitioner should always perform a thorough examination when one septic joint is discovered to rule out polyarthritis. Lameness may be severe (non–weight-bearing) and animals may remain recumbent. Affected animals are often febrile and anorexic. Other signs of systemic disease such as omphalitis, meningitis, and uveitis may be evident.

Diagnosis. A sterile aspirate of synovial fluid should be obtained and the fluid submitted for culture and cytology. The character of the synovial fluid varies according to the etiology and stage of disease. Synovial fluid from infected joints may be thin and watery (lacking normal viscosity) or thick and cloudy with purulent material. Infected synovial fluid often has characteristic pleocytosis and neutrophilia (more than 30,000 to 100,000 white blood cells/μl and more than 75% neutrophils), as well as an increased total protein. Not all aspirates from septic joints yield bacteria, but some do. Culture results may improve with the use of enhancement media or synovial membrane biopsy, particularly if the animal has been treated with antimicrobial agents. Radiography may be used to determine the severity of degenerative changes, although bony changes may not be visible for several days after the onset of disease. Radiography may be more important to monitor the progression of septic arthritis during therapy. Ultrasonography also may be useful in evaluating existing soft tissue pathology.

Treatment. The administration of antimicrobial agents and joint lavage are the mainstays of treatment of septic arthritis. Antimicrobials, which may be administered systemically or intraarticularly, should be chosen based on an assessment of specific pathogens (gram-positive bacteria are more likely) and culture results when available.[13] Lavage of the joint with sterile polyionic solution aids in removal of inflammatory products. Light sedation of the animal is usually indicated. The skin over the joint should be clipped and surgically prepared, and the clinician should adhere strictly to aseptic technique. The clinician inserts a needle (16- or 14-gauge) attached to a sterile syringe into the affected joint at the most obviously distended area and aspirates fluid (for culture and cytology). The joint is then distended with an isotonic solution (e.g., saline, lactated Ringer's). A second needle is placed in the joint on the opposite side of the joint. Between 0.5 to 1 L of fluid should be flushed through the joint. The joint should be distended several times during the lavage by occluding the egress needle. The joint should be flushed daily for 2 to 3 days; the need for subsequent flushings should be based on the presence of pain or swelling and cytologic evaluation of joint fluid. Removing inflammatory mediators by lavage can improve clinical signs, although such improvement is often temporary. Some cases have accumulated fibrin within the joint and over the articular cartilage that requires drainage and débridement by arthrotomy. Lavage of these joints may yield clear fluid after treatment, but any improvement is short-lived. Just after lavage, nonirritating antibiotics should be instilled into the joint. In general products for IV use are adequate for intraarticular use.

Regional limb perfusion with antibiotics is an adjunctive procedure that may be beneficial in some cases.[13] This technique entails instilling small volumes of antimicrobial agents in targeted locations to achieve high concentrations in infected areas. Regional perfusion can be accomplished with intramedullary administration of antimicrobial agents but is more easily and commonly performed by IV injection distal to a tourniquet. Sheep and goats generally should be sedated before this procedure. The skin over the peripheral vein is aseptically prepared. The clinician inserts a needle (20- or 21-gauge) into the vein in a proximal direction and infuses the antibiotic of choice (ceftiofur sodium 1 mg/kg or potassium or sodium penicillin 20,000 IU/kg). For repeated administration in chronic conditions, a catheter (22-gauge) can be placed in the vein and the leg wrapped to help maintain catheter patency.[14] The prognosis for septic arthritis is guarded and chronic lameness is a sequela in many cases.

Prevention. Ensuring adequate passive transfer in neonates helps prevent septicemia and septic arthritis resulting from hematogenous spread of bacteria to joints. Maintaining a clean environment for lambing and kidding and providing appropriate umbilical care also help prevent neonatal septicemia.

Chlamydial Polyarthritis

Chlamydial polyarthritis is a common contagious disease of feedlot lambs in the United States. The disease is suspected to occur in goats as well.[15] The causative agent was formerly considered to be a strain (immunotype 2) of *Chlamydia psittaci* but has been recently classified as *Chlamydophila pecorum*.[16,17] Economic losses associated with chlamydial arthritis result from weight loss and treatment costs. Disease occurs in 1- to 8-month-old lambs, with 3- to 5-month-old lambs most commonly affected.[18] In feedlots outbreaks often occur a few weeks after lambs are introduced.[18] Morbidity can be as high as 80%, with less than 1% mortality.[17]

Pathogenesis. *C. pecorum* is present in nasal and ocular secretions, feces, and urine of infected animals.[18] As many as half the lambs on some farms shed *C. pecorum* in feces without signs of clinical disease.[16]

Clinical signs. Affected lambs have fever (up to 108° F) and are reluctant to move, often appearing "tucked up" or becoming recumbent. Lameness is apparent in one or more limbs, and affected joints are typically enlarged.[15,18] Chlamydial conjunctivitis may occur concurrently.[18-20] The course of the disease is about 10 to 14 days without treatment. Most lambs recover, but some remain lame.[15] Significant necropsy findings include fibrinous exudate in joints and edema of surrounding tissue. The articular cartilage is minimally affected.[15,20]

Diagnosis. Joint fluid may contain fibrin but is not purulent. Elementary inclusion bodies may be seen on Giemsa-stained smears of synovial fluid (see Chapters 5, 6, and 11). Isolation of *Chlamydia* requires special media and is not routinely performed. The use of DNA-based tests should aid and improve the understanding of the epidemiology of different chlamydial infections.

Differential diagnoses for chlamydial polyarthritis include white muscle disease and nutritional osteodystrophy. These diseases lack fever and synovial effusion, however, and laboratory testing should help differentiate these conditions.

Treatment and prevention. Oxytetracycline (20 mg/kg SC or IM every 48 to 72 hours), erythromycin (3 to 5 mg/kg IM three times a day [TID] or BID), and tylosin (20 mg/kg IM BID) may be useful.[17] Treatment early in the course of disease speeds recovery.[15,20] During an outbreak, lame and febrile lambs should be isolated from healthy lambs to minimize the spread of infection. A vaccine is available for chlamydial abortion, but researchers have not determined whether it provides protection against *C. pecorum* arthritis (see Chapter 6).

Mycoplasmal Polyarthritis

Mycoplasmal arthritis is a highly fatal disease of goats marked by polyarthritis, septicemia, and mastitis. This disease is usually caused by *Mycoplasma mycoides* subspecies *mycoides (Mmm)*, although other mycoplasmas (*M. agalactiae, M. capricolum, M. putrefaciens*) cause similar syndromes.[21] Disease in goats is caused by the large-colony (LC) or caprine biotype of *Mmm*. This is distinct from the small-colony (SC) or bovine biotype that causes contagious bovine pleuropneumonia (CBPP), a disease eradicated from the United States in 1892. Sheep may be experimentally infected, and natural infection in sheep is suspected to occur.[22]

Mycoplasmal arthritis occurs as an epizootic condition in many countries throughout the world. In the United States, most outbreaks are in large goat dairies. Morbidity and mortality rates as high as 90% have been reported in kids.[23] *M. putrefaciens* was responsible for the loss of 700 goats in one California dairy.[24]

Mmm is usually introduced to a farm by an asymptomatic shedder. The bacteria are shed in the colostrum and milk of infected does, and ingestion is thought to be the primary source of infection of kids.[22-24] In one outbreak about half of the does shed *Mmm* in milk. Some animals were intermittent asymptomatic shedders, but most ultimately developed clinical mastitis.[25] Horizontal transmission was documented among kids housed together and is likely to occur among adults, especially in the milking parlor.[26] Illness often follows stresses such as castration, dehorning, concurrent disease, bad weather, and overcrowding.[24,25,27]

Pathogenesis. Infection leads to mycoplasmosis and involvement of numerous body systems, with fibrinous polyarthritis, pneumonia, peritonitis, mastitis, conjunctivitis, and pericarditis being among the more common presentations. If animals recover, the organism may be shed in ocular and nasal secretions and in milk.[28]

Clinical signs. Kids 3 to 8 weeks old are most susceptible, but animals of any age may be affected. Clinical signs include fever, warm swellings of numerous joints, mastitis, lameness, conjunctivitis, weight loss, and pneumonia. Three syndromes have been described in kids. A peracute form results in death in 12 to 24 hours with fever being the only sign. A second group of kids showed signs of brain disease (opisthotonos) and died in 24 to 72 hours. The third syndrome was characterized by fever, warm swollen joints, lameness, recumbency, and pneumonia. Many in this group died within a few days, but some lame kids recovered over a few weeks.[23] Adult females may develop acute or peracute mastitis, the latter causing death in 1 to 3 days. Does that recover may have udder fibrosis and may shed *Mmm* intermittently. Arthritis is a less common finding in adults compared with kids. Mastitis and severe lameness without fever were observed in an *M. putrefaciens* outbreak.[24]

Diagnosis. Laboratory work usually shows leukocytosis, neutrophilia, and hyperfibrinogenemia. Peracute cases may exhibit neutropenia with a left shift. Synovial fluid has an elevated cell count with neutrophilia and fibrin clots. *Mycoplasma* can be cultured using special media. The LC type of *Mmm* is considered less fastidious than other mycoplasmas.[23]

Postmortem findings include suppurative polyarthritis, osteomyelitis, fibrinous pleuritis, pneumonia, peritonitis, meningoencephalitis, and pericarditis.[23,25,27] The joints most commonly affected are the carpus, stifle, tarsus, hip, and elbow. Joint fluid is purulent and contains fibrin, and the joint capsules are thickened, with erosions of articular cartilage. *Mmm* can be cultured from synovial fluid and from many internal sites.[25]

Treatment. Antibiotic treatment does not eliminate infection in most cases. Some animals appear to improve only to relapse later. Tylosin is the antibiotic most commonly recommended (10 to 50 mg/kg TID), but its efficacy is uncertain.[28] The use of newer antibiotics (florfenicol) for mycoplasmal disease in goats has not been examined, but may be of value.

Prevention. Effective preventive measures for kids include the feeding of heat-treated colostrum and pasteurized goat milk. Disease in adults can be controlled by identifying carriers by milk culture and either culling carriers or isolating infected animals and milking them after uninfected animals. Cultures of individual does and the bulk tank should be performed periodically to identify newly infected animals or intermittent shedders, and colostrum should be cultured at the time of freshening. No vaccine is currently commercially available (see Chapter 5).

Osteomyelitis

Bone infections usually result from hematogenous spread of organisms or from direct inoculation associated with trauma to soft tissues covering the bone. The soft tissue damage may be from either an acute injury (trauma or surgical incision) or decubital ulcers in a recumbent animal. Occasionally the ulcers develop during normal recumbency when animals are housed on hard, rough surfaces and are not sequelae of debilitation. The infectious agents include *Corynebacterium*, *A. pyogenes*, *Rhodococcus equi*, and *E. coli*.

Clinical signs. Lameness, pain on palpation, and focal swelling are common clinical signs of osteomyelitis. Severe lameness may result in recumbency. Infection of vertebrae may produce signs of spinal cord dysfunction.[17]

Diagnosis. Radiographic changes usually cannot be seen before the infection has persisted for 10 to 14 days. When radiographic changes are present they consist of a combination of lysis and proliferation. Avascular fragments of dead bone and sequestra also may be seen. If the osteomyelitis is related to a surgical infection, the incision usually dehisces and the surrounding skin shows signs of inflammation or even vascular compromise. The site may be aspirated for culture. Laboratory tests may reveal leukocytosis, leukopenia, or hyperfibrinogenemia.

Trauma without bone infection must be considered as a differential diagnosis for this condition. These cases exhibit soft tissue inflammation but no osseous radiographic changes. The radiographic changes of lysis and proliferation also may resemble the changes seen in response to neoplasia. Osteomyelitis may predispose the animal to pathologic fracture if bone lysis becomes severe enough. The distinction must be made between a pathologic fracture related to neoplasia and a fracture that is infected or becoming a proliferative nonunion.

Treatment and prevention. The prognosis is guarded. Antimicrobial therapy alone is rarely successful because of its poor penetration of infected bone. Surgical débridement of infected tissue is an important component of therapy. Antibiotics, particularly those used based on culture and sensitivity patterns, should be continued for several weeks after surgical débridement. Regional perfusion of antibiotics may be useful in treating osteomyelitis. Amputation is the only possible way to rid the animal of infection in some cases. The possibility of control of infection varies with the cause of the infection. Environmental control is probably the most important mechanism to prevent trauma to the animal. Adherence to aseptic technique when performing any surgery on or near osseous structures decreases surgical infection.

Caprine Arthritis-Encephalitis

CAE is a chronic multisystemic disease of goats caused by a nononcogenic retrovirus. Infection with caprine arthritis-encephalitis virus (CAEV) is widespread and chronic polyarthritis is the most common clinical manifestation.[29] CAEV infection in sheep has been induced experimentally but not reported in nature.[30] Other lentiviruses that are closely related to CAEV include maedi-visna and ovine progressive pneumonia virus (OPPV).

The seroprevalence of CAEV in goats in the United States, Canada, and Europe ranges from 38% to 81%.[29,31,32] Seroprevalence in England, Australia, and developing countries is usually less than 10%.[33] Clinical arthritis is estimated to occur in less than 25% of seropositive animals but it may be more prevalent in some herds.[29,32] The prevalence of other clinical syndromes is not known. Infection occurs by transmission of fluids that contain infected macrophages from an infected animal to an uninfected animal. The most efficient manner of transmission is from dam to kid by ingesting colostrum or milk from infected does.[34] The presence of antiviral antibodies in colostrum is not protective. Feeding nonpasteurized milk increases the risk of infection.[31,32] Horizontal transmission of CAEV has been documented.[34,35] When uninfected goats are housed with infected goats for long periods a significant number seroconvert.[34] Uninfected does readily seroconvert when milked with infected does, presumably as a result of transfer of the virus during the milking process.[34] Venereal transmission is possible, especially if one of the animals is clinically infected.[36] Transmission from doe to kid before or during parturition has been documented.[35] No evidence supports transmission by an insect vector. Iatrogenic transmission (by dehorning equipment or needles) also is possible.

Pathogenesis. CAEV is a single-stranded ribonucleic acid (RNA) virus in the *Lentivirus* family that replicates by forming a reverse transcriptase–dependent deoxyribonucleic acid (DNA) intermediate that may become integrated into the host genome. CAEV infects monocytes and macrophages and induces a persistent (lifelong) infection despite host antibody production. "Restricted replication" allows the virus to remain latent in the host's monocytes and undetected by the immune system. Proposed mechanisms for persistence include latent infection by a DNA provirus, viral replication that waits for monocytes to differentiate into macrophages in tissue, low levels of neutralizing antibodies, and viral mutation of *env* genes. The virus localizes in the macrophages of the synovium, lung, central nervous system, and mammary gland. Initially the virus proliferates rapidly and induces a vigorous immune response that limits but does not eliminate the virus. Virus-infected macrophages may be more prone to activation and thereby induce proliferation of lymphocytes and macrophages. Lymphocyte proliferation is a hallmark pathologic lesion seen in CAEV infection. The important target tissues of CAEV include the joints, mammary glands, lungs, and brain. At these target sites CAEV induces chronic inflammation by invoking the host's immune responses. The virus is capable of making antigenic variants of itself to help it evade the host immune response. CAEV can often be isolated from the synovial fluid and milk of infected animals.[29,34] Disease results from inflammation elicited by the reaction of the immune system to the virus. Infected macrophages express viral proteins near major histocompatibility complex (MHC) antigens, which are recognized by T lymphocytes and stimulate cytokine production. Goats usually seroconvert in 2 to 8 weeks but can have a long clinical latency (years).

Clinical signs. CAEV can cause chronic disease in several body systems; however, most infected animals remain asymptomatic. Four clinical syndromes have been described for CAEV-infected goats: arthritis, leukoencephalomyelitis, interstitial pneumonia, and mastitis.

Chronic progressive arthritis is seen in goats older than 6 months and is usually characterized by swelling of one or both carpal joints. Arthritis of the hock, stifle, hip, and atlantooccipital joints occurs but is not usually detected clinically. In the initial stages, joint swelling may wax and wane, and lameness is minimal. Some animals experience a sudden onset of lameness. The time course is variable, with some animals deteriorating over a few years and others remaining stable for several years.[29] As the disease progresses, animals become lame or recumbent and debilitated. Effusion of the atlantooccipital and supraspinous bursae may be detected. Radiographs of joints show soft tissue swelling initially, and calcification of periarticular structures occurs in more advanced cases. The synovial fluid has a decreased protein concentration and an increased cell count comprised of 90% mononuclear cells, primarily lymphocytes.[29] Postmortem examination usually reveals pathology in numerous joints in addition to the carpus. The joint capsule is thickened, often with periarticular mineralization, but articular cartilage is usually intact. Histopathology shows chronic proliferative synovitis with infiltration by lymphocytes, macrophages, and plasma cells.

Diagnosis. No abnormalities are typically seen on hematology or blood chemistry except for mild anemia in some cases.[29] Routine diagnosis is based on serologic testing, although sensitivity and specificity are not well defined and tests are not standardized. The agar gel immunodiffusion (AGID) test is the most widely used test because of its low cost and rapid results. It has good specificity and fair sensitivity. Laboratories perform the test with either CAEV or OPPV. The enzyme-linked immunospecific assay (ELISA) test may detect infection earlier than the AGID.[36] Polymerase chain reaction (PCR) assays can detect viral proteins in blood, milk, and tissue and may prove useful in diagnosing early infection.[37] Virus isolation takes 3 to 4 weeks and sensitivity is poor.

A positive antibody test signifies infection, although animals may remain asymptomatic for years. The time to seroconversion varies and may not occur for months after infection. Therefore false negatives may occur early in the disease process. Intermittent negative AGID tests have been reported in seropositive animals.[38]

Treatment. No specific treatment exists or is likely to be developed. Affected animals are a source of infection to others and their symptoms worsen over time. Most symptomatic animals are ultimately culled or euthanized because of lameness, recumbency, weight loss, or poor production. Supportive care for affected goats consists of nutritional management and the provision of high-quality, easily digestible, readily accessible feed. Goats with the arthritic form of the disease require frequent proper foot trimming, administration of NSAIDs (phenylbutazone or aspirin 100 mg/kg PO BID), good pasture management, and soft and thick bedding to prevent trauma to the limbs. Treatment as described for degenerative joint disease may be of benefit.

Prevention. Attempts to induce immunity to CAEV with formalin-inactivated virus in adjuvants have not been successful. In fact, vaccinated goats develop more severe disease than unvaccinated controls when challenged.[39]

A program of periodic testing and culling of all positive animals should eradicate the virus from a herd. This method is not often chosen because of the large number of animals likely to be culled from herds with high infection rates.

The following management protocol should significantly reduce the prevalence of CAEV in a herd by eliminating the transmission of CAEV in colostrum and milk. Kids should be removed from the dam at birth to prevent nursing. They should be removed immediately because licking of the kid by the doe may allow transmission of CAEV, presumably via saliva.[36] Kids should be isolated from older animals and given colostrum that has been heat treated at 56° C (133° F) for 1 hour. At this temperature the virus is inactivated but the immunoglobulins remain intact.[36] Kids then are kept isolated and raised on pasteurized (74° C [165° F] for 15 seconds) goat or cow milk or milk replacer. At least every 6 months, keepers should test kids for CAEV and cull animals that test positive. Kids fed pasteurized milk are less likely to seroconvert than kids fed unpasteurized milk. However, cases presumed to result from horizontal transmission may continue to occur.[31,32] Contact transmission of CAEV infection has been demonstrated in goats of all ages, although the exact nature of the contract required for transmission is unknown. Transmission during breeding or gestation (transplacental) is unlikely. In a dairy herd, CAEV-infected does should be milked last. New additions should be quarantined and tested within 60 days of arrival. Under normal husbandry practices, transfer of CAEV from goats to sheep is unlikely.

Chemical disinfection of equipment between use with seropositive and seronegative animals should include the use of phenolic and quaternary ammonium compounds. Complete eradication of CAEV infection in a herd may be impossible without the culling of seropositive goats. Nevertheless, iatrogenic transmission by needles or instruments can be avoided through the use of aseptic technique. Segregation of seropositive and seronegative does by a solid wall or 2 m alley is advisable.[36]

Ovine Progressive Pneumonia

Ovine progressive pneumonia (OPP) is a chronic disease of sheep caused by a nononcogenic retrovirus. Predilection sites for this virus include the lung, udder, and, less commonly, joints. OPPV is similar to maedi-visna virus (MVV), and together the two are referred to as ovine lentivirus (OvLV).[40] OPPV also is closely related to CAEV, and arthritis caused by OPPV in sheep closely resembles that caused by CAEV in goats. Cross-infection with CAEV in sheep and OPPV in goats has been induced experimentally but not reported in nature.[30] Lentiviruses induce persistent infections (life-long) and replicate by integrating DNA into the host genome (see Chapter 5).

Clinical signs. The majority of sheep infected with OPPV are asymptomatic. Clinically apparent illness, which usually occurs years after infection, may involve one or more body systems. The lungs and udder are the sites most commonly affected, but chronic arthritis also occurs in association with OPPV infection.[41-43] In some sheep lameness is the chief clinical sign, although other body systems (typically lung or udder) may be concurrently affected.[41,42]

Because of OPP's long incubation period, clinical signs are observed in adults. Slowly progressive joint swelling, lameness, and weight loss despite good appetite are the typical musculoskeletal manifestations of OPPV infection. The carpi are the joints most commonly affected; the tarsi are affected less frequently.[40,42,43] Examination of the affected joints reveals firm soft tissue swelling.[41,42] Radiography may reveal mineralization of soft tissue and osseous proliferation of adjacent bones.[41] Sheep usually die within 1 year of developing clinical signs.[43] Postmortem examination reveals severe degenerative changes of the joints, with fibrosis of the joint capsule, proliferation of synovial membranes, and erosion of the articular cartilage. Histology reveals nonsuppurative lymphoid infiltration.[43] OPPV can frequently be isolated from the synovial fluid of affected joints.[42] The joint pathology is very similar to that reported in goats with CAEV infection.[42] Differential diagnoses include mycoplasmosis, chlamydial arthritis, and laminitis.

Diagnosis. Serologic tests are useful in diagnosing OPPV infection. The AGID test is the most widely used serologic test for OPPV because it is quick, inexpensive, very specific, and fairly sensitive. Other common serologic tests include ELISA, complement fixation (CF), serum neutralization, immunoblot, and immunoprecipitation. A diagnosis of OPP infection also may be made by virus isolation or identification of viral nucleic acid, but these methods are costly and rarely useful in clinical case management.

Because OPPV infection is lifelong, the presence of antibodies confirms infection, except in the instance of passive transfer of antibodies to a neonate from a positive dam. (Even in this instance, the lamb is likely to become infected by ingesting colostrum or milk from the infected ewe).[44] The majority of infected animals are asymptomatic, so the clinician should rule out other differential diagnoses before concluding that clinical signs are caused by OPP. Obviously, a negative test helps rule out infection. Reasons for false negative results include early infection (seroconversion may not take place for months after infection) and seroreversion, which is seen rarely in advanced stages of the disease.

Treatment. No specific treatment is available for OPPV. Palliative treatment with antiinflammatory drugs could be considered in certain cases; however, affected animals are a source of infection to others (see Chapters 5 and 14).

Lyme Disease

Lyme disease is a multisystemic infection caused by a spirochete, *Borrelia burgdorferi*. *Ixodes* species ticks transmit the organism from rodents such as the white-footed mouse *(Peromyscus leucopus)*, the primary reservoir species in the eastern United States, to larger mammals, including deer, human beings, cattle, horses, and sheep.

Clinical signs. Common clinical signs in human beings and dogs include arthritis, skin rash, neuritis, meningitis, and cardiac disease. Arthritis, abortion, poor milk production, and laminitis have been linked with *B. burgdorferi* infection in cattle.[45] Few cases of Lyme disease have been reported in sheep or goats. However, borreliosis has been suggested as a cause of arthritis in lambs even when *B. burgdorferi* could not be isolated.[46] A seroprevalence study using sheep from nine farms in Scotland revealed that 40% of 1-year-old ewes were seropositive although no clinical disease was reported. The tick *Ixodes ricinus* was present on these farms.[47] Experimental infection of lambs produced no signs of disease.[48]

Diagnosis. Ideally diagnosis depends on the identification of *B. burgdorferi* by culture, PCR, or other techniques, but the organism is difficult to culture and other techniques are not widely available. Serology is often used to confirm a diagnosis, but the high seropositive rate in the absence of clinical disease is a confounding factor. Frequently in endemic regions a clinical diagnosis is made based on clinical signs, elimination of other causes of lameness, and response to treatment.

Treatment. An optimal treatment for Lyme disease in ruminants has not been determined. A typical treatment regimen is a prolonged (2- to 4-week) course of oxytetracycline, ceftiofur, or penicillin. Prevention of the disease currently relies on eliminating the tick with insecticides. A vaccine has been developed for use in dogs, but none is available for large animals.

Clostridial Myonecrosis (Blackleg)

Clostridial myonecrosis is a highly fatal infection of muscle caused by the anaerobic spore-forming bacterium *Clostridium chauvoei*. Other clostridial species (chiefly *C. septicum* and *C. novyi*) have been isolated from cattle with blackleg, either alone or with *C. chauvoei*. The disease is most common in cattle, but sheep also may be affected. Goats appear less susceptible than sheep.[49]

Clostridial myonecrosis is not contagious, but often occurs in outbreaks in sheep because the predisposing conditions affect many animals simultaneously. Infection is usually associated with wounds from castration, dehorning, tail docking, shearing, dystocia, or injections.[50] Animals of any age, including fetal lambs, may be affected.[51] The mortality rate is close to 100%. *C. chauvoei* is ubiquitous and persistent in the soil and is frequently identified in the gastrointestinal tract.

Pathogenesis. In cattle most cases of blackleg arise when endogenous clostridial spores that have lodged in tissues after absorption through the gastrointestinal tract begin to proliferate and produce toxins. These cases do not usually have an associated break in the skin, although the animal may have a history of blunt trauma that might create a hypoxic environment conducive to clostridial growth in the muscle. In contrast, clostridial myositis in sheep most often develops after contamination of a wound by spores from the environment. The vegetative organisms liberate exotoxins that induce severe necrotizing myositis followed by systemic toxemia and death. Clostridial cardiac myositis has been reported in lambs.[50]

Clinical signs. Clostridial myonecrosis progresses very rapidly and animals are often found moribund or dead. Systemic signs observed early in the disease include fever, anorexia, and depression. Local signs depend on the site of infection. If a wound is infected, severe swelling and a malodorous discharge are often evident.[51] Blackleg is almost always fatal.

Diagnosis. Diagnosis is made based on culture of a clostridial pathogen from wounds or necrotic muscle as well as necropsy findings. Samples for anaerobic culture should be taken quickly because the normal proliferation of clostridial organisms in tissue after death can confound results. A Gram's stain of material from diseased muscle may show large gram-positive rods. On gross examination, affected muscle is darker than normal and has a rancid smell. Lesions tend to be deeper and have less associated gas than lesions typically found in cattle.[51] When external wounds are involved, edema is evident. Histology shows myonecrosis, edema, and neutrophilic inflammation; clostridial organisms can usually be visualized. Identification of *C. chauvoei* is aided by fluorescent antibody tests because culture of this organism may be difficult. Differential diagnoses include lightning strike and peracute infections such as anthrax and other clostridial diseases.

Treatment. The rapid death of most patients precludes treatment. However, if animals are detected by their early signs, high doses of penicillin (44,000 IU/kg IV every 4 to 6 hours) are indicated until the animal's condition stabilizes. Surgical incision of the skin and fascia over the affected area is thought to be beneficial. Supportive measures include IV fluids and NSAIDs.

Prevention. Vaccination against *C. chauvoei*, *C. novyi*, and *C. septicum* is recommended to reduce losses at lambing and shearing time. Ewes should receive two doses, the second being administered 1 month before lambing. Annual boosters before lambing are necessary to protect ewes and neonatal lambs. Some of the literature also recommends vaccinating older lambs before shearing. The efficacy of vaccination programs is unknown.

Carcasses should be buried deeply or burned to reduce contamination of soil.[51]

Sarcocystosis

Sarcocystis species parasites are coccidia that cycle between a carnivorous host and a herbivorous intermediate host. In ruminants, infection is often subclinical, but abortion, failure to thrive, and neuromuscular disease have been reported.[52] The development of clinical disease depends on the species of *Sarcocystis* as well as the dose ingested. *S. tenella* is considered the most pathogenic species for sheep, and *S. capracanis* is most pathogenic in goats.[52] The sarcocysts from some species (*S. gigantea, S. medusiformis*) are large enough to be seen macroscopically and result in carcass condemnation.

The prevalence of infection in sheep and goats is high, but clinical disease is uncommon. A postmortem survey of range goats in Texas revealed microscopic *Sarcocystis* species in 60% of the animals, with the tongue being the most commonly affected site.[53] The presence of working dogs that are fed raw meat is associated with sarcocystosis in a herd. Administration of monensin may predispose to the development of clinical disease.[54]

Pathogenesis. The definitive host, a carnivore, becomes infected by eating tissue from an intermediate host that contains sarcocysts. The parasite develops into a sporocyst that is passed in the feces of the definitive host. The intermediate herbivore host is infected by consuming contaminated feed or water. After ingestion, sporozoites penetrate the mucosa of the small intestine and lodge in the endothelial cells of the blood vessels. Damage to the vasculature results in hemorrhage and anemia. The parasites ultimately enter muscle and nerve cells, where they develop into sarcocysts.

Clinical signs. Common clinical signs in sheep include muscular weakness, ataxia, and flaccid paralysis. Poor growth and anemia also have been reported. Lambs are most susceptible. *Sarcocystis* infection also has been associated with esophageal dysfunction in sheep.[52] Experimental infection of two sheep with coyote-origin *Sarcocystis* produced fever, anorexia, and anemia; one sheep exhibited abnormal behavior. Myositis was found in many sites.[53,55]

Goats experimentally infected with *S. capracanis* showed a range of clinical signs. Goats receiving the smallest dose remained clinically normal, but goats receiving higher doses developed fever, depression, and weakness, and many died acutely in the first weeks after infection. Microscopically, stages of the parasite were detected in the endothelial cells of arteries in many organs. Myocardial necrosis was observed in many goats. Multifocal necrosis, gliosis, and vasculitis of the central nervous system was noted, and sarcocysts were found in the brain and spinal cord.[55]

Diagnosis. Laboratory findings reported in cattle include a regenerative anemia, and elevations of the muscle enzymes creatine phosphokinase (CPK), aspartate aminotransferase (AST), and lactate dehydrogenase (LDH). Similar results are expected in sheep and goats. Demonstration of a rise in titer after acute illness aids in diagnosis. Histology of skeletal or cardiac muscle reveals the presence of sarcocysts. Differential diagnoses include the numerous other causes of fever, anemia, and poor growth.

Treatment and prevention. No approved treatment exists for sarcocystosis. The use of amprolium (100 mg/kg/day) or salinomycin has been reported.[53] Carnivores should be kept away from sheep and goats and exposure to uncooked meat or carcasses should be minimized to help control this disease. However, removing carnivorous guard dogs may increase losses to predators. No vaccine is currently available.

Degenerative Joint Disease

Degenerative joint disease is a complex physiologic process that can destroy articular cartilage and cripple animals. Lameness is the most common clinical sign seen in animals with degenerative joint disease. This lameness results from normal destructive processes in the joint overriding the balancing repair processes normally present. This lack of balance in the joint leads to inflammation that produces heat, swelling, and pain. Degenerative joint disease in small ruminants is most often a sequela to infectious arthritis. However, trauma such as direct injury to a joint also can result in degenerative joint disease. Pet goats and sheep (particularly geriatric animals) tend to develop degenerative joint disease, and the condition can be exacerbated by CAE infection.[56] Other joints may be affected as well because of abnormal stresses resulting from aberrant gait or weight-bearing patterns used by the animal to compensate for the injured joint. Unfortunately, small ruminants function well with mild lameness and therefore degenerative disease is often quite advanced before an affected animal is brought to the attention of a veterinarian (Figures 9-11 through 9-13). If a clinician can examine an animal early in the process of degenerative joint disease, he or she may be able to address the etiology directly or at least change management procedures in order to slow the progression of the disease. Some affected animals refuse to walk or have a stiff gait; many often have overgrown feet.

Treatment. Several dietary supplements and chondroprotective agents are available to veterinary practitioners today. No scientific studies support the efficacy of these agents in small ruminants, but anecdotal reports suggest some may be beneficial.[56] Injections of a polysul-

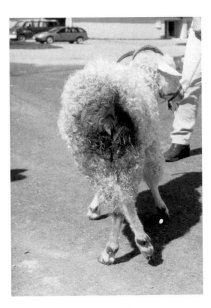

Figure 9-11   This photograph shows an animal with advanced degenerative joint disease. She had a history of an injury to the hip 3 years before this photograph was taken. By the time of presentation to the veterinary hospital this animal needed assistance to stand and would cross her hind legs as shown here.

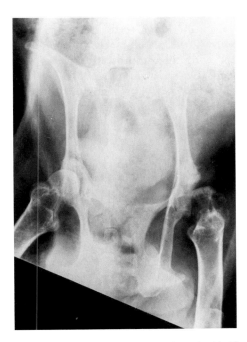

Figure 9-12   Ventrodorsal radiograph of the animal in Figure 9-11 showing extensive bone loss of the left femoral head, which most likely resulted from the reported injury to the hip.

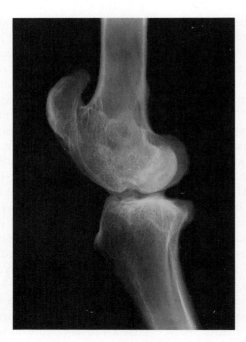

Figure 9-13 A lateral radiographic view of the right stifle of the goat in Figure 9-11. Note the osteophyte formation. The degenerative joint disease observed here is probably the result of abnormal stress in compensating for the chronic coxofemoral lesion.

fated glycosaminoglycan (Adequan) (125 mg/week for 4 weeks) have been suggested. Issues of expense and management regarding long-term treatment of individual animals must be addressed by the owner before instituting therapy with chondroprotective agents. Administration of NSAIDs (phenylbutazone 10 mg/kg PO SID, aspirin 100 mg/kg BID), provision of proper care, maintenance of good body condition scores (2 to 3) in animals, and avoidance of obesity are all valuable parts of the therapeutic plan.[56]

Foot and Mouth Disease

Foot and mouth disease (FMD) is a highly contagious viral disease of ruminants and swine characterized by fever and vesicles of the mouth, feet, and teats. Cattle and pigs are most severely affected, but sheep and goats are susceptible. FMD often produces a mild clinical syndrome in sheep and goats and therefore these species may be inapparent sources of the virus during outbreaks.[57,58] FMD has significant economic impact resulting from loss of production and limitations on movement of animals from affected areas. FMD is endemic in Asia, Africa, South America, and parts of Europe. North America, Central America, and Australia are currently free of FMD.[59] FMD usually occurs as an outbreak that spreads rapidly. All hoof stock except for horses are susceptible. Morbidity is high (close to 100%), although mortality is low. Most deaths are seen in young animals as a result of myocardial necrosis.[57,58]

FMD is readily spread by direct contact with affected animals; aerosolization of the virus is another important source of infection. Ruptured vesicles, respiratory secretions, saliva, milk, urine, and semen are sources of the virus. FMD also may be spread to new premises by human beings, animal products, fomites, and even wind currents.[59] Most animals stop shedding the virus within a few days of vesicle rupture, but cases of long-term (weeks to years) carriers have been reported.[57,58] The virus may persist in the environment for months, and it is not destroyed by common disinfectants. Wild hoof stock are susceptible to FMD and in some cases may act as reservoirs for the virus.

Pathogenesis. The FMD virus, an aphthovirus (family *Picornaviridae*), consists of seven serotypes (O, A, C, Asia 1, SAT 1, 2, and 3) and more than 60 subtypes that vary in virulence and species-specificity.[17] FMD virus gains access to the animal through the mucosal epithelium, viremia ensues, and the virus localizes to epithelial sites throughout the body. Lesions are most evident in the oral mucosa and feet. Necrotizing myocarditis has been reported to affect primarily young animals. Immunity conferred by infection is fairly short-lived (a few years), and cross-protection against other strains is poor.[17]

Clinical signs. In cattle infection with FMD virus produces fever, vesicles, erosions, and ulcers of the oral mucosa, teats, coronary band, and interdigital area. The lesions seem to be very painful, and the resulting clinical signs include anorexia, depression, salivation, agalactia, and lameness. Weight loss, mastitis, and secondary bacterial infections are common sequelae.[17] Most animals recover within 2 to 3 weeks. Sheep and goats usually show milder clinical signs than cattle; however, severe outbreaks have been reported in sheep. Oral lesions are usually mild and transient, and foot lesions and lameness are the predominant symptoms noted.[57,58] If the oral lesions are not detected, FMD may resemble infectious footrot.

Lesions detected on postmortem examination include vesicles, erosions, and ulcers of the mouth and feet. The udder, pharynx, trachea, esophagus, forestomachs, and intestines also may be affected. The myocardia of neonates often have pale streaks caused by necrosis, an appearance known as *tiger heart*.[17]

Diagnosis. Rapid confirmation of FMD is essential because of the far-reaching consequences of this disease. The clinical signs of FMD resemble those of other vesicular diseases such as bluetongue, vesicular stomatitis (which rarely causes disease in small ruminants), and poxvirus infection. If FMD is suspected, a state veterinarian should be contacted immediately.

Treatment. FMD has no specific treatment. Antiinflammatory agents and topical dressings may be used to alleviate discomfort.

Control. FMD-free regions maintain their status by restricting the entry of live animals and animal products from endemic areas. Outbreaks in nonendemic areas are generally controlled by quarantine and eradication of affected animals and those with which they have had contact. In endemic regions vaccination is employed to control FMD. Ideally the vaccine should contain local strains of virus. The immunity provided by killed vaccine is short-lived (6 to 8 months) and is protective against only a few strains of virus. Cattle are usually the focus of a vaccination program, but vaccination of sheep and goats in endemic regions is recommended.[57,58]

REFERENCES

1. Kaneps AJ: Orthopedic conditions of small ruminants, *Vet Clin North Am Adv Rumin Orthop* 12(1):211, 1996.
2. Nyack B, Padmore CL, White M: External fixation of carpal and metacarpal fractures in a goat, *Bovine Pract* 3(3):23, 1982.
3. Smith MC: Practice tips for small ruminant veterinarians, *Proceedings of the 1998 Symposium on Small Ruminants for the Mixed Animal Practitioner Western Veterinary Conference*, 1998, Las Vegas, NV.
4. Mbiuki SM, Byagagaire SD: Full limb casting: a treatment for tibial fractures in calves and goats, *Vet Med* 79(2):243, 1984.
5. Monin T: Tension band repair of equine mandibular fractures, *J Eq Med Surg* 1(10):325, 1977.
6. DeBowes RM: *Equine fracture repair*, Philadelphia, 1996, WB Saunders.
7. Nunamaker DM et al: A new skeletal fixation device that allows immediate full weight bearing application in the horse, *Vet Surg* 15(5):345, 1986.
8. Egger EL, Greenwood KM: *Textbook of small animal surgery*, Philadelphia, 1985, WB Saunders.
9. St-Jean G, Clem MF, DeBowes RM: Transfixation pinning and casting of tibial fractures in calves: five cases (1985-1989), *J Am Vet Med Assoc* 198:139, 1991.
10. Arnoczky SP, Blass CE, McCoy L: External coaptation and bandaging. In Slatter DH, editor: *Textbook of small animal surgery*, Philadelphia, 1985, WB Saunders.
11. Lamont MH: Arthritis. In Martin WS, editor: *Diseases of sheep*, Oxford, UK, 1983, Blackwell Scientific.
12. Watkins GH, Sharp MW: Bacteria isolated from arthritis and omphalitic lesions in lambs in England and Wales, *Vet J* 156:235, 1998.
13. Trent AM, Plumb D: Treatment of infectious arthritis and osteomyelitis, *Vet Clin North Am Food Anim Pract* 7:747, 1991.
14. Navarre CB et al: Ceftiofur distribution in plasma and joint fluid following regional limb injection in cattle, *J Vet Pharmacol Ther* 22:13, 1999.
15. Adams DS: Infectious causes of lameness proximal to the foot, *Vet Clin North Am Food Anim Pract* 5:499, 1983.
16. Everett KDE: Chlamydia and chlamydiates: more than meets the eye, *Vet Microbiol* 75:109, 2000.
17. Radostits OM et al: *Veterinary medicine*, ed 9, Philadelphia, 2000, WB Saunders.
18. Bulgin MS: Diagnosis of lameness in sheep, *Compend Contin Ed Pract Vet* 8:F122, 1986.
19. Stephenson EH, Storz J, Hopkins JB: Properties and frequency of isolation of *Chlamydia* from eyes of lambs with conjunctivitis and polyarthritis, *Am J Vet Res* 35:177, 1974.
20. Cutlip RC, Smith PC, Page LA: Chlamydial polyarthritis of lambs: a review, *J Am Vet Med Assoc* 161:1213, 1972.
21. DaMassa AJ, Wakenell PS, Brooks DL: Mycoplasmas of goats and sheep, *J Vet Diagn Invest* 4:101, 1992.
22. Rosendal S: Experimental infection of goats, sheep, and calves with the large colony type of *Mycoplasma mycoides* subsp. *mycoides*, *Vet Path* 18:71, 1981.
23. DaMassa AJ, Brooks DL, Adler HE: Caprine mycoplasmosis: widespread infection in goats with *Mycoplasma mycoides* subsp *mycoides* (large colony type), *Am J Vet Res* 44:322, 1983.
24. DaMassa AJ et al: Caprine mycoplasmosis: an outbreak of mastitis and arthritis requiring the destruction of 700 goats, *Vet Rec* 120:409, 1987.
25. East NE et al: Milkborne outbreak of *Mycoplasma mycoides* subspecies *mycoides* infection in a commercial goat dairy, *J Am Vet Med Assoc* 182:1338, 1983.
26. DaMassa AJ, Brooks DL, Holmberg CA: Induction of mycoplasmosis in goat kids by oral inoculation with *Mycoplasma mycoides* subsp *mycoides*, *Am J Vet Res* 47:2084, 1986.
27. Rosendal S: *Mycoplasma mycoides* subspecies *mycoides* as a cause of polyarthritis in goats, *J Am Vet Med Assoc* 175:378, 1979.
28. East NE: *Mycoplasma mycoides* polyarthritis in goats. In Smith BP, editor: *Large animal medicine*, ed 2, St Louis, 1996, Mosby.
29. Crawford TB, Adams DS: Caprine arthritis-encephalitis: clinical features and presence of antibody in selected goat populations, *J Am Vet Med Assoc* 178:713, 1981.
30. Banks KL et al: Experimental infection of sheep by caprine arthritis-encephalitis virus and goats by progressive pneumonia virus, *Am J Vet Res* 44:2307, 1983.
31. Rowe JD et al: Risk factors associated with the incidence of seroconversion to caprine arthritis-encephalitis virus in goats on California dairies, *Am J Vet Res* 53: 2396, 1992.
32. East NE et al: Serologic prevalence of caprine arthritis-encephalitis virus in California goat dairies, *J Am Vet Med Assoc* 190:182, 1987.
33. Adams DS et al: Global survey of serological evidence of caprine arthritis-encephalitis virus infection, *Vet Rec* 115:493, 1984.
34. Adams DS et al: Transmission and control of caprine arthritis-encephalitis virus, *Am J Vet Res* 44:1670, 1983.
35. East NE et al: Modes of transmission of caprine arthritis-encephalitis virus infection, *Small Rumin Res* 10:251, 1993.
36. Rowe JD, East NE: Risk factors for transmission and methods for control of caprine arthritis-encephalitis virus infection, *Vet Clin North Am Food Anim Pract* 13:35, 1997.
37. Smith MC, Cutlip R: Effects of infection with caprine arthritis-encephalitis virus on milk production in goats, *J Am Vet Med Assoc* 193:63, 1988.
38. Hanson J, Hydbring E, Olsson K: A long term study of goats naturally infected with caprine arthritis-encephalitis virus, *Acta Vet Scand* 37:31, 1996.
39. McGuire TC et al: Acute arthritis in caprine arthritis-encephalitis virus challenge exposure of vaccinated or persistently infected goats, *Am J Vet Res* 47:537, 1986.
40. de la Concha-Bermejillo A: Maedi-visna and ovine progressive pneumonia, *Vet Clin North Am Food Anim Pract* 13:13, 1997.

41. Oliver RE et al: Ovine progressive pneumonia: pathologic and virologic studies on the naturally occurring disease, *Am J Vet Res* 42:1554, 1981.

42. Cutlip RC et al: Arthritis associated with ovine progressive pneumonia, *Am J Vet Res* 46:65, 1985.

43. Cutlip RC et al: Ovine progressive pneumonia (maedi-visna) in sheep, *Vet Microbiol* 17:237, 1988.

44. Knowles DP: Laboratory diagnostic tests for retrovirus infections of small ruminants, *Vet Clin North Am Food Anim Pract* 13:1, 1997.

45. Parker JL, White KK: Lyme borreliosis in cattle and horses: a review of the literature, *Cornell Vet* 82:253, 1992.

46. Fridriksdottir V, Overnes G, Stuen S: Suspected Lyme borreliosis in sheep, *Vet Rec* 130:323, 1992.

47. Mitchell GBB, Smith IW: Lyme disease in Scotland: results of a serological study in sheep, *Vet Rec* 133:66, 1993.

48. Stuen S. Fridriksdottir V: Experimental inoculation of sheep with *Borrelia burgdorferi*, *Vet Rec* 129:315, 1991.

49. Guss SB: *Management and diseases of dairy goats*, Scottsdale, AZ, 1977, Dairy Goat Journal Publishing.

50. Radostits OM et al: *Veterinary medicine*, ed 9, Philadelphia, 2000, WB Saunders.

51. Glastonbury JR et al: Clostridial myocarditis in lambs, *Aust Vet J* 65:208, 1988.

52. Dubey JP, Livingston CW: *Sarcocystis capracanis* and *Toxoplasma gondii* infections in range goats from Texas, *Am J Vet Res* 47:523, 1986.

53. Jeffrey M, Low JC, Uggla A: A myopathy of sheep associated with *Sarcocystis* infection and monensin administration, *Vet Rec* 124:422, 1989.

54. Dubey JP, Fayer R, Seesee FM: *Sarcocystis* in feces of coyotes from Montana: prevalence and experimental transmission to sheep and cattle, *J Am Vet Med Assoc* 173:1167, 1978.

55. Dubey JP et al: Sarcocystosis in goats: clinical signs and pathologic and hematologic findings, *J Am Vet Med Assoc* 178:683, 1981.

56. Smith ME: Exotic disease of small ruminants. Geriatric medicine for small ruminants, *Proceedings of the 1998 Symposium on Small Ruminants for the Mixed Animal Practitioner Western Veterinary Conference*, 1998, Las Vegas, NV.

57. Sharma SK: Foot and mouth disease in sheep and goats, *Vet Res J* 4:1, 1981.

58. Barnett PV, Cox SJ: The role of small ruminants in the epidemiology and transmission of foot and mouth disease, *Vet J* 158:6, 1999.

59. Scott GR: Foot-and-mouth disease. In Sewell MMH, Brocklesby DW, editors: *Handbook on animal diseases in the tropics*, ed 4, Philadelphia, 1990, Bailliere Tindall.

METABOLIC AND NUTRITIONAL CONDITIONS

Nutritional Muscular Dystrophy

Nutritional muscular dystrophy (NMD), also known as *white muscle disease,* is a disease of all large animals caused by a deficiency of selenium and/or vitamin E. The disease affects skeletal and cardiac muscle and is most common in young, rapidly growing animals. Selenium and vitamin E deficiencies also produce syndromes of ill thrift and reproductive losses (see Chapter 2).[1]

NMD occurs in selenium-deficient areas throughout the world. It is a significant disease in North America, the United Kingdom, Europe, Australia, and New Zealand. In the United States the northeast, southeast, and northwest regions are deficient in selenium; the central region has sufficient selenium in its soil.[2] Even within a region the selenium content of soil and forage may vary depending on pH, season, and type of plants grown. For example, alkaline soils encourage selenium uptake by plants, whereas plants grown in areas of high rainfall and acidic soils are usually low or marginal in selenium content.[3] In most instances the selenium content of pasture is lowest in the spring. Nitrogen and to a certain degree phosphorus fertilization and irrigation may decrease selenium uptake by plants. Faster-growing plants have a lower selenium content; this condition is exacerbated when plants are grown on soils already marginal in selenium. Hay grown in drier areas tends to have a higher selenium concentration. Hay analysis is crucial in determining dietary selenium intake.

Selenium is absorbed, as are other minerals, in the small intestine. Therefore high concentrations of other minerals (e.g., calcium, sulfur, copper) may decrease its absorption. Also, certain feed contaminants (e.g., nitrate, unsaturated fats, sulfates) may further suppress selenium uptake and availability.[4] Forage with less than 0.1 ppm of selenium on a dry matter basis is deficient.

Vitamin E helps prevent peroxidation of cell membrane lipids, aiding in the maintenance of membrane integrity. It also is somewhat protective against selenium deficiency. Of the forms of vitamin E, the d-isomer of alpha-tocopherol has the greatest biologic activity. It also is absorbed in the upper small intestine.[5] Because bile acids are needed for proper absorption, derangements in small intestine function can decrease the absorption of vitamin E, even if dietary concentrations are adequate. Vitamin E–deficient sheep and goats probably absorb 50% to 75% of dietary tocopherol, whereas animals receiving adequate vitamin E absorb only 20% to 30%. Vitamin E activity is good in green pasture and good hay. Legumes often have less available vitamin E than grass.[3] Vitamin E can be destroyed by oxidative destruction, particularly if large amounts of unsaturated fats and certain minerals (e.g., copper, iron) are added to the same supplement or mineral mixture. Long-term storage of feedstuffs decreases vitamin E activity by as much as 50% per month.[3]

Deficiencies occur when animals are fed poor-quality hay or straw and lack access to pasture. Diets high in polyunsaturated fatty acids contribute to the development of NMD by increasing the requirement for vitamin E. Vitamin E requirements also are increased if vitamin C and/or carotenoids are deficient or if dietary nitrate intake is increased. However, adequate vitamin C and beta-carotene in the diet help lower vitamin E requirements. Adequate dietary selenium is almost completely protective against vitamin E deficiency.[6]

Limited vitamin E transport occurs across the placenta, but colostrum has a large quantity of vitamin E. Therefore lambs and kids deprived of colostrum need supplemental vitamin E.

NMD occurs most commonly in kids and lambs whose mothers were fed a selenium-deficient diet. Most cases occur in animals less than 6 months old, and NMD has been reported in neonates. Kids are believed to be more susceptible than lambs, possibly because they have a higher requirement for selenium. Further, sudden muscular activity in deficient animals unaccustomed to exercise often triggers episodes of NMD.[1]

Hydrogen peroxide and other free radicals are toxic byproducts of cell metabolism that have the ability to cause oxidative damage to biologic membranes. Selenium is a cofactor in several enzyme systems in the body, but much of the pathology associated with selenium deficiency is caused by an impairment of the enzyme glutathione peroxidase (GPx). GPx protects cell membranes against destruction by these endogenous peroxides by converting them to relatively benign hydroxy fatty acids. The lipid-soluble vitamin E molecule acts as a free radical scavenger within the cell membrane. High concentrations of dietary fat can overwhelm the vitamin E protection system.[6] Selenium and vitamin E act as antioxidants by separate mechanisms; diets that are deficient in selenium or vitamin E permit oxidative damage, which leads to muscle degeneration. The deficiency of these two nutrients result in a buildup of free radicals and increases in subsequent damage. Muscles with high metabolic activity are most susceptible (e.g., heart, diaphragm). This syndrome and other selenium-responsive diseases are most commonly encountered in young growing lambs, particularly those 2 to 4 months of age.[3,7] Selenium deficiency also may impair the body's immune system. In cattle and possibly in sheep and goats, deficient selenium intake can result in reduced neutrophilic response, a higher incidence of mastitis and metritis, and poor overall body condition. Because of their compromised immune systems, many of these lambs are more susceptible to other contagious diseases. Sheep consuming selenium-deficient diets produce low wool yields and may have an increased incidence of periodontal disease. Adults consuming a deficient diet may have these signs, whereas growing lambs and kids exhibit NMD.

Clinical signs.   Two syndromes of NMD are classically described: an acute to peracute cardiac form and the more common subacute skeletal muscle form. Animals with involvement of cardiac muscle show acute signs that include recumbency, respiratory distress, and death. Respiratory signs include tachypnea and frothy nasal discharge resulting from pulmonary edema. Tachycardia is common, sometimes accompanied by a heart murmur. Animals are often alert and their struggles to arise may be interpreted as seizures. A history of collapse after exercise is typical (see Chapter 15). Differential diagnoses include toxicities, fulminant infectious diseases, pneumonia, and neurologic disease such as polioencephalomalacia or tetanus.

Animals with skeletal muscle degeneration have a different appearance. These animals have a stiff gait and tremble while standing. Many prefer to remain in sternal recumbency. The muscles may feel firm. Signs described in this form of the disease include hunched appearance, stiff gait, and overall poor production.[3] Lambs and kids continue to weaken and eventually become unable to nurse.[7] Many young have aspiration pneumonia resulting from dysfunction of the glottis. Some adult animals continue to eat, but others are dysphagic because of involvement of the tongue. Skeletal and cardiac muscle disease may occur concurrently. Careful assessment of flock history and a through physical examination are required to determine the underlying cause of the pneumonia. Other diseases that may appear similar include enzootic ataxia, polyarthritis, and nutritional osteodystrophy. Vitamin E–associated NMD is most commonly encountered in lambs and yearling ewe lambs.[3]

Diagnosis.   Elevated creatine kinase (CK) is a good indicator of subclinical NMD.[3] Marked elevations in CK (10 to 50 ×) can occur in NMD. CK has a short half-life (2 to 4 hours), so elevations indicate recent or ongoing muscle damage. CK levels return to normal as the animal recovers. AST also is elevated with muscle injury; however, it is not specific to muscle disease—hepatic disease also may cause elevations in AST. AST has a longer half-life than CK, and concentrations are elevated for several days after an episode of NMD. Elevations in CK and AST are not specific for NMD, and these enzymes may be elevated in any recumbent animal. However, CK and AST generally occur in much higher serum concentrations in the presence of primary muscle disease such as NMD.

Selenium deficiency can be confirmed by measuring selenium levels in whole blood or tissues. In cases of flock problems, 10% of the flock or 7 to 10 ewes and/or lambs should have blood collected for selenium analysis.[3] Erythrocyte GPx concentrations are highly correlated with selenium concentration, and activity of this enzyme is a useful diagnostic test. However, GPx samples must be handled with care, and many diagnostic laboratories do not offer the test. Testing for serum selenium levels may be of value for flock assays if the diet has been maintained for weeks to months. It is of questionable value in assessing individuals, particularly those that have experienced any dietary changes. Obviously, most sick animals have undergone a diet change, and many have anorexia. Evaluating whole blood selenium is the easiest and most reliable test. Selenium concentrations in whole blood reflect the selenium concentration of the diet over the life of a red blood cell.[8] More than 95% of blood selenium is located inside the red blood cell and was placed there when the cell was manufactured. Vitamin E status can be assessed by measuring serum tocopherol. Some specialized laboratories offer a vitamin E assay. This chapter does not provide guidelines for adequate or deficient concentrations because of the variance in techniques and assays among laboratories. Instead, the clinician should inquire about normal values from the laboratory where samples are assayed.

At necropsy, affected muscles are friable and contain pale streaks that correspond with regions of degeneration and mineralization. The distribution is bilaterally symmetric. Similar changes are seen in the myocardium if animals have cardiac involvement. Histology of muscle shows hyaline degeneration, necrosis, and mineralization. Chronic infections (caused by depressed immune function) and aspiration pneumonia (resulting from compromised glottis-closing ability) also may be encountered.[1-3]

Treatment.   One injection of a vitamin E and/or selenium preparation should result in improvement within a few days. The treatment can be repeated in 24 hours. Following the label doses of some commercial products will provide adequate selenium but very little vitamin E, and supplementation may be required. If other animals show clinical signs, they also should be treated. The clinician should avoid exposing the animals to stress or exertion during treatment. Most animals respond to treatment; however, those with cardiac involvement have a poor recovery rate.

Prevention.   NMD can be prevented by supplementing the diet of susceptible animals with selenium and vitamin E. Supplementation of pregnant animals helps reduce disease in newborns because selenium is transferred across the placenta and also is present in colostrum and milk. Clinicians and keepers should pay careful attention to the proper dosage of selenium to prevent toxicosis in the animals and should adhere to withdrawal periods to limit concentrations in tissues at slaughter. Pasture, hay, and any grain supplements should be assayed to determine the amount of selenium to be added to a supplemental pellet, grain, or mineral mixture.

Selenium and vitamin E supplementation can take many forms. The dietary concentration of selenium should be more than 0.1 to 0.3 mg/kg.[1,7] Feed supplementation is commonly recommended. In some circumstances, higher levels of selenium are necessary to prevent NMD in lambs. Dietary supplementation appears to be the least expensive, most efficient method of ensuring selenium adequacy. Current regulations in the United States limit selenium supplementation for sheep to 0.7 mg/head/day or 90 ppm in the mineral mixture for free choice feeding.[3] Although the use of free choice mineral supplementation is an excellent mode of selenium supplementation, ensuring a complete diet or providing a dietary supplement of 0.2 ppm selenium ensures more consistent mineral intake.[7] Fresh legumes and grasses are good sources of vitamin E.[9] Silage, oil seeds, cereal grains, and dry hays tend to be poor sources of vitamin E.[5] Therefore, diets high in grain content should be supplemented with vitamin E.

Alternatively, selenium and vitamin E can be incorporated in mineral mixes that are fed free choice to pregnant and lactating ewes. If feedstuffs contain oxidizing agents (e.g., copper, iron), fats, or a high content of disulfide bonds (onions), vitamin E potency may be reduced, with resultant deficiency.[3] Whenever these dietary factors are encountered, supplemental vitamin E is indicated. Diets high in corn also may be associated with vitamin E deficiency because a lowered rumen pH reduces vitamin E activity. This condition can be clinically significant in the young growing lamb or kid.

If it is not practical to supplement the diet, monthly injections of a commercial vitamin E–selenium selenite compound may be useful, although they may need to be repeated more often in lambs.[1] Injecting the dam 30 days before birth can help prevent NMD.[3,7] Injecting lambs with selenium–vitamin E preparations at tail docking (1 mg selenium) and again at weaning (2 mg selenium) may be protective on some farms. In addition to injected supplements, another source of vitamin E should be provided because the amount in commercially available injectable compounds are too low to prevent disease in deficient animals. Access to pasture or quality forage should provide adequate levels of vitamin E.

Other options for selenium supplementation are practiced in some regions. A slow-release formulation of selenite can be given by SC injection. A dose of 1 mg/kg selenium given to ewes 3 weeks before lambing protects lambs for as long as 12 weeks after birth. An intraruminal selenium pellet also is available for sheep. Top-dressing of pasture with sodium selenite at a dose of 10 g selenium/hectare is practiced in some countries. This method is safe and prevents NMD for at least 12 months.[1] For bottle-fed lambs, the keeper should ensure an intake of adequate vitamin E in the milk replacer.

Rickets and Osteomalacia

Rickets is a disease of young animals caused by a failure of proper cartilage mineralization. Vitamin D deficiency is the most common cause, but rickets may occur as a result of deficiencies in phosphorus and calcium as well. In older animals the same deficiencies result in abnormal mineralization of osteoid, a condition known as *osteomalacia*.

Rickets occurs mostly in rapidly growing animals that have low vitamin D levels because of limited sun exposure. Animals housed indoors, those fed green (uncured) forage, and those living at high latitudes in winter are most prone. Animals that consume a diet low in calcium or phosphorus occasionally develop rickets. Ingestion of some poisonous plants, particularly those containing oxalates (which bind calcium in the intestine); chronic lead or flouride aluminum toxicity; and chronic parasitism can all produce or add to the pathogenesis of rickets.[6]

Pathogenesis.   The primary problem is failure of mineralization of cartilage and osteoid, which leads to persistence of cartilage and irregular osteoid deposition.[4] Irregular osteochondral junctions and widened physes result. The metaphyses at the costochondral junctions are noticeably affected. In the long bones the persistent soft tissue in the physis is deformed by weight bearing. In the diaphysis, osteoid is not properly mineralized.[10] Long-haired or woolly animals raised in latitudes closer to the earth's poles, those raised indoors, and those fed milk replacers with inadequate vitamin D concentrations may be particularly deficient in vitamin D and predisposed to NMD.

Clinical signs.   Affected animals are usually less than 1 year old and have a stiff gait, shifting legs, lameness, and recumbency. Joints and bones of the distal aspects of the limbs may be enlarged, and enlargements of the ribs at the costochondral junctions (rachitic rosary) are frequently seen. Limbs are frequently deformed and may be bowed. Teeth may be mottled and their eruption delayed. Animals may be thin as a result of failure to graze adequate forage.[8] Differential diagnoses include NMD and infectious arthritis.

Diagnosis.   Blood chemistry shows elevations in alkaline phosphatase greater than those seen in normally growing animals. Blood levels of calcium and phosphorus may be low. Serum vitamin D is low but usually within normal ranges. Radiographic changes include widened growth plates, bowing of long bones, and thinned cortices.[10] In adults with osteomalacia, radiographic examination reveals porous bone.

Postmortem examination reveals thickening of growth plates and epiphyseal enlargement of long bones. Rib fractures are often apparent. Histopathology of samples from the costochondral junction in live animals also may be useful.[10] Normal bone contains an ash–to–organic matter ratio of 3:2, whereas the ratio in rachitic bone is 1:2 to 1:3.

Careful investigation of feed content; access to sunlight; and vitamin D, calcium, and phosphorus levels aid in determining the underlying cause of rickets.

Treatment.   Vitamin D_3 injections (10,000 to 30,000 IU/kg) may be beneficial if dietary supplementation of calcium and phosphorus occurs concurrently.[10,11] Recov-

ered animals frequently maintain a short stature with limb deformities.

Prevention.   Rickets and osteomalacia can be managed by providing access to sunlight and properly cured forage. Dietary calcium and phosphorus levels should be adjusted if they are low, and a calcium-to-phosphorus ratio of 1:1 to 2:1 should be maintained. Any potentially toxic substances or plants should be removed from the diet.

Osteodystrophia Fibrosa

Osteodystrophia fibrosa is a metabolic disease of goats and sheep in which bone mineral is resorbed as a result of prolonged hypersecretion of parathyroid hormone (PTH). High phosphorus or low calcium levels in the diet frequently contribute to osteodystrophia fibrosa. Clinically, this disease is similar to rickets.

Osteodystrophia fibrosa is most commonly seen in animals consuming a high-phosphorus diet. Diets with a high proportion of bran or other cereal grains are often associated with this disease. Cereal grains have an inappropriate calcium-to-phosphorus ratio, and much of the phosphorus in cereal grains is in the form of phytic acid. High phytic acid content can further depress calcium absorption from the intestine. The dietary calcium–to–phosphorus ratio should be maintained at 1:1 to 2:1. Many cereal grains or byproduct feeds (bran) have a ratio of 1:6 or greater.

Pathogenesis.   Primary hyperparathyroidism caused by hyperplasia or neoplasia of the parathyroid gland is extremely rare. Most cases of hyperparathyroidism are sequelae of nutritional or metabolic conditions that produce hypocalcemia. Diets with low levels of calcium, high levels of phosphorus, or deficient amounts of vitamin D may result in hyperparathyroidism; frequently more than one factor is present. PTH stimulates vitamin D production, which in turn induces resorption of bone in the animal to maintain calcium homeostasis. Renal failure also may result in hyperparathyroidism, but this manifestation is uncommon in sheep and goats. All the bones of the body are affected, but the bones of the face and mandible are most obviously abnormal.

Clinical signs.   Bilateral enlargement of the mandible is typically the most obvious sign. The mandible feels soft and the animal may not be able to open its mouth properly. Lameness and stiffness are often observed as a result of pathologic fractures. Animals are often thin because of decreased food intake.

Diagnosis.   Radiographs show enlargement of the mandible, decreased bone density, and rotation of the cheek teeth with the occlusal surfaces pointed lingually. Fractures of other bones may be apparent.[12] Laboratory results may show low calcium or high phosphorus levels, but these tests often fall within the normal range. Alkaline phosphatase is sometimes elevated.[13] Postmortem examination shows the mandible to be quite soft and malleable. Histology of the mandible shows a lack of mineralization of bone and replacement of bone by an extensive fibrous matrix.

Caseous lymphadenitis (CL) commonly causes mandibular enlargement as a result of abscess formation in the submandibular and retropharyngeal lymph nodes. Palpation and radiographs should aid in distinguishing between CL and osteodystrophia fibrosa.

Treatment. Animals may recover if placed on a diet with a calcium-to-phosphorus ratio of 1:1 or 2:1. The enlarged mandible may not improve.[13] Formulation of a ration that ensures a calcium-to-phosphorus ratio of 1:1 or greater should prevent nutritional hyperparathyroidism and osteodystrophia fibrosa.

Epiphysitis

Epiphysitis is a condition of rapidly growing animals in which improper ossification of the physes occurs. The etiology is complex, with both genetic and dietary factors believed to play roles. It is seen in young rams being fed to maximize growth and is associated with pregnancy in about 1% of yearling dairy does.[14]

Clinical signs. Clinical signs reported in a pregnant yearling Nubian doe included insidious onset of lameness progressing to recumbency. Enlargement of the carpi, tarsi, and fetlock joints were observed, as was angular limb deformity. Radiographs revealed delayed maturation of cartilage and overgrowth of new bone. The animal's gait improved shortly after parturition, but a degree of limb deformity resulting from premature closure of a portion of the physes remained. The cause was attributed to trauma to the physes as a result of advanced pregnancy.[15] After noting epiphysitis in animals, the keeper should examine the diet to assess the adequacy of copper and maintain a proper calcium-to-phosphorus ratio of 4:1 to 6:1. Adequate calcium, phosphorus, protein, and energy should all be maintained. Proper foot trimming, the provision of pain relief (NSAIDs), and the removal of animals from hard surfaces may all be of benefit.[16,17]

Osteochondrosis

Osteochondrosis is a disease of abnormal endochondral ossification. It is common in pigs and chickens and occurs in most domestic animals, but it is rarely reported in small ruminants. However, osteochondrosis should not be omitted from a differential diagnosis list when animals that have been fed diets high in grain to produce rapid weight gain develop lameness or joint swelling. Radiographs of affected animals reveal osteochondrosis lesions as seen in other domestic animals.

REFERENCES

1. Radostits OM et al: *Veterinary medicine*, ed 9, Philadelphia, 2000, WB Saunders.
2. Edmondson AJ, Norman BB, Suther D: Survey of state veterinarians and state veterinary diagnostic laboratories for selenium deficiency and toxicosis in animals, *J Am Vet Med Assoc* 202:865,1993.
3. Maas J, Parish SM, Hodgson DR: Nutritional myodegeneration. In Smith BP, editor: *Large animal internal medicine*, St Louis, 1996, Mosby.
4. Jubb KVF, Kennedy PC, Palmer N: *Pathology of domestic animals*, ed 3, Orlando, FLA, 1985, Academic Press.
5. Bulgin MS: Diagnosing nutritional difficulties, *Proceedings of the 1998 Symposium on Small Ruminants for the Mixed Animal Practitioner Western Veterinary Conference*, 1998, Las Vegas, NV.
6. Smart ME, Cymbaulk: Trace minerals. In Naylor JM, Ralston SL, editors: *Large animal clinical nutrition*, St Louis, 1991, Mosby.
7. Naylor JM: Vitamins. In Naylor JM, Ralston SL, editors: *Large animal clinical nutrition*, St Louis, 1991, Mosby.
8. Ogilvie TH: Musculoskeletal disorders. In Ogilvie TH, editor: *Large animal internal medicine*, Baltimore, 1998, Williams & Wilkins.
9. Bretzlaff K, Haenlein G, Huston E: Common nutritional problems feeding the sick goat. In Naylor JM, Ralston SL, editors: *Large animal clinical nutrition*, St Louis, 1991, Mosby.
10. Maas J: Rickets in ruminants. In Smith BP, editor: *Large animal internal medicine*, St Louis, 1996, Mosby.
11. Bonniwell MA et al: Rickets associated with vitamin D deficiency in young sheep, *Vet Rec* 122:386, 1988.
12. Andrews AH, Ingram PL, Longstaffe JA: Osteodystrophia fibrosa in young goats, *Vet Rec* 112:404, 1983.
13. Hesters NL, Yates DJ, Hunt E: Nutritional secondary hyperparathyroidism. In Smith BP, editor: *Large animal internal medicine*, ed 2, St Louis, 1996, Mosby.
14. Guss SB: *Management and diseases of dairy goats*, Scottsdale, AZ, 1977, Dairy Goat Journal Publishing.
15. Bulgin MS: Diagnosis of lameness in sheep, *Compend Contin Ed Pract Vet* 8:F122,1986.
16. Hintz HF: Physitis (epiphysitis). In Smith BP, editor: *Large animal internal medicine*, ed 2, St Louis 1996, Mosby.
17. Anderson KL, Adams WM: Epiphysitis and recumbency in a yearling prepartum goat, *J Am Vet Med Assoc* 183:226, 1983.

TOXIC CONDITIONS

Selenium Toxicity

Selenium toxicity may result from grazing pastures with a high selenium content or from exogenous administration of selenium by injection or feed supplementation. Acute poisoning may result in death, but chronic overdose leads to hoof malformation and lameness. The toxic dose for sheep has been reported to be 2.2 mg/kg orally as a single dose or chronic ingestion of 0.25 mg/kg body weight.[1] Sheep are considered more susceptible to selenium toxicosis than cattle. Little information is available about the natural occurrence of selenium toxicosis in goats, but the administration of high doses of selenium can result in death.[2]

Soils in specific regions of North America, Ireland, Australia, and South Africa have a high selenium content because of the composition of the underlying rock.[1] Soils in areas of low annual rainfall often have an alkaline pH and are more likely to have high selenium levels. Plants extract selenium from the soil, and certain plants are concentrators of selenium. These plants are not highly palatable, but animals that graze in these areas may develop signs of toxicity if more palatable forage is lacking. Documented cases of naturally occurring selenium toxicity are uncommon.[3]

Selenium poisoning also occurs when incorrect doses of selenium are administered to flocks in an attempt to prevent NMD.

Organic selenium compounds (i.e., those found in plants) are considered more toxic than inorganic compounds such as selenite and selenium dioxide. This reported difference does not always correlate with clinical disease.[1]

Pathogenesis. Selenium concentrates in the kidney, liver, and keratinized tissue and has a dystrophic effect on skeletal muscle. Toxic concentrations of selenium may displace sulfur in some of the amino acids (methionine, cystine), preventing them from forming disulfide bonds and thereby weakening keratin formation. Hoof material has high concentrations of methionine and cystine. The mechanism of toxicity has not been determined, but selenium also may interfere with the function of certain enzymes. A high-protein diet is protective against selenium toxicosis in sheep.[1]

Clinical signs. Acute poisoning results in dyspnea, tachycardia, fever, depression, and death. Signs of chronic toxicity include poor hair coat, alopecia, ill thrift, abnormal appetite, respiratory failure, and lameness. Hoof lesions are apparent in all feet and include edema of the coronary bands and deformity or separation of hooves. Neonates may have hoof abnormalities apparent at birth.

Diagnosis. Diagnosis is based on identifying toxic levels of selenium in the animal. Selenium levels in blood, urine, and hair are all elevated. Anemia and low hemoglobin levels are characteristic of chronic selenium poisoning. Necropsy findings in chronic selenium poisoning show myopathy of skeletal and cardiac muscle and hoof and hair coat abnormalities as described previously. Lesions in many other organs also have been described.

Treatment. No specific treatment is effective. If possible the source of excess selenium should be removed.

Prevention. Selenium supplementation should be carefully monitored to ensure safe dosage. In regions with seleniferous soils, supplemental forage can be provided to reduce consumption of selenium-containing plants and increase dietary protein. Rich sources of sulfur-containing amino acids (soybean meal) in the diet are partially protective. Alternate grazing of areas with plants that do not accumulate toxic concentrations of selenium is another option. The addition of 0.01% arsanilic acid or 20 ppm copper to the ration also may be preventive, but these substances are potentially toxic.

Ergot Toxicosis

Ergot toxicity results from ingestion of alkaloid compounds produced by the fungus *Claviceps purpurea*. This fungus infects cereals and grasses, most commonly rye, wheat, and oats. The seeds of the plants turn dark as they are filled with the fungal sclerotia, and this grossly visible structure is referred to as an *ergot*. *C. purpurea* is the fungal species most frequently linked with ergotism, but *Acremonium coenophialum* may cause a similar syndrome.[1]

The pathology occurs in animals grazing ergot-infested pasture or eating grain or hay made from such plants. It is fairly common in cattle, but reports in sheep and goats are rare. In one report of goats and sheep cograzing a fescue pasture, only goat kids were affected.[4] The condition usually occurs after a warm wet season, conditions that favor growth of the fungus.

Pathogenesis. Ergots contain alkaloid compounds and other pharmacologically active compounds known as *ergotoxins*. The effects of this group of toxins, which includes ergotamine, ergotoxine, and ergometrine, include constriction of arterioles and endothelial damage leading to gangrene of the extremities.

Clinical signs. Clinical signs of ergotism include swelling, coolness, and hair loss, followed by drying and discoloration of the skin of the distal limbs, tail, and ears. A distinct demarcation between normal and gangrenous skin is observed, and affected tissue may slough. Lameness is evident, and animals may remain recumbent. Clinical signs reported in goats include lameness, most often in the hindlimbs, with separation of the hoof in the most severe cases.[5] Ulceration of the oral, ruminal, and intestinal mucosa has been reported in sheep.[1]

Diagnosis. Feed samples should be analyzed for ergot or similar compounds. Differential diagnoses include thrombosis secondary to sepsis and trauma.

Treatment. No specific treatment exists for ergot toxicity. Animals should be removed from the source of toxin.

Prevention. Feed should contain less than 0.1% infected seedheads.[1] Pastures with severe ergot infestations should not be used for grazing or hay.

Fluorosis (Fluorine Poisoning)

Chronic fluorine poisoning (fluorosis) occurs after the ingestion of toxic amounts of fluorine compounds by feed or water. The severity of disease depends on the fluorine compound ingested. Sodium fluoride is more toxic than rock phosphate; calcium fluoride or sodium fluorosilicate are much less toxic. Sheep and goats are reported to be less susceptible than cattle.[5]

Fluorine occurs naturally in rocks, usually in association with phosphate. Soils derived from these rocks and water that percolates through these rock formations may contain high levels of fluorine. Other sources of fluorine include industrial contamination (as far as 14 km downwind), deep water wells, volcanic ash, and phosphatic supplements given to combat hypophosphatemia.[1]

Pathogenesis. The mechanism of fluorine toxicity has not been determined. Excess fluorine is deposited in bones and teeth. Bony lesions may develop at any time in the animal, but dental lesions occur only if fluorine levels are high during the formation of the teeth. Urinary excretion of fluorine, accompanied by calcium and phosphorus, leads to mobilization of calcium and phosphorus and results in osteomalacia and osteoporosis. Many other sites, including the bone marrow, undergo degenerative changes.[1]

Clinical signs. Acute fluorine toxicity is marked by gastrointestinal signs, tetany, and death. Chronic ingestion leads to decreased feed consumption and unthriftiness. Dental lesions, which consist of surface pitting and increased wear caused by improper enamel formation, are the first to appear, although they may not be noticed. With time, rapid wear and tooth breakage occurs, leading to impaired mastication.[6,7]

Signs of osteofluorosis include ill thrift, stiffness, and lameness that is most prominent in the hindlimbs. Pathologic fractures, often of the third phalanx (P3), may occur in several animals in the group. The affected bones are painful to palpation and may be enlarged.[1]

Differential diagnoses include other causes of lameness on a herd or flock basis, including hypophosphatemia, vitamin D deficiency, selenium toxicity, and selenium deficiency.

Diagnosis. Serum fluorine levels are often elevated in toxicosis (the normal level for cattle is 0.2 mg/dl), but normal levels do not rule out toxicity because of the storage of fluorine in bone. Urinary fluorine is often elevated (16 to 68 mg/kg is normal for cattle). Serum alkaline phosphatase levels are usually elevated.[1,6]

Radiographic abnormalities include increased bone density, enlarged bones, narrowing of the marrow cavity, and spontaneous fractures that heal poorly.

Postmortem examination reveals chalky, brittle bones with diaphyseal exostoses. Histology shows abnormal calcification of bone. Hypoplasia of enamel is observed in animals with dental disease. Degenerative changes of many tissues, including bone marrow, are observed. The fluorine content of bones can be measured to confirm the diagnosis. The mandible and metacarpal and metatarsal bones are considered the most reliable sources of bone for fluorine assay.[1]

Treatment. Keepers should remove animals from the source of fluorine. Cases of acute toxicity can be treated with aluminum salts (to neutralize hydrofluoric acid in the stomach) and IV calcium salts to control tetany. Dental and bone lesions do not usually improve. Animals should be fed good-quality hay. The addition of calcium carbonate or aluminum sulfate to the diet at 1% of the dry matter intake may be beneficial in decreasing bone flouride content.

Prevention. Phosphate feed supplements for cattle should not contain more than 0.2% to 0.3% fluorine. A phosphorus-to-fluoride ratio greater than 100:1 should be maintained. Rock phosphate can be a source of fluorine, and deep water wells should be assayed for fluorine levels before use. Careful management of grassland and water in high-fluorine areas may reduce losses caused by fluorine toxicosis.[8] Some guidelines recommend feeding aluminum salts to bind fluorine and reduce accumulation in tissue, but these compounds are unpalatable.[1]

Plant Toxicity

Australian sheep eating lupine stubble infested with the fungus *Phomopsis (Diaporthe toxica)* developed a myopathy of skeletal muscle marked by stiff gait and recumbency.[9] Ingestion of *Cassia roemeriana* (twin-leaf senna) is believed to cause a similar syndrome in cattle and sheep in Texas, New Mexico, and Mexico.[10]

References

1. Radostits OM et al: *Veterinary medicine,* ed 9, Philadelphia, 2000, WB Saunders.
2. Ahmed KE et al: Experimental selenium poisoning in Nubian goats, *Vet Hum Toxicol* 32:249, 1990.
3. Edmondson AJ, Norman BB, Suther D: Survey of state veterinarians and state veterinary diagnostic laboratories for selenium deficiency and toxicosis in animals, *J Am Vet Med Assoc* 202:865,1993.
4. Hibbs CM, Wolf N: Ergot toxicosis in young goats, *Mod Vet Pract* 63:126, 1982.

5. Choubisa SL. Some observations on endemic fluorosis in domestic animals in southern Rajasthan (India), *Vet Res Comm* 23:457, 1999.
6. Botha CJ et al: Two outbreaks of fluorosis in cattle and sheep, *J S Afr Vet Assoc* 64:165, 1993.
7. Schultheiss WA, Van Niekerk JC: Suspected chronic fluorosis in a sheep flock, *J S Afr Vet Assoc* 65:84, 1994.
8. Wang JD, Hong JP, Li JX: Studies on alleviation of industrial fluorosis in Baotou goats, *Fluoride* 28:131, 1995.
9. Allen JG et al. A lupinosis-associated myopathy in sheep and the effectiveness of treatments to prevent it, *Aust Vet J* 69:75, 1992.
10. Rowe LD et al. Experimentally induced *Cassia roemeriana* poisoning in cattle and goats, *Am J Vet Res* 48:992, 1987.

NEOPLASIA

Neoplasia of the musculoskeletal system is extremely rare in sheep and goats. A study of 673 ovine neoplasms submitted to a veterinary laboratory in South Africa revealed that 21 of them were of connective tissue origin. Types of tumors included chondroma, chondrosarcoma, fibroma, fibrosarcoma, osteoma, rhabdomyosarcoma, leiomyoma, and fibrolipoma.[1]

Osteosarcoma and pathologic fracture developed in a 9-year-old Toggenburg goat 4 years after a comminuted humeral fracture had been repaired with an intramedullary pin. The animal also was reported to have pulmonary nodules, but these were not examined histologically.[2] Mandibular osteoma was diagnosed in a 10-year-old Toggenburg cross, and osteochondrosarcoma of the rib and sternum of a goat also has been described.[2,3]

A diagnosis of neoplasia is based ultimately on histopathology. Bony enlargement, lameness, and radiographic evidence of lysis or proliferation may suggest a diagnosis of neoplasia, especially in an older animal. Successful treatment of connective tissue tumors has not been reported.

REFERENCES

1. Bastianello SS: A survey on neoplasia in domestic species over a 40-year period from 1935 to 1974 in the republic of South Africa. II. Tumours occurring in sheep, *Onderstepoort J Vet Res* 49:205, 1982.
2. Steinberg H, George C: Fracture-associated osteogenic sarcoma and a mandibular osteoma in two goats, *J Comp Path* 100:453, 1989.
3. Cotchin E: Tumors of farm animals, *Vet Rec* 40:816, 1960.

TAIL DOCKING

Tail removal or "docking" is usually performed during the first 2 weeks of life.[1,2] Some lambs sold in niche markets do not have their tails docked, and in some breeds (e.g., Karakul) the tail should be left long because the fat at the base of the tail is considered a prized commodity. Still, in most environments in which lambs are kept, long tails can become soiled with loose stool or diarrhea (as a result of high-grain diets, lush pasture, or internal parasites), leading to flystrike or infestation of the wool with maggots. Furthermore, long tails in females appear to depress normal reproductive performance. For these and other reasons, tails are usually removed. If the lamb is less than 24 hours old, the stress associated with tail removal may decrease absorption of colostral antibodies and result in the diseases associated with failure or partial failure of passive transfer. Therefore lambs should be 2 to 3 days to 2 weeks old at docking. One of the authors (Dr. Pugh) prefers to dock tails at 3 days on alert, healthy animals that are being cared for by their dams. The docking can take place after the lambs and their dams are moved to a single family unit (jug) or holding area. Placing the new lamb and dam together helps prevent the ewe from wandering off or abandoning the lamb after the procedure. Anesthesia is seldom required, with the obvious exception of adult or pet animals (on owner's request). If anesthesia is required, either a sedative or a caudal epidural and ring block will suffice.[1] Some studies suggest that a tail ring block of a local anesthetic can reduce the stress associated with tail removal.[3] Still, Hooper[1] has suggested, and the authors of this chapter agree, that the neonatal lamb responds as much, or possibly more, to the injection of a local anesthetic as to the surgical removal of the tail without anesthesia.

The tail should be left long enough to cover the anus and may be extended to the dorsal aspect of the vulva on females.[2] The woolless distal attachment of the paired caudal skinfolds on the ventral tail surface provide a good landmark for the site of tail removal. Many owners of show or club lambs prefer to remove the tail as close to the body as possible. However, docking too close to the sacrum may result in an increased incidence of rectal and possibly vaginal prolapse.[1] The tail can be crushed, cut, cauterized, or removed with a combination of these methods.[2] Equipment used for tail removal includes an emasculator, an emasculatome, a hot chisel, a knife, or elastrator bands. Tails should be cleaned of dirt and feces. The lamb should be manually restrained as the clinician determines the exact spot of tail removal; the tail should not be excessively stretched. Leaving some skin proximal to the point of removal provides redundant skin to cover the spinal stump.[1] Use of a cautery unit (e.g., hot chisel, suture heated wedge, electric wedge, electric cautery) minimizes hemorrhage. If hemorrhage does occur, the ventral blood vessels can be clamped and sutured if needed. If cautery units are used and the wool is burned, some ewes may reject the lambs.[1] Removing wool over the docking site before the procedure and gently washing or cleansing the tail after removal can minimize ewe rejection. Ewe rejection caused by cautery docking is rare, and this method of docking is very acceptable. Cautery equipment should be used cautiously because of the possibility of burning the vulva, anus, or perineal skin. Regardless of the method, in the absence of complications the tail stump will heal within 2 weeks. Tetanus toxoid or antitoxin should be routinely administered on farms where tetanus is a problem; it also can be provided for all docked animals.

If an elastrator or rubber band is used, the tail sloughs because of ischemic necrosis. This procedure is controversial, and elastrator band use should always be accompanied by tetanus prophylaxis.

The tail of an adult sheep can be removed as it would be in other animals. The animal can be placed under general anesthesia or sedated, restrained, and given an epidural or ring block with local anesthetic. The surgical area is clipped and aseptically prepared, and the site for tail excision is determined. The clinician then makes a wedge-shaped skin incision distal to the intervertebral space where the tail is to be removed. This leaves enough skin to suture over the stump.[1] The clinician cuts the tail between the vertebrae, removes the tail, and closes the skin. If excessive hemorrhage occurs, the vessels can be cauterized or sutured with absorbable material. Animals can be placed on a broad-spectrum antibiotic and given tetanus prophylaxis.

REFERENCES

1. Hooper RN: General surgery techniques—Part I, *Proceedings of the 1998 Symposium on Small Ruminants for the Mixed Animal Practitioner Western Veterinary Conference*, 1998, Las Vegas, NV.
2. Johnson JH et al: The musculoskeletal system. In Oehme FW, Prier JE, editors: *Textbook of large animal surgery*, Baltimore, 1976, Williams & Wilkins.
3. Kent JE, Molong V, Graham MJ: Comparison of methods for the reduction of acute pain produced by rubber ring castrating or tail docking of week-old lambs, *Vet J* 155:39, 1998.

Chapter 10

Diseases of the Urinary System

ELLEN B. BELKNAP AND D.G. PUGH

EVALUATION OF THE URINARY TRACT

History

Obtaining a thorough history is crucial in diagnosing urinary tract disorders. In some instances a good history is as important as (if not more important than) the clinical examination. Knowledge of an affected animal's diet, use, onset and progression of disease, previous treatments, and responses to treatment is vital in making an accurate diagnosis. In addition, age at castration, time since parturition, and history of dystocia also may be relevant. The owner's interpretation of the clinical signs may be misleading and could suggest abnormalities of the gastrointestinal or reproductive tract. A selected list of plants associated with nephrotoxicity in sheep and goats is shown in Table 10-1.

Physical Examination

A general physical examination should be performed before the urinary system is evaluated. Close observation for signs of depression, hydration status, and systemic abnormalities is important. The clinician may wish to observe the animal as it urinates to detect stranguria, pollakiuria, dysuria, and abnormal urine color. Palpation and observation of the external urogenital structures should be performed routinely and followed by a digital rectal examination. Urethral rupture is relatively easy to determine in male sheep and goats. Most urethral ruptures occur at the distal sigmoid flexure, resulting in ventral fluid accumulation and edema. The preputial hairs should be examined for sand, calculi, and blood. Exteriorization of the penis can be accomplished by sitting the animal on the dorsum of its rump, grasping the penis through the sheath at the sigmoid flexure, and moving cranially while simultaneously (using the other hand) retracting the sheath caudally (Figure 10-1). An assistant should grasp the free portion of the penis with a piece of gauze. The urethral process can then be examined (and amputated if necessary) and the urethra catheterized. This procedure is more easily performed on rams than on bucks. Penile extension may be impossible in prepuberal males and those castrated before puberty. In the female the vulvar hair and perineal area should be examined for evidence of hematuria, pyuria, urine scalding, and crystalluria.

If the bladder is distended it can usually be palpated in the caudal abdomen. If it is not palpable, the bladder can be evaluated with real-time ultrasound. If the bladder has ruptured, bilateral symmetric ventral distention of the abdomen may be observed and a fluid wave may be appreciated with ballottement.

DIAGNOSTICS

Ultrasound

The urinary tract can be examined using real-time ultrasonographic equipment with either a 3.5- or 5-MHz transducer. Either a sector, curvilinear, or linear array transducer can be used rectally or transabdominally to visualize both kidneys (Figures 10-2 and 10-3) by scanning in the right paralumbar fossa; the bladder can be evaluated by scanning in the right inguinal area or transrectally.[1] In overconditioned or obese animals, visualization of the kidneys or urinary bladder may be difficult.

Excretory Program

A contrast radiographic evaluation of the bladder and urethra may be conducted after bladder or urethral surgery. Radiographic contrast material can be infused into the bladder through the catheter and the integrity of

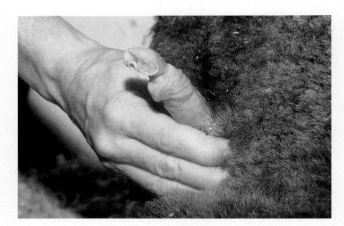

Figure 10-1   Exteriorization of a ram's penis. Note the urethral process.

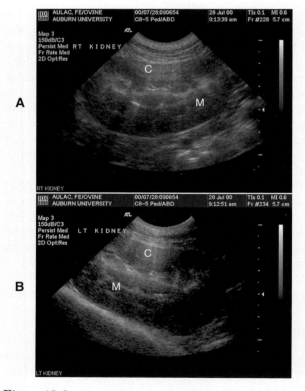

Figure 10-2   Ultrasound of a normal ovine kidney in the midsagittal plane using a variable-bandwidth, curvilinear, 5- to 8-MHz transducer. **A**, Right kidney. **B**, Left kidney. *C*, Cortex; *M*, medullary region. (Courtesy Dr. Margaret Blaik, Auburn, Alabama.)

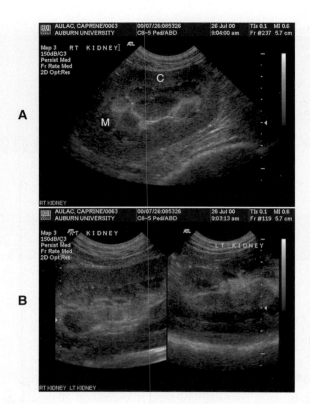

Figure 10-3   **A**, Ultrasound of a normal caprine right kidney in the dorsal plane using a variable-bandwidth, curvilinear, 5- to 8-MHz transducer. *C*, Cortex; *M*, medullary region. **B**, Split-screen ultrasound comparing the right and left sagittal planes of a caprine kidney. (Courtesy Dr. Margaret Blaik, Auburn, Alabama.)

the urethra can be evaluated (Figure 10-4). Lidocaine (1 ml of 2% lidocaine/10 ml of contrast media) can be added to the contrast media to prevent urethral spasms.

Renal Biopsy

To perform a renal biopsy in a sheep or goat, the clinician or an assistant clips and aseptically prepares the area over the last rib on the right side. Using a real-time ultrasound machine the clinician visualizes the kidney and advances a 14-gauge biopsy needle through anesthetized skin nicked with a #15 blade. Mild hematuria and subcapsular hematoma may result from this procedure. The resultant specimen is placed in 10% formalin and prepared for routine hematoxylin and eosin (H & E) staining. For immunofluorescent testing, samples should be placed in Michel's medium. If amyloidosis is suspected, special stains (Congo red) may be applied to subsequent sections.

Urinalysis

Along with serum creatinine assays, urinalysis is one of the most important diagnostic tests. Urine may be obtained from sheep by occluding the nostrils. Clinicians can easily catheterize female goats using a rigid Foley or metal urinary catheter (bitch catheter); they should avoid the suburethral diverticulum while passing the catheter toward the bladder. Obtaining urine from male goats is difficult, although they urinate frequently during the breeding season. Clinicians should make containers readily accessible when bucks lie down in case they urinate when

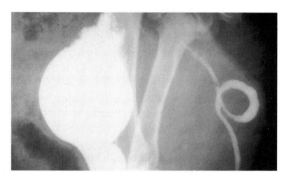

Figure 10-4 Contrast excretory urethrogram of a male pygmy goat. Note the filling defects in the urethra proximal to the sigmoid flexure.

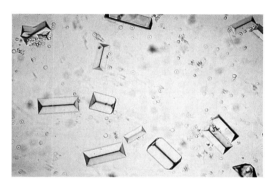

Figure 10-5 Photomicrograph of unstained urine sediment. Note the struvite crystals. (10× magnification.) (Courtesy Dr. Elizabeth Welles, Auburn, Alabama.)

TABLE 10-1

PLANTS ASSOCIATED WITH NEPHROTOXICITY*

PLANT	COMMENT
Vitamin D–containing plants *(Cestrum, Solanum)*	Contain vitamin D; cause soft tissue mineralization, glomerular fibrosis, and interstitial fibrosis (common in cattle)
Oxalate-containing plants	See Box 10-1
Amaranthus retroflexus (pigweed)	An oxalate and nitrate accumulator; causes perineal edema and nephrosis
Quercus species (oak)	Acorns and oak buds are most toxic; cause abdominal pain, extreme thirst, edema, elevated blood urea nitrogen, depressing edema, rough hair coat, and increases in serum creatinine and potassium; lesions include gastritis and nephritis, as well as hyaline and granular casts in the proximal controlled tubules; toxicity can be prevented by adding calcium hydroxide to the diet

*Fluid and supportive therapy are the treatments of choice for plant-associated nephrotoxicity. Before the onset of signs, administering oral charcoal and initiating emesis also may be of value.

they rise. Because of the presence of a urethral recess, catheterization of males is most often unsuccessful.[3]

Urinalysis can help localize disease, determine causes of discolored urine, identify inflammatory disease, and determine the kidneys' ability to concentrate urine. When present, urinary casts suggest tubular disease. A specific gravity greater than 1.025 and an alkaline pH make cast identification difficult. Urine should be analyzed promptly for sediment because casts, crystals, and other cellular elements degenerate or change configuration with time (Figure 10-5). Specific gravity can be measured with a hand-held refractometer. Specific gravity values between 1.007 and 1.012 (Table 10-2) indicate isosthenuria. These values should be interpreted with consideration of the animal's hydration status, degree of azotemia, and previous drug therapy. A specific gravity less than 1.007 or urine osmolality less than plasma values indicates renal medullary washout, polydipsia, or diabetes insipidus. However, diabetes insipidus is an extremely rare disease in sheep and goats (see Chapter 7). The urine pH of both sheep and goats is generally alkaline (greater

than 7.4) but may be acidotic as a result of paradoxic aciduria. This condition occurs in ruminants with hypochloremic, hypokalemic metabolic alkalosis as the kidney tries to reduce the bicarbonate load but cannot, resulting in the excretion of hydrogen ions into the urine.[2,4,5]

Urine protein concentration may be falsely elevated because of hemorrhage, inflammation, or colostral proteins in neonates less than 40 hours old. In the absence of hematuria or pigmenturia, marked proteinuria indicates glomerular disease. However, when dipsticks are used for evaluation, alkaline urine produces a falsely elevated protein value and a positive blood reaction can be caused by hematuria, hemoglobinuria, myoglobinuria, or contamination from fecal or reproductive blood. Glucosuria occurs when the renal threshold (100 mg/dl of glucose in peripheral blood) is exceeded. It can be caused by stress, xylazine or glucose administration, enterotoxemia, or renal disease and also is seen in moribund animals. Elevated levels of urinary gamma-glutamyl transferase (GGT) indicate proximal tubular dysfunction.

TABLE 10-2

URINALYSIS FOR SHEEP AND GOATS

TEST	NORMAL RESULTS
Color	Pale yellow
pH	7.2 to 8.0
Glucose	Negative
Specific gravity	1.015 to 1.045
Ketones	Negative
Protein	Negative to trace
Bilirubin	Negative
Turbidity	Clear
Red blood cells	Less than 5 (high power field)
White blood cells	Less than 5 (high power field)
Crystals	Rare
Casts	Occasional hyaline
Sperm	Variable
Epithelial cells	Occasional
Gamma-glutamyl transferase	Less than 40 U/L

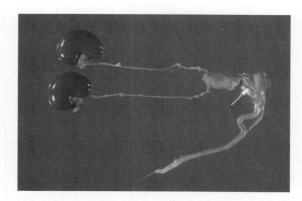

Figure 10-6   A dissected urogenital tract of a buck. The *arrow* points to the urethral diverticulum.

Fractional excretion (FE) of electrolytes may be useful to detect early renal dysfunction. To perform this test, the clinician should collect concurrent serum and urine samples. The percent FE is calculated by the urine electrolyte/urine creatinine concentration divided by the serum electrolyte/serum creatinine concentration, then multiplied by 100%. In sheep the normal FE of sodium is less than 1%; an FE of sodium greater than 1% indicates primary tubular disease or sodium toxicity.[2] Samples should be collected before fluid therapy is instituted.

Biochemistry Profile

Serum biochemistry profiles may be the easiest tests to perform to diagnose renal failure. Creatinine levels are the most reliable indicators of renal disease, although elevations also may result from prerenal and postrenal causes. Serum urea nitrogen levels may be altered because of the ruminant's ability to recycle nitrogen, so the authors of this chapter place more emphasis on serum creatinine levels. Hypochloremia is a consistent finding in renal failure. Depressed serum chloride concentrations may be caused by urinary loss and sequestration resulting from abomasal stasis. Hyponatremia also may be observed, whereas hyperkalemia is not consistently observed in postrenal obstruction cases. Magnesium is primarily excreted by the kidneys and may be elevated in renal disease. Phosphorous, which depends on the kidney as well as saliva for excretion, may be elevated. Hypocal-cemia is commonly identified as a sequela of reduced intake, gastrointestinal stasis, and hyperphosphatemia.

White Blood Cell Count

Leukocytosis, neutrophilia, and hyperfibrinogenemia are commonly reported in acute renal, bladder, and urethral infections. If the problem is chronic, globulin levels may be elevated, and if the inflammation is still active, hyperfibrinogenemia also may be present. Anemia caused by chronic inflammation may be observed in long-standing disease. Anemia of chronic inflammatory disease is nonregenerative and is characterized by low serum iron and a normal total iron-binding capacity.

Anatomic Considerations

Amputating the urethral process makes urethral catheterization easier. When attempting catheterization, the authors prefer to use polyethylene tubing. In many instances a catheter can be passed in a retrograde fashion to the point of the urethral diverticulum (recess) at the ischial arch (Figure 10-6).[3] Complete catheterization requires either an ischial urethrostomy or a cystotomy. During cystotomy, normograde catheterization of the urethra may be attempted and is often successful.

References

1. Braun U, Schefer U, Gerber D: Ultrasonography of the urinary tract of female sheep, *Am J Vet Res* 53:1734, 1992.
2. Garry F et al: Renal excretion of creatinine, electrolytes, protein, and enzymes in healthy sheep, *Am J Vet Res* 51:414, 1990.
3. Garett PD: Urethral recess in male goats, sheep, cattle, and swine, *J Am Vet Med Assoc* 191:689, 1987.
4. Lunn DP, McGuirk SM, Smith DF: Renal net acid and electrolyte excretion in an experimental model of hypochloremic metabolic alkalosis in sheep, *Am J Vet Res* (11):1723, 1990.
5. Michell AR, Moss P: Responses to reduced water intake, including dehydration natriuresis, in sheep excreting sodium predominantly in urine or in feces, *Exp Phys* 80:265, 1995.

UPPER URINARY TRACT PROBLEMS

Acute Renal Failure

Pathogenesis. Acute renal failure (ARF) is caused by a deterioration of renal function over a period of hours to days. This rapid onset can result from prerenal, postrenal, or intrinsic renal causes. Most intrinsic renal insults are ischemic or toxic in nature and can be caused by systemic disease, injury, and various therapeutic manipulations. Clinical situations that enhance the risk of ARF include dehydration, electrolyte abnormalities, systemic hypotension, hypoalbuminemia, vasculitis, fever, sepsis, prolonged surgery or anesthesia, and the use of potentially nephrotoxic drugs. The kidney is especially susceptible to toxic injury for several reasons. First, the kidneys acquire 20% of the cardiac output and thereby receive a relatively high proportion of blood-borne toxicants. The large glomerular capillary surface area provides a large contact area for toxicant interaction with epithelial cells. In the proximal tubule and thick ascending Henle's loop, high metabolic rates and transport functions make epithelial cells especially sensitive to intoxicants that disrupt their energy sources or membrane functions. Tubular epithelial cells also may actively resorb toxicants, which can accumulate to dangerous intracellular levels. The countercurrent mechanism and tubular concentrating function result in increased levels of toxic substances in the distal portions of the nephron.

Treatment. Treatment of ARF should be aimed at correcting electrolyte and acid-base imbalances and promoting diuresis. Furosemide (1 mg/kg intravenously [IV] every 2 to 3 hours) and dimethyl sulfoxide (DMSO, 1 g/kg IV as a 20% solution) may be given initially. If the animal remains anuric or oliguric, a dopamine drip (3 to 7 μg/kg/min IV) should be instituted. Close monitoring of hydration and plasma protein levels is important to prevent edema. After the animal is no longer oliguric, the clinician should maintain the animal on IV fluids until the serum creatinine level has returned to the normal range and the animal has begun to eat and drink again. Supportive care, maintenance of normal rumen flora, and nutritional support should be considered in these cases. Attitude is sometimes improved by having another sheep or goat nearby or moving the patient outside every day.

Acute Tubular Necrosis

Damage to the renal tubules may result in renal dysfunction. Ingestion or parenteral administration of toxins, renal hypoxia resulting from hypovolemia, and nephritis caused by endotoxemia or bacteremia may all damage the renal tubules. Proximal tubular toxins result in loss of solute in the more distal parts of the nephron. This can cause glucosuria, bicarbonaturia, natriuresis, proteinuria, and enzymuria. The taking of concurrent samples of urine and serum allow for the calculation of the FE rates of a particular solute, as shown here for sodium:

$$FE_{Na} (\%) = (U_{Na}/S_{Na} \div U_{Cr}/S_{Cr}) \times 100$$

where U_{Na} is the urine sodium level, S_{Na} is the serum sodium level, U_{Cr} is the urine creatinine level, and S_{Cr} is the serum creatinine level. Although it is affected by diet, the FE_{Na} can be used to assess proximal tubular damage, with elevations greater than 1% considered abnormal in sheep.[1] Urine GGT levels greater than 40 U/L are considered above normal.[2] Damage to the distal nephron often results in loss of potassium and hydrogen ions into the urine. Most nephrotoxins cause a decrease in the glomerular filtration rate (GFR) and tubular damage. If the GFR is not affected and uremia does not result, tubular toxicity may not be detected.

With acute tubular necrosis, anuria or oliguria are usually present; polyuria can occur in subacute or chronic cases. Identification of urine output and specific gravity is crucial to treatment of these cases. Because many of the clinical signs are nonspecific, determining a diagnosis can sometimes be difficult. Most animals have a hypochloremic metabolic alkalosis and experience proteinuria, hematuria, and granular casts in the urine early in the disease. An increased FE of electrolytes or urinary enzymes precedes these abnormalities.

Metal Toxicity

Goats are notorious for ingesting household items and zinc-containing objects such as pennies or sheet metal screws, both of which are potential sources of toxicity. Zinc is leached in the acid environment of the abomasum and may result in toxicity. Goat kids may become intoxicated by ingesting zinc sulfate–containing foot bath material, but this is rare. Serum, urine, or liver zinc concentrations may be diagnostic, and the clinician should collect samples from them in tubes designed for trace mineral analysis. Other metals that may cause acute tubular necrosis in ruminants include lead, mercury, cadmium, and arsenic.

Clinical signs. Clinical signs include anorexia, dehydration, diarrhea, weakness, jaundice, and death; hemolytic anemia and ARF may occur 2 to 3 weeks after ingestion. Arsenic also is known to cause gastrointestinal signs, including colic and hemorrhagic diarrhea. With mercury toxicosis, ulcerations of the mouth, esophagus, and gastrointestinal tract may lead to diarrhea.

Antibiotic Toxicity

Antibiotics known to induce acute tubular necrosis include aminoglycosides, tetracyclines, and sulfonamides.

Of these, tetracyclines and sulfonamides are frequently used in sheep and goats to treat many diseases. Their toxic effects on the kidney are enhanced by dehydration. Renal failure as a consequence of antibiotic overdose has been reported in cattle, but not in sheep and goats.[3,4] Nephrotoxicity results in part from inhibitory effects on the oxidative enzymes of tubule cells.[5] In addition, tetracycline inhibits the concentrating ability of the kidney,[6] and when given in a propylene glycol carrier results in systemic hypotension and decreased pulmonary and renal arterial blood flow.[7] Continued use of an antibiotic is contraindicated if adverse renal effects are noted. Concurrent use of nonsteroidal antiinflammatory drugs (NSAIDs) may predispose to renal tubular toxicity or cause problems by themselves.

Plant (Oxalate) Toxicity

Pathogenesis.   Ingestion of many plants may result in nephrotoxicity in sheep and goats. One of the most common problems is the continued ingestion of small amounts of oxalate. Oxalate is normally metabolized by the rumen, and oxalate tolerance increases with exposure. This helps to explain the observed decreased susceptibility over time of animals grazing pasture rich in oxalate-containing plants. Grazing pasture is most dangerous when a rapid growth of lush plants occurs in a warm fall after a dry summer.[8] Plants containing high concentrations of oxalate are listed in Box 10-1. The leaves contain

---

BOX 10-1

Plants Containing a High Oxalate Content

COMMON NAME	GENUS AND SPECIES
Halogeton	*Halogeton glomeratus*
Lamb's quarter or fat hen	*Chenopodium album*
Pokeweed	*Phytolacca americana*
Russian thistle	*Salsola kali*
Purslane	*Portulaca oleracea*
Bassia	*Bassia hyssopifolia*
Pigweed	*Amaranthus retroflexus*
Soursob	*Oxalis cernua* and *O. pes-caprae*
Greasewood	*Sarcobatus vermiculatus*
Dock and orchard sorrel	*Rumex acetosella* and *R. acetosa*
Cultivated rhubarb	*Rheum rhaponticum*
Sugar beet leaves	*Beta vulgaris*
Fungi	*Aspergillus niger* and *A. niger*

---

higher concentrations of oxalate than other parts of the plant.[9] The amount of oxalate required to cause toxicity is variable because mature animals that are gradually introduced to oxalate can experience a proliferation of oxalate-degrading rumenal microflora. Less than 1% of the body weight in soluble oxalate is toxic to a fasted sheep.[10] Abrupt introduction to pastures with an abundance of oxalate-containing plants is risky. This risk is magnified in animals who are thin and hungry. Sheep do not appear to adapt to the ingestion of plants in the *Brassica* family.

Clinical signs.   Signs of oxalate toxicity include lethargy, anorexia, recumbency, and death.[10,11] Pulmonary edema, muscle fasciculations, tetany, and seizures also may be observed. Oxalate has a strong affinity for calcium and produces insoluble calcium oxalate calculi in the urinary tract.[12] Hypocalcemia and azotemia are characteristic, and hyperphosphatemia and hypermagnesemia also may be observed.[11,13] A more chronic form of oxalate toxicity causes calcium oxalate deposition in renal tubules and vessels, renal fibrosis, renal insufficiency, and urolithiasis.

Diagnosis.   A history of access to toxic plants, the observation of increased renal cortical echogenicity on ultrasound, renal biopsy, and necropsy of dead animals may aid in establishing the cause of acute tubular necrosis.[14] Birefringent crystals may be observed in the renal cortex, papillary ducts, urine, and possibly in the rumen during histopathologic examination of tissues.[15] Rumenitis is a major lesion of oxalate toxicosis identified at necropsy.

Treatment.   Therapy should be aimed at promoting diuresis and eliminating the toxin source. IV fluids, calcium gluconate, oral magnesium hydroxide, and activated charcoal (1 to 2 g/kg by mouth [PO]) may all be beneficial. Oral calcium chloride or dicalcium phosphate can precipitate oxalate within the rumen and prevent its further absorption.[10] After ingestion but before the onset of clinical signs, survivability may be increased by administering large volumes of water and calcium salts orally.[12,15]

Prevention.   Prevention requires avoidance of forage that contains large quantities of soluble oxalate. If such forage cannot be avoided, gradual acclimation is indicated.[16]

Ethylene Glycol Toxicity

Pathogenesis.   Adult ruminants may be more resistant than monogastric animals or neonatal ruminants to the effects of ethylene glycol because of their ability to degrade oxalate, a metabolite of ethylene glycol, by rumen microorganisms.[16,17] Although they are relatively uncommon in sheep and goats because of their ability to metabolize oxalic acid, cases of ethylene glycol toxicity still occur, especially in pet or club lambs.[17] Sheep and goats seem to like the sweet taste of ethylene glycol and will drink it preferentially over water. As in other species, toxicity in sheep and goats is usually associated with the ingestion of antifreeze that contains ethylene glycol. For ruminants the median lethal dose (LD_{50}) of pure ethylene glycol is 5 to 10 ml/kg.[18]

Clinical signs. Clinical signs of ethylene glycol toxicosis include hypersalivation, bruxism, hindlimb ataxia, nystagmus, seizures, and death. A sweet odor may be detected on the animal's breath. A diagnosis may be based on a history of ingestion, analysis of rumen contents for ethylene glycol, or glycolic acid levels in urine, serum, or ocular fluid.[17] Metabolic acidosis, azotemia, and hyperosmolality are likely findings. Birefringent crystals arranged in sheaves or rosettes typical of oxalate crystals may be observed in the renal tubules on histopathologic examination.[17] Unlike in monogastric animals that absorb ethylene glycol within 48 hours, the rumens of sheep and goats may act as reservoirs for continued absorption.

Treatment. Therapy may include activated charcoal (0.11 kg PO). Aggressive fluid therapy, including 20% ethanol at 50 ml/hour is reported to prevent conversion of ethylene glycol to glycolic acid, a metabolic intermediate.[19]

Oak (Acorn) Toxicity

Pathogenesis. Sheep are much more susceptible to the effects of oak (*Quercus* species) leaf, bud, twig, or acorn toxicity than goats because goats reportedly have greater concentrations of tannase enzymes in their ruminal mucosae.[8] However, acorns are palatable and readily consumed by goats.[20] Gallotannic acid is thought to be the toxic component in young oak leaves or acorns; it is hydrolyzed in the rumen to produce gallic acid, pyrogallol, tannic acid, and other compounds.[20] Tannins bind to the proteins of epithelial cells, resulting in ulcerations, and hydrolyzed tannins bind to plasma proteins and endothelial proteins, resulting in fluid loss from the intravascular fluid compartment and hemorrhage.[20] Toxicity is observed more commonly in the spring and the fall when other feed sources are limited and acorns are abundant. The concentration of toxic compounds is higher in immature, green acorns than in mature, ripe acorns.[21] Oak forage must comprise a large portion of the diet for clinical signs to be present. Concurrent protein deficiency may contribute to disease predisposition and development. Poorly fed, heavily parasitized animals are therefore most susceptible. The organs and tissues most commonly affected are the mouth, esophagus, gastrointestinal tract, and kidneys.

Clinical signs. Clinical signs may appear 3 days after ingestion of the oak source. Initially the animal may be listless, anorectic, and weak. Polyuria, ventral edema, perineal and vulvar edema, abdominal pain, and constipation followed by the excretion of mucus-covered feces and hematochezia may be observed. As uremia progresses the scleral vessels become engorged, and a smell of ammonia may become apparent on the animal's breath. Azotemia, hyponatremia, hyperkalemia, hypochloremia, hyperphosphatemia, hypocalcemia, metabolic acidosis, and an elevated anion gap are found initially.[22] Affected animals also may exhibit anuria, isosthenuria, proteinuria, and glucosuria. Death is generally attributable to renal failure, although ulcerations of the mouth, esophagus, and gastrointestinal tract may be evident.

Diagnosis. The most characteristic lesions at necropsy include edema and hemorrhagic enteritis. The kidneys may be normal or enlarged with hemorrhages on the surface in acute cases or roughened, pitted, and pale in more chronic cases.[14,22] Hydrothorax, hydroperitoneum, perineal edema, and hemorrhage may accompany these lesions. Histopathologic lesions include multifocal, proximal convoluted tubular necrosis with proteinaceous casts and dilated tubules. Glomerular degeneration and fluid in Bowman's capsule also are seen.[14,20]

Treatment. Treatment is aimed at correcting electrolyte abnormalities and base deficits and promoting diuresis. If the animal survives the acute stage and begins to eat, recovery may occur, although 5 to 10 weeks may elapse before renal function returns to normal.[22]

Prevention. Prevention is more successful than treatment and includes good pasture management, the provision of supplemental alfalfa hay, or administration of a 10% to 20% calcium hydroxide (slake lime) and grain concentrate mixture. A mixture of 491 kg (1080 lb) of cottonseed or soybean meal, 272.7 kg (600 lb) of dehydrated alfalfa, 54.5 kg (120 lb) of vegetable oil, and 90.0 kg (200 lb) of hydrated lime, fed at a rate of 0.1 to 0.2 kg/head/day (0.25 to 0.5 lb/head/day) may protect against acorn toxicity.

INFECTIOUS DISEASES

Enterotoxemia

Enterotoxemia caused by epsilon toxin–producing *Clostridium perfringens* type D (pulpy kidney disease) is an important syndrome in the sheep and goat industries. Grain-fed lambs on a high-concentrate diet are most susceptible, but adult sheep and goats also may be affected.[8,23] Goats are more commonly affected with the hemorrhagic enterocolitis form of enterotoxemia.[24] The epsilon toxin is produced when the animal's diet provides adequate substrate for proliferation of the type D organism in the intestine. The epsilon toxin increases vascular permeability, leading to edema in the pulmonary system and kidneys and explaining the name *pulpy kidney disease.*[25]

Clinical signs. Lambs are generally found dead within 12 hours and ewes within 24 hours of the onset of disease. The body conditions of the dead animals are usually good, glucosuria is a consistent finding, and within a few hours of death the kidneys become soft and pulpy. Other lesions include excess pericardial fluid, pulmonary edema, and hemorrhage on serosal surfaces.

Prevention. Vaccination with the bacterin-toxoid is imperative in preventing disease in lambs; antitoxin (200 units/kg IV) may be given during an outbreak. The vaccine is not as effective in goats as it is in lambs.[25] Oral sulfa and tetracycline drugs can reduce the proliferation of bacteria in the intestine and are occasionally placed in diets for this purpose (see Chapter 14).

Leptospirosis

Leptospirosis can have a variety of clinical manifestations depending on the serovar of *Leptospira interrogans*, the immune status of the animal, and various virulence factors. *L. pomona, L. icterohemorrhagica,* and *L. hardjo* more commonly infect sheep,[10,26] whereas *L. pomona, L. icterohemorrhagica,* and *L. grippotyphosa* are more commonly identified in goats.[27] The organism is very infectious, a quality that is enhanced by its ability to penetrate intact mucous membranes. Only a few organisms are required to infect an animal, but as many as 10^5 organisms/ml of urine can be shed within the first few weeks of infection.

Pathogenesis. The most important mode of transmission is by contaminated urine,[28] and therefore the likelihood of infection increases after periods of heavy rainfall, especially in poorly drained environments. Reservoir hosts persist as infection sources within a species, but accidental infection can occur in non–host-adapted species. Nonadapted serovar infections can cause severe hemolytic disease, interstitial nephritis, and tubular nephrosis. After the organism gains entrance to the body, a period of septicemia and leptospiremia results, followed by dissemination to most tissues.

Clinical signs. Clinical signs of leptospirosis may include fever, anorexia, depression, anemia, hemoglobinuria, and icterus. Sudden death also may occur in sheep.[29] Outbreaks of abortion and stillbirth may be seen in the flock concurrently with the urogenital form of the disease.

Diagnosis. Leptospirosis can be diagnosed by serology (microscopic agglutination test or enzyme-linked immunospecific assay [ELISA]), the polymerase chain reaction (PCR) test, dark-field microscopy, immunofluorescent antibody tests, culture, and phase-contrast microscopy of urine or urine sediment samples.[30] The kidneys are usually dark and swollen. Renal lesions during the chronic phase include enlarged kidneys, pale foci in the renal cortices, and a diffuse, chronic interstitial nephritis on histopathologic examination. Kidney lesions result from damage caused by hemolysis, lipase, and urease.[31]

Treatment. Dihydrostreptomycin (12.5 mg/kg every 12 hours intramuscularly [IM]) and oxytetracycline (10 to 15 mg/kg every 12 hours IM) are potentially nephrotoxic antibiotics, and controversy exists regarding their efficacy in the treatment of other species (cattle).[32,33] No reports have been published concerning their use in sheep and goats with leptospirosis.

Prevention. The most effective means of preventing leptospirosis is vaccination, but limiting contact with carrier cattle, wild animals, and rodent populations and blocking access to standing water can help prevent transmission. Multivalent vaccines should be used for animals older than 3 months of age and should be administered two to four times annually, depending on the prevalence of leptospirosis in the area.

Adenovirus

Adenovirus particles have been identified in the endothelia of renal interstitial blood vessels in a lamb.[34] They were observed during routine histopathologic examination of several 8-month-old Merino lambs. Experimental infection with some strains of ovine adenovirus in lambs resulted in degeneration of epithelial cells in the proximal convoluted tubules.[35] Prevention requires good management practices; no adenovirus vaccines are available.

CHRONIC RENAL DISEASE

Mesangiocapillary Glomerulonephritis

Mesangiocapillary glomerulonephritis occurs primarily in Finnish Landrace lambs less than 4 months of age, although reports exist of it in cross-bred lambs sired by Finnish Landrace rams.[36,37] Immunofluorescent studies demonstrate subendothelial deposits of immunoglobulin M (IgM), immunoglobulin G (IgG), immunoglobulin A (IgA), and third component of complement (C3) and neutrophil infiltrates in the glomerular capillary walls. Affected lambs are born with a C3 deficiency involving a complex mode of inheritance that does not necessarily imply that all lambs in a litter from a carrier ewe mated to a known transmitting sire will be affected.[38]

Clinical signs. Clinical signs of glomerular disease become apparent within weeks after birth. Initially the lambs become isolated from the flock and appear anorexic. Some develop signs of central nervous system disturbance, then progress to display signs of abdominal pain. Transabdominal ultrasonographic evaluation often reveals enlarged kidneys that may be painful on palpation. The lambs are azotemic, with hypocalcemia, hyperphosphatemia, hypoalbuminemia, and albuminuria.[36,37]

Diagnosis. The diagnosis is based on observed expansion of the mesangial region of the glomeruli with cellular infiltrates; the peripheral capillary walls are swollen, refractile, and infiltrated with neutrophils.[39] Grossly, the kidneys appear greatly enlarged with red or yellow spots in the cortex. Concurrent neuronal lesions have been reported.[37] To control this condition, the sire and ewe that gave birth to the affected lambs should be culled.

Glomerulonephritis

Pathogenesis. Glomerulonephritis of sheep tends to be nonprogressive and asymptomatic, with no glomerular lesions identified in lambs younger than 3 months of age.[40] Immune-mediated mechanisms cause deposition of antigen, immunoglobulins, and complement along the basement membranes of the glomerular capillaries. The complexes become trapped at the basement membranes of the glomerular capillaries, where they form subendothelial or subepithelial electron-dense deposits. Membranous glomerulonephritis is the most common form in sheep and results when the subepithelial deposits stimulate overgrowth of the capillary basement membranes, which thicken and form projections to enclose packets of the complexes. The disease is usually sporadic and associated with some chronic inflammatory or infectious process, usually chronic lung or liver abscesses.[38]

Clinical signs and diagnosis. Affected animals appear unthrifty and may have ascites or hydrothorax, but the disease is not rapidly progressive.[41] Goats may acquire a spontaneous membranous glomerulonephritis but seldom display clinical signs.[27,41] Definitive diagnosis is achieved by renal biopsy. The kidneys are pale and contracted. On histopathologic examination most or all of the glomeruli are shrunken and fibrosed, the capillaries are occluded, the tubules are atrophic, and the interstitium is thickened and fibrous. In addition, glomerulonephritis has been described in ewes with concurrent pregnancy toxemia.[42] Clinical signs are typical of pregnancy toxemia, with concurrent azotemia, proteinuria, and ketonuria.

Treatment. No successful treatment is available for glomerulonephritis in goats and sheep. Glucocorticosteroids may help reduce the inflammation produced by the disease, but the prognosis is poor.

Pyelonephritis

Pathogenesis. Pyelonephritis in sheep and goats has been reported to be caused by *Escherichia coli*[43] and *Corynebacterium renale*.[44-46] The pili of *C. renale* are important in attaching to the animal's tissues and establishing infection.[47] *Chlamydia psittaci* also can cause pyelonephritis.

Clinical signs and diagnosis. Weight loss, anorexia, dysuria, and anuria are occasionally observed. The history may reveal recent parturition. Urinalysis can aid in diagnosis and may reveal proteinuria, hematuria, and pyuria. Renal enlargement, echogenic material within the renal pelvis, and dilation of the renal calyces are ultrasonographic findings supportive of a diagnosis of pyelonephritis. At necropsy the kidneys may appear swollen with thickened capsules. Purulent material is found in the renal pelvis and ureters, and some animals may have chronic cystitis. The condition may be unilateral or bilateral, and hydronephrosis or hydroureter may accompany the lesion.

Treatment. Where possible, therapy should be based on bacterial culture and antibiotic sensitivity. When urine bacterial culture is unavailable, therapy should include the administration of procaine penicillin G (22,000 IU/kg every 12 hours IM or subcutaneously [SC]) for at least 1 week. Favorable results also may be obtained by administering ceftiofur sodium (2.2 mg/kg SC every 24 hours) for at least 1 week. Urinalysis should be repeated to confirm the absence of pyuria before antibiotics are discontinued. Good sanitation practices at parturition may help decrease the incidence of this condition.

Amyloidosis

Pathogenesis. Amyloidosis is a chronic wasting disease of animals caused by the tissue deposition of fibrils formed by the polymerization of protein subunits arranged in a specific beta-pleated sheet biochemical conformation.[48] Reactive systemic amyloidosis may occur as a sequela to chronic inflammatory or neoplastic disease, although in some instances no predisposing cause is identified.[48] It most commonly occurs in sheep and goats used for research or production of antisera and in chronic cases of caseous lymphadenitis.[49,50]

Clinical signs and diagnosis. The signs of amyloidosis depend on the organs involved; the most commonly affected organs are the kidneys, and the condition can lead to renal failure and death. A nephrotic-like syndrome occurs and produces chronic weight loss, ventral edema, ascites, pleural and pericardial edema, hypoproteinemia, and proteinuria. Diarrhea may accompany these findings as a sequela of the hypoproteinemia or because of infiltration of the intestine with amyloid. Affected animals are generally anorexic. Diagnosis is confirmed by renal biopsy or at necropsy. Histologic evaluation of Congo red–stained renal tissue reveals amyloid deposition in the glomeruli and medulla.

Treatment. The treatment for amyloidosis is limited and therefore an accurate diagnosis is important. In pet animals the administration of DMSO may prevent the formation of some of the affecting proteins and promote the solubility of myeloid fibrils. If the disease is associated with chronic infection, appropriate antibiotics can be administered. However, the prognosis is poor.

Interstitial Nephritis

Adenovirus has been isolated from the kidney tissue of lambs with acute interstitial nephritis, hepatocellular necrosis, and enteritis.[34] The precise role of adenovirus in disease in lambs is not known, but it usually accompanies another disease. Often interstitial nephritis is diagnosed at necropsy rather than as a cause of clinical disease. In countries in which sheep pox is endemic, renal lesions caused by direct viral damage may be observed in addition to skin and pulmonary lesions.[38] Focal dense interstitial infiltrates of lymphoid cells have been reported in renal lesions of lambs persistently infected with border disease virus.

Parasites

A nephrosis thought to be associated with *Nematodirus battus* infestation of grazing lambs in the spring and early summer has been reported, primarily in the United Kingdom; it has no particular breed, sex, management, or feeding predisposition.[51] Other reports have identified nephrosis in lambs that were too young to suffer from clinical nematodiriasis.[48,52] The exact mechanism for the nephrosis is unknown, although histologic and biochemical abnormalities suggest an acute nephrotoxic renal failure.[38] Most affected lambs are less than 1 month old and only 1% to 2% of a flock may be affected. The lambs develop a progressive illness characterized by dullness, anorexia, weakness, and staggering proceeding to recumbency and coma. Diarrhea and/or dehydration occurred in approximately half of the lambs surveyed in one study.[52] Abnormalities include azotemia, hyperglobulinemia, hypoalbuminemia, metabolic acidosis, proteinuria, and hyperphosphatemia. N-acetyl-β-glucosaminidase is elevated in urine, indicating proximal tubular damage.[53] Most affected lambs die within a few days. Enlarged, pale, soft kidneys are observed at necropsy. Histopatho-

logic examination reveals distended cortical tubules containing casts of serous protein-like or fibrin-like material and lined with undifferentiated, low cuboidal cells. Although nephrosis was the predominant finding in one survey of 48 lambs, the authors were unable to explain the etiology of the condition.[52] Any treatment attempted should be aimed at rehydration and correction of acid-base abnormalities. Management practices do not appear to play a role in the progression of this disease.[52]

A *Toxoplasma*-like organism was reported to cause renal disease in a 4-year-old goat. Before death the goat showed signs of depression, weight loss, and tenesmus.[54] The kidneys were enlarged and hemorrhagic, with cortical white streaks. Cortical tubular necrosis with vasculitis was observed, as were large numbers of parasites, individually or in clumps, in the affected areas. These organisms were identified as *T. gondii* by electron microscopy. Protozoa also were observed within the bile duct, and portal fibrosis, hepatic necrosis, and vasculitis were reported. Prevention of transmission of the organism to sheep and goats is best accomplished by reducing contamination of feed by feline feces.

A protozoal parasite, *Nosema (Encephalitozoon) cuniculi*, was reported to produce numerous white spots in the renal cortex of a goat that showed no clinical signs of disease before death.[55] Focal tubular atrophy and replacement with fibrous connective tissue and mononuclear cells were observed, and schizont-like structures were visualized in the medullary tubular epithelium and free in the lumen of the tubules. This latter finding is most significant because of its zoonotic potential to cause meningoencephalitis in human beings.

Abscesses

Corynebacterium pseudotuberculosis infection and subsequent abscess formation throughout the body can cause severe economic losses in flocks and herds. Rarely, abscesses may form on or in the kidneys of infected animals in a flock or herd. Other organisms that can cause renal abscesses and embolic nephritis include *Staphylococcus*, *Salmonella*, *Chlamydia*, and *Streptococcus* species.[38] Embolic nephritis and abscesses are generally discovered at necropsy. The kidneys may be enlarged and uniform foci may be noted on the cortex and in the parenchyma when the kidney is opened on its longitudinal plane. The clinician should document these lesions and look for other focal areas of infection or lesions indicative of a septic process. Treatment varies depending on the underlying problem. Other animals in the flock should be observed for signs of sepsis, swollen joints, and other signs of illness.

Caprine Cloisonné Lesions

A condition reported in castrated male white Angora goats causes pigmented thickening of the proximal convoluted tubular basement membrane and is termed *cloisonné kidney*.[56] All of the affected goats are from a specific area of Texas; herds and flocks in that area report an incidence of about 2% for this subclinical condition.[57,58] The proposed etiology is repeated intravascular hemolytic episodes.[56] Because the condition is usually subclinical no treatment has been described. All goats in this area appear susceptible, but no preventive measures have been reported.

Copper Toxicity

Sheep are much more susceptible to copper toxicity than goats,[59,60] and young lambs and kids are more vulnerable than adults.[61] Potential sources of excess copper include swine, equine, or cattle rations; trace mineral supplements; liquid from foot baths containing copper sulfate ($CuSO_4$); pastures fertilized with $CuSO_4$ or swine or chicken manure; and feed with an improper copper-to-molybdenum ratio. Calf milk replacers may be a source of excess copper for bottle-fed lambs and kids.[62] Depending on the dosage and duration of exposure to copper, the toxic effects can be acute or chronic. When the dietary copper-to-molybdenum ratio exceeds 10:1, copper accumulates in the liver and binds to the metalloprotein ceruloplasmin. After the liver is saturated, stress can precipitate the release of free copper. The non-bound or free form of copper is potentially hemolytic. Simple, hepatogenous, and phytogenous copper poisoning are the most common mechanisms of chronic copper toxicity. In the simple form of copper toxicity the animal ingests excess copper from an identifiable source, whereas in the hepatogenous form the liver has been damaged by toxic alkaloids and has an increased affinity for expanded storage of copper.[63] The phytogenous form of chronic copper toxicity occurs when animals graze pastures with normal copper concentrations (10 to 20 ppm dry weight) but deficiencies in molybdenum and/or an excess of sulfates. Whole blood copper levels are maintained at a steady level during the accumulation phase, but just before a hemolytic crisis the levels double. Stressors such as shearing, handling, and parturition may precipitate a hemolytic crisis. During such a crisis the liver releases massive amounts of copper, which induces oxidation of red blood cell membranes. This in turn causes membrane compromise, rupture of the red blood cell, and release of "free" hemoglobin into the circulation.

Clinical signs and diagnosis. During a hemolytic crisis, anemia, methemoglobinemia, hemoglobinuria, muddy mucous membranes, dehydration, and weakness may be observed. The sheep are depressed, anorectic, and reluctant to move. Deposition of hemoglobin in the renal tubules may contribute to renal impairment. Serum, liver, or kidney copper levels may be used to diagnose the condition. Serum copper concentrations during the he-

molytic crisis are 5 to 20 μg/ml, with liver and kidney levels exceeding 500 μg/g dry weight and 80 to 100 μg/g dry weight, respectively. In sheep, dietary copper concentrations higher than 25 mg/kg may lead to chronic toxicosis, but intake as low as 8 mg/kg may be harmful if molybdenum is low (0.5 mg/kg).[61] Blue-black kidneys are observed at necropsy along with splenomegaly and an orange-yellow liver. When cut longitudinally, the renal cortex may not be demarcated well from the medulla.[64]

Treatment and prevention. Ammonium tetrathiomolybdate (1.7 mg/kg IV or 3.4 mg/kg SC) removes copper from the lysosomes and cytosol of copper-loaded hepatic cells. The chelating agent D-penicillamine (50 mg/kg daily for 7 days) also may be effective. Fluid therapy is important to maintain diuresis and avoid renal damage. The daily addition of ammonium molybdate to the feed at 50 to 500 mg/animal may help prevent hemolytic crises if chronic copper toxicity is suspected.[63] Maintaining the copper content of the diet at 7 to 11 ppm and achieving a copper-to-molybdenum ratio of 6:1 are effective preventive methods (see Chapters 2 and 4).

REFERENCES

1. Garry F et al: Renal excretion of creatinine, electrolytes, protein, and enzymes in healthy sheep, *Am J Vet Res* 51:414, 1990.
2. Garry F, Chew DJ, Hoffsis GF: Enzymuria as an index of renal damage in sheep with induced aminoglycoside nephrotoxicosis, *Am J Vet Res* 51:428, 1990.
3. Vaala WE, Ehnen SJ, Divers TJ: Acute renal failure associated with administration of excessive amounts of tetracycline in a cow, *J Am Vet Med Assoc* 191:1601, 1987.
4. Lairmore MD et al: Oxytetracycline-associated nephrotoxicosis in feedlot calves, *J Am Vet Med Assoc* 185:793, 1984.
5. Fox SA, Berenyi MR, Straus B: Tetracycline toxicity presenting as a multisystem disease, *Mt Sinai J Med* 43:129, 1976.
6. Cox M: *Nephrotoxic mechanisms of drugs and environmental toxins*, New York, 1982, Plenum Press.
7. Gross DR, Kitzman JV, Adams HR: Cardiovascular effects of intravenous administration of propylene glycol and of oxytetracycline in propylene glycol in calves, *Am J Vet Res* 40:783, 1979.
8. Radostits OM et al: *Veterinary medicine*, Philadelphia, 2000, WB Saunders.
9. Adair HS, III, Adams WH: Ascorbic acid as suspected cause of oxalate nephrotoxicosis in a goat, *J Am Vet Med Assoc* 197:1626, 1990.
10. Kimberling CV, Arnold KS: Diseases of the urinary system of sheep and goats, *Vet Clin North Am Food Anim Pract* 5(3):637, 1983.
11. Andreasen CB: Clinical chemistry manifestations of toxicologic and nutritional problems in large animals, *Proceedings of the 12th American College of Veterinary Medicine Forum*, 1994, San Francisco.
12. James LF, Johnson AE: Prevention of fatal *Halogeton glomeratus* poisoning in sheep, *J Am Vet Med Assoc* 157:437, 1970.
13. James LF: Serum electrolyte, acid-base balance, and enzyme changes in acute *Halogeton glomeratus* poisoning in sheep, *Can J Comp Med* 32:539, 1968.

14. Burrows GE, Tyrl RJ: Plants causing sudden death in livestock, *Vet Clin North Am Food Anim Pract* 5(2):263, 1989.

15. Panciera RJ et al: Acute oxalate poisoning attributable to ingestion of curly dock *(Rumex crispus)* in sheep, *J Am Vet Med Assoc* 196:1981, 1990.

16. Crowell WA et al: Ethylene glycol toxicosis in cattle, *Cornell Vet* 69:272, 1979.

17. Boermans HJ, Ruegg PL, Leach M: Ethylene glycol toxicosis in a pygmy goat, *J Am Vet Med Assoc* 193:694, 1988.

18. Hovda LR: Toxicologic problems of small ruminants, *Proceedings of the Twelfth American College of Veterinary Medicine Forum*, 1994, San Francisco.

19. Plumlee KH: Toxicology of organic compounds. In Smith BP, editor: *Large animal internal medicine*, St Louis, 1996, Mosby.

20. Smith BP: Oak (acorn) toxicosis. In Smith BP, editor: *Large animal internal medicine*, St Louis, 1996, Mosby.

21. Basden KW, Dalvi RR: Determination of total phenolics in acorns from different species of oak trees in conjunction with acorn poisoning in cattle, *Vet Human Toxicol* 29(4):305, 1987.

22. Spier SJ et al: Oak toxicosis in cattle in northern California: clinical and pathologic findings, *J Am Vet Med Assoc* 191:958, 1987.

23. Menzies P et al: Death due to *Clostridium perfringens* type D enterotoxemia in adult ewes, *Can Vet J* 34:58, 1993.

24. Blackwell TE et al: Differences in signs and lesions in sheep and goats with enterotoxemia induced by intraduodenal infusion of *Clostridium perfringens* type D, *Am J Vet Res* 52:1147, 1991.

25. Michelsen PGE: Diseases caused by toxins of *Clostridium perfringens*. In Smith BP, editor: *Large animal internal medicine*, St Louis, 1996, Mosby.

26. Gerritsen MJ et al: Sheep as maintenance host for *Leptospira interrogans* serovar *hardjo* subtype *hardjo-bovis*, *Am J Vet Res* 55:1232, 1994.

27. Smith MC, Sherman DM: Urinary system. In Smith MC, Sherman DM, editors: *Goat medicine*, Philadelphia, 1994, Lea & Febiger.

28. Heath SE, Johnson R: Leptospirosis, *J Am Vet Med Assoc* 205:1518, 1994.

29. Gordon LM: Isolation of *Leptospira interrogans* serovar *hardjo* from sheep [letter], *Aust Vet J* 56:348, 1980.

30. Heath SB: Leptospirosis in cattle: a new look at an old disease, *Proceedings of the Tenth American College of Veterinary Medicine Forum*, 1992, San Diego, CA.

31. Bolin CA, Zuerner RL, Trueba G: Comparison of three techniques to detect *Leptospira interrogans* serovar *hardjo* type *hardjo-bovis* in bovine urine, *Am J Vet Res* 50:1001, 1989.

32. Thiermann AB: Leptospirosis: current developments and trends, *J Am Vet Med Assoc* 184:722, 1984.

33. Gerritsen MJ et al: Effective treatment with dihydrostreptomycin of naturally infected cows shedding *Leptospira interrogans* serovar *hardjo* subtype *hardjo-bovis*, *Am J Vet Res* 55:339, 1994.

34. Finnie JW, Swift JG: Adenovirus infection in ovine kidney and liver, *Aust Vet J* 68:184, 1991.

35. Belak S et al: Isolation of a pathogenic strain of ovine adenovirus type 5 and a comparison of its pathogenicity with that of another strain of the same serotype, *J Comp Path* 90:169, 1980.

36. Angus KW et al: Mesangiocapillary glomerulonephritis in lambs. I. Clinical and biochemical findings in a Finnish Landrace flock, *J Comp Path* 84:309, 1974.

37. Frelier PF et al: Spontaneous mesangiocapillary glomerulonephritis in Finn cross lambs from Alberta, *Can J Comp Med* 48:215, 1984.

38. Angus KW: Nephropathy in young lambs, *Vet Rec* 126:525, 1990.

39. Angus KW et al: Mesangiocapillary glomerulonephritis in lambs. II. Pathological findings and electron microscopy of the renal lesions, *J Comp Path* 84:319, 1974.

40. Lerner RA, Dixon FJ: Spontaneous glomerulonephritis in sheep, *Lab Invest* 15:1279, 1966.

41. Lerner RA, Dixon FJ, Lee S: Spontaneous glomerulonephritis in sheep. II. Studies on natural history, occurrence in other species, and pathogenesis, *Am J Path* 53:501, 1968.

42. Ferris TF et al: Toxemia of pregnancy in sheep: a clinical, physiological, and pathological study, *J Clin Invest* 48:1643, 1969.

43. Mahaffey LW: Diffuse suppurative pyelonephritis in a sheep, *Aust Vet J* 17:109, 1941.

44. Allen RW, Mestanza WF, Van Dresser WR: Nephritis in a sheep—a case report, *J Am Vet Med Assoc* 134:235, 1959.

45. Higgins RJ, Weaver CR: *Corynebacterium renale* pyelonephritis and cystitis in a sheep, *Vet Rec* 109:256, 1981.

46. Gajendragad MR, Kumar AA, Biswas JC: Unilateral pyonephrosis in a pashmina goat, *Ind Vet J* 60:494, 1983.

47. Honda E, Yanagawa R: Attachment of *Corynebacterium renale* to tissue culture cells by the pili, *Am J Vet Res* 36:1663, 1975.

48. DiBartola SP, Benson MD: The pathogenesis of reactive systemic amyloidosis, *J Vet Intern Med* 3:31, 1989.

49. Rings DM, Garry FB, Rings DM: Amyloidosis associated with paratuberculosis in a sheep, *Comp Cont Ed Pract Vet* 10:381, 1988.

50. Farnsworth GA, Miller S: An unusual morphologic form of hepatic amyloidosis in a goat, *Vet Path* 22:184, 1985.

51. Benson JA, Williams BM: Acute renal failure in lambs, *Br Vet J* 130:475, 1974.

52. Angus KW et al: Acute nephropathy in young lambs [published erratum appears in *Vet Rec* 124(3):62, 1989], *Vet Rec* 124:9, 1989.

53. Angus KW, Hodgson JC: Recognition and management of nephrosis in lambs, *In Pract* 12(1):3, 1990.

54. Hartley WJ, Seaman JT: Suspected *Toxoplasma* infection in an adult goat, *Vet Path* 19:210, 1982.

55. Khamma RS, Iyer PKR: A case of *Nosema cuniculi* infection in a goat, *Ind J Med Res* 59:993, 1971.

56. Grossman IW, Altman NH: Caprine cloisonné renal lesion. Ultrastructure of the thickened proximal convoluted tubular basement membrane, *Arch Path* 88:609, 1969.

57. Thompson SW, Bogdon TR, Yost DH: Some histochemical studies of "cloisonné kidney" in the male Angora goat, *Am J Vet Res* 22:757, 1960.

58. Altman NH, Grossman IW, Jernigan NB: Caprine cloisonné renal lesion. Clinicopathological observations, *Cornell Vet* 60:83, 1970.

59. Adam SEI, Wasfi IA, Magzoub M: Chronic copper toxicity in Nubian goats, *J Comp Path* 87:623, 1977.

60. Auza NJ et al: Diagnosis and treatment of copper toxicosis in ruminants, *J Am Vet Med Assoc* 214:1624, 1999.

61. Lofstedt J: Comparative aspects of copper metabolism in ruminants and horses, *Proceedings of the Seventh American College of Veterinary Internal Medicine Forum*, 1989, San Diego, CA.

62. Humphries WR, Morrice PC, Mitchell AN: Copper poisoning in Angora goats, *Vet Rec* 121:231, 1987.

63. Bostwick JL: Copper toxicosis in sheep, *J Am Vet Med Assoc* 180:386, 1982.

64. Gopinath C, Hall GA, Howell JM: The effect of chronic copper poisoning on the kidneys of sheep, *Res Vet Sci* 16:57, 1974.

LOWER URINARY TRACT PROBLEMS

Urolithiasis

Urolithiasis is a common and frustrating problem for both owners and veterinarians of male sheep and goats. It is less commonly seen in females and is most common in feedlot lambs and pet goats.[1] The composition of urinary calculi (uroliths) varies according to geographic location, but they are commonly composed of calcium salts and phosphatic complexes (e.g., calcium apatite, calcium hydrogen phosphate dihydrate, calcium carbonate, magnesium ammonium phosphate).[2,3]

Pathogenesis. Phosphatic calculi are formed in response to high-concentrate, low-roughage, low calcium-to-phosphorus ratio, high-magnesium diets and alkaline urine.[4] Lambs fed a diet high in phosphorus and magnesium have a high incidence of calculi on postmortem examination. High-grain diets result in the excretion of large amounts of phosphorus in the urine as a result of an overwhelmed salivary excretion mechanism. Certain breeds of sheep (Texel) are predisposed to increased urinary excretion of phosphorus.[5]

Silicate calculi also are occasionally diagnosed.[1,5] They occur more often in sheep fed plants grown in sandy soil or water containing high levels of silica, conditions that are common in western North America.[6] Diets high in silica with high calcium-to-phosphorus ratios that are supplemented with sodium bicarbonate may predispose to the formation of silica calculi.[7]

Oxalate calculi are caused by the ingestion of excessive quantities of oxalate-containing plants. Oxalates bind calcium in the rumen, but bacteria in a healthy rumen may (over time and with continued exposure) adapt enzyme systems that more effectively degrade oxalates. All uroliths are composed of salts and minerals in a crystal lattice surrounding an organic matrix (nidus) of proteinaceous material. Nidus formation occurs when urine mucoproteins coalesce and precipitate with crystals in supersaturated urine.[8] Urinary mucoprotein production is increased by estrogenic compounds, inadequate levels of vitamin A, and high-concentrate diets.[8] Uroliths can be formed in either the upper or lower urinary tract; by obstructing urine flow, they cause the clinical signs of stranguria, dysuria, hematuria, uremia, and possibly death.

Because of the length and diameter of the urethra, urolithiasis is more commonly identified in males. Early castration can decrease the urethral diameter and therefore increase the incidence of obstruction. The most common sites of obstruction are the urethral process and distal sigmoid flexure, although the trigone of the bladder, ureter, and renal pelvis also may become obstructed.[9]

A complete dietary history is crucial. It should include hay, grain, pasture, and toxic plant ingestion; trace mineral availability; water sources; and any supplemented feeding. In addition, information about previous health, current medications, age at castration, and duration of the problem is important in determining the cause and prescribing proper therapy. Initial observations by the owner may include anorexia and depression, with later reports of urine dribbling, abdominal pain, and stranguria and tenesmus in some animals.

Risk factors for urolithiasis include dietary imbalances, limited availability of water, abnormal urinary pH, age of the animal at time of castration, and possibly genetic predisposition. High-grain, low-roughage diets decrease the formation of saliva and increase the amount of phosphorus excreted in the urine. As a general rule the calcium-to-phosphorus ratio should be maintained between 1:1 and 2:1. Cereal grains have an abnormal calcium-to-phosphorus ratio of 1:4 to 1:6. High-grain diets overwhelm the salivary excretion mechanism and cause excessive urinary excretion of phosphorus. High-calcium diets are effective at reducing the absorption of phosphorus from the gastrointestinal tract. Legumes (e.g., alfalfa, clover, kudzu) have much more calcium than phosphorus. Increased levels of magnesium in diets with normal calcium and phosphorus concentrations can cause an increased incidence of urolithiasis in feedlot lambs.[10] Acidic urine (pH less than 7.0) predisposes to the formation of silicate calculi. Alkaline urine (pH greater than 7.0) favors the formation of phosphate, carbonate, and struvite calculi. Oxalate calculi may form in either acidic or alkaline urine. Some oxalate-containing plants are listed in Box 10-1. Forage-based diets commonly contain excessive amounts of potassium, which can result in an alkaline urinary pH. Genetic factors may play a role; excretion of salts by the kidney and the production of crystal-inhibiting compounds appear to differ among animals.

Clinical signs and diagnosis. Dysuria and stranguria with dribbling of urine and vocalization (especially in goats) are the two most common signs. Forceful contraction of the abdominal musculature ("heaving") may be observed. Hematuria, prolonged urination, flagging of the tail, apparent abdominal pain (e.g., stretching out, kicking at the abdomen, looking at the side), and bruxism are additional clinical signs. Exteriorization of the penis and examination of the urethral process is the most important step in the evaluation of these cases. In severe cases the urethra can be ruptured along the penile shaft, resulting in fistula formation. The urethral process or appendage may be necrotic from lodged calculi. Scalding of the perineal region or rear legs may be observed, possibly with concurrent prolapse of the prepuce or rectum. Careful examination of the preputial hairs or vulvar region may reveal attached crystals. The signs exhibited in cases of urolithiasis may vary depending on the duration and severity of the obstruction.

Abdominal palpation reveals a distended bladder. Transrectal or transabdominal real-time ultrasonography can be used to visualize the enlarged urinary bladder in some cases.[11] Echogenic material in the kidney, ureters, bladder, or urethra cannot always be visualized. The normal size of the bladder is 5 cm and 8 cm or larger in diameter in pygmy goats and other goat and sheep breeds, respectively.[10] Digital rectal palpation may reveal increased urethral pulsation. However, the clinician should exercise caution when interpreting this sign because some intact males contract the crura of the penis normally on digital palpation of the anus.[9] Renal calculi and occlusion of the ureter may lead to hydronephrosis, which can be visualized with ultrasonography.

Radiographs can demonstrate the presence of calcium oxalate or calcium carbonate calculi, whereas struvite, apatite, and silicate crystals may not be visible radiographically. Rupture of the bladder (discussed later in this chapter) is likely if ascites can be appreciated. In the case of urethral obstruction or rupture, pulsations, swelling, and pain may be appreciable on palpation.

Blood collected for a complete blood count and biochemistry profile may reveal stress leukograms, azotemia, and hyperkalemia depending on severity. Urine for urinalysis may be difficult to obtain, but testing can reveal hematuria, crystalluria (see Figure 10-5), and proteinuria.

Medical treatment. Amputation of the urethral process at its base near the glans penis is a commonly performed procedure to treat urolithiasis. Urine flow is restored in as many as 66% of cases.[12] If this procedure fails to allow normal urination, catheterization of the urethra and retrograde flushing may dislodge some calculi. Stones can form and adhere to any portion of the urinary tract. The male is sedated (with acepromazine 0.03 to 0.1 mg/kg IV) and positioned on his rump. The clinician exteriorizes the penis by simultaneously pulling the sheath and prepuce caudally, straightening the sigmoid flexure, and forcing the penis cranially. The urethra can then be catheterized for retrograde urethral lavage. A lidocaine-saline flush solution (1 part 2% lidocaine to 3 parts saline) may be beneficial. This initial flush can be followed with administration of a weak acetic acid solution (1 part vinegar to 1 to 4 parts sterile water) to help dissolve urethral and bladder stones. When flushing the urethra the clinician should take care not to become overly aggressive because excessive inflammation or rupture of the urethra may occur. Acepromazine maleate (0.03 to 0.1 mg/kg IV) has been used with some success to reduce urethral smooth muscle spasms and relax the retractor penis muscle.[13-15] If the urethra is not completely occluded and urine can be seen dribbling from the prepuce, ammonium chloride (300 mg/kg PO) can be administered to dissolve stones and NSAIDs (flunixin meglumine 1 to 2 mg/kg

IV) can be provided to reduce urethral irritation and swelling; this is a relatively successful nonsurgical management method. In some instances, these medical treatment techniques combined with dietary changes may be useful. However, because urolithiasis often causes sludge-like calculi to form in the bladder, the problem tends to recur in the majority of cases.

Surgical treatment. Several surgical techniques can be used to manage these cases, including urethrostomy, urethrostomy, and cystotomy. The following paragraphs describe surgical techniques for perineal urethrostomy, tube cystotomy, and bladder marsupialization.

Perineal urethrostomies have been performed in many sheep and goats, but surgical failure, poor long-term survival rates (because of strictures), and decreased reproductive function limit this method to a salvage only procedure.[12,16,17] The animal can be heavily sedated, given epidural anesthesia, or placed under general anesthesia. The perineal area is scrubbed and aseptically prepared. The clinician then makes a midline skin incision between the scrotum and anus and identifies the retractor penis muscles and the penis. The penis should be exteriorized and rotated to expose the dorsal blood supply, which can then be double ligated before the penis is incised near the ligatures.[14,17-19] As much of the penis as possible should be freed of surrounding tissue in order to place the urethra in close proximity to the skin. The urethra is incised and the urethral mucosa and tunica albuginea are pulled up and sutured to the skin under as little tension as possible. The urethra is then sutured with a simple interrupted pattern and a monofilament, nonabsorbable material.[14] The skin incision should be closed with two layers of nonabsorbable monofilament suture placed in the skin using a simple interrupted pattern. A Foley catheter can be passed through the urethral opening into the urinary bladder and kept there for 3 to 4 days.[14] Animals should be placed on an antibiotic (procaine penicillin G 22,000 IU/kg twice a day [BID]) before surgery and for 3 to 5 days after surgery. The clinician or keeper can remove the sutures in 10 to 14 days. Animals that have undergone urethrostomy can no longer be used for breeding. If strictures develop after surgery, they can be treated with a prepubic urethrostomy or bladder marsupialization.[6,10] The prognosis for long-term survival after urethrostomy is guarded to poor because of stricture formation.

Cystotomy and tube cystotomy are the authors' preferred methods of surgical correction. They allow for the longest survival and return to normal breeding function. Unfortunately, the cost of cystotomy may relegate its use to pets or breeding animals. The animal is anesthetized and placed in dorsal recumbency, the skin is clipped and surgically prepared, and a right paramedian incision is made. The incision should be 2.0 to 3.0 cm off midline extending cranially approximately 6 cm from the teats. The clinician then opens the abdomen and visualizes the urinary bladder. Placement of stay sutures at either end of the cystotomy site allows for greater stabilization of the bladder.[18,19] The clinician then performs the cystotomy, empties the bladder, and lavages the bladder to remove all calculi. Light massage of the bladder during lavage may help remove any calculi attached to or imbedded in the bladder wall. Mild normograde urethral flushing with an isotonic solution can be attempted. Some practitioners report greater success combining normograde and retrograde flushing.[19] Intraoperative flushing of the urethra with a vinegar/distilled water solution (1:1 to 1:4) can help dissolve the stones.[14] The authors do not make more than three or four attempts to relieve obstructions in order to minimize urethral damage.

After the urethra is clear and the bladder is cleaned of all visible stones, the cystotomy and abdominal incision are closed. However, if the urethra cannot be cleared, a tube cystotomy should be performed. The bladder incision is closed using an inverting pattern with absorbable suture. Occasionally, a two-layer closure is necessary. Placement of a Foley (16 to 24 French) or mushroom catheter into the bladder and exiting through the ventral abdomen (Figure 10-7) allows for continual drainage of urine. By routing urine flow through the catheter, the clinician permits the urethra to rest, allows inflammation to subside, and promotes healing.[16] The clinician makes a small skin incision lateral to the paramedian incision and inserts the catheter subcutaneously, where it enters first the abdomen and then the bladder. To position the Foley catheter, a purse-string suture is placed in the bladder wall. A small stab incision is made in the middle of the purse-string, and the balloon end of the Foley catheter is threaded into the bladder, after which the purse-string suture is tightened. After inflating the Foley catheter or placing the mushroom catheter, the clinician tacks the

bladder with minimal tension to the body wall in multiple sites. Alternatively, the omentum may be "pleated" around the purse-string site, after which the catheter is sutured to the skin and the paramedian incision is closed. If a Foley catheter is to be used, the clinician should check for proper bulb air or saline retention before inserting it. The authors of this chapter prefer to fill the Foley's bulb with saline. A one-way valve can be made from the finger of a latex glove and placed over the end of the catheter to create a crude Heimlich valve (Figure 10-8). This helps decrease the incidence of ascending infection.[16,18,19]

Regardless of the procedure (cystotomy or tube cystotomy) employed, the celiotomy sites should be closed in three layers with an appropriately sized absorbable suture. The authors prefer to close the abdominal fascia with a simple continuous pattern and the skin with a Ford interlocking suture or a horizontal mattress pattern. The skin should be closed with appropriately sized nonabsorbable suture; the stitches should be removed in 10 to 14 days. Many goats attempt to pull or chew the tubes, so belly bandages, Elizabethan collars, and close observation should be employed to help maintain catheter placement (see Figure 10-8). Ammonium chloride (2 to 4 g daily

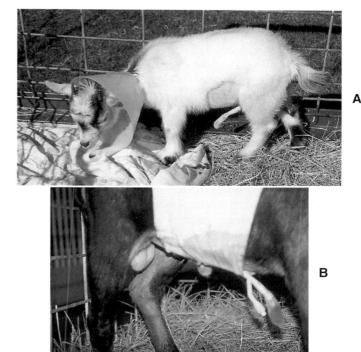

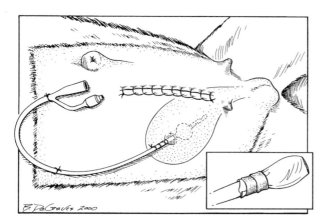

Figure 10-7   Illustration of a tube cystotomy. Note the location of the incision and the placement of the catheter into the bladder. The catheter is secured to the body wall at several sites. *Inset* shows Heimlich valve.

Figure 10-8   **A,** An Elizabethan collar is used to prevent the male from chewing or pulling on the catheter; a belly band **(B)** helps maintain the catheter. When using belly bands, the clinician or keeper should examine the animal's underlying skin daily. Applying antibiotic ointment (triple antibiotic) at the catheter exit site may help minimize infection. Note the modified Heimlich valve at the end of the Foley catheter in **B.**

PO) is generally given to maintain urine pH between 6 and 6.5. Because of its bitter taste, ammonium chloride should be mixed with syrup and given with a syringe. Animals should be closely monitored for signs of depression, anorexia, and abdominal pain. If a belly band is used to support the Foley catheter, the bandage should be changed at least every other day and the underlying skin examined daily. Clamping of the catheter should be instituted on the fourth day after surgery to allow for normal urination. This should be done in a dry stall and with an increasing duration until full-stream urination is achieved.[16] Normal urination should occur for 1 to 2 days before the catheter is deflated and removed. The Foley catheter should not be removed before day 7 after surgery. By waiting more than 7 days to remove the catheter, the clinician reduces the chances of urine leaking from the bladder.[16] The bladder defect is allowed to heal spontaneously. Normograde contrast cystourethrography through the tube cystotomy catheter can help the clinician evaluate the extent and healing of urethral lesions.[20]

Bladder marsupialization also has been described[18, 21] as an alternative to urethroscopy and lithotripsy techniques.[10] It may be used as a primary surgical procedure for urolithiasis or as a salvage technique in cases in which perineal urethrostomy has been previously performed but had scarred to the point of urethral closure. The laparotomy portion of the marsupialization technique is similar to that used in tube cystotomy or cystotomy. The animal is anesthetized and placed in dorsal recumbency, the site is surgically prepared, and an 8- to 12-cm paramedian incision made in the caudoventral abdomen parallel and 2 to 4 cm lateral to the prepuce (Figure 10-9). The clinician carefully exteriorizes the bladder apex, decompresses the bladder, places stay sutures 4 to 5 cm apart, and makes a cystotomy incision between them. A second abdominal incision is made on the opposite side of the prepuce. The site for the second abdominal incision is chosen to minimize urine scalding of the surrounding skin. The bladder apex should be pulled or lifted into the second abdominal incision by the stay sutures. Undue tension on the bladder should be minimized as it is pulled into this incision site.[18,21] The clinician then sutures all four corners of the bladder to the abdominal wall and sutures the bladder's seromuscular layer in a circumferential fashion to the abdominal fascia using a horizontal mattress pattern and absorbable suture. The bladder margins are sutured in a circumferential fashion to the skin with absorbable suture. A simple interrupted, horizontal mattress, or other pattern may be used. The original abdominal incision is closed in three layers as described for tube cystotomy.[18,21] Urine is voided from the bladder through the marsupialized site. Therefore after suturing the incision should be large enough to allow urine flow but not large enough to allow bladder eversion or prolapse. Animals should be placed on antibiotics, preferably preoperatively

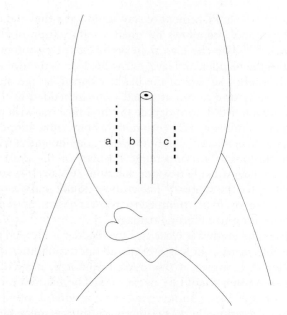

Figure 10-9 An 8- to 12-cm celiotomy incision *(a)* is placed 2 to 4 cm lateral to the prepuce *(b)*. The smaller incision site for marsupialization *(c)* should be chosen to minimize bladder tension and urine scalding.

and for as long as 14 days postoperatively (procaine penicillin 20,000 to 30,000 IU/kg IM BID, ceftiofur 2.2 mg/kg IM once a day [SID] to BID).[21] Virginia researchers described excellent long-term survival. Of the cases of marsupialization they studied, 7 of 19 goats had undergone urethrostomy before referral for marsupialization. Short-term complications of marsupialization include bladder prolapse and cystitis; over time fibrotic stomal closure of the marsupialization site may occur.[21] No instances of fatal cystitis or upper urinary tract infection were reported. This technique is a good alternative procedure, particularly for non-breeding animals and those whose perineal urethrostomy sites have strictured to the point of preventing urine flow.

Regardless of the surgical technique, fluid therapy (0.9% saline) is warranted for animals that are at least moderately dehydrated or uremic. Potassium and calcium may be supplemented as indicated. Postoperative diuresis is crucial. Antiinflammatory drugs and broad-spectrum antibiotics should be given as needed. Despite alleviation of the urinary obstruction, possible sequelae include erectile failure resulting from vascular occlusion of the corpus cavernosum penis.[22] If one animal in a flock or herd is treated for urolithiasis, preventative measures should be put in place to reduce the incidence in the rest of the group.

Prevention. Access to fresh, clean water encourages consumption, decreases the supersaturation of minerals in the urine, and decreases the incidence of urolith formation. In the winter, warming the water may increase consumption.[5] Sodium chloride added at the rate of 3% to 5% of the dietary dry matter intake increases water consumption, and the chloride ions may reduce supersaturation of calculus-forming salts.[23,24] Chloride has the ability to prevent phosphates from binding to the mucoprotein matrix that forms part of the struvite molecule. The addition of salt can help prevent phosphate-, magnesium-, and silicate-based calculi. An anionic diet increases the urinary excretion of hydrogen ions, decreases urinary pH, increases urinary excretion of calcium, and decreases the precipitation of struvite. Conversely, diets and feedstuffs rich in cations (e.g., alfalfa, molasses) should be avoided. Grass hays should be considered the primary forage source for males because grass has a better cation-to-anion balance than legumes for struvite prevention. To avoid precipitation of magnesium and calcium phosphate, urine pH should be maintained at or below 6.8.[25]

Balancing levels of calcium, phosphorus, and magnesium in the diet is important to prevent urolithiasis. If the magnesium content of the diet is greater than 0.6%, struvite uroliths may be encountered even if a normal calcium-to-phosphorus ratio exists. Adding calcium to the diet may help reduce intestinal uptake of phosphorus and magnesium. Therefore analyzing the diet and adding calcium carbonate or calcium chloride to the diet to attain a 2:1 calcium-to-phosphorus ratio are excellent techniques to reduce the incidence of urolithiasis. The addition of ammonium chloride to the diet decreases the incidence of silica uroliths.[1] The potential for the formation of phosphatic calculi increases when pelleted rations are fed because lowered saliva production limits phosphate excretion by the gastrointestinal tract and increases the excretion of phosphorus by the urinary tract.[13] Pelleted rations also are associated with increased mucoprotein excretion in the urine. Cereal grains (e.g., corn, oats, milo) are all high in phosphorus and relatively low in calcium; their consumption should be minimized. If cereal grains are fed, calcium should be added to the diet to maintain the proper calcium-to-phosphorus ratio (2:1).

The addition of chlortetracycline or tetracycline to complete diets, mineral mixtures, or feed supplements also can be helpful in some cases. Including beta-carotene or vitamin A in the diet can help prevent urolithiasis. Diets containing 30% green forage probably are sufficient in beta-carotene content.

When uroliths are discovered, submission of the stones for laboratory analysis can aid in the development of a preventative plan for the rest of the flock. In cases in which calcium oxalate or calcium carbonate calculi are identified, the feeding of legumes (e.g., alfalfa, clover, kudzu) should be limited or avoided. If silicate calculi are identified, the calcium-to-phosphorus ratio is greater than 2:1, and sodium bicarbonate has been added to the diet, adding phosphorus and ammonium chloride to the diet may help decrease the incidence in the flock or herd. Oddly, attaining a calcium-to-phosphorus ratio of 0.7:1 to 1:1 and acidifying the urine may be the best methods of preventing silicate calculi. Silicates are associated with the feeding of oats, oat straw, and some native grasses. When silicate stones are discovered, the consumption of these feedstuffs should be reduced or avoided. The plants listed in Box 10-1 are all associated with oxalate calculi and therefore their ingestion should be avoided or minimized.

The intake of excessive protein, which is common in feedlot lambs, can result in an increased urinary output of the mucoprotein that is the "backbone" of most uroliths. Therefore dietary protein should be fed to meet but not greatly exceed requirements for maintenance or growth. Diets high in estrogenic compounds and some growth-promoting implants can increase secondary sex gland size and increase the output of urinary mucoprotein; their consumption should be avoided. Many legumes (e.g., white clover) have estrogenic compounds, inappropriate calcium-to-phosphorus ratios, and a larger than necessary protein content, contributing to some forms of stones. Although legumes in hay and forage may improve growth and productivity, they should be used and fed to males with caution.

Whenever acidifying products are fed, urine pH should be monitored. For pet or valuable breeding males, the owner can be instructed to collect urine once or twice weekly and measure urine pH (pH paper is acceptable for this purpose). Urine pH should be maintained at or slightly under 6.8. Ammonium chloride (200 to 300 mg/kg/day or 2% of the total diet) appears effective in maintaining proper pH, but it is extremely unpalatable. The ammonium chloride can be added to the feed, mixed with honey, and sprayed onto forage to ensure adequate intake. However, if animals consume too much of it, ammonium chloride can produce a metabolic acidosis. Signs of toxicity include inappetence, depression, and diarrhea. Vitamin C (3 to 4 mg/kg/day) also can help maintain pH balance, but administering the vitamin often enough for it to be of practical value may be difficult.[14]

If left untreated, urolithiasis will progress to rupture of the urethra or bladder. The primary sign of urethral rupture is a large, fluctuant, ventral swelling at the level of the distal sigmoid flexure[14] caused by urine diffusing into the subcutaneous tissue of the perineum and ventral abdomen. The clinician should take care to differentiate urethral rupture from preputial or penile injury or abscess and abdominal hernia. He or she can facilitate the drainage of the fluid by making numerous stab incisions (0.5 to 1.0 cm in length) into the fluctuant area, taking care to avoid superficial epigastric vessels. Affected animals should be treated with procaine penicillin G (22,000 IU/kg IM every 12 hours) for 5 to 7 days. The use of NSAIDs should be considered.

Ruptured Bladder

Pathogenesis. Bladder rupture more commonly occurs in males as a sequela of urolithiasis. However, improper castration with an elastrator band can result in urethral occlusion and cause bladder rupture. Because ruminant urine contains high concentrations of potassium and low concentrations of sodium and chloride, a diffusion of blood sodium and chloride into the peritoneal cavity may be noted. After rupture of the bladder a concurrent movement of water from the intracellular and extracellular fluid compartments occurs as a result of the greater intraabdominal osmolality. The release of aldosterone secondary to hyponatremia leads to reabsorption of sodium by the gastrointestinal tract and increased potassium secretion by the salivary glands. The reabsorbed sodium causes competitive inhibition of potassium absorption by the gastrointestinal epithelium and thereby increases the fecal elimination of potassium. Therefore hyperkalemia may have a slower onset in ruminants than in other species with ruptured urethras or bladders. If the rupture is preceded by signs of urinary obstruction, immediately after rupture the animal acts normal and may even eat.

Clinical signs. Mild colic, depression, anorexia, abdominal distention, dehydration, and production of little or no urine are common clinical signs. After the first signs are noted, the animal's condition deteriorates over the next 2 to 5 days.[26] The ventral abdomen is often distended and may assume a pear-shaped contour.

Diagnosis. Blood collected for serum biochemistry and electrolyte analysis may reveal azotemia, hyperphosphatemia, hyperkalemia, hyponatremia, and hypochloremia, depending on the duration of the problem. A fluid wave is appreciated with abdominal ballottement in some cases. Excessive abdominal fluid can be confirmed by real-time ultrasonography. A definitive diagnosis is most easily achieved by demonstrating elevated peritoneal creatinine levels more than two times higher than serum levels (collected by paracentesis), by performing retrograde flushing of dye (methylene blue) into the bladder and recovering it in the peritoneal fluid, and by surgical exploration. Peritoneal potassium levels also may be higher than 10.0 mEq/L.

Treatment. Stabilization of the patient with IV physiologic saline (0.9%) or 0.45% saline in 2.5% dextrose is imperative as urine is drained slowly from the peritoneal cavity. Surgical exploration of the abdomen by paramedian celiotomy can be performed as described previously. The clinician identifies the rent or necrotic area and débrides the edges before closing the site. Thorough lavage and removal of calculi should be performed. Occasionally bladder tears heal spontaneously, with those in the dorsal area of the bladder being more likely to heal than those in the ventral area.

URETHRAL HEMORRHAGE AND OTHER URETHRAL PROBLEMS

As a sequelae to dystocia, an obstructive uropathy can develop and result in stranguria, pollakiuria, and enlarged kidneys with a distended pelvis.[6] In these cases, palpation of the abdomen should reveal a firm mass cranial to the pelvic brim.

Urinary Incontinence

Pathogenesis. Urinary incontinence may result from a number of primary problems. If it is a sequela to a neurologic problem, the clinician should determine whether the primary lesion is affecting the detrusor muscle or the urethral sphincter muscles of the bladder.

Clinical signs. Sheep and goats with dysuria and lower motor neuron disease usually have bladders that are extremely distended. Gentle transabdominal pressure usually results in the voiding of urine. Affected animals may display ataxia of the rear limbs and have depressed rear limb, tail, and perineal reflexes. Upper motor neuron lesions can result in a distended bladder that does not empty on firm palpation because of the increased tone of the urethral sphincter. Localization of the lesion and determination of the underlying cause are crucial in making a prognosis and outlining treatment options for these patients.

Treatment. Catheterization of the female bladder with a Foley catheter is helpful in supporting does or ewes with urinary incontinence. For temporary relief, cystocentesis of the urinary bladder may be indicated, particularly in males. Ultrasound guidance is helpful in this procedure. The use of pharmacologic agents to promote micturition has not been reported in sheep and goats, but cholinergic agents such as bethanechol (0.04 to 0.08 mg/kg SC three times a day [TID] or 4 mg/kg PO four times a day [QID]) may be given to stimulate smooth muscle activity and detrusor contraction. Drugs used to decrease smooth muscle activity of the urethra are generally given orally; the authors of this chapter have not used them in ruminants. The prognosis depends on the primary cause of the incontinence.

Cystitis

Pathogenesis. Cystitis may develop as a sequela to problems at lambing or kidding; the infection may ascend and become a pyelonephritis.[27] C. renale is the most commonly reported causal organism. Other causal organisms include Proteus, E. coli, Staphylococcus, and Streptococcus.

Clinical signs. Pollakiuria, hematuria, restlessness, and pyuria are frequently associated with cystitis. The condition is observed in females more commonly than in males because of the closer proximity of the female bladder to the external environment.

Diagnosis. Cytologic evaluation of either a mid-stream voided or catheterized urine sample may be diagnostic for pyuria. Occasionally, bacteriuria occurs. External palpation or ultrasonic evaluation of the bladder can help define the thickness of the bladder wall. A thickened wall suggests cystitis. Cystitis should be differentiated from upper urinary tract infection, and bacterial causes should be distinguished from neoplastic conditions that can cause cystitis (enzootic hematuria).

Treatment. Urine should be properly collected for bacterial culture and antibiotic sensitivity patterns because any therapy is based on these results. In cases in which cost considerations preclude bacterial culture, broad-spectrum antibiotics (ceftiofur sodium 2.2 mg/kg SC every 12 hours) should be given for at least 10 to 14 days. With aggressive therapy most affected animals improve within 2 weeks.

Prevention. Prevention is best accomplished by avoiding situations that compromise normal urine flow or may lead to ascending infection of the lower urinary tract.

NEOPLASTIC CONDITIONS

Enzootic Hematuria

Pathogenesis. Chronic ingestion of bracken fern (*Pteridium aquilinum*) causes hemorrhagic cystitis initially and progresses to neoplastic involvement of epithelial, mesenchymal, and mixed cell populations. Enzootic hematuria is generally a condition of adults that results from grazing the plant or ingesting contaminated hay. The fern is concentrated in open areas of forest in well-drained, fertile soils. All parts of the plant are toxic, and no single component has been identified to be the inciting cause of clinical disease.[28] Some reports state that bovine papilloma virus may work in concert with bracken fern to produce neoplastic lesions in the bladder.

Clinical signs and diagnosis. Usually affected animals have a history of ingesting the fern or contaminated hay and often numerous animals are involved. Initial signs reported by owners include hematuria and even clots of blood. With time, a decrease in body condition, productivity, and exercise tolerance occurs. As a result of anemia, pale mucous membranes, tachycardia, and tachypnea are reported. Infiltration of the bladder leads to dysuria, pollakiuria, and possibly obstruction. Thickening of the bladder wall results, and papillomas develop after 1 year, with invasive carcinoma occurring 2 to 6 years later.[28,29] Transabdominal ultrasonographic evaluation of the bladder may aid in identifying excessive bladder wall thickness and asymmetry. The disease may persist for months or years depending on the magnitude and duration of ingestion of bracken fern.[9,19] One flock of Merino wethers had access to bracken fern for at least 18 months, and 5% to 8% appeared to have bladder tumors.[30]

Prevention. The condition can be limited by reducing or eliminating bracken fern in the diet.

Leiomyoma

The primary tumor type known to invade the bladder of sheep and goats is leiomyoma. Leiomyomas may be solitary or multiple, and the animal may have other primary neoplasms.[31] Most often, these tumors are incidental findings at necropsy.

Renal Neoplasms

The multicentric form of lymphosarcoma caused by ovine leukemia virus may involve the kidneys in sheep.[24] A nephroblastoma has been reported in a 3-month-old ovine fetus that was aborted by an adult ewe.[32] The report suggested that infectious causes of abortion acted as a teratogenic factor and altered normal renal embryogenesis. Only 6% of neoplasms occurring in sheep affect the kidneys.

Congenital Defects

Hypospadias is a common congenital defect observed in newborn male lambs or kids. It is caused by failure of closure of the urethra and results in a visible opening on the ventral aspect of the penis and prepuce.[33] The kids are usually genetically female intersexes.[34,35] Concurrent diaphragmatic hernia, brachygnathia, and atresia ani are reported.[36] Urethral dilatation with a hypoplastic distal urethral tip is described in an intersex Nubian/French Alpine goat.[37] These goats also may have hypospadias[38] (see Chapter 6). A congenital urethral diverticulum has been reported in male kids with a ventral swelling of the prepuce caused by accumulation of urine in the urethral outpockets.[39]

Polycystic kidneys are frequently diagnosed in sheep and goats at the slaughterhouse or at birth if the condition is bilateral or severe enough to result in death.[35] A congenital cystic disease of the liver, pancreas, and kidney has been diagnosed in a 3-week-old Nubian goat.[40] In Canary goats, renal dysplasia results in signs of chronic renal failure.[41] The kidneys are smaller than normal and have irregular surfaces with numerous small cysts. Lambs have been reported to suffer from renal agenesis, hydronephrosis, cystic renal dysplasia, and patent urachus; all with concurrent defects.[42-45] Again, the use of transabdominal real-time ultrasonography may be useful in identifying these conditions.

Ulcerative Posthitis (Pizzle Rot)

Pathogenesis. Rams, bucks, and wethers are all susceptible to bacterial posthitis-balanoposthitis.[46] The most common bacterial infection of the prepuce is referred to as *ulcerative posthitis, pizzle rot,* or *sheath rot.* This condition is caused by an interaction of the local bacterial flora (most commonly *C. renale*) with excess urinary urea and typically occurs when animals consume high-protein diets. Diets rich in legumes may contain more than 18% protein, resulting in an alkaline urine that generally has a larger than normal concentration of urea. Whenever protein is fed above the maintenance requirement for a particular animal, ulcerative posthitis may occur. Excess dietary protein is usually deaminated by the body, its carbon chains used as an energy source, and the amino groups converted to urea. In the presence of the urease enzyme–producing *C. renale,* excess urea can be converted to ammonia. The ammonia may damage mucosal surfaces and result in pizzle rot. It occurs more commonly during wet springs and when animals graze lush legume or legume-grass pastures. Young male feedlot lambs, club or show lambs and kids, wethers kept for wool or mohair production (e.g., Merino sheep, Angora goats), and animals raised and maintained for blood or the production of blood products are all predisposed to this condition because they are all fed high-protein diets. Pre-sale and breeding diets for rams and bucks typically contain more than 12% protein and are often fed in confinement settings. However, diets as low as 12% protein have been associated with this condition. Castration before puberty also can be a predisposing factor because castrated animals have a decreased ability to extend the penis and tend to urinate in the sheath. Confinement rearing concentrates animals in smaller areas and is conducive to *C. renale* survival. Pizzle rot may be detected as early as 2 weeks after an increased protein intake. The condition has some similarities to and on occasion can be confused with the viral disease ulcerative dermatosis. A differential diagnosis can be based on the location of lesions. With ulcerative dermatosis the lesions occur on the penis, sheath, vulva, legs, lips, and eyes. The gram-negative coccobacillus *Actinobacillus seminis* is occasionally associated with posthitis in rams. This organism is rare in North America. *C. renale* can be transmitted by asymptomatic ewes, does, and possibly cows and insects. However, clinical disease rarely appears without a concurrent protein intake that exceeds the animals' requirements.

Clinical signs. Ulcerative posthitis is characterized by straining during urination, swelling of the prepuce, necrosis and ulceration of the preputial mucosa, and occasionally stenosis of the preputial orifice. In severe cases affected animals may show signs of abdominal discomfort or colic and a stiff-stilted gait. The urine of affected animals is usually malodorous and appears thick or semi-solid.

Treatment and prevention. Treatment includes reducing the protein content of the diet; débriding necrotic tissue; applying astringents, antiseptics, or antibiotics to skin lesions (e.g., gentian violet, iodine, triple antibiotic ointment); and possibly irrigating the sheath. In extreme cases in which the preputial orifice is scarred to the point that normal urine flow is partially or completely impeded, the sheath should be opened surgically to allow for urine escape. This salvage procedure entails making a 2- to 4-cm ventral incision through the ventral skin and into the sheath as aseptically as possible. The incision allows urine to drain from the sheath during or after urination. The incision and sheath can be infused with antiseptics (e.g., organic iodine solution) and the animal can be placed on broad-spectrum antibiotics (e.g., tetracycline 2 to 10 mg/kg SID to 20 mg/kg every 48 to 72 hours).

Affected animals should be sheared of their preputial wool or mohair, and the sheared fiber should be burned or disposed of in a manner to prevent the spread of the causal organism. An unlimited supply of fresh, clean water should always be available. In cases in which management conditions are favorable for this disease but dietary changes are difficult to make, the feeding of urine acidifiers (e.g., ammonium chloride) and/or antimicrobial agents (e.g., chlortetracycline) may be of benefit. Still, decreasing the dietary protein intake is the best method of treatment and prevention. If such procedures are possible, treating sheep wethers with 70 to 100 mg of testosterone propionate or implanting zeranol (12 mg) may help decrease the incidence of this disease.[46]

Ulcerative Dermatosis

Pathogenesis. Ulcerative dermatosis is a contagious disease of sheep caused by a parapoxvirus. This condition also is referred to as *lip and leg ulceration* and *ovine venereal disease.* The lesions may be contaminated by *Fusobacterium necrophorum* or other bacteria, which may affect the severity of the clinical signs. The virus typically gains access into the skin through cuts, scrapes, shearing or other wounds, and breeding trauma. This disease has been associated with breeding unshorn sheep, which can cause abrasions around the vulva and penis.

Clinical signs. Lesions associated with ulcerative dermatosis include circular crusty ulcers (typically 5 to 30 mm in diameter and 3 to 5 mm deep) on the skin of the prepuce, penis, vulva, nostrils, eyes, legs, and hooves. The ulcers may contain a viscous, odorless, purulent exudate. Penile lesions typically involve the glans penis and may cause scarring of the glans and/or the formation of urethral fistulas. Penile damage can result in a loss of breeding ability and possibly depressed libido. In severe cases inflammation associated with these lesions may lead to both phimosis and paraphimosis. The course of the disease may be from 2 to 6 weeks.

Treatment. Treatment is aimed at reducing pain and applying astringents or antibiotic ointments to the cleaned lesions. All affected animals should be isolated until their lesions are healed.

Prevention. Preventive methods include improved hygiene, isolation of affected animals until the wounds are healed, and quarantine of all new flock additions for as long as 4 weeks. During the quarantine period the animals should be examined to ensure they are free of disease before they are placed with the rest of the flock.

Caprine Herpes Virus

Venereally transmitted viral forms of vulvovaginitis and balanoposthitis have been reported in breeding age goats.[34,47-50] The causative herpesvirus can produce hyperemia and focal erosion of the preputial, penile, or vulvar epithelium, with a slight vulvar or preputial discharge. The lesions usually heal within 2 weeks, but the condition occasionally recurs. Prevention entails closing the flock, isolating or removing all infected animals, and retaining only noninfected animals for breeding.[34] Kids born of seronegative does that are themselves seronegative after weaning are good candidates for flock replacements.[34] As with ulcerative dermatosis, biosecurity protocols should be in place to prevent the introduction of this and other diseases to naive flocks.

REFERENCES

1. Stewart SR, Emerick RJ, Pritchard RH: Effects of dietary ammonium chloride and variations in calcium to phosphorus ratio on silica urolithiasis in sheep, *J An Sci* 69:2225, 1991.
2. McIntosh GH: Urolithiasis in animals, *Austr Vet J* 54:267, 1978.
3. Osborne CA et al: Analyzing the mineral composition of uroliths from dogs, cats, horses, cattle, sheep, goats, and pigs, *Vet Med* 750, 1989.
4. Hooper RN, Taylor TS: Urinary surgery, *Vet Clin North Am Food Anim Pract* 11:95, 1995.
5. Anderson DE: Urolithiasis in small ruminants, *Proceedings of the North American Veterinary Conference*, 1998, Orlando, FL.
6. Bailey CB: Silica metabolism and silica urolithiasis in ruminants: a review, *Can J An Sci* 61:2199, 1981.
7. Stewart SR, Emerick RJ, Pritchard RH: High dietary calcium to phosphorus ratio and alkali-forming potential as factors promoting silica urolithiasis in sheep, *J An Sci* 68:498, 1990.
8. Divers TJ: Diseases of the renal system. In Smith BP, editor: *Large animal internal medicine*, St Louis, 1996, Mosby.
9. Holland S, Phelps M, House JK: New methods to treat and prevent obstructive urolithiasis in small ruminants and pot-bellied pigs, *Proceedings of the Eighteenth American College of Veterinary Medicine Forum*, 18:268, Seattle, 2000.
10. Poole DBR: Observations on the role of magnesium and phosphorus in the aetiology of urolithiasis in male sheep, *Irish Vet J* 42:60, 1989.
11. Morin DE, Badertscher RR: Ultrasonographic diagnosis of obstructive uropathy in a caprine doe, *J Am Vet Med Assoc* 197:378, 1990.
12. Van Metre DC et al: Obstructive urolithiasis in ruminants: medical treatment and urethral surgery, *Comp Cont Ed Pract Vet* 18(3):S317, 1996.
13. Hay L: Prevention and treatment of urolithiasis in sheep, *In Pract* 12:87, 1990.
14. Hooper RN: Management of urinary obstruction in small ruminants, *Proceedings of the 1998 Symposium on Small Ruminants for the Mixed Animal Practitioner Western Veterinary Conference*, 1998, Las Vegas, NV.
15. Murray MJ: Urolithiasis in a ram, *Comp Cont Ed Pract Vet* 7(4):S269, 1985.
16. Rakestraw PC et al: Tube cystostomy for treatment of obstructive urolithiasis in small ruminants, *Vet Surg* 24:498, 1995.
17. Noordsy JL: *Food animal surgery*, Trenton, NJ, 1994, Veterinarian Learning Systems.
18. Moll HD, May KA: Urolithiasis in small ruminants. In Wolfe DF, Moll HD, editors: *Large animal urogenital surgery*, Philadelphia, 1998, Williams & Wilkins.
19. Van Metre DC et al: Obstructive urolithiasis in ruminants: surgical management and prevention, *Comp Cont Ed Pract Vet* 18(10):S275, 1996.
20. Palmer JL et al: Contrast radiography of the lower urinary tract in the management of obstructive urolithiasis in small ruminants and swine, *Vet Radiol Ultrasound* 39:175, 1998.
21. May KA et al: Urinary bladder marsupialization for treatment of obstructive urolithiasis in male goats, *Vet Surg* 27:583, 1998.
22. Todhunter P, Baird AN, Wolfe DF: Erection failure as a sequela to obstructive urolithiasis in a male goat, *J Am Vet Med Assoc* 209:650, 1996.
23. Gohar HM, Shokry M: Efficacy of sodium chloride in prevention of sheep urolithiasis, *Bull Anim Health Prod Afr* 29:321, 1981.
24. Kimberling CV, Arnold KS: Diseases of the urinary system of sheep and goats, *Vet Clin North Am Food Anim Pract* 5(3):637, 1983.
25. Hoar DW, Emerick RJ, Embry LB: Influence of calcium source, phosphorus level and acid-base-forming effects of the diet of feedlot performance and urinary calculi formation in lambs, *J An Sci* 31:118, 1970.
26. Baird AN: Surgery of the urinary bladder. In Wolfe DF, Moll HD, editors: *Large animal urogenital surgery*, Philadelphia, 1998, Williams & Wilkins.
27. Higgins RJ, Weaver CR: *Corynebacterium renale* pyelonephritis and cystitis in a sheep, *Vet Rec* 109:256, 1981.
28. Hopkins NC: Aetiology of enzootic haematuria, *Vet Rec* 118:715, 1986.
29. Madewell BR, Theilen GH: Tumors of the urogenital tract. In Theilen GH, Madewell BR, editors: *Veterinary cancer medicine*, Philadelphia, 1987, Lea & Febiger.
30. Pamukcu AM, Price JM, Bryan GT: Naturally occurring and bracken-fern-induced bovine urinary bladder tumors. Clinical and morphological characteristics, *Vet Path* 13:110, 1976.
31. Lairmore MD, Knight AP, DeMartini JC: Three primary neoplasms in a goat: hepatocellular carcinoma, phaeochromocytoma and leiomyoma, *J Comp Path* 97:267, 1987.
32. Raperto F, Damiano S: Nephroblastoma in an ovine foetus, *Zentralbl Vet Med* 28:504, 1981.
33. Dennis SM: A survey of congenital defects of sheep, *Vet Rec* 95:488, 1974.

34. Smith MC, Sherman DM: Urinary system. In Smith MC, Sherman DM, editors: *Goat medicine,* Philadelphia, 1994, Lea & Febiger.

35. Singh AP: Congenital malformations in ruminants—a review of 123 cases, *Ind Vet J* 66:981, 1989.

36. Dennis RJ: Hypospadias in Merino lambs, *Vet Rec* 105:94, 1979.

37. Karras S, Modransky P, Welker B: Surgical correction of urethral dilatation in an intersex goat, *J Am Vet Med Assoc* 201:1584, 1992.

38. Nair NR: Congenital urethral anomaly in a kid and its surgical correction, *Ind Vet J* 66:762, 1989.

39. Gahlot TK et al: Congenital urethral diverticulum in male goat *(Capra hircus)*—surgical management, *Ind J Vet Surg* 3:95, 1982.

40. Krotec K et al: Congenital cystic disease of the liver, pancreas, and kidney in a Nubian goat *(Capra hircus)*, *Vet Path* 33:708, 1996.

41. Gomez-Villamandos JC, Carmona JM, Castellano J: Possible renal dysplasia in two related, juvenile goats, *Small Rumin Res* 13:311, 1994.

42. Dennis SM: Urogenital defects in sheep, *Vet Rec* 105:344, 1979.

43. Dennis SM: Patent urachus in a neonatal lamb, *Cornell Vet* 59:581, 1969.

44. O'Toole D et al: Pathology of renal dysplasia and bladder aplasia-hypoplasia in a flock of sheep, *J Vet Diagn Invest* 5:591, 1993.

45. Jones TO et al: A vertically transmitted cystic renal dysplasia of lambs, *Vet Rec* 127:421, 1990.

46. Kimberling K: *Diseases of sheep,* ed 3, Philadelphia, 1980, Lea & Febiger.

47. Benies PE, McKercher DG: Characterization of a caprine herpes virus, *Am J Vet Res* 36:1755, 1975.

48. Horner GW, Hunter R, Day AM: An outbreak of vulvovaginitis in goats caused by caprine herpes virus, *N Z Vet J* 30:150, 1982.

49. Grewal AS, Wells R: Vulvovaginitis of goats due to a herpes virus, *Aust Vet J* 63:79, 1986.

50. Tarigan S, Webb RF, Kirkland D: Caprine herpes virus from balanoposthitis, *Aust Vet J* 64:321, 1987.

Chapter 11

Diseases of the Neurologic System

MARGO R. MACHEN, BRYAN M. WALDRIDGE, CHRISTOPHER CEBRA, MARGARET CEBRA, ELLEN B. BELKNAP, LISA HELEN WILLIAMSON, AND D.G. PUGH

NEUROLOGIC EXAMINATION AND LOCALIZATION OF LESIONS

The purpose of a neurologic examination is to determine the anatomic portion of the nervous system responsible for the clinical signs an animal is demonstrating. In sheep and goats a thorough general physical examination followed by a specific neurologic examination similar to that used in small animals allows the clinician to make an accurate diagnosis and provide a prognosis to the client. Localizing neurologic pathology requires the categorization of clinical signs the animal is demonstrating to either the lower motor neuron (LMN) or upper motor neuron (UMN) pathways. The LMNs can be further divided into the peripheral spinal nerves and spinal cord. Pathology of the LMN results in typical segmental physical abnormalities such as paralysis of the muscles innervated; areflexia; muscle atrophy and flaccidity; loss of resistance to passive manipulation; and anesthesia, hypoesthesia, or hyperesthesia of the affected area.[1] UMN functions are performed by the cranial nerves, brainstem, cerebellum, and cortex. Pathology of the UMN or lesions in a portion of the tract from the brain to the spinal cord result in poor postural performance, normal or hyperactive spinal reflexes, increased tone in extensor muscles, abnormal reflexes, loss of consciousness, and interruptions in sensory processing.[1,2] Clinical signs such as conscious proprioceptive deficits and ataxia make localizing lesions difficult.[3]

Signalment

Breed distinctions within species of goats and sheep as well as age and sex can be important clues in the diagnosis of neurologic disease. Many infectious agents that can cause neurologic signs are species-specific to sheep or goats. In addition, certain breeds of animals within a species may have a hereditary predisposition to develop a particular pathology. Young animals are more likely to have congenital, inherited, or infectious disorders, whereas older animals tend to develop neoplastic and degenerative diseases.[4]

History

The clinical history of an animal should be included in a database that also records the results of a complete physical examination. Important items such as the animal's diet, housing, purpose, vaccination history, and previous individual disease history (as well as herd health history) should all be part of the initial information gathered from the client. Construction of a sign-time graph allows the clinician to plot the severity of the clinical signs against time and is a useful diagnostic tool.[5] The course of disease begins with the owner's initial observation of the presenting complaint. The clinician and owner should take care not to overlook early behavioral abnormalities that could be interpreted as unrelated to the present problem. Acute disease processes can be either progressive or nonprogressive; however, chronic diseases are usually progressive.

The history combined with an appropriate neurologic examination can provide the clinician and owner with an accurate prognosis. A slow, progressive disease carries a poorer prognosis than one that has passed its peak of severity and is now improving.[4] Neurologic deficits that manifest themselves as sensory and motor deprivations are associated with a poorer prognosis than those that just produce motor losses. The duration that clinical signs are observed also can be used as a prognostic indicator because nervous tissue is fairly intolerant of long-term insults.

Initial Observations

The sheep or goat should initially be observed unrestrained so that the clinician can adequately assess locomotive deficits, postural abnormalities, unilateral conformational and musculoskeletal alterations, and the mental status of the animal. The clinician should give the animal sufficient time to calm down if it is not in its normal environment.

Mental status.   During the period of initial observation the animal's mental status can be assessed. For animals to be alert and oriented two basic components of the nervous system must be functioning—the cerebral cortex and the ascending reticular activating system.[2] The reticular activating system receives sensory information from the spinal cord and cranial nerves and diffusely projects this information through thalamic relays into the cerebral cortex. Therefore external stimulation from light, touch, sound, smell, and temperature helps to maintain consciousness in the brain.

An animal's mental status can be categorized as *hyperexcited, alert, depressed, stuporous,* and *comatose.* Table 11-1 describes each category and lists an example of atypical behavior. Normally an animal should appear as sensitive to its environment as its herd mates. If the animal has been removed from its habitat, it should be aware of the examiner and follow the examiner's movement with its head, eyes, and ears. All animals should avoid painful stimuli and appear alert and wary of new situations. Other signs related to abnormal behavior may include yawning, head pressing, compulsive walking, circling, and gazing.[4]

Behavioral disorders are hard to localize because abnormalities in the limbic system, which includes the hypothalamus, hippocampus, amygdala, and portions of the cerebral cortex, are all associated with complex behavior.[6,7]

Cranial nerves.   Abnormalities in the function of the twelve cranial nerves result from localized lesions of the brainstem or specific cranial nerves (CNs).[8]

OLFACTORY NERVE—CN I: The olfactory nerve (CN I) consists of chemoreceptors in the nasal mucosa that transmit impulses through axons that penetrate the cribriform plate to synapse on the olfactory bulb.[1] From there axons of the olfactory bulb travel ipsilaterally to the olfactory cortex, which is part of the rhinencephalon and limbic system.

Assessment of the sense of smell in sheep or goats is difficult; however, because they must have a sense of smell in order to have a strong appetite, if they are eating the assumption is that CN I is intact.[9] Substances such as alcohol, cloves, and benzol can be used to elicit a reaction from an animal, but smoke and ammonia should not be used because they are irritants that also stimulate trigeminal nerve endings. The most likely cause of anosmia is bilateral nasal passage disease because both halves of the brain participate in the interpretation of smell. Tumors and polyps in the nasal passages of sheep and maxillary

TABLE 11-1

CATEGORIES AND DESCRIPTION OF DIFFERENT LEVELS OF CONSCIOUSNESS

LEVEL OF CONSCIOUSNESS	DEFINITION	DESCRIPTION OF BEHAVIOR
Hyperexcitability	Rage, mania, frantic motor activities	Striking with front limbs, kicking, charging, excessive vocalization, violent struggling, possibly normal behavior
Alertness	Conscious, observant, responding appropriately to stimuli	
Dementia	Inappropriate responses to external stimuli	Afraid of feed, running into walls, self-mutilation
Stupor	Unresponsive to external stimuli; responsive to painful stimuli	Droopy ears, holding head low, reluctant to move
Depression	Reduced responses to external stimuli and pain	Unwillingness to rise, lack of recognition, inappetence, head pressing, propulsive walking
Coma	No response to external or painful stimuli	Recumbent, convulsions
Narcolepsy	Episodic condition in which animals exhibit stupor without motor activity	Rapid eye movement; after the episode animals return to normal

tooth root abscesses in both sheep and goats also can cause disturbances in the sense of smell.

OPTIC NERVE—CN II: The optic nerve (CN II) transmits sensory impulses from electrochemical receptors in the retina to the optic chiasm. In sheep and goats, 90% of optic nerve fibers cross at the chiasm to enter the contralateral optic tract, which transmits the impulses to the lateral geniculate nucleus and visual cortex in the occipital lobe via the optic radiation.[2] The brain is then able to recognize the object in the visual field.

Several methods can be used to assess the function of CN II. The first is observing the animal maneuver through an obstacle course. This is the least reliable method, especially if the animal has other neurologic deficits.[1] The menace response is the most reliable and easiest method to use for evaluation; it also assesses the facial nerve CN VII, which is responsible for blinking. The examiner moves his or her hand toward the animal's eyes or drops an object into the animal's visual field from above, which should elicit a blink response from the animal. The optic nerve is responsible for the afferent pathway and the facial nerves are responsible for the efferent pathway. The examiner should be careful not to generate air currents that may stimulate deficits in the trigeminal nerve endings.[1] Another method is the direct pupillary light reflex, which also assesses the oculomotor nerve CN III, which mediates pupillary constriction. The clinician examines the eyes for symmetry before the test and then shines a light directly into one eye. The direct response should be constriction of the pupil, and the opposite eye also should constrict as a result of the consensual pupillary reflex.

Unilateral lesions in the optic tract, which includes the lateral geniculate nucleus, optic radiation, and occipital lobe cortex, cause contralateral visual deficits and failure of the menace response with normal pupil light response.[10] However, affected animals retain consensual pupillary light reflexes when the opposite eye is stimulated. Lesions that occur in the retina and optic nerve cause ipsilateral visual deficits and failure of both the direct pupillary and consensual light reflexes. Depending on the severity of the lesion in the optic chiasm, the resulting clinical signs can include bilateral fixation of pupils, no response to light, and loss of vision.

OCULOMOTOR NERVE—CN III: The oculomotor nerve (CN III) is responsible for constriction of the pupils; the sympathetic system is responsible for dilation. After the optic nerve fibers pass through the optic chiasm, they synapse on the pretectal nucleus, which sends its neurons to the contralateral oculomotor nucleus; some innervate the ipsilateral nucleus of CN III too. The neurons of CN III leave the ventral midbrain medial to the crus cerebri, extend across the edge of the tentorium

cerebelli, and penetrate the dura mater.[1] The fibers of CN III are then joined by nerve fibers from the trochlear nerve (CN IV) and abducent nerve (CN VI), which work together to move the eyeball. After the CN III fibers reach the eyeball, they synapse on the ciliary ganglion, and the postganglionic fibers of the ciliary nerves innervate the ciliary muscles and pupillary constrictor muscles. Dilation of the pupils is mediated through the sympathetic nervous system, which originates from the hypothalamus. The sympathetic nerve fibers descend to the spinal cord in the lateral lectomertospinal pathway to synapse on the cell bodies of preganglionic neurons in segments T1 through T3. The preganglionic neurons then ascend in the vagosympathetic trunk to the cranial cervical ganglion, which is located ventromedial to the tympanic bulla. The postganglionic fibers then form a nerve plexus that follows the internal carotid artery through the middle ear and enters the skull at the base, eventually exiting through the orbital fissure and innervating the ciliary body and iris dilator muscles of the eye.

As previously stated the direct and consensual pupillary light reflex is one of the methods used to assess CN III's role in pupil function. After performing an initial assessment of pupil size for symmetry and to rule out primary ocular disease, the examiner should place the animals in a dark area so that external light does not influence the examination. Pupils that are very small are considered miotic, and dilated pupils are mydriatic. Occasionally the pupil size is unequal. If it is not extremely pronounced this may be a normal finding for the animal, but severe asymmetry is called *anisocoria*.[2] To determine if there is any irregularity in pupil size, the clinician should place the animal in the dark and then in a bright area. A sympathetic lesion will keep the affected pupil from dilating in the dark, and a CN III lesion will prevent the pupil from constricting in the bright light. The direct pupillary light reflex is more powerful than the consensual reflex, so the eye that the light is being directed toward constricts more than the opposite eye.

Examining the animal's eye position in relationship to its head at rest and during lateral movement of the head can help the examiner assess the motor function of CN III. If the motor function of CN III is abnormal, the eye is dilated and deviated to a fixed ventrolateral position known as *strabismus*. In addition, CN III is responsible for innervation of the levator palpebrae muscle, which when affected results in a drooping upper eyelid, known as *ptosis*. Ptosis is not commonly noted in sheep or goats because they also have a frontalis muscle that can lift the upper eyelid. Lateral motion of the head should cause the animal's eye to try to remain focused straight ahead and therefore result in the eye moving in the opposite direction of head movement. However, as the head continues to turn, the eye begins to move quickly in the same direction because of vestibular influences. This is a normal oculovestibular response.

Unilateral lesions of the oculomotor nucleus or nerve produce mydriasis of the ipsilateral pupil without loss of vision in either eye.[9] The ventrolateral strabismus noted with lesions of CN III is fixed regardless of the position of the animal's head. These types of clinical signs can be observed in animals with otitis media and otitis interna because of the relationship of the cranial cervical nerve fibers to the middle ear.

TROCHLEAR NERVE—CN IV:

The trochlear nerve (CN IV) is responsible for the motor pathway to the dorsal oblique muscles of the eye. The trochlear nucleus originates in a position similar to that of the oculomotor nucleus. The axons of the nerve run dorsally then cross before exiting the caudal colliculus. The fibers then run along the side of the midbrain before they join CN III at the cavernous sinus, where both nerves exit the orbital fissure.[11]

Assessment of CN IV is easier to do in animals such as goats and sheep because they have horizontal pupils. Damage to this nerve results in a dorsomedial strabismus. Bilateral dorsomedial strabismus occurs in several diffuse encephalopathies in sheep and goat such as polioencephalomalacia and listeriosis, but it is unclear whether this is the result of a true bilateral trochlear lesion.[2]

ABDUCENT NERVE—CN VI:

The last of the three nerves responsible for eye movement is the abducent nerve (CN VI), which innervates the lateral rectus and retractor bulbi muscles of the eye. The nerve originates in the rostral medulla and its axons run ventrally out of the medulla and lateral to the pyramid. It joins CN III and CN IV in the cavernous sinus, where it exits the orbital fissure to innervate the eye muscles.

The methods previously described for use in assessing CN III function can be used to assess the function of CN VI. Lesions in CN VI result in an inability of the eye to be moved laterally, producing a ventromedial strabismus. The abducent nerve also controls the animal's ability to retract its eyeball for protection. Stimulation of the corneal reflex by touching the eyeball should result in the retraction of the eye and extrusion of the third eyelid. Lesions in CN VI that do not involve CN III or CN IV are very rare.[1]

Lesions affecting CN III, CN IV, and CN VI can only be clinically assessed by moving the animal's head and observing the ocular position. Cerebellar and vestibular diseases also produce nystagmus, but the strabismus changes whenever the head and neck are moved. Complete ophthalmoplegia occurs when all the muscles responsible for eye movement are paralyzed. Lesions on the floor of the skull affect CN III, CN IV, and CN VI as well as sympathetic innervation as they leave the cavernous venous sinus and enter the orbital fissure. Diagno-

sis of such a lesion requires the examiner to force the animal's head into an abnormal orientation in which the head is extended and the nose is elevated. Sheep and goats should drop their eyes as the head is lifted. If one or both eyes deviate from the normal position, the condition is termed *positional nystagmus*. Most commonly the abnormal eye deviates ventrally; this is most easily appreciated by observing the more prominent dorsal sclera of the affected eye.[2]

TRIGEMINAL NERVE—CN V:

The trigeminal nerve (CN V) supplies sensory innervation to the head and motor innervation to the muscles of mastication. The nerve is divided into three branches: the ophthalmic, maxillary, and mandibular. The motor nucleus of the trigeminal nerve lies in the pons, and its axons run in the mandibular branch of CN V. The mandibular nerve innervates the masseter, temporal, rostral digastric, pterygoid, and mylohyoid muscles.[12] The cell bodies of the sensory fibers are in the trigeminal ganglion, which is located in the canal housing the trigeminal nerve in the petrosal bone.[1] The sensory fibers enter the brainstem and run to the first cervical spinal cord segment as the trigeminal nerve. A second set of sensory neurons receives information from mechanoreceptors and transmits nociceptive information through the maxillary branch to the pontine and spinal nucleus. Their axons travel to the thalamus associated with the contralateral medial lemniscus and to the facial nucleus.[1] From the thalamus, the axons project diffusely into the cerebral cortex and are closely associated with the respiratory centers in the brain. Axons from the spinal and pontine nucleus also run to the facial nucleus through the ophthalmic branch, which allows for the completion of the palpebral and corneal reflex.

To access all the functions of CN V, the examiner must assess several areas of the face. Initiating the palpebral reflex by touching the cornea of the eye is part of the assessment of the ophthalmic branch, which innervates the eye and surrounding skin and is responsible for the maintenance of corneal epithelium. If the medial canthus of the eye is touched the animal should close its eye. If the cornea is touched the animal should retract the eye and close the lids; this reflex also involves the facial nerve. A deficient palpebral reflex with a normal menace response suggests a lesion in the trigeminal nerve or ganglion.[9] Loss of CN V innervation to the corneal epithelium can result in neurotropic keratitis.

The maxillary branch supplies sensory innervation to the maxillary portions of the face and external nasal mucosa. Touching the lateral canthus of the eye or stimulating the external nares should elicit two responses if the axons are intact. The first is a subconscious localized reflex from CN V to CN VII that causes the skin to twitch. The second is a consciously mediated action in which the animal moves its head away from the annoying stimulus; this involves the contralateral thalamus and parietal cortex.

The mandibular branch of CN V supplies both sensory and motor innervation to the mandibular muscles of the face. Interruptions in motor innervation result in muscle atrophy of the temporal and masseter muscles and decreased jaw tone. Often the animal's tongue protrudes from the mouth, but the animal can withdraw it when stimulated. If bilateral involvement of the nerve has occurred, the animal is unable to close its mouth and may drool excessively, losing bicarbonate in the saliva. The nerve also supplies sensory innervation to the skin covering the mandibular area, which when stimulated should produce a behavioral response similar to that evoked in the maxillary area.

Damage to any branch of the trigeminal nerve results in sensory losses to the areas it innervates. Sensory losses to the facial skin are usually unilateral and can be attributed to peripheral lesions of CN V. Diffuse loss of sensation in the face is rare, although it may result from bilateral cerebral cortical disease.[9] An animal with forebrain disease should have an intact reflex component for CN V but will not consciously move away from facial stimulation.[2] If the damage occurs to the motor portion of the mandibular branch, marked muscle atrophy can be noted 2 to 3 weeks after the lesion occurs.

FACIAL NERVE—CN VII: The facial nerve (CN VII) innervates a number of facial muscles responsible for expression and provides parasympathetic innervation to the lacrimal, mandibular, and submandibular glands. The nucleus of CN VII originates in the ventral medulla oblongata. Its axons course through the lateral brainstem and enter the petrosal bone at the internal acoustic meatus, where CN VII divides into several nerve branches. The major petrosal nerve branches off first and travels to the lacrimal ducts, where it is responsible for tear film production. The sensory geniculate ganglion receives fibers from the rostral two thirds of the tongue and is responsible for detecting taste. These fibers follow the trigeminal nerve back into the cortex. The next branch is the chorda tympani nerve, which innervates the mandibular and submandibular salivary glands. In addition a small branch of this nerve also innervates the stapedius muscle in the middle ear. As the facial nerve exits the stylomastoid foramen, its fibers fan out and provide motor function to a number of muscles responsible for facial expressions and closure of the palpebral fissure.

Damage to CN VII can be localized according to the clinical signs. Lesions in the brainstem can result in a number of discrete or diffuse clinical signs in affected animals. Listeriosis in sheep and goats can cause discrete lesions throughout the brainstem, which may result in abnormal function of the facial muscles and stapedius muscle and variable effects on taste and lacrimation.[2] Because of the close proximity of the vestibulocochlear nerve (CN VIII) and CN VII, vestibular signs often are noted in affected animals; however, Horner's syndrome does not occur. Inner ear infections can damage the facial sympathetic nerves and cause vestibular signs, resulting in Horner's syndrome.[1]

Lesions in the petrosal bone that occur between the internal acoustic meatus and stylomastoid foramen can result in keratoconjunctivitis sicca (dry eye) and loss of taste. Loss of taste is difficult to assess in sheep or goats, but placing a noxious stimulus on the animal's rostral tongue should result in head shaking, rapid tongue movement, and salivation. A Schirmer's tear test can be used to assess lacrimal gland function (see Chapter 12).

Lesions in CN VII that occur distal to the stylomastoid foramen or damage the motor fibers affect the facial muscles, but not the ability of the animal to taste and form a tear film. In goats and sheep with compromised motor function, alterations occur in ear, eyelid, lip, muzzle, and nares carriage. The facial nerve maintains facial muscle tone. Goats and sheep that have erect ears should hold them erect; those with pendulous ears should be able to move the base of the ear canal to follow external stimuli. Animals with CN VII paralysis have droopy ears and are unable to move them in response to external stimuli. The animals should have a palpebral and menace response that results in them closing the palpebral fissure when stimulated. Simultaneous loss of the menace response and the palpebral reflex suggests a lesion in the facial nerve of the orbicularis oculi muscle.[9] The palpebral fissure also should remain open when the animal is alert, and the upper eyelid should not droop. An interruption in tone results in deviation of the muzzle to the normal side and loss of the ability of the nares to retract and dilate during inspiration and expiration. The tongue may protrude out of the affected side of the mouth and the animal may drool. Affected animals often have feed packed into the cheek pouch of the affected side. If CN VII becomes irritated, it can cause facial muscle spasms, which can be observed in animals that have tetanus.

VESTIBULOCOCHLEAR NERVE—CN VIII: The vestibulocochlear nerve (CN VIII) has two divisions, the cochlear division, which mediates hearing, and the vestibular division, which is responsible for providing information about the orientation of the head in relation to gravity.[4] The receptors of the vestibular division lie in the inner ear and are located in the petrosal bone. The vestibulocochlear nerve has three semilunar canals that are oriented at right angles to each other. They contain the crista ampullaris receptors that relay information related to the detection of motion in three directions. The utriculus is oriented horizontally and the sacculus is oriented vertically; both have receptors called *maculae* that signal the static position of the head in relation to gravity.[1] When all of these receptors are stimulated by the animal moving, signals are sent to the bipolar cell bodies of the vestibular neurons in the petrosal bone. The axons of the cell bodies, along with those of the cochlear nucleus, ascend through the petrosal bone via the internal acoustic meatus into the brainstem and terminate in one of four vestibular nuclei and the cerebellum.

After information has been delivered to the brainstem, the lateral vestibular nuclei maintains postural tone by sending out ipsilateral signals through the vestibulospinal tract to stimulate extensor muscles and inhibit flexor muscles. The lateral, medial, and rostral nuclei all send axons to CN III, CN IV, and CN VI to mediate vestibular eye movement.

The assessment of unilateral hearing loss in large animals is difficult; it requires the use of sophisticated equipment modified to assess brain stimulation from noises generated in each ear (brainstem auditory evoked response [BAER]). Animals that have bilateral hearing losses are easier to assess because they do not respond to loud environmental noises that do not generate vibrations.

Brainstem lesions must be differentiated from peripheral lesions in the inner ear to aid in prognosis and treatment. Table 11-2 lists clinical signs associated with central and peripheral vestibular lesions. Clinical signs associated with vestibular lesions include ataxia, staggering, head tilt, nystagmus, and ocular deviations. They usually occur in groups according to the portion of the nervous tract affected. A thorough otoscopic examination should be performed on all animals demonstrating vestibular signs; radiographs of the tympanic bulla also may be warranted. The assessment of the vestibular system involves observing the animal's head orientation as well as the

gait, posture, ocular movement, and extensor tonus. Most animals have unilateral vestibular signs that include ataxia, nystagmus, and a head tilt toward the origin of the lesion.[7] Recumbent animals with vestibular lesions lie on the affected side. If they are rotated to the opposite side, they spontaneously reposition themselves with the affected side down. The limbs on the affected side are hyperreflexic and hypotonic. The animal may circle or exhibit ataxia and is prone to falling frequently. If the animal remains standing, it assumes a wide-based stance to maintain balance. The head tilt should be obvious and can be accentuated if the animal's eyes are covered to eliminate visual compensation. Paradoxic vestibular syndrome resulting from central vestibular damage causes the animal's head to tilt away from the side of the lesion.

The direction of the nystagmus varies depending on the location of the lesion in the vestibular system.[9] To assess an animal's nystagmus, the examiner should first place the animal standing with its head in a normal position and then move the animal's head in all four directions, observing their eye movement after the head has stopped. Normally sheep keep the optic plane parallel to the ground when their heads are moved and goats maintain their eyes in the center of the palpebral fissure in all head positions.[9] Nystagmus is spontaneous eye movement that can occur as a fast or slow phase. The fast phase returns the eye to its resting location, and the slow phase moves the eye in the direction of the lesion. Nystagmus is characterized by the direction in which movement occurs in the fast phase—horizontal, vertical, or rotatory.[2] Rotatory and horizontal nystagmus can indicate peripheral or central vestibular lesions. It occurs when the animal's head position changes. Vertical nystagmus indicates cen-

TABLE 11-2

SIGNS OF VESTIBULAR DISEASE

CONDITION	PERIPHERAL NERVOUS SYSTEM	CENTRAL NERVOUS SYSTEM
Mental status	Normal	Frequently depressed
Gait	Asymmetric ataxia, may cause increased extensor tone contralaterally, falling, rolling	Asymmetric ataxia, paresis
Postural reactions	Normal	Abnormal
Cranial nerves	May have deficits in CN V, VII, Horner's syndrome, head tilt	May have deficits in CN VI, VII, IX, X, or XII
Nystagmus	Horizontal or rotatory, not altered in direction with changes in head position; fast phases away from the side of the lesion; positional ventral strabismus	Horizontal, rotatory, or vertical; may change direction with position of the head
Bilateral peripheral vestibular Disease	No nystagmus or vestibular eye movements, symmetric ataxia, crouching posture with jerky swinging movements of the head, deafness	

tral vestibular disease and is constant regardless of the animal's head movement or position.

GLOSSOPHARYNGEAL NERVE AND VAGUS NERVE—CN IX AND CN X: The glossopharyngeal nerve (CN IX) carries sensory information from the rostral pharynx, larynx, and tongue through the solitary tract to the nucleus of the medulla. The motor nerves of CN IX arise from the nucleus ambiguus in the ventrolateral medulla and innervate the pharynx and palate. The glossopharyngeal nerve also has a parasympathetic component that innervates the parotid and zygomatic salivary glands. The vagus nerve (CN X) provides motor innervation to the pharynx, larynx, palate, and striated muscles of the esophagus by the recurrent laryngeal nerve. The parasympathetic branch of CN X arises from the vagal nucleus in the medulla and innervates all the abdominal and thoracic viscera with the exception of the pelvic viscera.

Damage to CN IX and CN X results in clinical signs related to laryngeal and pharyngeal function. Affected animals have difficulty swallowing. The examiner can assess the gag reflex of sheep and goats by placing a tongue depressor in the back of the mouth. Normally the animals should gag, pushing the stimulating object out of the area with the caudal aspect of the tongue.[2] A small tube also can be gently passed into the pharynx to see whether the animal will swallow and allow it to enter into the rumen. The examiner should exercise caution in handling these animals if rabies is suspected. Often affected sheep and goats have stertorous breathing resulting from unilateral or bilateral paresis of the larynx. Animals with pharyngeal paralysis can regurgitate food through the nose.[9] Functional examination of CN IX and CN X should include auscultation of the larynx for stertorous airway sounds, passage of an oral gastric tube to evaluate pharyngeal activity, and palpation of the cricoarytenoid dorsalis muscle for atrophy.[9] Loss of vagal innervation of the rumen in goats and sheep results in uncoordinated rumen contractions and the inability to have a primary rumen contraction.

ACCESSORY NERVE—CN XI: The accessory nerve (CN XI) innervates the trapezius and parts of the brachiocephalic and sternocephalic muscles.[1] The nerves arise from the ventral roots of cervical vertebrae C1 to C7 and the medulla, run cranially as the spinal root, and emerge from the skull at the tympanooccipital fissure. The muscles that CN XI innervates allow the forelimb of the animal to be elevated and advance and stabilize the neck laterally.

Observation of conformational abnormalities and palpation of the trapezius, brachiocephalic, and sternocephalic muscles for atrophy are used to assess damage to CN XI. A decrease in resistance to the movement of the head and neck contralateral to the side of the lesion also may be noted. Electromyography (EMG) can be used to measure the electroconductivity of the affected areas. Damage to the accessory nerve is rare because it is well protected from the overlying muscle; injury to the spinal canal or base of the skull is often accompanied by more profound neurologic deficits that may mask clinical signs of accessory nerve damage. The most common pathologic conditions associated with injury to the nerve include skull fractures, penetrating wounds (such as those caused by goring with a horn), injection site infections, and contusions.

HYPOGLOSSAL NERVE—CN XII: The hypoglossal nerve (CN XII) is the motor pathway to the intrinsic and extrinsic muscles of the tongue and geniohyoideus muscle.[4] The nucleus of the nerve lies in the caudal medulla and its axons run from the ventral medulla lateral to the pyramids as they exit into the hypoglossal canal and innervate the muscles of the tongue. The nerve allows the animal to protrude and retract its tongue. The tongue is innervated on each side by CN XII.

Animals that have damage to CN XII often have a history of difficulty apprehending and masticating their food. The owners may observe the animals dropping feed and cuds out of their mouths while eating and ruminating. To assess the function of the tongue, the examiner places a palatable substance on the animal's lips and nose; it should be able to protrude its tongue and lick the substance off of the area. In addition, the clinician can gently grasp the animal's tongue with gauze and assess the strength with which its tries to retract it. Often unilateral damage to CN XII causes the tongue to deviate or protrude toward the affected side. Atrophy of the lingual muscles can occur as early as 1 week after an insult to the nerve.

LOCALIZATION OF NEUROLOGIC LESIONS

Sensorium

The somatic afferent system is responsible for transmitting signals related to pain, touch, and temperature. The receptor organs, both encapsulated and nonencapsulated, are classified as mechanoreceptors, thermoreceptors, and nociceptors. They are stimulated by physical contact with the external environment.[12] Two types of responses can occur in animals that have these receptors stimulated. The first is a subconscious localized reflex withdrawal from a stimulus or skin twitching, and the second is a conscious reaction that may include vocalization, aggression, or movement of the animal away from the stimulus.

Strips of skin along the surface of an animal are innervated by one pair of spinal nerves in a distinct pattern referred to as a *dermatome*. Each strip receives overlapping innervation from three different spinal roots.[4] Sensory fibers from the dermatome enter the spinal cord at the dorsal root and have one of two fates. The first involves them synapsing on interneurons in the dorsal horn of the gray matter, which then sends short axons to the alpha motor neurons to stimulate a reflex withdrawal. This reflex pathway requires an intact LMN reflex arc to function. Therefore if the spinal cord is transected cranial to an area being stimulated, the animal maintains an intact reflex reaction to stimulation. The cutaneous or panniculus response to stimulation of the skin covering the trunk also relies on a reflex arc. The sensory fibers from the skin enter the dorsal root of the spinal cord and then ascend to the C8 and T1 segments, where the motor neurons of the lateral thoracic nerve are located. Therefore a transection of the spinal cord caudal to T1 may result in a decreased or absent cutaneous response in the area caudal to the transection.

Two types of pathways are responsible for transmitting painful stimuli to the brain. The first transmits superficial pain sensations primarily from the nociceptors but also can carry information from the other two types of receptors. The axons of these receptors are small myelinated and unmyelinated fibers that enter the dorsal root of the spinal tract and ascend through a series of ipsilateral and contralateral synapses. The second pathway relays information about deep pain and involves proprioceptive fibers that enter the spinal cord and ascend by ipsilateral dorsal columns and the contralateral spinothalamic tract.

Conscious proprioceptive information is carried in the dorsal columns and spinomedullothalamus tract in the dorsolateral fasciculus of the spinal cord through the brainstem to the sensorimotor cortex.[4] The information is processed to determine the orientation of an appendage in relation to an environmental stimulus.

Compromises to the spinal cord result in loss of function in the following order of severity:

1. Proprioception
2. Voluntary motor function
3. Superficial pain sensation
4. Deep pain

Therefore an animal with a loss of pain sensation has a graver prognosis than an animal with a loss of conscious proprioception and motor function. A positive response to painful stimuli may result in the animal vocalizing, moving its head in the direction of the stimulus, moving its entire body away from the stimulus, or kicking at the offending object. However, limb withdrawal should not be interpreted as a behavioral response to a stimulus because of the local reflex arcs in the spinal cord. Superficial pain is most easily assessed by using a needle to prick the surface of the skin lightly or by using a pair of hemostats to pinch the skin.

Deep pain assessment requires a more aggressive approach to evaluate the animal's response. To elicit a deep pain response, the examiner must stimulate the periosteum of the bone. Placing a large pair of hemostats above the coronary band across the dorsal surface of P1 and pinching aggressively can elicit a deep pain response in the limbs of sheep and goats. Determining the animal's sensitivity to deep pain is important because of the grave prognosis that accompanies its loss. Fibers that carry deep pain perception are less susceptible to the effects of pressure, and because their tracts cross and re-cross widely in the spinal cord, a complete transection of the cord is generally required to produce loss of pain sensation.[2]

Hyperesthesia indicates an increased sensitivity to stimuli in an area that is palpated; it can result from spinal cord or nerve root lesions. Diffuse hyperesthesia also can result from infectious agents that cause meningitis.

Although the dermatomes have not been mapped in sheep and goats, they have been in horses, cats, and dogs. These areas are relatively similar among species and can be used to help localize lesions to areas of the spinal cord. In assessing the superficial pain responses of an animal the clinician must be able to accurately determine the boundaries of the loss of sensation and hyperesthesia.

Gait

Goats and sheep walk by first flexing the hindlimb on one side and then the forelimb on the same side; the process is then repeated on the opposite side. Animals must integrate a number of neural processes to be able to ambulate. Spinal cord reflexes are responsible for maintaining the limbs in extension, supporting the animal's weight, and initiating stepping motion. These functions are locally mediated at C6 to T1 and L4 to S2. The organization of stepping motion is performed at the brainstem in the reticular formation. The cerebellum is responsible for smooth locomotion and coordination of the muscle movement. The vestibular system maintains balance and helps anticipate alterations in the animal's center of gravity so it can compensate appropriately. The cerebral cortical functions control both voluntary and fine movement of learned functions.

To assess an animal's gait the examiner should observe it walking in a straight line as well as turning in a tight circle. Animals can be led through a maze of obstacles to assess their cranial nerve integration with the ability to coordinate movement. Gait abnormalities include conscious proprioceptive deficits, paresis, circling, ataxia, dysmetria, spasticity, stiffness, and myotonia. Musculoskeletal and other systemic abnormalities should be ruled out with a thorough physical examination before the animal is diagnosed with a neurologic problem. The animal's stride should be assessed to determine whether the length is normal, increased, or decreased.

Conscious proprioceptive deficits can result in several clinical signs, including knuckling over, stumbling, adduction or abduction, and interference of the limbs. The examiner tests the conscious proprioception of a limb either by placing the dorsum of the distal limb down and seeing whether the animal rights it or by crossing one limb over the other and observing the animal reposition the limb correctly. Walking an animal up and over an obstacle such as a curb while taking care to prevent visual stimulus helps the examiner evaluate proprioception. The proprioceptive pathway runs in the dorsolateral columns and projects into the cerebellum (unconscious) and cerebral cortex (conscious).[4] Slight compression of the spinal cord often causes deficits in proprioception, as do lesions in the cerebral cortex.

Paresis is a decrease in the ability of the animal to move a limb properly. The term *paresis* is usually preceded by the prefix *mono-*, *para-*, *tetra-*, or *hemi-*, which indicates the number of limbs involved. Dragging a limb while walking or scuffing the surface of the hoof wall is often noted. Usually paresis is noted while the animal is moving; however, abnormal hoof wear or growth also can provide clues. Paresis can result from a UMN or LMN lesion but is confined to the voluntary motor pathway that includes the cerebral cortex, brainstem, lateral column, spinal cord, and LMN.

Circling occurs primarily in animals that have brainstem lesions; the direction of circling is usually toward the lesion. Tight circling is associated with brainstem lesions, and rostral midbrain lesions may cause the animal to circle away from the affected side. Twisting or tilting of the head also indicates involvement of the vestibular system.

Ataxia is a lack of coordination without spasticity, paresis, or involuntary movements, although each of these conditions may have ataxia associated with them.[4] Affected animals often have jerky leg movements and sway as they walk; lesions in the cerebellum, vestibular system, and spinal cord sensory pathways often first appear this way. Truncal ataxia results in animals swaying constantly when they are not in motion. They also may stand with their limbs crossed. If the animals appear to have a loss of conscious proprioception without muscle weakness, the lesion is usually of cerebellar origin. All of these clinical signs can be exaggerated by lifting the animals' heads while they are walking or leading them up a slope.

Dysmetria occurs when an animal overshoots or undershoots its intended target. Hypermetria results in a high-stepping gait when the animal is walking (goose-stepping), whereas hypometria results in a stiff, shortened stride that is pronounced in the forelimbs. Both of these gait abnormalities are observed with lesions in the cerebellum or spinocerebellar pathway; they can be accompanied by tremors and ataxia. In hypermetria the loss of cerebellar input that normally dampens the flexion phase of gait results in exaggerated movement.[2]

Spasticity is unnatural increased muscle tone in a limb. The resulting clinical signs are similar to those seen in dysmetria but also include a notable increase in muscle tone when the limb is manipulated or palpated. Lesions in the white matter of the brainstem and spinal cord often cause this type of gait abnormality.

Stiffness is associated with a decrease in stride length and is commonly seen in diseases of the peripheral neuromuscular apparatus (motor neuron cell body, nerve roots, peripheral nerve, neuromuscular junction, and muscle).[2] Animals with orthopedic abnormalities may have similar clinical signs and maintain conscious proprioception.

Myotonia is persistent muscle contraction after the initiation of a voluntary muscle movement. The alternating contraction and relaxation of muscle groups that are stimulated when the animal tries to initiate voluntary movement cause intention tremors. Affected animals often have a stiff gait and prolonged muscle contractions in the affected area. Cerebellar lesions can cause myotonia.

In general, cerebellar lesions result in an animal being able to walk, but without precision. Lesions in the brainstem and cervical spinal cord often prevent the animal from walking or dramatically affect the gait. Often affected animals exhibit increased spinal reflexes in the affected limbs. Several LMN lesions also can cause alterations in gait. Table 11-3 describes the results of lesions in several LMNs of the limbs.

TABLE 11-3

EFFECTS OF DAMAGE TO PERIPHERAL NERVES

DAMAGED NERVE	EFFECT	MANIFESTATION
Femoral nerve, caudal spinal cord	Bunny hopping and a shortened stride	Difficulty in bringing both rear or one rear limb forward
Obturator nerve	Limbs slide laterally without the animal replacing them	Inability to abduct the limb; gait is normal
Sciatic nerve	Rear foot is thrown forward by proximal trunk muscles	Hock is overflexed
Radial nerve	Inability to extend the carpus	Shoulder lifts in an exaggerated motion to advance the limb
Medial and ulnar nerve	Carpus is overextended	Same as for radial nerve

Posture and Postural Reactions

Posture is normally assessed at rest at the same times as the animal's head carriage and limb and trunk orientation are examined. The most common abnormality in head carriage is a tilt to one side. After otitis has been ruled out, the most likely cause is a lesion in the vestibular system. Animals that exhibit not only a head tilt but also a rotation of the neck and thoracic area may have a lesion in the brainstem or cerebellum. To diagnose or rule out cervical lesions, the animal's head should be rotated back to its normal position so the examiner can assess its reaction. An animal with neuromuscular damage or cervical pain may resist head movement and arch its thoracic vertebrae or display a painful response.

Limb posture should be assessed with the animal standing, but if the animal is recumbent the orientation should be noted and the muscle tone of the legs should be carefully palpated. Animals that are ataxic often assume a wide-based stance. Lesions in the cerebellum, vestibular system, and spinal cord can produce this appearance. Preferential distribution of the animal's weight also should be noted because it may indicate pain or weakness on the non–weight-bearing limbs. Spasticity can be observed at rest or while the animal is moving; it is usually indicative of a central nervous system motor pathway lesion. Decerebrate rigidity is manifested as extreme opisthotonos, extension of all four limbs, and loss of consciousness. It is caused by a loss of descending input from supratentorial structures in the medullary centers, which are normally responsible for flexion of the limbs, and is seen in severe brainstem lesions.[2] This is a common presentation for sheep and goats afflicted with tetanus. Decerebellate rigidity is characterized by front limb extension and opisthotonos, but the rear limbs are flexed and the animal is mentally alert. Cerebellar disease that does not involve the ventral aspects of the cerebellum produces this posture. Decreased muscle tone and the ability of an examiner to manipulate the animal's limbs passively are associated with LMN disease. Affected animals also may stand knuckled over on the dorsum. Increased muscle tone is usually the result of UMN disease. Schiff-Sherrington syndrome is associated with spinal cord lesions between T3 and L3; affected animals exhibit thoracic limb extension and normal tone and reflexes in their pelvic limbs. This is a rare finding in large animals.

Trunk posture should be assessed after a thorough examination of the vertebral column. Deviations in the vertebral column such as scoliosis, lordosis, and kyphosis may cause abnormal muscle tone and posture because of malformation of the vertebral disk spaces.

Postural reactions are responsible for maintaining an animal in a normal upright orientation. They involve the integration of the LMN and UMN pathways, and therefore localization of lesions can be difficult at times. Postural reactions are hard to assess in large animals because of size limitations; however, in assessing sheep and goats the examiner can conduct many of the tests used in dogs and cats.

Assessment of the righting response involves placing an animal on its side; the normal response should be for the animal to roll over into sternal recumbency and then rise up, rear limbs first. This action requires the integration of the vestibular labyrinths and proprioceptive receptors in the joints, tendons, and muscles.[9] Information is relayed to the thalamus and sensory cortex for processing and then transmitted to the motor cortex, brainstem, spinal cord, and LMN. It is then relayed to the musculature. Deviations from the normal righting response can help the examiner localize lesions in the nervous system. An animal that is reluctant to rise but does so eventually may have a lesion in the cerebral cortex or diencephalon. An animal that is unable to lift its head may be lying with the affected side up or have a lesion cranial to C4. If the animal is able to rise after it has been rotated to the opposite side, the lesion can be localized to that side. Incomplete lesions in the C5 to T2 area result in a recumbent animal that can lift its head; if the lesion is located from T3 to L3, the animal may be able to assume a "dog-sitting" position.

Forcing the animal to hop primarily on one leg tests strength, proprioception, and voluntary movement.[2] Animals with cerebellar lesions make exaggerated hopping motions when forced to bear their weight on primarily one limb. Lifting one of the forelimbs or hindlimbs and pushing the animal's weight over to the opposite limb should force the animal to hop as its center of gravity shifts over the weight-bearing limb. Animals that have cerebellar lesions may fall over or lean their weight against the examiner.

Conscious proprioceptive deficits can result from lesions in several locations because the pathway responsible for relaying proprioceptive information to the brain runs ipsilaterally up the spinal column, but then crosses over to the contralateral side of the cortex at the level of the caudal mesencephalon and rostral pons. Lesions in the contralateral brain or ipsilateral spinal cord cause deficits on the same side. In addition, LMN lesions and somatic lesions prevent neuromuscular movement.

Spinal Reflexes

Spinal reflexes are used to evaluate the integrity of LMNs. To have a clear knowledge of the way the information gained from spinal reflexes can be used, the examiner must understand the differences between UMNs and LMNs. Primarily UMNs are responsible for dampening or inhibiting spinal reflexes. Their axons and cell bodies remain within the central nervous system and influence LMN activities. As a result, when interruptions occur in UMN influence, animals often have hyperreflexia or hypertonia. If muscle atrophy occurs as a sequela to a lesion of the UMN, it generally results from improper use of the affected muscle caused by poor nervous system control.[2] The afferent fibers that relay information to the cerebral cortex ascend the spinal tract ipsilaterally, then cross at the level of the caudal mesencephalon, which means that lesions in the UMN cause contralateral neuromuscular deficits. The resulting muscle atrophy takes longer to develop and is not as pronounced as in LMN disease.

Before examining LMN reflexes the clinician should first understand the way the nerves relay and process information locally to elicit a muscular reaction. The reflex arc consists of an afferent receptor that relays information into the gray matter of the spinal cord, which consists of a varying number of interneurons that can stimulate inhibitory and excitatory neurons and alpha motor neurons. Alpha motor neurons exit the spinal cord and innervate the motor end plates of the ipsilateral and contralateral muscle bundles. The information also is relayed to the cortex by the lateral spinothalamic, fasciculus cuneatus, and gracilis tracts. In turn, UMN influences are relayed back to the LMN by way of the rubrospinal and reticulospinal tracts. Several different responses can be observed during testing of spinal reflexes. The first is a normal response indicating that both sensory and motor components are intact. The second is an exaggerated response, which indicates an abnormality in the UMN pathways. The third is a depressed or absent response, which indicates LMN disease in either the sensory or motor components. Animals that have LMN lesion exhibit muscle atrophy, hyporeflexia, areflexia, hypotonia, atonia, and paresis.

Before the examination begins the animal should be placed in lateral recumbency. The musculature and tone should be assessed by palpation to determine any obvious signs of atrophy. Usually the pelvic limbs are examined first. The examiner should identify any musculoskeletal injuries before beginning the neurologic examination. Passive extension and flexion of the limb can be used to assess muscle tone. Animals with LMN disease exhibit depressed or absent resistance to the flexion, whereas those with UMN disease display increased tone of the extensor muscles as the limb is manipulated. Normally reflexes have two phases: the first is rapid movement of the limb, which is LMN-mediated; and the second is conscious recognition of the stimulus, which is UMN-mediated. An interruption in the sensory tract of the LMN system prevents or decreases both phases, and a lesion in the UMN system may prevent conscious recognition of the stimulus—the reflex may still be intact but may be inappropriate. Animals with lesions in the LMN motor pathway may consciously recognize the stimulus but be unable to form a reflex reaction. This is rare because damage to the motor pathway usually results in damage to the sensory pathway too; however, in some instances an animal recovering from an injury to the LMN system may regain sensory innervation before motor control is restored.

Stimulating stretch receptors in muscle spindles assesses myotatic reflexes, which stem from a two-neuron system. The reflexes are basic to the regulation of posture and movement.[4] The muscle belly contains stretch receptors composed of muscle spindle fibers that detect the amount of tension placed on the muscle. Sudden changes in the amount of tension in the muscle spindle cause it to discharge and elicit a reflex reaction through the LMN pathway. Absence or depression of the reflex suggests a lesion in the LMN pathway. The bilateral absence of reflexes indicates a segmental spinal cord lesion. Exaggerated reflexes or increased muscle tone indicate a lesion in the UMN pathways descending from the cortex or in the cortex itself. A UMN lesion in the spinal cord is ipsilateral to the affected limb; additional clinical signs of neurologic abnormalities in the cranial limbs or trunk can be used to determine the exact level of the spinal cord lesion. If the lesion occurs in the cortex, the contralateral side of the animal displays hyperresponsive activity diffusely.

The patellar reflex is assessed by laying the animal on its side as the examiner supports the femur with the stifle slightly flexed as seen in Figure 11-1. When the patellar ligament is sharply tapped with a plexor, the normal response is for the animal to extend the stifle quickly. This test measures the function of the peroneal and ischiatic nerves and spinal cord segments L6 to S2.

The cranial tibial reflex test is performed if the patellar reflex is abnormal or a sciatic nerve lesion is suspected. Supporting the rear leg behind the stifle, the examiner strikes the belly of the tibial muscle right below

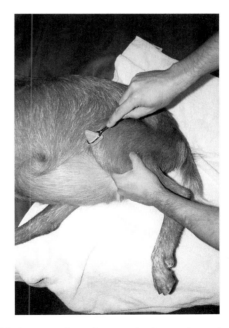

Figure 11-1   A patellar reflex examination can be performed on a goat to assess the function of the peroneal and ischiatic and spinal cord segments L6 to S2. This goat is lying on its side and the clinician is supporting the femur with the stifle slightly flexed.

the stifle. The hock should flex in response. The response is very subtle in small ruminants and the examiner should be careful not to place too much emphasis on the results. This test measures the function of the femoral nerve, quadriceps femoris muscle, and L4 to L6 spinal cord segments.

The gastrocnemius reflex test can be performed after the tibial reflex is assessed; it requires the examiner to support the limb from behind the leg at the level of the stifle and slightly flex the hock while striking the tendon of the gastrocnemius muscle above the hock, which should extend in response. The tibial branch of the sciatic nerve innervates the muscle and originates from L6 to S2.

To perform the extensor carpi radialis reflex test the examiner supports the animal's elbow from behind, maintaining flexion of the elbow and carpus. The extensor carpi radialis muscle is then struck just distal to the elbow; the carpus should extend. The muscle is innervated by the radial nerve, which originates from C5 to T2.

To perform the triceps reflex test the examiner restrains the animal as in the extensor carpi radialis flexion test with the elbow in flexion. The triceps brachii muscle is struck above the olecranon, which should cause the elbow to extend. The muscle is innervated by the radial nerve, which originates from C5 to T2.

The biceps reflex test is conducted with the animal's leg in flexion at the carpus and the examiner's hand or fingers placed over the insertion of the biceps muscle above the elbow, maintaining the elbow in slight extension. The muscle belly of the biceps is lightly struck, which should cause flexion in the elbow and extension of the carpus. This tests the function of the musculocutaneous nerve and spinal segment C6 to C8.

Several other reflex tests that can be used to assess LMN function do not involve myotatic reflexes. One such test involves the cutaneous or panniculus reflex; it was previously discussed in the Sensorium section of this chapter.

Another test is the flexor withdrawal reflex of a limb to a noxious stimulus. The minimal amount of noxious stimulus necessary to elicit a response from the sole of the claw or an area right above the coronary band should be used. A normal response is for the animal to flex its forelimb and hindlimb fully away from the stimulus. If used on the forelimb this test assesses the motor components of the axillary, median, musculocutaneous, ulnar, and long thoracic nerves, as well as spinal cord segment C5 to T2.[9] The sensory components are the median nerve, which innervates the cranial, palmar, and medial sides; and the ulnar nerve, which innervates the cranial lateral aspect of the digit.[9] Proximal portions of the forelimbs are innervated through the axillary, musculocutaneous, ulnar, and radial nerves. In the rear limb the motor component of the flexion arises from the peroneal, tibial, and ischiatic nerves, as well as spinal segments L6 to S2. The sensory innervation to the rear limb arises from the peroneal and tibial nerves. Unilateral absence or depression of the flexor test may indicate damage to any of the peripheral nerves responsible for the reflex reaction; bilateral deficits indicate a spinal cord lesion.

The crossed extensor reflex can be observed when the flexor reflex is being evaluated. When one of the forelimbs or hindlimbs is being tested, the opposite limb should not extend if the animal is recumbent. Normally the UMN pathways inhibit this reaction in a recumbent animal. When an animal is standing, the flexor reflex sensory fibers send collaterals to interneurons on the opposite side of the spinal cord, which excite the extensor motor neurons.[4] This prevents the animal from falling over as it flexes its limbs and shifts weight to the opposite side.

The perineal reflex is elicited by pinching the skin around the anus (Figure 11-2).[9] The reflex is mediated by S1 to S5 and should result in a tightening of the anal sphincter, clamping of the tail, and possibly aggressive kicking of the hindlimbs. A lesion in this area can cause several complications, including absent anal tone and a relaxed anal sphincter. The animal's tail does not raise when it defecates, and fecal pellets dribble out of the anus as the colon becomes full. Often bladder atony is caused by an interruption in parasympathetic innervation, resulting in a flaccid full bladder and urine dribbling. The animal's perineal and inguinal area may show signs of urine scalding when examined.

LESION LOCALIZATION

To localize a lesion in the nervous system, the examiner must first determine whether the animal is displaying UMN or LMN clinical signs. After this the examiner should assess all the clinical findings to determine which portions of the pathways are involved. The UMN system is composed of the cerebrum, basal nuclei, telencephalon, diencephalon, mesencephalon, metencephalon, myelencephalon, thalamus, hypothalamus, midbrain, cerebellum, pons, and medulla oblongata. The UMN system is re-

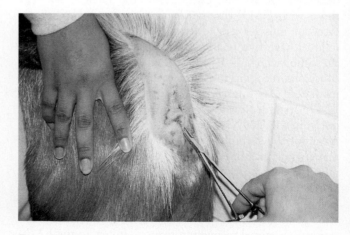

Figure 11-2   Assessing the perineal reflex in a goat by pinching the skin around the anus. The animal should respond by clamping its tail and tightening the anal sphincter. This test assesses spinal cord segments S1 to S5.

sponsible for initiation and maintenance of normal movement and for maintenance of tone in the extensor muscles to support the body against gravity.[4] The LMN system is divided into segments from which two spinal nerves emerge to innervate each side of the body. The LMN system is responsible for relaying sensory information to the UMN system, relaying motor control information from the UMN system, and maintaining local reflexes.

Tables 11-4 through 11-6 contain information that can aid the clinician in determining whether a lesion is of

---

TABLE 11-4

SUMMARY OF LOWER AND UPPER MOTOR NEURON SIGNS

PARAMETER	LOWER MOTOR NEURON SEGMENTAL SIGNS	UPPER MOTOR NEURON LONG TRACT SIGNS
Motor function	Paralysis—loss of muscle power, flaccidity	Paresis to paralysis—loss of voluntary movements
Reflexes	Hyporeflexia to areflexia	Normal to hyperreflexia (especially myotatic reflexes)
Muscle atrophy	Early and severe: neurologic; contracture after several weeks	Late and mild: disuse
Muscle tone	Decreased	Normal to increased
Electromyographic changes	Abnormal potentials (fibrillation, positive sharp waves) after 5 to 7 days	No changes
Associated sensory signs	Anesthesia of innervated area, paresthesia or hyperesthesia of adjacent areas	Decreased proprioception; decreased perception of superficial and deep pain

From Oliver JE, Jr, Lorenz MD: *Handbook of veterinary neurologic diagnosis,* Philadelphia, 1983, WB Saunders.

TABLE 11-5

LOWER MOTOR NEURON LESION LOCALIZATION CHART

VERTEBRAE	AFFECTED MUSCLE OR CONDITION	CLINICAL SIGNS
C1 to C6	C6 to C8—Biceps brachii	Ipsilateral ataxia and paresis in all four limbs; hyperreflexia (worse in the rear); hopping; cutaneous sensation loss to innervated areas
C6 to T2	C6 to C8—Biceps brachii C5 to T2—Triceps brachii C5 to T2—Extensor carpi radialis C8 to T1—Cutaneous trunci C6 to T2—Brachial plexus T1 to T3—Sympathetic nerve damage C1 to C6—Flexor withdraw of forelimb	Both the forelimbs and hindlimbs can be weak and ataxic; hyporeflexia in forelimbs; hyperreflexia in hindlimbs; myotic pupils; Horner's syndrome; radial nerve paralysis
T2 to L3	T2 to L3—Schiff-Sherrington syndrome	"Dog sitting;" hopping; normal forelimbs; hyperreflexia of hindlimbs; polyuria; loss of cutaneous sensation in the area innervated
L4 to S2	L4 to S2—Lumbosacral plexus L4 to L5—Quadriceps L6 to L7—Cranial tibial L6 to S2—Gastrocnemius L6 to S2—Patellar L6 to S2—Flexor withdraw	Dog sitting; normal forelimbs; hyporeflexia in the hindlimbs; loss of cutaneous sensation
S1 to S3	S1 to S3—Pelvic plexus	Flaccid bladder; urine dribbling; no anal tone; tail will not lift or move

TABLE 11-6

SIGNS OF LESIONS IN THE BRAIN

LESION LOCATION	MENTAL STATUS	OCULAR	CONSCIOUS PROPRIOCEPTION	GAIT	POSTURE
Cortical	Depression, abnormal behavior, seizures	Normal vision	Deficits	Ataxia, stumbling knuckling over	
Cerebrocortical				No gait abnormality if in a straight line	
Frontal lobe		Normal palpebral response			
Diencephalon				Normal, but hemiparesis and tetraparesis can occur	Normal
Thalamus Lateral geniculate		Ocular deviation toward the lesion			
Limbic	Behavioral changes				
Reticular activating	Depression, coma, convulsions				
Ventral hypothalamus	Abnormal appetite				
Mesencephalon	Depression, coma	Mydriasis, dorsomedial strabismus	Deficits	Spasticity	Delayed return to normal
Metencephalon (pons, cerebellar peduncles)	Depression, coma	Corneal reflexes present	Deficits	Ataxia; hemiparesis and tetraparesis can occur	Decerebrate rigidity
Myelencephalon (medulla oblongata, lower brainstem)	Severe depression and coma	Medial strabismus, inability to retract the eye	Deficits	Ataxia, hemiparesis (ipsilateral), tetraparesis	Deficits ipsilateral to the lesion
Cerebellum	Normal		Normal	Truncal ataxia	Intention tremors
Rostral cerebellar (vermis, cerebellar cortex)				Opisthotonos	

POSTURAL REACTION	CRANIAL NERVES	SPINAL REFLEXES	MUSCLE TONE	ADDITIONAL
Deficits (contralateral)				
				Problems with complicated movements
				Poor response to stimulation
Deficits (contralateral)	Optic nerve loss of vision, loss of menace response, normal pupillary light reflex			Unilateral lesion contralateral signs
				Head tilt
				Polyuria and polydipsia, bradycardia
Deficits (contralateral)	Trochlear, oculomotor	Spasticity, hyperreflexia	Clonus, hypertonia	Unilateral lesion, contralateral signs, crossed extensor reflex present
Deficits (ipsilateral or contralateral)	Trigeminal	Hyperreflexia	Hypertonia, muscle atrophy of the masseter, tongue may protrude	Depressed sensorium, head tilt away from lesion, salivation
Deficits (ipsilateral or contralateral), poor righting response if the lesion side is up	Abducent, ambigmus, contralateral), poor vestibular, accessory, glossopharyngeal	Hyperreflexia facial, vagus,		Unilateral lesion, ipsilateral signs
Normal to dysmetria		Hyperreflexia	Hypertonia, especially of the extensor muscles	Uncoordinated movements

UMN or LMN origin and pinpointing the likely location of the lesion.

Peripheral Neuropathies

Peripheral neuropathies can be classified according to their cause, which may be congenital, inflammatory, metabolic, toxic, idiopathic, traumatic, degenerative, vascular, or neoplastic. The clinical findings in neuropathy vary according to the dysfunction of the structures innervated by the afferent and efferent nerve fibers affected.[1] Clinical signs include muscle atrophy, hypotonia or atonia, hyporeflexia or areflexia, and decreases in sensory innervation to the affected area. The peripheral neuropathies may involve a single nerve (mononeuropathy) or several nerves (polyneuropathy). Histologically the primary pathology that is observed is axonal degeneration or demyelination.[1] Diagnosis of affected animals is based on neurologic examination findings, age, breed, and EMG studies. Several peripheral neuropathies have been documented in sheep and goats and are reviewed in the following paragraphs.

Horner's syndrome is a combination of clinical signs seen in animals that have lesions in the gray matter of the thoracic spinal cord cranial to T3. Lesions in this area injure the sympathetic nerve fibers that form the sympathetic trunk.[4] The clinical signs include miosis, enophthalmos, ptosis, and increased warmth on the affected side of the face. Enophthalmos and extrusion of the third eyelid results from paralysis of the periorbital smooth muscle that helps maintain the eye in its normal position. Myosis is a result of the loss of sympathetic innervation to the ciliary muscles that dilate the pupil. Horner's syndrome is often associated with dramatic injuries to the brachial plexus, so in addition to the ocular abnormalities, paresis of the forelimb and loss of the cutaneous trunci reflex also may occur. Compressive lesions such as those resulting from caseous lymphadenitis abscesses, esophageal perforations, and otitis interna or otitis media also can damage T1 to T3.

Radial nerve paralysis can result from rib or humerus fractures or brachial plexus avulsion. The location of the injury determines the severity of clinical signs. In general the more distal the injury on the limb, the less the animal's gait is affected. Often affected animals extend their elbows but knuckle over onto the dorsum of their hooves because of paralysis of the extensor muscles of the carpus and digits. A loss of sensory innervation to the dorsum of the leg below the elbow also may be evident. The animals may have scuffed or abnormally shaped hooves as well as abrasions on the front of the fetlocks.

Femoral nerve paralysis results in an animal dragging or carrying its rear limb and hopping on the unaffected hindlimb. The femoral nerve arises from L4 to L6 and supplies motor pathways to the major extensor muscles in the hindlimb that are responsible for weight bearing. Sensation in the medial skin surfaces is preserved through the saphenous branch of the femoral nerve. Injury to this nerve often results from extreme rear-leg extension or injection sites that have become infected.

Obturator nerve paralysis occurs as a result of extreme adduction of the rear limb or as a lambing or kidding injury. When the nerve is damaged, the animal is unable to adduct its rear limb, and as a result the limb may slide laterally on slippery surfaces. Unilateral involvement of the obturator nerve causes fewer gait abnormalities than bilateral involvement. The examiner should take radiographs of the pelvis of any animal with these clinical signs to rule out pelvic fracture.

Sciatic nerve paralysis most commonly occurs as a sequel to a pelvic or lumbosacral fracture. The nerve arises from L6 to S2 and travels in the vertebral canal after the spinal cord has ended but before its fibers exit the canal. Branches of the nerve supply the muscles responsible for extending the hip and flexing the stifle. At the level of the hip the nerve divides into two branches—the peroneal and tibial nerves—that are responsible for innervating the majority of the motor and sensory functions of the lower limb. Lumbosacral fractures usually cause bilateral hindlimb paresis or paralysis. After damage to the proximal sciatic nerve, which can be caused by proximal acetabular and femur fractures, only the extensor muscles of the stifle remain functional, allowing the animal to bear weight but not flex the stifle. The animal will exhibit a dropped hock and the limb will be knuckled over. The animal's flexor response is greatly inhibited. If the medial claw is pinched, the animal flexes its hip but cannot flex the rest of the limb. This occurs because the medial side of the limb still has sensory innervation intact through the saphenous branch of the femoral nerve. Many of these injuries resolve if given time, but a poor prognosis is associated with the complete loss of deep pain.

The peroneal nerve supplies the muscles that flex the hock and extend the claws and provides cutaneous sensory innervation to the dorsal aspect of the foot and cranial surface of the hock and tibia.[4] Improperly administered injections often injure this nerve, resulting in knuckling over onto the dorsum of the fetlock and overextension of the hock. Animals appear to be able to compensate fairly well with this type of injury, flexing the hip and extending the stifle more to walk. The flexor response is depressed when the dorsum of the fetlock is stimulated; however, if the sole of the hoof is stimulated the animal flexes its leg but keeps the hock fixed.

References

1. Oliver JE, Mayhew IG: Neurologic examination and diagnostic plan. In Oliver JE et al, editors: *Veterinary neurology*, Philadelphia, 1987, WB Saunders.

2. Bagley R, Mayhew I: Clinical examination of the nervous system. In Radostits OM et al, editors: *Veterinary clinical examination and diagnosis*, Philadelphia, 2000, WB Saunders.

3. Tyler JW: Practical food animal neurology: the black box approach, *Proceedings of the American College of Veterinary Internal Medicine Eighteenth Annual Meeting*, 2000, Seattle, WA.

4. Oliver JE, Lorenz MD: Neurologic history and examination. In Oliver JE et al, editors: *Handbook of veterinary neurology*, Philadelphia, 1993, WB Saunders.

5. Oliver JE: Neurologic examinations: taking the history, *Vet Med Small Anim Clin* 67:433, 1972.

6. Chrisman CL: *Problems in small animal neurology*, Philadelphia, 1982, Lea & Febiger.

7. Jenkins TW: *Functional mammalian neuroanatomy*, ed 2, Philadelphia, 1978, Lea & Febiger.

8. Brewer BD: Examination of the bovine nervous system, *Vet Clin North Am Food Anim Pract* 3(1):13, 1987.

9. George LW: Localization and differentiation of neurologic disease. In Smith BP et al, editors: *Large animal internal medicine*, St Louis, 1996, Mosby.

10. de Lahunta A: Small animal neurology examination, *Proceedings of the American College of Veterinary Internal Medicine Eighteenth Annual Meeting*, 2000, Seattle, WA.

11. Liebman M: Cranial nerves. In Liebman M, editor: *Neuroanatomy made easy and understandable*, Gaithersburg, MD, 1983, Aspen.

12. de Lahunta A: Cranial nerve-lower motor neuron: general somatic efferent system, special visceral efferent system. In de Lahunta A, editor: *Veterinary neuroanatomy and clinical neurology*, Philadelphia, 1983, WB Saunders.

ANCILLARY TESTS

A number of diagnostic tests are available to help determine the cause of a neuropathic condition and localize the lesion. Most of these procedures are cost-prohibitive for small ruminant medicine and may not be widely available; however, their use can be considered when appropriate. After a lesion has been localized, plain survey films may be helpful to identify luxations of the vertebral column, osteomyelitis, or fractures of the pelvis. Survey radiographs of the skull can be used to diagnose fractures or assess involvement of the tympanic bulla in cases of otitis. Radiographic techniques used in medium to large dogs are applicable to sheep and goats. For UMN disease of the forebrain, brainstem, or cerebellum, several diagnostic imaging procedures can be performed. The structural integrity of the UMN anatomy can be evaluated through the use of computed tomography (CT) and magnetic resonance imagery (MRI) (see Chapter 7). Myelography can be used to identify compressive or expansive lesions in the spinal cord. Electromyography also can be used to determine whether specific neurons are responsible for neuromuscular disease by measuring the electrical activity of the muscle after a neuron is stimulated. Electroencephalography can be used to assess the electrical activity present in various parts of the brain. It is primarily used in cases that are manifested by seizures, narcolepsy, and encephalopathy.

Cerebrospinal fluid (CSF) can be easily collected from the lumbosacral site. The animal can be manually restrained in sternal recumbency or mildly sedated. The lumbosacral space at the cranial aspect of the tuber sacrale should be clipped and aseptically prepared. A palpable divot should be felt at this space and 2% lidocaine (0.5 ml) should be used to subcutaneously infiltrate this site. A 5-cm, 20-gauge stylet-type spinal needle or disposable needle is then slowly introduced at a slight caudal angle to enter the subarachnoid space. If bone is encountered, the needle should be redirected either cranially or caudally. A "pop" can be heard or felt as the needle passes through both the interarcuate ligament and the subarachnoid membrane. The examiner should frequently remove the stylet and check for CSF because subtle changes are often difficult to appreciate and the examiner may miss the subarachnoid space and advance the needle too far. Approximately 1 ml of CSF per 10 lb of body weight may be safely removed. Gently and slowly aspirating CSF or allowing it to flow freely from the needle prevents excessive movement and blood contamination. In addition, applying digital pressure over both jugular veins causes engorgement of the ventral venous plexus, resulting in increased CSF pressure and greater flow (see Appendix III).

NEUROLOGIC DISEASES

Scrapie

An important member of the slow infectious group of diseases known as *transmissible spongiform encephalopathies* in sheep and goats is scrapie. Scrapie is an afebrile, chronic, progressive, degenerative disorder of the central nervous system of sheep and occasionally goats.[1,2,3] The causative agent is poorly characterized, and several hypotheses attempt to link the concept of genetic susceptibility and an infectious agent. Three theories have been put forth regarding the nature of the infectious agent that causes scrapie:

1. The agent is a filamentous virus.
2. The agent is a self-replicating protein (prion).
3. The agent is a very small nucleic acid with a protective protein coat encoded in the host DNA.

The discovery of a glycoprotein termed *PrP^c* on the neuronal surface of normal sheep that also has been identified within the neurons of scrapie-affected sheep (PrP^{sc}) has led to the most recently accepted hypothesis regarding the infectious nature of scrapie. The PrP^{sc} protein is a rod-shaped protein that has in the past been referred to as a *scrapie-associated fibril (SAF)*; its identification has been correlated 100% with scrapie infections in sheep.[3] The PrP^{sc} proteins are unique because they are not autolyzed and can be readily recovered in fresh-frozen or formaldehyde-fixed tissues.

Pathogenesis. Sheep and goats to a lesser degree are the natural hosts for scrapie. The transmission has been documented to occur both horizontally and vertically. The majority of sheep with clinical signs of scrapie are 3½ years of age.[4] Although the offspring of infected ewes and rams are objectively more susceptible to scrapie infection, the exact mechanism of transmission is unknown. The general belief is that most sheep are infected at birth, and therefore the age of clinical presentation is a reflection of the incubation period.[2] The primary mode of transmission is believed to be oral. These observations indicate that an infectious agent is responsible for the transmission of the disease and that transmission occurs after birth, not in utero.[5,6] After the causative agent enters the host it goes into a quiescent phase in which no virus can be detected in tissues for as long as 8 months or more. The replication of the infectious agent takes place in the lymphoreticular system during this time and can last for 2 to 5 years. The end of the incubation period is marked by the presence of detectable virus in the nervous system and by the conversion of the PrP^c protein to PrP^{sc} protein. Researchers have not yet determined how the wild form of the protein is converted to the mutant form. Experiments have demonstrated that the PrP^{sc} protein content in neuronal cells can increase without the synthesis of new protein.[4] Moreover, PrP^{sc} may act as an infectious agent and catalyze the conversion of PrP^c in uninfected cells. The PrP^{sc} protein itself is believed to be toxic to cells, and as it accumulates within the cells it causes the neurodegenerative lesions histologically observed in scrapie-affected sheep.[1,7,8]

Host genetic factors and the strain of the infectious agent are important in determining susceptibility to the development of natural scrapie infections. Currently several genetic variants have been identified in sheep breeds that predispose to scrapie. Studies have confirmed that eight polymorphisms result in six amino acid variations at three different codon positions in the sheep genome: 136, 154, and 171.[4] Two of these positions, 136 and 171, are associated with increased susceptibility to scrapie and a decrease in survival time. Certain breeds of sheep are more inclined to have a particular genetic composition at these two new positions and therefore appear to be more susceptible to scrapie.[4] Not all breeds of sheep have the same genotype at the three different codon positions, and certain genotypes appear to be more prevalent among specific breeds.[9] Scrapie occurs primarily in Suffolk, Cheviot, Southdown, and Hampshire breeds. Suffolk sheep that have the genetic composition of A_{136}, R_{154}, Q_{171} are more susceptible to developing scrapie. All breeds of sheep appear to be more susceptible to scrapie if they have a genotype encoding QQ_{171}.[4] The valine breeds (particularly Cheviot, Swaledale, and Shetlands) have the amino acid valine at position 136, which confers susceptibility.[1,9,10] However, these breeds also must have the haplotype of valine, glutamine, and arginine (VQR) to develop clinical scrapie.

The amino acid variations that occur in sheep at these three positions influence the incubation period. The strain of scrapie infecting the animal and the specific position it targets influence the rate of conversion or resistance to conversion of PrP^c to PrP^{sc}.

Clinical signs. In the United States, scrapie is diagnosed most commonly in Suffolk sheep. Most of the clinical signs indicate the locations that are damaged in the central nervous system. The onset of disease is marked by subtle changes in behavior such as mild apprehension, staring or fixed gaze, failure to respond to herding, and aggressiveness towards objects and people[2] (Figure 11-3).

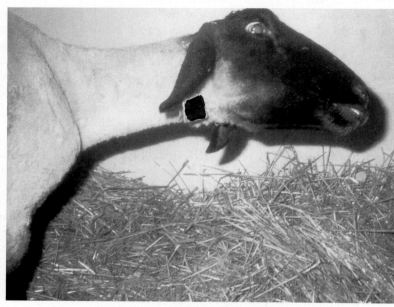

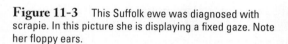

Figure 11-3 This Suffolk ewe was diagnosed with scrapie. In this picture she is displaying a fixed gaze. Note her floppy ears.

Several months later the animals often become intolerant to exercise and develop a clumsy, unsteady gait and floppy ears. The fleece may develop whitish tips over the lumbar region. Some affected sheep have intense pruritus that causes them to self-mutilate by rubbing immobile objects.[2] Wool loss is most prevalent around the base of the tail, the sides of the body, and above the elbow and lateral neck (Figure 11-4). When affected sheep have their lumbar regions rubbed, they often compulsively nibble their legs below the carpus and hock and may extend their heads and slap their lips together. Fine body and head tremors, wide-based stance, and severe progressive ataxia and paresis of the limbs may be present. If these animals are encouraged to run they will high-step with their forelimbs and bunny-hop with their hindlimbs. During the ensuing 3 to 4 months the animals lose weight and become extremely difficult to handle. In the terminal stages sheep are recumbent and have hypertonic limbs. They may develop blindness, seizures, and an inability to swallow just before death.

Goats may exhibit signs similar to those seen in sheep. They can develop the disease without direct contact with sheep. The hallmarks of scrapie in both species are intense pruritus, ataxia, and wasting.

Diagnosis. No specific lesions are characteristic of scrapie. No detectable host humoral or cellular immune responses are evoked by the scrapie organism because it contains no antigens that are recognized by the host. Histologically the only consistent lesions are degenerative changes in the central nervous system consisting of bilaterally symmetric vacuolation of the neurons in the brainstem and spinal cord. Astrocyte proliferation precedes the vacuolization of neurons, and demyelination does not occur.[11] Most of these changes occur in the gray matter of the medulla, pons, midbrain, and thalamus.[3] These histopathologic changes are not pathognomonic because other diseases can cause the same types of pathologic changes.

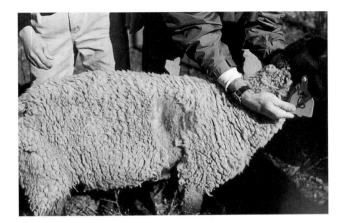

Figure 11-4 This 3-year-old Suffolk ewe displayed pruritus and wool loss on her mid-thorax, at the level of her elbow.

Immunohistochemical (IHC) staining and microscopic examination of brain tissue currently is considered the standard for clinical diagnosis of scrapie in sheep. This postmortem test is highly specific and sensitive. Recently a technique has been developed to examine IHC-stained lymphoid tissue from the nictitating membrane as an antemortem test. This test may aid in diagnosing animals in the quiescent phase, during which the protein is replicating in the lymphoreticular system. A live assay also is available. It involves injecting mice with suspension brain tissue from suspected sheep to observe whether they develop clinical disease.

Attempts have been made to adapt a human assay used to detect a specific protein that increases in concentration in the CSF in patients that have spongiform encephalopathies. If it is approved, this test could be performed as an antemortem diagnostic tool in sheep demonstrating clinical neurologic signs. The sensitivity and specificity of the immunoassay in sheep has yet to be determined.

Treatment. No effective treatment is available for scrapie, and the condition is considered fatal. It also is a reportable disease that results in depopulation of affected flocks.

Prevention. Scrapie costs the United States sheep industry $20 million annually in direct losses and millions more in lost potential markets and flock productivity. A number of control programs have been instituted since scrapie was first recognized as a problem in 1952. To date all of these programs have fallen short of their goal of eliminating scrapie from the sheep industry because of the economic constraints that culling and depopulating impose and the lack of a reliable antemortem diagnostic test. One federal program that sheep producers can voluntarily participate in is called the *Scrapie Flock Certification Program.* It requires flocks to be assessed for 5 years to determine that they do not contain any scrapie-infected sheep. This program has four levels of clearance and when the final level is attained, the producers are able to export and sell sheep both within the United States and internationally without restrictions.[12] Currently the United States is reviewing the federal Scrapie Flock Certification Program to ensure that it is consistent with advances in diagnostic techniques.

Some individual states and European countries are developing programs to classify herds according to genetic susceptibility and flock health history. Although these classifications are not based on the detection of scrapie-infected animals, their purpose is to eliminate susceptible animals within a breed to eradicate the disease.[13]

The zoonotic potential of scrapie to humans is unknown. Evidence indicates that some variants of Creutzfeldt-Jakob disease are caused by ingestion of bovine products contaminated with scrapie or scrapie-like organisms.

References

1. Hunter N: Scrapie, *Mol Biotech* 9:225, 1998.
2. Linnabary RD et al: Scrapie in sheep, *Comp Cont Ed Pract Vet* 13:511, 1991.
3. Detwiler LA: Scrapie, *Rev Sci Tech Off Int Epiz* 11:491, 1992.
4. Machen MR: Scrapie: deciphering its pathophysiology and cause, *Comp Cont Ed Pract Vet*, 23:S52, 2001.
5. Woolhouse MEJ et al: Epidemiology and control of scrapie within a sheep flock, *Proc R Soc London B* 265:1205, 1998.
6. Hoinville LJ: A review of the epidemiology of scrapie in sheep, *Rev Sci Tech Off Int Epiz* 15:827, 1996.
7. Chaplin MJ, Aldrich AD, Stack MJ: Scrapie associated fibril detection from formaldehyde fixed brain tissue in natural cases of ovine scrapie, *Res Vet Sci* 64:41, 1998.
8. Stack MJ et al: The distribution of scrapie-associated fibrils in neural and non-neural tissues of advanced clinical cases of natural scrapie in sheep, *Res Vet Sci* 64:141, 1998.
9. Hunter N: PrP genetics in sheep and the implications for scrapie and BSE, *Trends Microbiol* 5:331, 1997.
10. Bossers A et al: Scrapie susceptibility-linked polymorphisms modulate the in vitro conversion of sheep prion protein to protease-resistant forms, *Proc Natl Acad Sci USA* 94:4931, 1997.
11. Dandoy-Dron F et al: Gene expression in scrapie, *J Biol Chem* 273:7691, 1998.
12. Detwiler LA: Scrapie control in the United States: a review of the past with emphasis on the present flock certification program, *Dev Biol Stan* 80:109, 1993.
13. Dawson M et al: Guidance on the use of PrP genotype as an aid to the control of clinical scrapie, *Vet Rec* 142:623, 1998.

Caprine Arthritis-Encephalitis

Caprine arthritis-encephalitis (CAE) is a retroviral infection of goats that is similar to ovine progressive pneumonia in sheep. The disease takes several forms—neurologic, arthritic, and mastitic (hard udder). It is primarily transmitted from dam to kid through colostrum.

Clinical signs. The neurologic form of the disease usually affects kids 1 to 4 months of age but is occasionally seen in adults. The clinical signs include a secondary ataxia and paresis progressing to tetraplegia. As the disease progresses, kids may become blind and develop a head tilt, facial paralysis, and opisthotonos. The clinical course of disease can last from 1 to 2 weeks.[1,2]

Diagnosis. The antemortem diagnosis of CAE is based on agar gel immunodiffusion (AGID) for CAE antibodies. CSF has an elevated protein content and mononuclear pleocytosis. Postmortem examination reveals widespread perivascular foci and demyelination of the white matter of the brain and spinal cord.

Prevention. No treatment is available. To prevent this disease, kids should not be fed colostrum from infected dams. This can be aided by inducing parturition of the dam or performing a Cesarean section and removing the kids before the ingestion of colostrum. If colostrum from an unknown or infected source is all that is available, it can be heated (56° C for 1 hour).[1,2] Infected animals should be culled or quarantined from the flock. CAE can be spread by fomites such as needles; they should be used only once and then discarded. Proper sterilization of surgical equipment also is warranted (see Chapters 9, 13, and 14).

References

1. Dawson M: Caprine arthritis-encephalitis. In Boden E, editor: *Sheep and goat practice*, London, 1991, Bailliere Tindall.
2. Pringle J: Neurologic disorders. In Ogilvie TH, editor: *Large animal internal medicine*, Baltimore, 1998, Williams & Wilkins.

Rabies

Rabies is a fatal disease of animals and humans. Rabies virus belongs to the genus *Lyssavirus* from the family *Rhabdoviridae*. Outbreaks in domestic animals appear to be associated with a "spillover" from epizootic spread in affected wildlife populations.[1,2] These wild reservoir hosts include the skunk (Midwest to North Central United States), raccoon (Southeastern and East Coasts), coyote (South Texas), and gray fox (Southern Arizona, mid-Texas). Of these wild species, foxes and coyotes seem to be the most susceptible to rabies, with skunks, raccoons, bats, and bobcats showing an intermediate susceptibility. Opossums and armadillos appear fairly resistant to infection. In areas where foxes and/or skunks are the predominant wildlife reservoir hosts, the disease usually has a seasonal incidence. An increased incidence has been associated with the migratory patterns of the reservoir host and changes in population densities. The susceptibility of the sheep or goat to rabies increases in proportion to the quantity of inoculum (usually saliva from a bite) placed into a wound, the number of nerves in the area around the wound (rabies virus migrates along nerves), the vaccination history of the bitten animal, and the location of the wound. The closer the wound is to the central nervous system, the more susceptible to infection the animal becomes. The virus spreads along the peripheral nerves from the site of the wound to the central nervous system and then systematically, including the salivary glands. The incubation period is from 2 weeks to several months. Shorter incubation periods are associated with bites near the central nervous system (head or neck).[2] In the United States between 5 and 20 cases of rabies are reported annually in sheep and goats.

Clinical signs. Sheep and goats can have a variety of clinical signs, including depression or excitation, anorexia, nystagmus, and muscle spasms. Rams may exhibit sexual excitement. Goats or sheep also can become aggressive and attack objects and handlers.[3] The course of disease usually progresses as an ascending paralysis that initially may appear as a proprioceptive deficit (rear-end paralysis, knuckling), ataxia, and tail and penile paralysis. Pharyngeal paralysis results in excessive salivation.[1-3] The disease progresses to recumbency, convulsions, and death over a 7- to 10-day period.

Diagnosis. Rabies should be part of the rule-out list in all neurologic cases. Whenever it is suspected because of clinical signs, history, or animal death, regulatory authorities should be notified and the brain and salivary glands of the animal submitted for laboratory testing. In cases of suspected rabies, collection of CSF should be avoided because of the zoonotic potential of this disease. If CSF is nevertheless collected, it will have an increase in total protein, mononuclear cells, and neutrophils. Tissues shipped to a diagnostic laboratory should be cooled but not frozen. The disease produces a nonsuppurative encephalitis. If formalin-fixed tissues are to be evaluated, no more than half the brain should be fixed. A confirmed diagnosis can be made by fluorescent antibody (FA) tests of impression smears of the hippocampus, cerebellum, medulla, or salivary glands.

Prevention. Several killed vaccines are available and approved in the United States for use in sheep. Although they are not specifically approved for goats, they appear to be efficacious.[3] In endemic regions, vaccination should begin at 3 months of age and be followed by an annual booster.[2] However, vaccination may not be cost effective in many instances.[3] Post-exposure vaccination protocols appear less useful in sheep than in other species. If permitted, exposed animals should be quarantined for 6 months and vaccinated immediately with a second, and possibly third booster at 2, 4, and 6 weeks after exposure. Because of the zoonotic potential of this disease, clinicians should use extreme caution when handling suspected animals and tissues.

REFERENCES

1. Pringle J: Neurologic disorders. In Ogilvie TH, editor: *Large animal internal medicine,* Baltimore, 1998, Williams & Wilkins.
2. George LW: Rabies. In Smith BP, editor: *Large animal internal medicine,* ed 2, St Louis, 1996, Mosby.
3. Biggs DJ: Rabies in food animals. In Howard JL, Smith RA, editors: *Current veterinary therapy 4, food animal practice,* Philadelphia, 1999, WB Saunders.

Pseudorabies

Pseudorabies is rarely documented in sheep and goats and infected swine are the most common reservoirs of infection. This herpes virus infects sheep or goats through the respiratory tract or open wounds. After the virus has gained entrance, it invades the central nervous system.[1,2] Pseudorabies also can be transmitted to sheep by syringes previously used to vaccinate hogs with modified live pseudorabies virus.[3]

Clinical signs. Infected sheep or goats have extreme pruritus in localized areas.[1] They may vocalize, circle, and self-mutilate by licking and scratching the skin (hence the name *mad itch*). Additional clinical signs include ataxia, paralysis, and death within 72 hours of the onset of signs.[2]

Diagnosis. Grossly, a meningoencephalitis is seen at necropsy.[1] Histologically perivascular cuffing and focal necrosis of the gray matter occurs, along with eosinophilic intranuclear inclusion bodies of the dorsal horn and dorsal nerve rootlets.[1,2] The diagnosis can be confirmed with virus isolation.

Treatment and prevention. No treatment exists. Contact with infected animals should be prevented. Barns and paddocks where infected animals are housed should be thoroughly sanitized (with quaternary ammonium or compounds containing phenol).[4]

REFERENCES

1. Pringle J: Neurologic disorders. In Ogilvie TH, editor: *Large animal internal medicine,* Baltimore, 1998, Williams & Wilkins.
2. George LW: Pseudorabies. In Smith BP, editor: *Large animal internal medicine,* ed 2, St Louis, 1996, Mosby.
3. Van Alstine WG, Andersen TD, Reed DE: Vaccine induced pseudorabies in lambs, *J Am Vet Med Assoc* 185:409, 1984.
4. Brown TT: Laboratory evaluation of selected disinfectants as virucidal agents against porcine parvovirus, pseudorabies virus, transmissible gastroenteritis virus, *Am J Vet Res* 42:1033, 1981.

Bacterial Meningitis

Suppurative meningitis or neuritis can occur as a sequela to surgical procedures (dehorning, tail docking), failure of passive transfer (septicemia), pneumonia, gastroenteritis, omphalophlebitis, otitis, and mastitis.[1-3] *Escherichia coli, Streptococcus,* and *Pasteurella haemolytica* are common bacterial causes of meningitis in neonates. *Pseudomonas aeruginosa* can cause meningitis in some adult goats secondary to mastitis. *Mycoplasma mycoides* subsp. *mycoides* can cause disease in goat kids that ingest milk or colostrum from infected dams.[3]

Clinical signs. Meningitis associated with tail docking can be a progressive ascending paralysis.[1] Cases of meningitis resulting from neonatal septicemia can present with diarrhea, fever, stiff neck, nystagmus, convulsions, depression, and death.[1,3] Many affected animals resist or display signs of pain on manipulation of the neck.[3]

Diagnosis. A tentative diagnosis can be based on clinical signs and history. Analysis of the CSF shows a turbid, possibly clotted sample with increased leucocytes and protein. Sometimes bacteria can be identified in Gram's-stained CSF.[3] Gross examination of the carcass at necropsy reveals congested meningeal vessels, swollen meninges, and petechiation.[3]

Treatment. Treatment should be based on culture and sensitivity patterns, antibiotic patterns, or Gram's stain findings of the CSF.[3] However, in most situations laboratory results are not available when therapy is initiated. A cephalosporin (ceftiofur 4 to 5 mg/kg intravenously [IV] four times a day [QID]) can provide excellent antimicrobial therapy.[2,3] Concurrently, glucocorticosteroids (dexamethasone 1 mg/kg IV) and/or dimethyl sulfoxide (DMSO, 1 mg/kg in a 5% solution IV) can be administered to help reduce inflammation.[2,3] Diazepam should be considered if the animal is convulsing, at a dosage of 0.01 to 0.4 mg/kg.[3] Aggressive therapy for 10 to 14 days may yield satisfactory results if therapy is initiated early in the course of the disease. As inflammation of the meninges subsides, some antibiotics (aminoglycosides) may have difficulty reaching therapeutic concentrations in the meningeal space.[3] This can result in relapse, localized infection, or abscess formation. In cases of failure of passive transfer, plasma (intraperitoneal [IP] or IV) should be given.

Prevention. Prevention is best achieved by ensuring ingestion of adequate colostral antibodies; avoiding excessive damage to tissues during tail docking, dehorning, or disbudding; using sterile equipment; and employing aseptic technique.

References

1. Smith MC: Inflammatory neurologic diseases of small ruminants. In Smith RA, editor: *Current veterinary therapy 3, food animal practice,* Philadelphia, 1993, WB Saunders.
2. Divers TJ: Diseases of the nervous system. In Howard JL, Smith RA, editors: *Current veterinary therapy 4, food animal practice,* Philadelphia, 1999, WB Saunders.
3. George LW: Meningitis (suppurative meningitis). In Smith BP, editor: *Large animal internal medicine,* ed 2, St Louis, 1996, Mosby.

Listeriosis

Listeriosis is a disease caused by the bacterium *Listeria monocytogenes*. The most common form of the disease in ruminants is a focal encephalitis; however, septicemia, abortion, and visceral infection also may occur. The organism survives for long periods in a wide variety of environmental conditions and latently in carrier animals. It is shed in feces, milk, tears, and uterine fluid of sick as well as apparently healthy goats. *L. monocytogenes* is a small, motile, aerobic and facultative anaerobic gram-positive rod. It has 16 serotypes, of which each has a variety of subtypes.[1-3] It is widely distributed in nature and can survive for years in soil, feces, and vegetation over a broad range of temperatures and pH. Although listeriosis is commonly associated with silage feeding, it also can occur in animals on pasture. *L. monocytogenes* is resistant to freezing conditions but cannot survive if the environmental pH is less than 5 (e.g., in properly packed silage). Rotting forage, spoiled silage, silage at the end of trench silos, and the bottoms of round bales of hay are all sources of infection.

Small ruminants are apparently more susceptible to listeriosis than cattle, and goats are reportedly more susceptible than sheep. The disease is more common in winter but may be seen throughout the year. Listeriosis is most commonly observed in animals grazing or browsing in areas with boggy soils.

The organism is thought to invade the host through breaks in the buccal membrane and ascend the trigeminal nerve roots. This form is most common in adults fed contaminated silage. The breaks in the mucosa associated with shedding and replacing incisor are associated with infection of the cranial nerves.[3] Therefore the condition is most common in animals older than 6 months. Stress; the introduction of hard feeds, pellets, or browse in the diet; and concurrent damage to the oral cavity can predispose to listeriosis.[4] Clinical signs may vary according to the location of multifocal microabscesses throughout the braistem. Unilateral deficits of CN V (dysphagia, pseudoptyalism, dropped jaw, facial anesthesia), CN VI (medial strabismus of the opposite eye), CN VII (lip or ear droop, ptosis, absent menace and palpebral reflexes, exposure keratitis), CN VIII (head tilt, circling, nystagmus), CN IX and CN X (pharyngeal paresis, dysphagia, upper respiratory obstruction, stertor), and CN XII (unilateral tongue paresis, dysphagia) are most common. Multiple nerves may be affected, but bilateral lesions are infrequent. The organism has zoonotic potential and can cause abortion and sepsis in people.[1-3]

Clinical signs. Sheep and goats with listeriosis exhibit depression from brainstem involvement or concurrent meningitis and encephalitis. Loss of the ability to eat and drink, dehydration, and acid-base disturbances may contribute to the degree of depression. Often animals with early cases of listeriosis exhibit only depression and a failure to eat; therefore the clinician must be able to recognize early neurologic deficits and have a degree of suspicion. Fever is an inconsistent finding and when present is often only seen during the first 3 or 4 days of illness. In sheep the morbidity is low, but mortality is high. When first examined by the clinician, many goats are recumbent and comatose, with a head tilt.[4] Corneal ulceration resulting from keratoconjunctivitis is a common finding in goats.

Specific neurologic signs are usually associated with pathology in CN V through CN XII. The bacteria ascend up the trigeminal nerve, causing weakness of the muscles of mastication (dropped jaw), inability to eat, and loss of saliva (Figure 11-5). Facial and vestibular lesions are common, as are lesions of the glossopharyngeal and vagus nerves, which result in dysphagia. Other neurologic deficits resulting from CN damage include a medial strabismus from paresis of CN VI and an inability to retract the tongue from changes to CN XII.

Diagnosis. No specific antemortem diagnosis for the encephalitic form of listeriosis is available. Diagnosis depends on an accurate neurologic examination and identification of multifocal brainstem disease. Supporting evidence can be obtained from analysis of CSF. The fluid may have an elevated protein (more than 40 mg/dl) and white blood cell (WBC) count (more than 5 cells/μl); the CSF white cell differential is often 50% or more mononuclear cells and the remainder neutrophils. However, these findings are not consistent. Culture on blood agar of the CSF is usually unrewarding because the organisms are not present in the CSF unless meningitis has developed. Culture of the blood and milk in cases of septicemia may identify systemically ill animals and persistent shedders. The organism can be isolated more efficiently by employing microaerophilic techniques. On postmortem examination, *L. monocytogenes* can be identified with an FA test. This test is the most specific for all nonsurviving cases.[1-4]

Treatment. *L. monocytogenes* is a facultative intracellular organism, and therefore intensive antibiotic treatment is necessary to reach minimal inhibitory concentrations in macrophages and to cross the blood-brain barrier. The organism is sensitive to a variety of antibiotics. However, because of cost and practicality, penicillin (22,000 to 44,000 units/kg IM BID), oxytetracycline (5 to 10 mg/kg IV twice a day [BID]), and florfenicol (20 mg/kg intramuscularly [IM] every 48 hours) are the most commonly used antibiotics. Therapy is recommended for a minimum of 10 to 14 days; if further antibiotic treatment is necessary, IM or subcutaneous medication can be administered. Antiinflammatory therapy is recommended as well (flunixin meglumine 1.0 mg/kg). If the patient is dehydrated or has electrolyte and acid-base disturbances, these should be addressed at the initiation of therapy. In cases of conjunctivitis or keratitis, broad-spectrum ophthalmic antibiotics (tetracycline) and ophthalmic atropine may be indicated. Orally administered fluids can be used to soften rumen contents and aid in rumen contraction. Feeding an alfalfa slurry or other nutritional supplement via oral gastric tube may be necessary.[3] Patients should be kept by themselves in a stall with thick bedding. Recumbent animals should be turned often, supported in sternal recumbency, and given adequate supportive care.[1-3]

Animals that are treated before becoming recumbent have a fair to good prognosis if appropriate antibiotic and supportive therapy are provided. Therapy appears to be less effective in sheep than in goats.[2]

Prevention. Most inactivated (heated or formol-treated) vaccines are of limited value. Good immunity, however, is reported in sheep with some attenuated vaccines.[1,5] All infected animals should be isolated, animals that die should be disposed of quickly, and all barns and contaminated equipment should be sanitized. Silage with a pH higher than 5.5 or with a foul odor should be discarded. In farms that have pastures with boggy, high-pH soils; in areas where rough browse is consumed; and in contaminated feedlots or paddocks, the continuous feeding of chlortetracycline (6 to 12 mg/kg by mouth [PO] daily) may be beneficial.[1] *L. monocytogenes* can be found in the feces of many healthy sheep. Therefore feeders should be designed to prevent animals from defecating in them, and fecal contamination of feed-handling equipment should be avoided.

Public health concerns. *L. monocytogenes* causes a variety of diseases in people, including bacterial meningitis. *Listeria* may be shed by sick, recovering, or clinically normal animals in milk and feces for prolonged periods. It has been reported to survive during low-temperature pasteurization in milk and in the milk products of goats. Veterinarians and handlers should use caution when handling the secretions of affected animals. Unpasteurized milk and milk products should not be consumed.

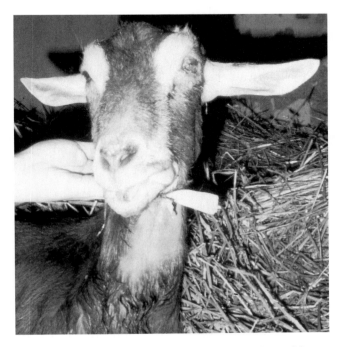

Figure 11-5 This goat has listeriosis. Its jaw has dropped, its tongue is not functioning, and it is exhibiting excessive salivation.

REFERENCES

1. Finley MR: Listeriosis (circling disease, silage sickness). In Howard JL, Smith RA, editors: *Current veterinary therapy 4, food animal practice,* Philadelphia, 1999, WB Saunders.
2. Dennis SM: Listeriosis (circling disease, silage sickness). In Smith RA, editor: *Current veterinary therapy 3, food animal practice,* Philadelphia, 1993, WB Saunders.
3. Smith MC: Inflammatory neurologic disease of small ruminants. In Smith RA, editor: *Current veterinary therapy 3, food animal practice,* Philadelphia, 1993, WB Saunders.
4. Bulgin MS: Central nervous system disorders of sheep, *Proceedings of the 1998 Symposium on the Health and Disease of Small Ruminants,* 1998, Las Vegas, NV.
5. Gudding R, Gronstal H, Larson HJ: Vaccination against listeriosis in sheep, *Vet Rec* 117:89, 1985.

Brain Abscesses

Brain abscesses result from seeding of the nervous tissue by pyogenic bacteria from septicemia. Bacteria can spread from localized infections (dehorning) and areas of existing disease (caseous lymphadenitis). Abscesses in the nervous system are commonly caused by *Actinomyces (Corynebacterium) pseudotuberculosis, A. pyogenes, Staphylococcus,* or aberrant migration of nasal bots *(Oestrus ovis).*[1-3]

Clinical signs. Clinical signs depend on the location and size of the lesion. Animals may be febrile with alterations in the heart and respiratory rates. Circling, depression, drooping ears, ataxia, and blindness also may be noted. Abscess ruptures result in acute death.[1]

Diagnosis. A presumptive diagnosis can be based on clinical signs. Analysis of CSF shows an increase in protein concentrations and the presence of inflammatory cells. A complete blood count may yield normal findings or leukocytosis. Definitive diagnosis is made by identifying the abscess in the brain.

Treatment. Affected animals have a grave prognosis. Antibiotics (penicillin 22,000 IU/kg IV or IM BID, oxytetracycline 10 mg/kg IV BID), nonsteroidal antiinflammatory drugs (NSAIDs, flunixin meglumine 1 to 2 mg/kg IM or IV), and glucocorticosteroids (dexamethasone 1 to 2 mg/kg) should be used.[4]

Prevention. The major differential diagnosis for brain abscess is listeriosis (Figure 11-6). Clinicians should identify the causative agent for the abscess and address any managerial considerations. In the rare event of an outbreak of affected animals, the inclusion of oral antimicrobial agents (chlortetracycline, tetracycline, sulfamethazine) in a complete feed, protein-energy supplement, or mineral mixture may help control the disease.

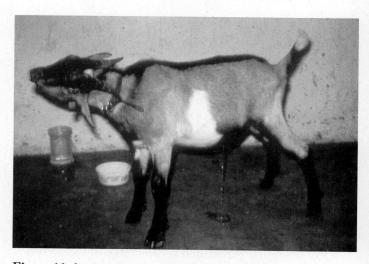

Figure 11-6 This goat has a brain abscess and is displaying a head tilt and a wide-based stance. This condition should be differentiated from listeriosis.

REFERENCES

1. Linkleter KA, Smith MC: *Color atlas of diseases and disorders of sheep and goats,* Aylesbury, UK, 1993, Wolfe Publishing.
2. Bulgin MS: Central nervous system disorders of sheep, *Proceedings of the 1998 Symposium on the Health and Disease of Small Ruminants,* 1998, Las Vegas, NV.
3. Pringle J: Neurologic disorders. In Ogilvie TH, editor: *Large animal internal medicine,* Baltimore, 1998, Williams & Wilkins.
4. Smith MC: Inflammatory neurologic disease of small ruminants. In Smith RA, editor: *Current veterinary therapy 3, food animal practice,* Philadelphia, 1993, WB Saunders.

Otitis Externa, Otitis Interna, and Otitis Media

Little is known about otitis in goats and sheep compared with the information available on cattle and horses. *Otitis* is defined as inflammation of the auditory structures and is divided into anatomic regions. Otitis externa involves the external auditory meatus, otitis media the tympanic bulla, and otitis interna the vestibulocochlear nerve, semilunar canals, utricle, saccule and cochlea.

Etiology

BACTERIA: Bacterial infections in the ear canal and external auditory canal have been reported as causes of injury or rupture of the tympanic membrane; they can result in otitis media and otitis interna. Several case reports in lambs indicate that otitis media and otitis interna may result from respiratory infections by bacterial migration via the auditory tubes. All ages and both sexes of sheep and goats can be affected, but young animals and those placed under great stress during processing are more susceptible.

The most common bacterial isolates identified in cases of otitis media in lambs with intact tympanic membranes are *P. haemolytica* and *P. multocida;* their isolation has coincided with the animals also having pneumonia caused by the same organisms.[1,2] A number of commensal bacterial organisms also have been isolated from sheep suffering from otitis media and otitis interna. These include *Neisseria catarrhalis;* coagulase-positive, hemolytic, and mixed hemolytic *Staphylococcus;* and hemolytic *Streptococcus.*[2] In cases in which the tympanic membrane of the animal has ruptured, a wide variety of bacteria may be involved. One case report from Britain cited consistent isolation of *Pseudomonas aeruginosa* from an outbreak of severe necrotic dermatitis and otitis media/otitis interna in a flock of sheep after dipping.[3]

PARASITES: Parasitic infestation of the external auditory meatus is common in goats and sheep. Infestation with ticks, biting flies, and gnats can cause inflammation and irritation to the external ear canal. Although the aforementioned are common etiologic agents in external ear canal pathology, mite infestation can cause more severe economic and pathologic complications.

Psoroptic mange mites are non-burrowing parasites that feed on the superficial skin of the host, causing inflammation at the site of infestation.[4] The mites have a 2-week life cycle on the host but can live off the host for as long as 3 weeks.[5] Mite infestation can occur in all ages and both sexes of animals. Horizontal transmission can occur rapidly in a herd, and animals can be affected unilaterally or bilaterally. Most affected animals go undetected unless they show severe clinical signs. The mites appear to congregate around the tympanic membrane, making diagnosis difficult. A variety of psoroptic mites affect sheep; their classifications are based on the sites occupied on the host and morphology.[4] *Psoroptes cuniculi* causes ear infestations in goats and rabbits; another variant, *P. ovis,* is capable of causing sheep scab in the ears and throughout the body.[4,6]

In goats two different mites have been identified as causative agents of otitis: *P. cuniculi* and *Raillietia manfredi.* Dual infestations have been found in affected herds, and the majority of the mites infest the base of the external ear canal around the tympanic membrane.[7] Although infestation with ear mites is common in goats, it rarely produces clinical signs, with the exception of head shaking and ear twitching.[8]

Sarcoptes scabiei is a contagious mite that initially manifests itself around the external ear canal. It can affect both sheep and goats but is difficult to diagnose, even though it causes severe pruritus. The mite has a 10- to 17-day life cycle; it burrows under the skin to deposit its eggs.[5] *Sarcoptes* mite infestations are reportable in the United States.

Otitis Externa

Pathogenesis.   Many factors can predispose sheep and goats to otitis externa. The first is the anatomic orientation of the ear canal itself. The vertical canal slopes medially into a horizontal orientation on the outside of the tympanic membrane. This prevents drainage of debris as it accumulates. The skin lining the external ear canal has a large number of glands; these include modified apocrine glands called the *ceruminous glands.*[9] These glands produce a large amount of secretions, setting up an environment that is favorable for irritation and infection. Pendulous-eared breeds of goats and sheep that have hair within the ear canal are predisposed to moisture collection within the canal. As the moisture content of the stratum corneum increases, its protective immunologic defenses are compromised.[10] Furthermore, a number of yeast and bacterial species commonly inhabit the ear canal and can become secondary opportunistic invaders when conditions are favorable. In addition to the commensal organisms in the canal, parasites and foreign objects can initiate an inflammatory condition.

Clinical signs.   The most common presenting complaint of sheep and goats with otitis externa is excessive head shaking, ear twitching, and scratching of the ears with the hindlimbs. Often the animals do not have any gross indications of parasite infestation or infected lesions.[8] The only abnormality that is consistently reported is excessive accumulation of earwax at the base of the ear canal that forms a cast.[4,8,11] When animals develop gross clinical lesions they initially appear as small sores and dry, flaky scabs in the external auditory meatus. Ear mite infestation in sheep or goats rarely leads to rupture of the tympanic membrane and consequent otitis media or otitis interna.

More chronically affected animals may display gross distortion of the pinnae caused by excessive rubbing; this may cause the pinnae to appear crumpled. The epidermis of the pinnae and external auditory meatus also is grossly thickened, and histologic examination of the tissues reveals hyperparakeratosis, acanthosis, and infiltration of the dermis with neutrophils, plasma cells, lymphocytes, and histiocytes.[7] Numerous small abscesses resulting from infection by secondary opportunistic bacterial invaders may be evident.

Otitis Media and Otitis Interna

Pathogenesis.   Otitis media and otitis interna can result from bacterial, viral, or fungal infection; parasitic infestation; tumors; vascular lesions; and immune disorders.[12] Otitis media occurs when the inner ear canal medial to the tympanic membrane becomes involved in an infectious process. Otitis interna is the result of involvement of the vestibulocochlear nerve and usually is accompanied by peripheral vestibular clinical signs such as a head tilt and ipsilateral facial nerve paralysis. Infectious agents can follow three routes of entry to cause inner ear pathology. The first is hematogenous, in which the tympanic membrane remains intact. Affected animals exhibit a systemic disease process that has its nidus elsewhere. The second is colonization of the middle ear by bacteria in the pharynx through the pharyngeal ostia of the auditory tubes.[1] This is believed to be the primary route of infection in sheep that have respiratory infections. The most common bacterial isolates from otitis media and interna in sheep are *P. haemolytica, P. multocida, Pseudomonas aeruginosa*, coagulase-positive hemolytic and mixed hemolytic *Staphylococcus*, and hemolytic *Streptococcus*.[1,2] In most case studies the tympanic membrane appeared intact and showed no evidence of exudate in the external ear canal. These findings are similar to those seen in otitis in horses, but are unlike the findings in cattle, in which the membrane is usually ruptured.[12,13] Two defined stages of infection for otitis media have been documented grossly and histopathologically. In the acute stage a small amount of yellow-tinged fluid can be visualized in the tympanic bulla, and the mucous membranes are swollen, hyperemic, and hemorrhagic.[1] Histologically the mucosae of the bulla are edematous, thrombosed, and have a large accumulation of neutrophils; however, the tympanic membrane often appears intact. In more advanced chronic stages, inspissated pus is present and can extend into the eustachian tubes; the mucous membranes are thickened and rough.[2] Histologically the mucosae of the bulla and tympanic membrane appear hemorrhagic and fibrosed, and the architecture of the epithelial cells appears more cuboidal.

The third route of entry is through the external auditory meatus after the tympanic membrane has ruptured. This is an uncommon sequela to parasitic infestation of sheep and goat ears by *Psoroptes cuniculi*. It is believed that the accumulation of secretions and mites places excessive pressure on the tympanic membrane, causing it to rupture.[4]

Clinical signs. Otitis media is often diagnosed as an incidental finding during postmortem examination of sheep.[2,3] Antemortem clinical signs are not reported unless the infection progresses into the inner ear. This also is believed to be the case in goats. Otitis interna as a sequel to otitis media is the most common cause of peripheral vestibular disease in farm animals. The majority of sheep and goats have ipsilateral peripheral vestibular signs, including head tilt toward the lesion, droopy ears, stumbling, and progressive weakness that can lead to recumbency and death.[3] Neurologic signs are a result of decreased drainage through the auditory tubes because of swelling in the mucosa and clogging exudate, which can lead to persistent infection and damage to the facial nerves.[1]

Diagnosis. A thorough history and physical and neurologic examination is necessary for goats or sheep that display head shaking and deficits of the facial and vestibulocochlear nerves.[12] The pinnae and external auditory meatus should be examined and cartilage of the ear palpated for pain. Otoscopic examination of the ear canal for foreign bodies and assessment of mucosal inflammation and integrity of the tympanic membrane also should be performed.[14] If mites are suspected, skin scrapings of the epidermis at the base of the ear canal may be necessary to diagnose *Sarcoptes scabiei*. Diagnosing psoroptic mites with cytologic preparations on swabs taken from the ear canal is difficult. The mites have been repeatedly demonstrated to congregate around the tympanic membrane deep in the ear canal and out of reach of most swabs.[4,8] Flushing the ears gently with warm saline for examination may be more diagnostic than swabbing.

Culture and sensitivity testing of exudate from external abscesses in the ear canal is unrewarding diagnostically except in the following conditions[14]:

1. Bacterial infection persists in spite of appropriate antibiotic treatment
2. The animal has a history of frequent topical antibiotic therapy, suggesting the possibility of a resistant gram-negative bacterial or fungal organism
3. Otitis media or otitis interna is suspected.

Radiographic examination of the skull in sheep or goats with neurologic signs helps the examiner rule out skull fractures that could account for the neurologic signs. The tympanic bullae also can be assessed for increased density. In dogs, calcification of the auricular cartilage is an indication for surgical intervention.[14] Endoscopy can be used to examine the ear canal and tympanic membrane and remove any foreign objects.

Ancillary tests such as complete blood counts, chemistry profiles, and CSF analyses may be warranted if animals show signs of systemic illness, display neurologic signs, or do not respond to treatment.

Treatment of otitis externa. The goal of treatment for otitis externa is to remove ceruminous accumulation and the inciting cause, clean and dry the ear, reduce inflammation, and resolve any secondary infections.[14] This may be as simple a task as removing a foreign object and thoroughly cleaning the ear; however, it also may require the application of topical antiinflammatory agents and antibiotics. External scabs can be removed with warm water and mild soap. Any solutions that are used to help flush and cleanse the ear canal must be selected with the knowledge of whether the tympanic membrane is intact because many flushing solutions are ototoxic. Ceruminolytic agents contain surfactants and emulsifiers to liquefy earwax and aid in its removal. They should be applied to the ear canal 5 to 15 minutes before the canal is

TABLE 11-7

BACTERICIDAL SOLUTIONS THAT CAN BE USED TO FLUSH THE EXTERNAL AUDITORY MEATUS

SOLUTION	CONCENTRATION	TOXICITY	SUSCEPTIBLE ORGANISMS	RESISTANT BACTERIA
Chlorhexidine	2%, 0.05%	Ototoxic	Gram-negative and gram-positive bacteria; fungi	*Pseudomonas*
Povidone iodine	0.1% to 1%; smaller concentrations are more effective	Ototoxic	Gram-negative and gram-positive bacteria; fungi	Gram-negative bacteria
Acetic acid	1:1, 1:2, or 1:3 dilution of a 5% stock	Ototoxic	*Pseudomonas, Staphylococcus, Streptococcus, Escherichia coli,* and *Proteus*	Very few bacteria are resistant at 5% concentration but it is irritating to the mucosa

cleaned.[10] Flushing solutions are then used to remove the ceruminolytic agents and debris. Saline is the safest solution to use, although a variety of bactericidal solutions with a broad spectrum of activity also may be used (Table 11-7). After flushing the ear canal should be dried thoroughly; astringents such as aluminum acetate and boric acid can be applied to enhance drying.[10] If the canal is severely inflamed, the animal may benefit from topical corticosteroids or systemic dexamethasone administration.

In cases in which the inciting cause has been identified as a psoroptic or sarcoptic mite, ivermectin can be used as an acaricide. In addition to treating the affected sheep or goats, all in-contact animals should be treated as well.

Treatment of otitis media and otitis interna. If the tympanic membrane is ruptured, the clinician must take care to select ear-cleansing solutions that are not ototoxic. In general broad-spectrum antibiotics should be administered to eliminate bacterial infections. Systemic antiinflammatory agents may be warranted if neurologic signs are present. If the animals are unresponsive to treatment and adequate drainage of the canal cannot be achieved, a lateral ear resection may be necessary to provide access to the horizontal ear canal.

REFERENCES

1. Jensen R et al: Middle ear infection in feedlot lambs, *J Am Vet Med Assoc* 181:805, 1982.
2. Macleod NSM, Wiener G, Barlow RM: Factors involved in middle ear infection (otitis media) in lambs, *Vet Rec* 91:360, 1972.
3. Davies IH, Done SH: Necrotic dermatitis and otitis media associated with *Pseudomonas aeruginosa* in sheep following dipping, *Vet Rec* 132:460, 1993.
4. Morgan KL: Parasitic otitis in sheep associated with *Psoroptes* infestation: a clinical and epidemiological study, *Vet Rec* 130:530, 1992.
5. Bates PG: Ear mites in sheep, *Vet Rec* 128:555, 1991.
6. Evans AG: Psoroptic mange. In Smith BP, editor: *Large animal internal medicine*, St Louis, 1996, Mosby.
7. Cook RW: Ear mites (*Raillietia manfredi* and *Psoroptes cuniculi*) in goats in New South Wales, *Aust Vet J* 57:72, 1981.
8. Williams JF, Williams CS: Psoroptic ear mites in dairy goats, *J Am Vet Med Assoc* 173:1582, 1978.
9. Fraser G: The histopathology of the external auditory meatus of the dog, *J Comp Path* 71:253, 1961.
10. Griffin CE: Otitis externa, *Comp Cont Ed Pract Vet* 3:741, 1981.
11. Littlejohn AI: Psoroptic mange in the goat, *Vet Rec* 82:148, 1968.
12. Blythe LL: Otitis media and interna and temporohyoid osteoarthropathy, *Vet Clin North Am Equine Pract* 13:21, 1997.
13. Jensen R et al: Cause and pathogenesis of middle ear infection in young feedlot cattle, *J Am Vet Med Assoc* 182:967, 1983.
14. Rosychuk RAW: Management of otitis externa, *Vet Clin North Am Small Anim Pract* 24:912, 1994.

Cerebrospinal Nematodiasis

Etiology and pathogenesis. The larvae from *Parelaphostrongylus tenuis* (North America)[1-6] and *Setaria* species (India, Japan, Korea, and Russia)[7,8] can aberrantly migrate into the central nervous system in many small ruminant species.

Setaria is found in the connective tissue and peritoneal cavities of adult cattle.[8] Adult worms produce blood-borne microfilaria that are picked up by blood-sucking insects and occasionally transmitted to sheep and goats.[7] The larvae can migrate into the spinal cord and cause disease by destroying nervous tissue during their migration.

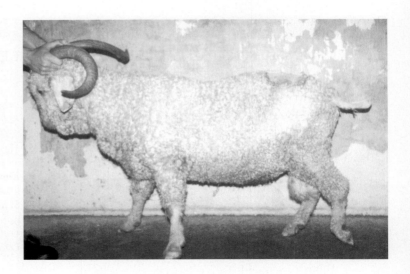

Figure 11-7 This Angora goat with *P. tenuis* infection has rear limb ataxia. The CSF contains an increased number of leucocytes, with more than 50% eosinophils. Other breeds of goats can become infected with *P. tenuis,* but most of the reported cases have been in Angora goats.

P. tenuis is a meningeal worm commonly found in white-tailed deer *(Odocoileus virginianus);* it rarely causes serious pathology and clinical disease in this specie.[1] In the white-tailed deer the adult *P. tenuis* lives in the meninges, predominantly in the cranial regions. Adults lay eggs in the venous sinuses, where they are carried to the lungs. The eggs become lodged in small capillaries, hatch, and migrate into the alveoli. The larvae are then coughed up, swallowed, and passed into the feces.[1] The intermediate hosts are species of slugs and snails that become infected by *P. tenuis* larvae when they feed on deer feces. Sheep and goats accidentally ingest these gastropod intermediate hosts while grazing and become infected. The larvae is freed of the gastropod during digestion in the abomasum. The *P. tenuis* larvae migrate along peripheral nerves toward the spinal cord. On reaching the spinal cord of the host, the larvae migrate along the nervous tract, causing inflammation.

Clinical signs.   Clinical signs depend on the migration pattern of the parasite through the central nervous system. *Setaria* larvae movements are apparently random, whereas *P. tenuis* larvae migrate in a cranial direction. Animals usually display an acute onset of signs. If lesions occur only in the spinal cord, the affected animal remains bright and alert, may have a good appetite, and will make attempts to rise. Depression, ataxia, and paralysis of the hindlimbs or of all four limbs may occur. Signs tend to be symmetric, but a vertically oriented strip of self-excoriation may be evident as a result of pathology of the dorsal nerve roots.[8] Occasionally lesions occur in the brain and the animal may be depressed, become blind, or die; the animal also may exhibit opisthotonos, circling, and a head tilt.[1] All breeds appear susceptible, but anecdotally Angora goats may be more likely to become infected (Figure 11-7).[2] In one outbreak (attended by one of the authors, Dr. Pugh) in which 80 Angora, Nubian, Spanish, and cross-bred goats were grazing and browsing

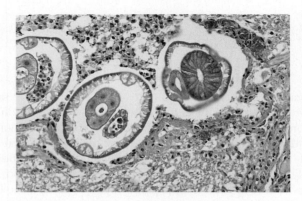

Figure 11-8   This cross-section of the spinal cord shows both an increase in inflammatory cells and the parasite. (Courtesy Dr. Christine Navarre, Auburn, AL.)

low-lying, wet areas, 8 goats showed clinical signs. In this outbreak only the Angoras were affected. The diagnosis was confirmed on necropsy. Angora goats may be more prone to infection because of their grazing versus browsing behavior. *P. tenuis* signs usually appear during the fall and winter months in North America, and then only in areas that have white-tailed deer and the gastropod intermediate hosts.[1]

Diagnosis.   A definitive diagnosis is made by identifying the larvae on histologic examination of the spinal cord (Figure 11-8). Diagnosis depends on the entire spinal cord and brain being removed at necropsy, cooled (not frozen), and quickly delivered to a suitable diagnostic laboratory. Good presumptive evidence of this disease is a bright and responsive animal that nevertheless has an increased number of white blood cells, mostly eosinophils, in the CSF and exhibits some degree of rear-limb paralysis or ataxia.[3] Reports suggest that 70% of goats with *P. tenuis* infestations have increased eosinophils in the CSF.[8] Trauma, spinal cord abscess, spondylitis, and enzootic ataxia must be ruled out.[7] Complete blood count results are usually normal, but serum chemistry findings usually reveal an elevation of muscle-specific enzymes (e.g., lactate dehydrogenase [LDH], creatine phosphokinase [CPK]). Gross lesions are usually undetectable; however, small hemorrhagic areas may be seen in the spinal cord. Histologic lesions include demyelination, axonal degeneration, and malacia. Infiltration of eosinophils, lymphocytes, and macrophages often occurs around any larvae that may be found on histologic sections.

Treatment and prevention.   Treatment with anthelmintics (ivermectin 500 μg/kg subcutaneously [SC] once a day [SID], followed by 200 μg/kg SC SID for 5 days and/or fenbendazole 15 mg/kg PO SID for 3 to 5 days), NSAIDs (flunixin meglumine 1mg/kg IV or IM as needed) or glucocorticosteroids for nonpregnant animals, and other antiinflammatory drugs (DMSO) has been employed in other species susceptible to infestation.[1,8] Recovery depends on the site of the lesion(s), the onset of treatment with respect to the occurrence of clinical signs, and the diligence of nursing care. Ivermectin is thought to be unable to pass the blood-brain barrier, but in areas where the worm has caused a localized inflammatory response, ivermectin may cross into the inflamed area.[8] However, ivermectin's effect may be relegated to preventing any larvae remaining in peripheral tissues from reaching the spinal cord.

Prevention of infestation with *Setaria* is difficult, but minimizing biting insects may be of value. To minimize *P. tenuis* infestation, suppressive deworming programs have been used in llamas.[1] However, suppressive deworming may be too expensive to use in sheep and goats and can result in anthelmintic resistance of other nematode (HOTC complex) parasites (see Chapter 4). Still, the use of a short-term monthly suppressive deworming program (late fall and winter) with ivermectin (200 μg/kg SC) appeared to be of value in stopping an explosive outbreak (8 of 80 animals in a 1-week period).[9] Susceptible animals should be removed from low-lying or moist pastures, particularly those adjacent to habitats where a white-tailed deer population exists. If alternative pastures are unavailable, frost or freezing temperatures may alleviate some of the risk. Fencing off damp areas and instituting snail and slug control measures (often done with geese) may reduce the incidence of clinical disease. Such pastures should first be grazed by less susceptible species (cattle). Minimizing contact with white-tailed deer and/or intermediate hosts is an excellent, yet difficult, method of prevention.

References

1. Pugh DG et al: Clinical parelaphostrongylosis in llamas, *Comp Cont Ed Pract Vet* 17:600, 1995.
2. O'Brien TD et al: Cerebrospinal parelaphostrongylosis in Minnesota, *Minn Vet* 26:18, 1986.
3. Kopcha M et al: Cerebrospinal nematodiasis in a goat herd, *J Am Vet Med Assoc* 194:1439, 1989.
4. Jortner BS et al: Lesions of spinal cord parelaphostrongylosis in sheep: sequential changes following intra medullary larval migration, *Vet Path* 22:137, 1985.
5. Alden C et al: Cerebrospinal nematodiasis in sheep, *J Am Vet Med Assoc* 166:784, 1975.
6. Mayhew IG, deLahunta A, Georgi JR: Naturally occurring cerebrospinal parelaphostrongylosis, *Cornell Vet J* 66:56, 1976.
7. Kimberling C: *Diseases of sheep*, ed 3, Philadelphia, 1988, Lee & Febiger.
8. Smith MC: Inflammatory neurologic diseases of small ruminants. In Smith MC, editor: *Current veterinary therapy 3, food animal practice*, Philadelphia, 1993, WB Saunders.
9. Pugh DG, personal communication.

Tetanus

Tetanus is caused by *Clostridium tetani*. The organism is a common inhabitant of the herbivore intestinal tract and its spores may be present in large numbers in feces. *C. tetani* spores appear to have a long extra-intestinal life span and may remain viable in soil for years. Infection in sheep and goats is most commonly through a contaminated skin break (injury, umbilicus, tail docking, castration) but also can occur as part of postpartum metritis. The organism proliferates and produces toxins under acidic, anaerobic conditions; therefore it is most common in deep, necrotic wounds. The organism can remain dormant as a spore in tissue until a favorable environment for replication develops. Therefore clinical tetanus is often seen several weeks after the original injury.[1,2]

Pathogenesis.   The organism produces three toxins, the most important of which is the plasmid-derived tetanospasmin. Tetanospasmin binds to gangliosides in nerves and is carried by retrograde axoplasmic flow through the smooth endoplasmic reticulum to the central nervous system, where it prevents the release of the inhibitory neurotransmitter glycine. The toxin can initially bind to nervous tissue near the site of infection, in which case local neurologic signs develop before the disease becomes generalized (ascending tetanus). Alternatively, it can circulate in the blood and bind to nervous tissue near the head, in which case head and neck signs are seen before limb signs (descending tetanus). In both cases the effect of the toxin on the central nervous system is to prevent inhibition of muscular contraction, resulting in continuous tetanic contraction of muscle groups. Postural and facial muscles are most commonly affected.

The other two toxins are tetanolysin and a nonspasmogenic neurotoxin. Tetanolysin is thought to encourage necrosis and thereby create a favorable site for proliferation of the organism. The second neurotoxin appears to cause neuromuscular blockage and activate the sympathetic nervous system. Tetanus occurs worldwide. Sheep and goats are generally considered more susceptible to tetanus than cattle.

Clinical signs. With ascending tetanus the clinical signs first noted are often stiffness or perceived lameness in one leg. Within 24 hours generalized stiffness, a stilted gait, raised tail head ("pump-handle"), saw-horse stance, trismus ("lockjaw"), and retraction of the lips from the teeth ("sardonic grin") may be noted. Stimulation can cause tetanic muscular spasms, particularly of postural and facial muscles and the third eyelid. The infected animal may appear restless and have pyrexia. Severely affected animals are recumbent and display rigid, uncorrectable extension of the neck and all four limbs (Figure 11-9). Bloat and aspiration also are common findings. Rigid paralysis of the muscles of respiration induce hypoxemia and severely limit the animal's ability to function. Clinical signs are present for several weeks in animals that recover; however, death is the usual outcome.

Diagnosis. Stress leukograms and marked increases in muscle enzymes are the most typical antemortem abnormalities. The clinician may determine the original route of entry for the organism and attempt to isolate the organism from that area. Diagnosis is by characteristic signs with or without isolation of the organism.

Treatment. The clinician must keep several goals in mind when treating small ruminants with tetanus. They include muscle relaxation; supportive care, including the provision of good footing; fluid and nutritional support; elimination of the infection; neutralization of unbound toxin; and provision of active antitoxic immunity. Extremely high doses of penicillin (20,000 to 40,000 IU IV

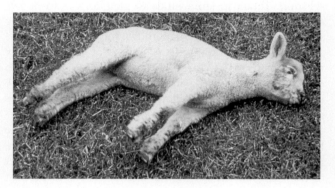

Figure 11-9 This lamb developed tetanus as a sequela of tail docking. Any wound, particularly one in which tissue trauma and depressed oxygen tension are evident, is susceptible to *C. tetani* infection and elaboration of the neurotoxin. The first signs occur by 3 weeks after an injury or surgical procedure (tail docking, dehorning, castration). Death usually occurs as a result of respiratory failure. On farms and ranches with a high incidence, tetanus antitoxin (150 to 300 IU) and tetanus toxoid should be given at the time of any surgical procedures.

BID to QID) are the antibiotics of choice to kill *C. tetani.* Tetanus antitoxin can be administered with tetanus toxoid (at different sites) to help neutralize unbound toxin and provide active immunity. Slings and deep, soft bedding are important to prevent decubital ulcers and maintain circulation in the extremities. A rumenotomy may be necessary in some sheep and goats that are anorexic and suffering from ruminal tympany. Animals should be kept in a dark, quiet place with minimal stimulation to reduce muscle spasms and stress. Sedation also may be beneficial.

Prevention. In addition to general matters of hygiene, especially during surgical procedures, the administration of tetanus toxoid may help prevent this disease. A two-dose course in the first year of life followed by annual boosters is recommended. Additional boosters may be given to individual animals after injuries.[2]

REFERENCES

1. Hagan WA, Bruner DW, Timoney JF: *Hagan and Bruner's microbiology and infectious diseases of domestic animals,* ed 8, Ithaca, NY, 1988, Comstock Publishing.
2. George LW: Tetanus (lockjaw). In Smith BP, editor: *Large animal internal medicine,* ed 2, St Louis, 1996, Mosby.

Botulism

Clostridium botulinum is the cause of botulism. The organism proliferates and produces toxin under neutral or alkaline, anaerobic conditions. Spoiled feedstuffs, moist alkaline silage, brewer's grains, decaying vegetation, and animal carcasses are common sites of proliferation. Feed-related outbreaks are common and often are associated with contamination of a feedstuff with a decaying animal carcass. Factors that promote pica (such as hypophosphatemia and starvation) may promote outbreaks by encouraging animals to consume sources of the toxin they would otherwise not eat. Several strains of *C. botulinum* have been identified. Strain C is the most common cause of disease in sheep. Botulism occurs worldwide.

Pathogenesis. In sheep and goats, botulism is almost always caused by ingestion of preformed toxin, rather than production of the toxin by viable bacteria within the intestinal tract (toxicoinfectious botulism) or a wound. Adult ruminants are less susceptible than neonates and animals that lack a fermentative stomach because most ingested botulism toxin is degraded by rumen microbes and therefore ingestion of large doses of toxin is necessary to cause disease. Toxin that survives the rumen is absorbed across the intestinal wall, where it enters the circulation. It binds gangliosides at the neuromuscular junction and thereby prevents the fusion of acetylcholine vesicles with the presynaptic membrane. Flaccid paralysis results, usually within a week of ingestion of the toxin.[1-3]

Clinical signs.   Generalized muscle weakness is the most common clinical sign. Affected animals move slowly and reluctantly, often dragging their feet or swaying from side to side. Once they become recumbent, they often have difficulty rising. The head is usually held low, and protrusion of the tongue may cause pseudoptyalism and dysphagia. Bloat, regurgitation, rumen hypomotility, and a distended, hypomotile bladder may occur.[3]

Diagnosis.   No clinicopathologic abnormalities or postmortem lesions are specific to botulism. Transudates may be found in body cavities and tissues may be edematous. Cardiac disease must be ruled out as a cause for these lesions. Diagnosis is made by characteristic signs and identification of the toxin in feed, blood, or gastrointestinal contents. Identification of the specific strain is made by use of a live animal assay or an enzyme-linked immunospecific assay (ELISA).

Treatment.   Therapy consists of fluid and nutritional support, general nursing care (including wound management), and supportive ventilation if warranted. Penicillin-class antibiotics are effective, but intramuscular procaine penicillin should be avoided if possible because it can exacerbate the neuromuscular blockage. Metronidazole also is effective, especially if wound contamination has occurred, but it should not be used in ruminants that may be slaughtered for food. Polyvalent antitoxin may be effective in the early stages of the disease and in animals at risk of contracting botulism. A beneficial effect may be achieved by administering anticholinesterase (neostigmine methylsulfate 0.01 to 0.02 mg/kg SC).

Prevention.   Proper handling and avoiding the feeding of contaminated feedstuffs are the best methods of prevention. This includes proper fermentation of silage, rodent control, and removal of carcasses from feeds before processing. A vaccine is available in the United States against type B botulism, but not against type C.[3]

References

1. Hagan WA, Bruner DW, Timoney JF: *Hagan and Bruner's microbiology and infectious diseases of domestic animals,* ed 8, Ithaca, NY, 1988, Comstock Publishing.
2. Allison MJ, Maloy SE, Matson RR: Inactivation of *Clostridium botulinum* toxin by ruminal microbes from cattle and sheep, *Appl Environ Microbiol* 32:685, 1976.
3. Smith MO: Botulism. In Smith BP, editor: *Large animal internal medicine,* ed 2, St Louis, 1996, Mosby.

Tick Paralysis

Tick paralysis is a rapidly progressive LMN paralysis that occurs in both sheep and goats. The tick, probably the female, releases a toxin in its saliva that blocks or decreases the release of acetylcholine at the neuromuscular junction, resulting in paresis.[1,2] Ticks of the genus *Dermacentor* are associated with this disease. Tick paralysis occurs in North America west of the Rocky Mountains. A similar condition is reported in Australia and is caused by the tick *Ixodes holocyclus.* However, in the Australian strain of the disease animals usually do not recover even if the tick is removed.

Clinical signs.   A progressive paralysis and weakness occurs. If left untreated, it results in death by respiratory paralysis.

Diagnosis.   Diagnosis is based on clinical signs and finding ticks. This condition must be differentiated from botulism.

Treatment and prevention.   Animals can be sprayed with pyrethrins or given ivermectin; however, ticks should be removed. Animals should be sheared if necessary in order for the examiner to find the tick(s). Animals quickly recover after the tick has been removed. Applying tick or insect repellents is helpful in some high-risk areas.[1,2]

References

1. Schofield LN, Saunders JR: An incidental case of tick paralysis in a Holstein calf exposed to *Dermacentor andersoni, Can Vet J* 33:190, 1992.
2. Fowler ME: Tick paralysis, *Cal Vet* 39(2):25, 1985.

Organophosphate Toxicosis

Some sheep have a familial predisposition to chronic organophosphate toxicity,[1] although all sheep and goats are susceptible. Organophosphates inhibit cholinesterase, and toxicosis caused by the compound may be cumulative.

Clinical signs.   Acute signs include hypersalivation, depression, incoordination, and death. This slow, progressive condition is characterized by dyspnea, weakness, rear-limb ataxia, apparent loss of proprioceptive ability, and bloat. With chronic organophosphate toxicosis, animals become recumbent and lose tail, rectal, and bladder function. However, most maintain a good appetite.[1,2]

Diagnosis.   Red blood cell cholinesterase concentrations are depressed at the onset but soon return to normal. No gross lesions are noted on postmortem evaluation. Histologic examination reveals demyelination, swelling, and Wallerian degeneration that progresses from the periphery to more central areas of the central nervous system.

Treatment.   No treatment is available for the chronic form of the disease. Acute cases may be treated with high doses of atropine (0.2 to 0.4 mg/kg IV) or pralidoxime (2 PAM, 20 mg/kg).

REFERENCES

1. Williams JF, Dade AW: Posterior paralysis associated with anthelmintic treatment of sheep, *J Am Vet Med Assoc* 169:1307, 1976.
2. Linklater KA, Smith MC: *Color atlas of diseases and disorders of the sheep and goat,* Aylesburg, UK, 1993, Wolfe Publishing.

Lead Toxicity

Lead toxicity (plumbism) in sheep and goats is most likely to result from a single accidental ingestion of harmful amounts of lead.[1,2] Common sources of lead exposure include lead-containing paints, petroleum products, and discarded batteries.[1-4] Lead is believed to produce neurologic disease by a direct toxic effect on the vasculature of the central nervous system that causes capillary edema and hemorrhage. Goats are more resistant to lead toxicity than other species[5] and lethal doses of lead vary widely among goats.[4] Sheep were experimentally fed lead at 4.5 mg/kg for 27 weeks without developing any apparent clinical signs of plumbism.[6]

Clinical signs. Clinical signs of plumbism in sheep include cortical blindness, dullness, anorexia, circling, and gait abnormalities.[3] In contrast to other species, blindness did not occur in goats with experimental lead toxicity.[4] Clinical signs of lead toxicity in goats include anorexia, diarrhea, weight loss, and death.[4]

Diagnosis.   Diagnosis of plumbism is based on consistent clinical signs and blood lead concentrations. Background blood lead concentrations vary geographically, and therefore the normal range of blood lead concentrations differs among diagnostic laboratories.[2] If exposure to lead is chronic, anemia may result. CSF analysis may show an increase in protein concentration and in the number of neutrophils and monocytes. At necropsy, affected goats have cerebral edema, microscopic lesions of meningeal and perineuronal edema, neuronal degeneration, and vascular congestion of medullary and cerebellar white matter.[4] The kidneys and livers of suspected cases should be measured for lead concentration.

Treatment.   Treatment of lead toxicity involves the administration of lead chelating agents such as ethylenediamine tetra-acetic acid (EDTA).[5] In goats, 110 mg/kg EDTA (6.6% solution) is administered IV twice a day at 12-hour intervals for 2 days. Alternatively, EDTA (70 to 75 mg/kg IV) can be administered slowly for 3 to 5 days, followed by 2 days of no treatment and then 5 more days of therapy. The 2-day rest allows bone lead stores to equalize with the soft tissues.[7] Thiamine administration as described for treatment of polioencephalomalacia also

is beneficial.[2,3,5] A combination of thiamine (5 mg/kg IM SID or TID) and EDTA appears to give the best results.[7] The administration of oral magnesium sulfate may help decrease the absorption of lead salts in sheep and goats, as it does in other species.[8] Nutritional (oral or total parenteral nutrition) and fluid support are required. If convulsions occur, they can be controlled with diazepam (0.5 to 2 mg/kg IV).

REFERENCES

1. Allcroft R: Lead poisoning in cattle and sheep, *Vet Rec* 63:58, 1951.
2. Baker JC: Lead poisoning in cattle, *Vet Clin North Am Food Anim Pract* 3:137, 1987.
3. Radostits OM, Blood DC, Gay CC: Diseases caused by inorganic and farm chemicals. In Radostits OM, Blood DC, Gay CC, editors: *Veterinary medicine,* ed 8, London, 1994, Bailliere Tindall.
4. Davis JW et al: Experimentally induced lead poisoning in goats: clinical observations and pathologic changes, *Cornell Vet J* 66:490, 1976.
5. Smith MC, Sherman DM: Nervous system. In Smith MC, Sherman DM, editors: *Goat medicine,* Philadelphia, 1994, Lea & Febiger.
6. Carson TL et al: Effects of low level lead ingestion in sheep, *Clin Toxicol* 6:389, 1973.
7. George LW: Diseases of the nervous system. In Smith BP, editor: *Large animal internal medicine,* ed 2, St Louis, 1996, Mosby.
8. Pringle J: Neurologic disorders. In Ogilvie TH, editor: *Large animal internal medicine,* Baltimore, 1998, Williams & Wilkins.

Sodium Toxicosis and Water Deprivation

Sodium toxicosis and water deprivation (salt toxicity) occur under the following conditions[1-3]:

1. Excessive sodium ingestion with adequate water intake
2. Consumption of normal amounts of sodium with limited access to water
3. Consumption of water with a high sodium concentration
4. The administration of hypertonic oral electrolyte solutions

Feeding salt-limited diets, particularly during periods of water deprivation or weather changes, may result in salt toxicity. Prolonged hypernatremia causes an increase in CSF and brain sodium concentrations. As an additional response to hypernatremia, iodogenic osmoles accumulate inside neurons. Both of these protective mechanisms increase osmolality and retain water within the CNS. Neurologic disease results from cerebral edema when the animal is rehydrated too quickly and water follows an osmotic gradient into the CNS.[1,4]

Clinical signs and diagnosis.   Clinical signs reported in affected sheep include increased thirst, somnolence, hyperthermia, tachycardia, tachypnea, muscle fasciculation, rumen stasis, diarrhea or mucus-coated feces, regurgitation, nasal discharge, convulsions, and death.[3] Affected lambs may have serum and CSF concentrations of sodium in excess of 180 mEq/liter.[3,4]

Treatment. Treatment of sodium toxicosis and water deprivation initially involves restricting water intake to frequent, small quantities and reducing cerebral edema with corticosteroids (dexamethasone 1 to 2 mg/kg IV), mannitol (0.25 to 1 mg/kg IV), or possibly furosemide (1 to 2 mg/kg IV). Severely affected animals may require IV fluid replacement to gradually restore sodium and water homeostasis.[1,3]

Prevention. Fresh, clean water should be made available. If salt-limited feeds are offered, changes in water intake associated with weather should be anticipated. Owners should be instructed in the proper use of oral electrolyte solutions for rehydration.

REFERENCES

1. Miller PE: Neurogenic vision loss. In Howard JL, Smith RA, editors: *Current veterinary therapy 4, food animal practice,* Philadelphia, 1999, WB Saunders.
2. Kopcha M: Nutritional and metabolic diseases, *Vet Clin North Am Food Anim Pract* 3:119, 1987.
3. Divers TJ: Diseases of the nervous system. In Howard JL, Smith RA, editors: *Current veterinary therapy 4, food animal practice,* Philadelphia, 1999, WB Saunders.
4. Scarratt WK, Collins TJ, Sponenberg DP: Water deprivation-sodium chloride intoxication in a group of feeder lambs, *J Am Vet Med Assoc* 186:977, 1985.

Urea (Ammonia) Toxicity

Urea (ammonia toxicity) is seen in animals fed non-protein nitrogen (e.g., urea, ammoniated feeds). It is more common in animals newly introduced to such diets (see Chapter 2). Excess non-protein nitrogen, particularly at a high rumen pH, is catabolized to ammonia. If adequate carbon chains from readily fermentable feeds are lacking (corn, oats) or if the rumen pH is high because of poor-quality forage intake (resulting in enhanced function of the urease enzyme), bacterial production of protein from the released ammonia is overwhelmed, resulting in alkalosis and encephalopathy.

Clinical signs. Trembling, facial twitching, incoordination, blindness, recumbency, and death are all encountered. Animals also may become bloated, dyspneic, and hyperesthetic.

Diagnosis. The clinical signs coupled with a history of an abrupt introduction to non-protein nitrogen are useful for a presumptive diagnosis. Blood and CSF ammonia concentrations are usually elevated.

Treatment. Infusing a cold 2% acetic acid solution (1 mg/kg PO) into the rumen improves the blood acid-base status and slows bacterial production of ammonia. Oral charcoal (0.5 kg PO) also may be helpful in decreasing ammonia absorption.[1]

Prevention. Slow introduction of sources of non-protein nitrogen is a good method of prevention (see Chapter 2).

REFERENCE

1. Divers TJ: Diseases of the nervous system. In Howard JL, Smith RA, editors: *Current veterinary therapy 4, food animal practice,* Philadelphia, 1999, WB Saunders.

Polioencephalomalacia

Polioencephalomalacia (PEM), or cerebrocortical necrosis, is most commonly diagnosed in 2- to 6-month-old lambs and kids that are typically being fed high-concentrate diets.[1-4] However, PEM can occur in animals of any age. Other nutritional factors associated with PEM include sudden changes in diet, feeds high in molasses (horse feed), moldy hay, rumen acidosis, and the dietary stress of weaning.[4] In ruminant animals the ruminal bacteria normally produce sufficient thiamine (vitamin B_1) to meet their requirements. Rumen acidosis (most commonly caused by feeding excess concentrates) predisposes animals to the development of PEM in several ways: the population of thiamine-producing bacteria decreases, bacterial thiaminase production increases, and ruminal thiaminase activity is potentiated by acidic conditions.[2,5] Bracken fern *(Pteridium aquilinum)* also contains thiaminase and experimental feeding trials in sheep have produced clinical signs and necropsy lesions consistent with PEM.[6] Overdosage of thiamine analogs such as amprolium has caused PEM in sheep by competitive inhibition.[7] Thiamine is a necessary cofactor for enzymes involved in glucose metabolism, including transketolase and pyruvate decarboxylase. The brain derives energy from glucose through the pentose phosphate pathway, which requires thiamine diphosphate as a coenzyme for transketolase. When energy production in the neurons is impaired as a result of thiamine deficiency, cellular osmotic gradients cannot be maintained and neuronal swelling results in PEM.

High dietary sulfate also may cause clinical signs and necropsy lesions consistent with PEM. Excessive dietary sulfur intake may result from mixing errors, high-sulfur water sources, feed intake limiters such as gypsum (calcium sulfate), and urinary acidifiers such as ammonium sulfate.[8] Sulfur-induced PEM also has occurred in sheep allowed to graze areas that were recently sprayed with an elemental sulfur solution.[9] The neurotoxic mechanism of sulfur is not completely understood but may result from the production of large amounts of hydrogen sulfide in the rumen. High concentrations of sulfides interfere with energy production in the brain by inhibiting cytochrome oxidase, which participates in the electron transport chain to eventually produce ATP. Dietary sulfur concentrations of 0.43% and greater have caused PEM in sheep.[10,11]

Clinical signs. Clinical signs of PEM include central blindness, dorsomedial strabismus, depression, incoordination, head pressing, recumbency, opisthotonos, and convulsions[1-9] (Figure 11-10). Diarrhea and anorexia may be noticed before clinical signs occur or soon after onset.[1,4] Severely affected animals can become comatose and die. PEM caused by thiamine deficiency usually only affects a few individuals in the herd or flock, but sulfur toxicity may involve a large number of animals.[10]

Diagnosis. Diagnosis of PEM is most often based on the animal's clinical signs and response to therapy.[1,2,4] Blood thiamine concentration and erythrocyte transketolase activity can be measured, but these tests are not routinely available. Using high-pressure liquid chromatography, normal blood thiamine concentrations have been reported to be between 75 and 185 nmol/l and 66 to 178 nmol/l in sheep[12] and goats,[13] respectively. The most useful assay of transketolase activity determines the thiamine diphosphate (TPP) effect, which is a measure of the percentage increase in transketolase activity after the addition of excess TPP to a sample.[5] In sheep affected with PEM, transketolase activity increases from 96% to 158% when they are tested for the TPP effect.[14] Blood thiamine concentration and transketolase activity are normal in animals with sulfur-induced PEM.[8] CSF analysis is usually normal, but

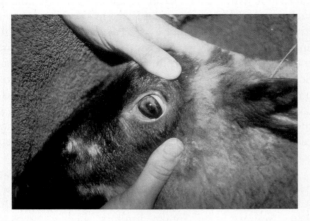

Figure 11-10 A lamb with polioencephalomalacia resulting from a diet deficient in forage and rich in cereal grains. Note the characteristic dorsomedial strabismus. Feedlot animals, club lambs and goats, and pet animals fed diets rich in energy or sulfate and low in forage are at high risk to develop this disease.

slight elevations may occur in protein concentration or mononuclear cell count.[2,4] If sulfate-induced PEM is suspected, the sulfate content of the ration and water sources should be determined. Examination of rumen contents reveals an increased number of gram-positive bacilli and decreased numbers of gram-positive cocci organisms.[15]

Necropsy lesions of PEM are limited to the brain and include a softened, edematous cerebral cortex that often has a gray to yellowish discoloration. The cerebral gyri may appear flattened and the cerebellum may be herniated through the foramen magnum in severe cases.[3,4] If transverse sections of the cerebrum are examined with an ultraviolet light, the necrotic areas fluoresce because of the presence of lipofuscin pigment. Histopathologic findings include laminar necrosis in affected cerebral gyri, with separation of the white and gray matter. The neurons have an eosinophilic cytoplasm and may appear degenerated and shrunken. Pericellular edema, nuclear chromatolysis, and vacuolization may occur.[3,4]

Treatment. Treatment most importantly involves thiamine replacement at a dosage of 10 mg/kg. The initial dose should be given IV; additional injections can be IM or SC and should be administered every 6 hours for the first day of therapy.[1,4,5] Thiamine injections (10 mg/kg every 6 to 12 hours IM, SC, or IV) should be continued for at least 2 days. The frequency of injection may be gradually reduced as the animal improves and regains a normal appetite.[1,3,4] Many affected animals exhibit significant improvement within 24 hours of the first thiamine injection. In severe cases, cerebral edema can be reduced with furosemide, mannitol (1 to 2 g/kg IV), or dexamethasone (0.1 mg/kg IV, IM, or SC).[1,4] Seizures may be controlled with diazepam (0.5 to 1.5 mg/kg IV) as needed.[1,4] Euthanasia should be recommended for animals not responding to therapy within 3 days; however, some animals may take as long as 1 week to fully recover.[1] Blindness is usually permanent in severely affected animals because of extensive cerebrocortical necrosis.[3,4] In contrast with animals affected by PEM of different etiologies, animals affected with PEM because of excess dietary sulfur usually do not respond well to thiamine administration.[8-10]

Prevention. Sudden dietary changes to more energy-dense feeds should be avoided. The addition of thiamine (3 to 10 mg/kg/day) to the diets of animals prone to this condition and thiamine administration before weather changes may be preventative.[16] Other measures to reduce the incidence of PEM include allowing free access to a good-quality trace mineral salt, paying careful attention to animals fed a diet with calcium sulfate as a component and to those offered water with a high sulfate content, and providing free access to good-quality forage.

REFERENCES

1. Miller PE: Neurogenic vision loss. In Howard JL, Smith RA, editors: *Current veterinary therapy 4, food animal practice,* Philadelphia, 1999, WB Saunders.
2. Smith MC: Polioencephalomalacia in goats, *J Am Vet Med Assoc* 174:1328, 1979.
3. Pierson RE, Jensen R: Polioencephalomalacia in feedlot lambs, *J Am Vet Med Assoc* 166:257, 1975.
4. Smith MC, Sherman DM: Nervous system. In Smith MC, Sherman DM, editors: *Goat medicine,* Philadelphia, 1994, Lea & Febiger.
5. Rammell CG, Hill JH: A review of thiamine deficiency and its diagnosis, especially in ruminants, *N Z Vet J* 34:202, 1986.
6. Evans WC et al: Induction of thiamine deficiency in sheep, with lesions similar to those of cerebrocortical necrosis, *J Comp Path* 85:253, 1975.
7. Loew FM, Dunlop RH: Induction of thiamine inadequacy and polioencephalomalacia in adult sheep with amprolium, *Am J Vet Res* 33:2195, 1972.
8. Jeffrey M et al: Polioencephalomalacia associated with the ingestion of ammonium sulfate by sheep and cattle, *Vet Rec* 134:343, 1994.
9. Bulgin MS, Lincoln SD, Mather G: Elemental sulfur toxicosis in a flock of sheep, *J Am Vet Med Assoc* 208:1063, 1996.
10. Low JC et al: Sulfur-induced polioencephalomalacia in lambs, *Vet Rec* 138:327, 1996.
11. Gooneratne SR, Olkowski AA, Christensen DA: Sulfur-induced polioencephalomalacia in sheep: some biochemical changes, *Can J Vet Res* 53:462, 1989.
12. Hill JH, Rammell CG, Forbes S: Blood thiamine levels in normal cattle and sheep at pasture, *N Z Vet J* 36:49, 1988.
13. Rammell CG, Hill JH, Orr M: Blood thiamine levels in clinically normal goats and goats with suspected polioencephalomalacia, *N Z Vet J* 36:99, 1988.
14. Edwin EE et al: Diagnostic aspects of cerebrocortical necrosis, *Vet Rec* 104:4, 1979.
15. Haven TR, Caldwell DR, Jensen R: Role of predominant rumen bacteria in the cause of polioencephalomalacia (cerebrocortical necrosis) in cattle, *Am J Vet Res* 44:1451, 1983.
16. George LW: Diseases of the nervous system. In Smith BP, editor: *Large animal internal medicine,* ed 2, St Louis, 1996, Mosby.

Enzootic Ataxia

Enzootic ataxia, or swayback, is a neurologic condition seen in newborn and growing lambs and kids. Pregnant ewes and does that graze pastures or are fed diets deficient in copper can give birth to lambs with swayback. Conditional copper deficiency (secondary to excess molybdenum, sulfate, iron, or other contaminants, and minerals such as cadmium) also may predispose to the condition.

Clinical signs. Lambs affected in utero may be stillborn; those that live are weak and ataxic and may die within the week. Lambs and kids that develop the condition after birth display ataxia between 2 weeks and 3 months of age. Adults can be affected by many forms of copper deficiency (e.g., anemia, fever, diarrhea) (see Chapter 2).

Diagnosis. Antemortem diagnosis is based on clinical signs, dietary deficiency of copper (4 ppm), and deficient serum or liver concentrations of copper (deficient concentration in the liver is less than 0.5 ppm; serum concentrations less than 0.6 ppm are deficient). CSF values are unremarkable.

Treatment and prevention. Affected animals should be given copper either orally (copper wire, copper particles) or parenterally. However, much of the developmental pathology (hypomyelinogenesis, demyelination, of lower motor neurons) appears irreversible. Increasing the dietary copper to 5 to 15 ppm and maintaining a copper-to-molybdenum ratio of 6:1 in pregnant females is usually protective.

Spinal Trauma, Abscesses, and Tumors

Trauma to the spinal cord can result from injuries caused by other animals (e.g., predators, other goats or sheep, horses), cars, and hunting accidents, among other causes. Young growing animals occasionally have vertebral fractures secondary to dietary or metabolic calcium disorders. These fractures occur in animals consuming diets deficient in calcium and vitamin D and/or rich in phosphorus. Spinal cord tumors (e.g., lymphosarcoma) are space-occupying lesions that compress the spinal cord. Vertebral abscesses may be a component of caseous lymphadenitis or may result from omphalophlebitis or septicemia.[1]

Clinical signs. The clinical signs depend on the location of the injury and the degree of severity of damage to the spinal cord. The signs are usually symmetric and vary from paresis and stiffness to paralysis. In some cases of spinal tumors or vertebral abscesses the signs may either be progressive or appear to have an acute onset. In cases of spinal trauma the onset is acute.

Diagnosis. In cases of trauma a complete physical examination may reveal cuts, punctures, abrasions, and hemorrhages. Palpation of the spinal cord may indicate displacement of the spine in the area of the fracture. Radiographs are useful in aiding the diagnosis of demineralization, spinal cord abscess, osteomyelitis, or fractures.[2] In these cases, serum calcium and phosphorus concentrations are normal, but urinary calcium clearance is depressed and phosphorus clearance is increased (see Chapters 2 and 10). Serum vitamin D concentrations may be depressed. With spinal cord abscesses a complete blood count may show a normal leukogram, an elevated white count, and/or elevations in fibrinogen concentrations. In most instances of trauma the CSF reveals xanthochromia and an increase in total protein.[2] Occasionally spinal cord tumors are indicated by the presence of exfoliated cells on cytologic examination of collected CSF. One of the authors of this chapter (Dr. Pugh) has encountered this in one case each of melanoma and lymphosarcoma.

Treatment. In cases caused by trauma, the use of NSAIDs (flunixin meglumine 1 to 2 mg/kg IV or IM BID, phenylbutazone 5 to 10 mg/kg IV SID) and DMSO (1 mg/kg in 5% dextrose IV SID or BID) is indicated.[2] In cases of vertebral abscesses, antibiotic therapy is indicated (penicillin 22,000 IU/kg BID) but is rarely rewarding.[2]

References

1. Smith MC: Inflammatory neurologic diseases of small ruminants. In Smith RA, editor: *Current veterinary therapy 3, food animal practice*, Philadelphia, 1993, WB Saunders.
2. Sweeney RW: Spinal cord diseases. In Howard JL, Smith RA, editors: *Current veterinary therapy 4, food animal practice*, Philadelphia, 1999, WB Saunders.

Hydrocephalus and Hydranencephaly

Hydrocephalus results from fluid accumulating in excessive amounts in the ventricular system of the cranium. Compensatory hydrocephalus results from destruction of neural tissue and replacement of that space with CSF. This form of hydrocephalus also is referred to as *hydranencephaly,* and is discussed separately. Obstructive hydrocephalus can occur as an internal accumulation of CSF in the ventricular system or an external accumulation of CSF in the subarachnoid space. In addition, two classifications are used to describe the cause of hydrocephalus: *normotensive* (in which the pressure of the CSF is normal, as it is in the case of hydranencephaly) and *hypertensive.* Hypertensive hydrocephalus results from an increase in the amount of CSF because it cannot be absorbed properly as a consequence of a blockage or partial obstruction in the ventricular system. The obstruction can be communicating or noncommunicating, acquired or congenital. Most forms of hydrocephalus recognized in sheep and goats are congenital. Communicating hydrocephalus results from an extraventricular obstruction and is associated with an inability of the arachnoid villi to absorb CSF. Noncommunicating hydrocephalus results from an intraventricular obstruction that prevents the flow of CSF from the ventricular system to the cerebellomedullary cistern of the subarachnoid space.[1]

Hydranencephaly is the complete or almost complete absence of the cerebral hemisphere and basal ganglia in a cranium of normal size.[2] The cavity that remains is filled with CSF and surrounded by a thin layer of cerebrum. This condition also is termed *normotensive hydrocephalus* and results from the neurologic tissue not developing as it should in the fetus. The causative agent is usually an in utero infection in the fetus caused by a virus during a specific stage of gestation. A fetal cerebrovascular insult also may result in massive necrosis and reabsorption of tissue.[3] The extensive loss of neural tissue results in the limbs of the affected fetus being severely contracted (arthrogryposis).

Hydrocephalus

The pathophysiology behind hydrocephalus is still not completely known. In congenital forms the obstruction results from stenosis during fetal development. The sites of obstruction are most commonly the lateral apertures, mesencephalic aqueduct, lateral ventricles, interventricular foramina, and fourth ventricles.[4] A genetic predisposition for the development of hydrocephalus in Suffolk sheep along with cerebellar hypoplasia is called *Dandy-Walker syndrome.*[5] Some poisonous plants such as *Veratrum californicum* and *Conium maculatum* can cause teratogenic defects that result in hydrocephalus if they are ingested in large enough quantities by ewes during pregnancy.[6] Acquired hydrocephalus is rare in small ruminants but can potentially result from inflammation of the arachnoid villi. This can occur as a result of vitamin A deficiency and meningitis because these conditions interfere with the absorption of CSF by the arachnoid villi. Trauma resulting in obstruction and neoplastic masses also are potential causes of hydrocephalus. In obstructive hydrocephalus, pressure from accumulating CSF and ventricular enlargement may result in disruption of the pellucid septum; atrophy of associated structures, including subcortical white matter; and optic radiations.[7]

Hydranencephaly

The pathophysiology behind hydranencephaly is not completely understood. The disease has several recognized causes, including bony malformation with hypoplasia of tissue, degeneration associated with ischemia, and inflammation or injury that results in the destruction of neural tissue.[1] Whatever the cause, the effects on the neural tissue result in a loss of dorsolateral ventricular ependyma, thinning of the white matter, and porencephalic cyst formation. The space that is left from the absent tissue is then filled with CSF. Because CSF pressure (normotensive) in the cranium does not increase during fetal development, affected animals rarely have enlarged craniums. Many viral organisms that infect sheep and goats during pregnancy produce in utero infections that cause degenerative changes in neuronal tissues during their development.

Akabane virus belongs to a family of single-stranded ribonucleic acid (RNA) viruses that are transmitted by arthropods. It is responsible for causing arthrogryposis with hydrocephalus and hydranencephaly in lambs. The virus is considered exotic to North America but is present in Australia, Japan, Israel, and Korea. The virus multiplies in extra-fetal tissues in the host, producing viremia of 1 to 9 days' duration.[8] During this time an arthropod can bite the host and transmit the virus to another if sufficient viremia is present. After the host is infected and develops viremia, transplacental infection of the endothelial cells of the placenta occurs, followed by sustained replication in the trophoblastic cells of the fetus.[8] The placentome appears to be an essential route for hematogenous spread of virus from the dam to the fetus,[9] and the timing of infection seems to be an important factor in determining whether the fetus develops congenital abnormalities.

If the dam is infected with Akabane virus around day 30 or 31 of gestation (before the fetus develops immunocompetence at days 65 to 70), the fetus will develop neurologic damage. At day 30 the chorioallantoic membrane is formed, as is the interdigitation of the fetal cotyledon with the maternal caruncle. The virus appears to spread rapidly to the fetus at this time. The most severe lesions are found in a fetus that is infected during the early stages of organogenesis after placental attachment and before the development of immunocompetence. During this time vulnerable cell populations are dividing rapidly, especially in the central nervous system.[10] The extent of fetal malformation determines whether the fetus can be sustained in utero to term. The virus has a predilection to accumulate in neural tissue and skeletal muscle. Neonates tend to exhibit primarily nonsuppurative encephalomyelitis and polymyositis. Hydranencephaly results from necrosis of the subventricular zones in the cerebrum that prevent the outward migration of neuroblasts; the areas of necrosis then quickly become filled with CSF. Because sheep attain immunocompetence at day 70 of gestation, they are often born without the virus. Arthrogryposis appears to be a consequence of a primary necrotizing polymyositis, with viral replication occurring in the myotubule during the early stages of gestation and myofiber development.[9]

Bluetongue virus is a double-stranded RNA virus that is a member of the genus *Orbivirus* and family *Reoviridae*. Vaccination of pregnant ewes with modified live vaccines and natural infections during gestation are responsible for cerebral malformations, including hydranencephaly. An arthropod vector, most notably *Culicoides* species, transmits the virus. It is primarily endemic in tropical areas, where warm, moist climates prevail; however, it has been reported in the United States in association with vaccination using modified live virus.[11] A variety of clinical signs can occur in infected sheep, but the discussion here is confined to the deformities it produces in the fetus.

The type of fetal deformity observed depends on the stage of gestation during which the ewe becomes infected. Fetal lambs that are between 55 to 60 days of gestation do not have neurons or glial cells, only precursor cells in the subependymal plates that begin to migrate to the peripheral cortex.[12] Bluetongue virus causes cytotropic changes in the undifferentiated cells and results in a necrotizing encephalopathy with cavitation hydranencephaly and retinal dysplasia. Infections that occur between 70 and 80 days of gestation result in porencephaly or cerebral cysts, but no ocular lesions. After 100 days of gestation, infection results in focal areas of meningoencephalitis without destructive lesions.

Pestivirus infections in pregnant ewes also have been implicated in causing hydranencephaly in fetuses. Both border disease (BD) and bovine viral diarrhea virus (BVDV) belong to this family. BD and BVDV in sheep cause several pathologic problems that result in abortions, infertility, and deformities in lambs. Sheep that are infected with BD virus develop a short transitory viremia that apparently is self-limiting and then become immune to reinfection. It is transmitted both vertically and horizontally by the secretions of infected seronegative animals that act as reservoirs in a flock.

Hydranencephalic lambs affected with BD are born with normal-sized heads, fine fleece, and no obvious tremors; some may have arthrogryposis. Grossly the cerebral hemispheres are composed of a thin, delicate membrane that is filled with fluid and attached to the meninges. The olfactory lobes, basal ganglia, hippocampus, and mesencephalon may all be normal.[13] The lesions that occur in BD-infected fetuses with hydranencephaly result from necrosis and inflammation in ependyma. Histopathologically, BD is associated with hypomyelination, which is believed to result from the virus somehow diverting glial cell precursors away from myelin-forming oligodendroglial cells.[13] BD also inhibits the thyroid gland from producing thyroid hormone, which is necessary for proper myelin formation. Thyroidectomized fetal lambs have been experimentally demonstrated at parturition to have hydranencephaly.[14]

Cache valley virus (CVV) causes outbreaks of lambs born with congenital arthrogryposis and hydrocephalus or hydranencephaly throughout the United States. It is a bunyavirus and is spread by arthropods in a similar manner to Akabane virus. Although the clinical signs exhibited by animals infected with CVV are similar to those seen in BD and infection with BVDV, arthrogryposis is a consistent feature of this disease that is rare in animals infected with the other two types of viruses.[15] The lesions observed both grossly and histologically are indistinguishable from those caused by Akabane virus.

Sporadic reports implicate a variety of factors that can result in hydranencephaly. Nutritional deficiencies of copper and thiamine produce hydranencephaly in fetuses. In sheep and goats with PEM, thrombosis of the middle cerebral artery leads to infarction of a large portion of the cerebrum, which causes CSF to accumulate in the area of necrotic tissue.[1] One report describes a concurrent in utero infection of a fetal lamb with *Toxoplasma gondii* and *E. coli* that resulted in hydranencephaly.[16]

TABLE 11-8

PLANTS ASSOCIATED WITH NEUROLOGIC DISEASES*

DISEASE	PLANT	SYMPTOMS
Paralysis	*Astragalus, Oxytropis*—locoweed	Emaciation, proprioceptive deficits, staggering, paralysis
	Delphinium—larkspur	Rapid onset, nervous muscle twitching, paralysis, death
Seizures or central nervous system stimulation	*Apocynum*—Indian hemp	Convulsions, weakness, coma
	Asclepias—milkweed	Convulsions, coma, death
	Cicuta—water hemlock	Rapid onset, extremely toxic, convulsions, muscle spasms, grinding teeth, coma, death
	Conium—poison hemlock	Trembling, incoordination, respiratory paralysis
	Corydalis—fitweed	Rapid onset, ataxia, seizures, twitching facial muscles, chewing movements
	Delphinium—larkspur	Excitability, staggering, vomiting, convulsions
	Lupinus—lupines	Nervousness, convulsions, coma
Central nervous system stimulation and depression or mixed central nervous effects	*Aesculus*—buckeye, horse chestnut	Vomiting, ataxia, trembling, convulsions, hyperesthesia, excitement or depression
	Datura—Jimson weed	Ataxia, tremors, hallucinations, mydriasis, tachycardia, tachypnea
	Eupatorium—white snakeroot	Trembling in the muzzle and legs after exercise, weakness, difficulty breathing
	Haplopappus—rayless goldenrod	Depression, stiff gait, trembling, weakness, recumbency, coma, death
	Kalmia, Rhododendron—mountain laurel, rhododendron, azaleas	Convulsions, vomiting, weakness, paralysis, death
	Leucothoe—fetterbush	Incoordination, vomiting, weakness, spasm, coma, death
	Lupinus—lupines	Nervousness, depression, twitching, convulsions, death
	Ricinus—castor bean	Diarrhea, dullness, weakness, trembling, incoordination
	Solanaceae—ground cherry, nightshade, horsenettle, soda apple	Depression, mydriasis, bradycardia, incoordination
	Veratrum—false hellebore	Vomiting, arrhythmias, weakness, convulsions, coma
	Zigadenus—death camus	Weakness, staggering, convulsions, coma, excess salivation
Depression or weakness	*Halogeton*	Rapid and shallow breathing, coma
	Helenium—sneezeweed, bitterweed	Depression, weakness, chronic vomiting
	Hymenoxys—rubberweed	Depression, weakness, bloat, green nasal discharge
	Oxytenia—copperweed	Depression, weakness, coma
	Sarcobatus—greasewood	Dullness, nasal discharge, drooling, weakness
	Tetradymia—horsebrush	Depression, weakness, swelling around head, peeling skin

*Cyanogenetic plants such as *Triglochin* (arrowgrass) and *Prunus* (wild cherry), as well as plants that contain nitrates, may cause signs that mimic neurologic deficits. Treatment of animals that have ingested any of these toxic plants should include oral charcoal (0.5 kg PO) and diazepam (0.25 to 0.5 mg/kg) to control seizures, maintenance of hydration status, and nutritional support.

Clinical signs. The clinical signs in animals with hydrocephalus and hydranencephaly are similar and can vary depending on severity and whether the animal has bilateral or unilateral cerebral involvement. Neonates are often born dead or die shortly after birth. If they are born alive and are unable to stand, the animals often succumb to septicemia because of an inability to nurse. If they survive more than a few months, they display poor growth characteristics and have difficulty keeping up with the herd and socializing. The mental status of the animals can range from depressed to comatose, and the animals' craniums may be grossly enlarged with open fontanelles. Motor disturbances include spastic paresis, strabismus, conscious proprioceptive deficits, ataxia, tremors, and blindness. Unilateral involvement of one cerebral hemisphere results in a head tilt, circling, and unilateral hyperreflexia.

REFERENCES

1. de Lahunta A: Cranial nerve—lower motor neuron: general somatic efferent system, special visceral efferent system. In de Lahunta A, editor: *Veterinary neuroanatomy and clinical neurology,* Philadelphia, 1983, WB Saunders.
2. Leipold HW, Dennis SM: Examination of the bovine nervous system, *Vet Clin North Am Food Anim Pract* 3:163, 1987.
3. Icenogle DA, Kaplan AM: A review of congenital neurologic malformations, *Clin Pediatr* 20:565, 1981.
4. George LW: Diseases of the nervous system. In Smith BP, editor: Large animal internal medicine, St Louis, 1996, Mosby.
5. Pritchard GC et al: Multiple cases of Dandy-Walker malformation in three sheep flocks, *Vet Rec* 135:163, 1994.
6. James LF et al: Effect of natural toxins on reproduction, *Vet Clin North Am Food Anim Pract* 10:587, 1994.
7. Braund KG: Neurologic examination and diagnostic plan. In Oliver JE et al, editors: *Veterinary neurology,* Philadelphia, 1987, WB Saunders.
8. Charles JA: Akabane virus, *Vet Clin North Am Food Anim Pract* 10:525, 1994.
9. Parsonson IM, Della-Porta AJ, Snowdon WA: Akabane virus infection in the pregnant ewe. 2. Pathology of the fetus, *Vet Micro* 6:209, 1981.
10. Kirkland PD et al: The development of Akabane virus–induced congenital abnormalities in cattle, *Vet Rec* 122:582, 1988.
11. Osborn BI, Silverstein AM: Hydranencephaly, porencephaly, cerebral cyst, retinal dysplasia, CNS malformations, *Am J Path* 67:211, 1972.
12. Osborn BI: Bluetongue virus, *Vet Clin North Am Food Anim Pract* 10:547, 1994.
13. Barlow RM: Morphogenesis of hydranencephaly and other intracranial malformations in progeny of pregnant ewes infected with pestiviruses, *J Comp Path* 90:87, 1980.
14. McIntosh GH: Foetal thyroidectomy and hydranencephaly in lambs, *Aust Vet J* 54:408, 1978.
15. Edwards JF et al: Ovine arthrogryposis and central nervous system malformations associated with in utero cache valley virus infection: spontaneous disease, *Vet Path* 26:33, 1989.
16. Woods LW, Anderson ML: Scoliosis and hydrocephalus in an ovine fetus infected with *Toxoplasma gondii, J Vet Diagn Invest* 4:220, 1992.

OTHER NEUROLOGIC DISEASES

Neurologic diseases seen in small ruminants have many other causes. These include lidocaine toxicity (see Chapter 16), hypermagnesemia and hypocalcemia (see Chapter 2), hypovitaminosis A (see Chapter 12), and heat stress (see Chapter 6). Toxic plants also can cause neurologic dysfunction. Some of these are listed in Table 11-8. Grasses associated with staggers or ataxia are described in Table 11-9. Table 11-10 covers many of the inherited storage diseases seen in sheep and goats.

TABLE 11-9

GRASS STAGGERS

PLANT	TOXIN	SIGNS	CONTROL
Perennial ryegrass (*Lolium perenne*)	Fungus produces tremorgenic toxin	Trembling, stiff gait, hypermetria of limbs; worsens when excited; animals collapse, struggle, and then recover	Remove from toxic pasture; ammoniation of hay cut from affected pasture may reduce toxicity
Annual ryegrass (*Lolium rigidum*)	Corynetoxin (?)	Trembling, stiff gait, hypermetria of limbs; worsens when excited; animals collapse, stagger, and then recover	Toxin concentrated in seed head and during warm season; therefore mowing or burning reduces toxicity
Bermuda grass (*Cynodon dactylon*)	Alkaloid	Tremors	Mow
Dallas grass, Bahia (*Paspalum* species)	Ergot ("honey rust" on seed head)	Head tremors, muscle fasciculations, ataxia	Toxin concentrates on seed head; mow or burn pastures that have seeded out

TABLE 11-10

INHERITED LYSOSOMAL STORAGE DISEASES OF SHEEP AND GOATS

DISEASE	BREEDS	INHERITANCE AFFECTED	CLINICAL	DIAGNOSIS
β-Mannosidosis	Nubians, Nubian crosses	Autosomal recessive	• Unable to stand • Carpal contraction • Hindlimb extension • Pastern hyperextension • Intention tremors • Nystagmus • Deafness • Bilateral Horner's syndrome • Domed head • Thickened skin	• Reduced plasma β-mannosidase activity • Abnormal oligosaccharides in urine • Histopathology • Vacuolization of neurons and other cells • Demyelinization
GM_1 gangliosidosis Generalized glycogenosis β-Galactosidase deficiency	Suffolks	Autosomal recessive	• Normal at birth • Ataxic at 4 to 6 months • Prostrate within 2 months	• Histopathology • Vacuolization • Marked distension of neuronal cytoplasm, periportal hepatocytes, and renal epithelial cells
Globoid cell leukodystrophy Krabbe's disease Galactocerebrosidosis	Polled Dorsets	Believed to be autosomal recessive	• Pelvic limb incoordination progressing to tetraplegia destruction	• Decreased brain galactocerebrosidase activity • Histopathology • Myelin • Loss of oligodendroglia • Astrogliosis • Accumulation of PAS*-positive globoid cells

Modified from Kumar K et al: Caprine β-mannosidosis: phenotypic features, *Vet Rec* 118:325, 1986; Smith MC, Sherman DM: Nervous system. In Smith MC, Sherman DM, editors: *Goat medicine,* Philadelphia, 1994, Lea & Febiger; Jolly RD: Lysosomal storage diseases in livestock, *Vet Clin North Am Food Anim Pract* 9:41, 1993; George LW: Diseases of the nervous system. In Smith BP, editor: *Large animal internal medicine,* ed 2, St Louis, 1996, Mosby; Murnane RD, Ahern-Rindell AJ, Prieur DJ: Ovine GM_1 gangliosidosis, *Small Rumin Res* 6:109, 1991; Pritchard DH, Napthine DV, Sinclair AJ: Globoid cell leukodystrophy in polled Dorset sheep, *Vet Path* 17:399, 1980.
*Periodic acid–Schiff reaction.

Chapter 12

Diseases of the Eye

BRYAN M. WALDRIDGE AND CARMEN M.H. COLITZ

OCULAR ANATOMY

Understanding the normal anatomy of the eye is important when attempting to identify abnormalities. Few phylogenetic differences occur among species. Eyes have largely retained the same basic components and embryologic development over the course of evolution. Variations are additive to the basic design and have occurred largely because of ecological factors such as light intensity and duration and feeding habits.[1] Goats and sheep are arrhythmic ruminants—they are equally active diurnally and nocturnally.

Adnexa

Orbit. Sheep and goats have an enclosed orbit, typical of most grazing animals. Both species have lacrimal, zygomatic, frontal, sphenoid, and palatine bones comprising the bony fossa of the orbit. In addition, sheep have a maxillary bone and goats have an ethmoid bone that forms part of the orbit. The size, shape, and position of the orbit are closely associated with visual activity and feeding behavior.[1] In general, prey species such as sheep and goats have eyes that are located more laterally on the skull and have mostly monocular vision.[1] Nerves and blood vessels travel into the orbital region by the rostral alar, ethmoidal, lacrimal, orbital, ovale, optic, rotundum, and supraorbital foramina or fissures. The pterygopalatine region has nerves and vessels associated with the orbit as well, including the caudal palatine, maxillary, and sphenopalatine foramina. Glands of the infraorbital sinus are present only in sheep and are better developed in rams than in ewes. These are specialized cutaneous glands that produce pheromones; their secretions exit from the infraorbital sinus in a depression just rostral to the eye.[2]

Orbital fascia and fat. The globe is surrounded by three fascial layers. The periorbita is the most external layer and is attached near the optic foramen and the apex of the muscle cone at the exit of the optic nerve from the orbit.[3] The superficial muscular fascia lies within the periorbita and encloses the lacrimal gland and the levator palpebrae superiors. The deep muscular fascia is more fibrous than the other two fascial layers and originates at the superior and inferior palpebrae and from the limbus. It sheaths the extraocular muscles and optic nerve.[3] The orbital fat fills the orbital dead space and provides a cushion that protects the globe and extraocular muscles.

Extraocular muscles. Seven extraocular muscles suspend the globe and move the eye. The four rectus muscles include the dorsal, ventral, medial, and lateral recti; they move the globe in the direction indicated by their names. The recti originate from the orbital apex. The dorsal oblique originates from the medial orbital apex, passes anteriorly on the dorsomedial wall of the orbit, and is then deflected around the trochlea to insert on the dorsolateral aspect of the globe beneath the tendon of the dorsal rectus muscle.[3] The trochlea is a cartilaginous pulley that is attached to the anterior aspect of the medial wall of the orbit.[4] The dorsal oblique muscle rotates the dorsal aspect of the globe medially and ventrally. The ventral oblique muscle originates from a depression in the ventromedial wall of the orbit, specifically the anterolateral margin of the palatine bone. It passes laterally beneath the globe, crossing the ventral rectus tendon before inserting on the ventrolateral aspect of the globe.[1,3] The ventral oblique muscle moves the globe medially and dorsally. The retractor bulbi muscle originates from the orbital apex and inserts posterior to the equator beneath the recti muscles, forming an almost complete cone around the optic nerve. The retractor bulbi muscle retracts the globe for additional protection. The oculomotor nerve (cranial nerve III) innervates the dorsal, ventral, and medial recti. The dorsal oblique is innervated by the trochlear nerve (cranial nerve IV), and the lateral rectus and retractor bulbi muscles are innervated by the abducens nerve (cranial nerve VI).

Eyelids and conjunctiva. The superior and inferior palpebrae (eyelids) are two musculofibrous folds of thin skin continuous with the facial skin. The superior eyelid is more mobile than the inferior eyelid. The opening formed by the free edges of the eyelids is the palpebral fissure.[1,3,4] Histologically, the eyelids have four tissue layers: the skin, the orbicularis oculi muscle, the tarsus and stromal layer, and the palpebral conjunctiva. The palpebral skin is thin and elastic and is covered by a dense coat of short hairs with small tubular and sebaceous glands. The superior palpebrae have a row of cilia, and vibrissae are present a short distance from the superior and inferior palpebral margins in goats and sheep. The arrectores ciliorum are bundles of smooth muscle fibers that extend from the eyelash follicles toward the tarsus and are present in ruminants, but not in carnivores.[1] The superior palpebral skin receives sensory innervation by the ophthalmic branch of the trigeminal nerve (cranial nerve V), and the inferior palpebral skin is innervated by the maxillary branch of the trigeminal nerve. The orbicularis oculi muscle encircles the entire palpebral fissure and functions to close the palpebral fissure. It receives motor innervation by the palpebral branch of the facial nerve (cranial nerve VII). The superior eyelid is elevated by the levator palpebrae superioris muscle, which receives motor innervation from the oculomotor nerve. The levator palpebrae superioris originates at the orbital apex and extends along the dorsal half of the mid-stroma. The sympathetically innervated Müller's muscle complements the function of the levator palpebrae superioris. Other muscles that are associated with eyelid function include the corrugator supercilii muscle, which assists in elevating the superior eyelid, and the retractor anguli oculi muscle, which lengthens the lateral palpebral fissure. Both of these muscles are innervated by the facial nerve. The tarsus is a poorly developed narrow layer of dense collagenous connective tissue that separates the eyelid muscles from the palpebral conjunctiva. The tarsus is continuous with the septum orbitale in both the superior and inferior palpebrae. The septum orbitale is attached to the periosteum of the bony orbital rim.[5] Near the margin of both eyelids are the tarsal gland openings. The tarsal glands are sebaceous glands that produce the lipid component of the preocular tear film. These glands open onto the edge of both eyelids through small openings arranged longitudinally. The tarsal glands are parasympathetically innervated by the oculomotor nerve.[1] The palpebral conjunctiva is the mucous membrane that lines the inner aspect of the eyelids. It consists of stratified columnar epithelium that becomes more stratified and squamous as it nears the eyelid margin. The stratified columnar epithelia have numerous goblet cells that contribute to the mucus

layer of the preocular tear film. The palpebral conjunctiva continues onto the globe as the bulbar conjunctiva where it meets and is continuous with the corneal epithelium. The palpebral and bulbar conjunctivae meet at the fornix, and this region is lined with stratified cuboidal epithelium. The potential space created by the conjunctivae is the cul-de-sac. The palpebral, bulbar, and nictitans conjunctivae are named based on their anatomic locations, but they are continuous. The vascular supply to the conjunctiva is from the anterior ciliary arteries (branches of the external ophthalmic artery).[1] Ventromedially, the lacrimal caruncle is seen as a small mucosal elevation that may or may not be pigmented.

The nictitating membrane (third eyelid, nictitans) is located ventromedially between the lacrimal caruncle and the globe. It is completely lined by conjunctiva and contains a T-shaped cartilaginous plate with a gland (gland of the nictitating membrane or nictitans) at its base. The horizontal part of the T lies at the free edge of the fold. The gland of the nictitating membrane surrounds the stem of the cartilage. The anterior and posterior aspects of the nictitating membrane are lined with nonkeratinized stratified squamous epithelium. The nictitating membrane moves passively over the eye in a dorsolateral direction when the globe is retracted by contraction of the retractor oculi muscle and displacement of the orbital fat.[1]

Lacrimal and Nasolacrimal Systems

The lacrimal system consists of the lacrimal gland, the gland of the third eyelid, the accessory glands of Krause and Wolfring, the glands of Zeis, the tarsal glands, and the nasolacrimal duct system.[1,3,4] The lacrimal gland lies in the dorsolateral wall of the orbit between the dorsolateral wall of the orbit and the globe. Histologically, the lacrimal gland of the sheep and goat is a compound tubuloalveolar mixed gland.[6,7] The lacrimal gland receives its blood supply from the lacrimal artery. The lacrimal nerve sends sensory innervation to the gland, and the secretory portion of the gland is sympathetically innervated by postganglionic fibers from the cranial cervical ganglion. Two large and four to five small excretory ducts originate from the central surface of the lacrimal gland in both sheep and goats.[7] The lacrimal fluid drains into the dorsal fornix of the conjunctival sac and mixes with the secretions of the accessory glands.[3] The glands of Zeis and the tarsal glands produce the outer lipid layer of the preocular tear film. The lacrimal gland, the gland of the third eyelid, and the accessory glands of Krause and Wolfring produce the middle aqueous component of the preocular tear film. The inner mucin layer is produced by the conjunctival goblet cells.[1] The three layers of the preocular tear film are continuously spread across the eye's surface by the eyelids and nictitating membrane during blinking. Unlike cattle, sheep and goats have lysozyme, an antibacterial enzyme, in their tears.[8] Excess preocular tear film pools in the lacrimal lake at the ventromedial angle of the eye. Mechanical pumping action draws the tear fluid into the superior and inferior puncta lacrimale (lacrimal puncta). The puncta are located on the palpebral conjunctiva, just inside the edge of the eyelid and medial to the last tarsal gland.[1] Smooth muscle in the puncta contract during blinking to remove pooled tear fluid. The superior and inferior lacrimal puncta continue as the superior and inferior canaliculi. The canaliculi coalesce at the nasolacrimal sac located in the lacrimal fossa of the lacrimal bone.[1] The lacrimal sac empties into the nasolacrimal duct, which initially continues rostrally through the osseous lacrimal canal and the osseous lacrimal groove of the maxilla. It then parallels the mucous membrane of the middle meatus and opens on the nasal mucous membrane at the junction of pigmented and nonpigmented skin.[7]

Vascular Supply of the Eye

In domestic mammals the majority of the ocular and adnexal vascular supply is from the external ophthalmic artery, a branch of the maxillary artery. The arteries supplying the globe originate from the external ophthalmic and the malar artery, a smaller branch of the maxillary artery. The nasal and lateral long posterior ciliary arteries (LPCAs) branch off of the external ophthalmic arteries. The lateral and nasal LPCAs branch to the choroid and ciliary processes; in the periphery, each LPCA divides again into dorsal and ventral branches that form the major arterial circle of the iris. The LPCAs give off the short posterior ciliary arteries (SPCAs). The SPCAs penetrate the globe adjacent to the optic nerve to supply the inner layers of the retina and then ramify into the choroidal vasculature. The SPCAs also branch to the perilimbal region and the anterior ciliary body. The smaller internal ophthalmic artery supplies the optic nerve and anastomoses with the external ophthalmic artery or one of its branches.[1] The external ophthalmic artery then gives off two muscular branches: the ventral and the dorsal branches. These branches supply the extraorbital muscles, the gland of the nictitating membrane, the lacrimal gland, and the levator palpebrae superiors.

Globe

The globe (bulbus oculi) is nearly spherical in shape. The average anterior to posterior axis of the sheep globe is 26.85 mm; that of the goat globe has not been reported. The globe is composed of three tunics or coats: the fibrous, vascular, and nervous tunics. The external fibrous tunic is made up of dense collagenous connective tissue that resists the eye's internal pressure and gives the globe its round shape. The fibrous tunic is composed of the cornea and sclera, which coalesce at the corneoscleral junction or limbus. The middle vascular tunic is comprised of the uvea, which includes the iris, ciliary body,

and choroid. The inner nervous tunic includes the retina and optic nerve. The three tunics surround the aqueous humor, lens, and vitreous humor.

Fibrous Tunic

Cornea.   The cornea is the transparent, avascular, and colorless anterior 20% of the fibrous tunic. It is composed of dense collagenous connective tissue arranged in a regular lamellar pattern. This lamellar pattern, combined with the physiologic pump of the posterior epithelium, maintains the cornea's transparency and deturgescence. The nonkeratinized anterior surface epithelium and the small diameter of the collagen fibrils also contribute to the cornea's transparency.[9]

The cornea is the most powerful refractive surface of the eye. In sheep and goats the shape of the cornea is elliptical, with its horizontal diameter greater than its vertical diameter. In sheep the average width of the cornea is 22.4 mm and the average height is 15.4 mm.[1] The sheep cornea is thickest at its center (0.8 to 2.0 mm) and thinnest at its edge (0.3 to 0.5 mm).[1] The cornea is innervated by the long ciliary nerves, which derive from the ophthalmic branch of the trigeminal nerve.

In domestic animals the cornea has four layers. The anterior, nonkeratinized, stratified, squamous epithelium (epithelium corneae) covers the outermost corneal surface and is continuous with the conjunctival epithelium. The most posterior layer of the anterior epithelium consists of a monolayer of columnar basal cells that lie on a thin basement membrane. The basement membrane of the anterior epithelium is made up of primarily types IV, VI, and VII collagen.[1] Anterior to the basal layer are numerous layers of polyhedral or wing cells, and anterior to these are numerous layers of nonkeratinized squamous epithelial cells. Hemidesmosomes, arranged in a linear manner, attach the basal cells to the basal lamina of the basement membrane (lamina limitans).[1,4] The stroma (substantia propria) forms the bulk of the cornea (90%). The stroma is composed of extracellular matrix and a lamellar arrangement of collagen fibrils oriented in parallel lamellae positioned at oblique angles to each other and separated by less than a wavelength of light.[10] Interwoven between the collagen fibrils and extracellular matrix are keratocytes. Keratocytes possess cellular extensions that help maintain the stromal lamellae. After a deep corneal injury, keratocytes can differentiate into fibroblasts and contribute to scar formation.[1] Descemet's membrane (lamina elastica), located on the posterior aspect of the cornea, is homogeneous and acellular and functions as a protective boundary within the cornea. It is produced throughout life by the corneal endothelium and is made up of types I, III, IV, V, VI, and VIII collagen. Descemet's membrane terminates at the apex of the trabecular meshwork in the area of the limbus.[1] The endothelium is a monolayer of flattened polygonal cells lining the most posterior aspect of the cornea. In the adult the endothelium rarely undergoes mitosis and has an age-dependent loss of endothelial cells.

Lens. The lens further focuses light entering the eye to allow for sharp focus of visualized images. The lens is a transparent, biconvex, almost spherical structure that is located posterior to the iris and anterior to the vitreous. It is held in position by the zonular ligaments (zonula ciliaris) that arise from the ciliary epithelium and are composed of fibrillin.[11] Other structures that support the lens include the patellar fossa of the vitreous and the iris. Herbivorous animals have a marginally functional accommodative mechanism and therefore have poor near vision.

The lens is transparent and avascular and receives the majority of its nutrients from the aqueous humor. The lens grows throughout life at a slow, regulated rate because of continued division and differentiation of the lens epithelial cells into lens fiber cells. The average diameter of the sheep lens is between 14.5 to 15.53 mm; it weighs approximately 2.3 g.[1]

The lens is enveloped in a basement membrane of primarily type IV collagen. The anterior lens capsule is significantly thicker than the posterior lens capsule and thickens with age. The lens capsule is produced by the lens epithelial cells, which are only present on the anterior aspect of the lens. The lens epithelial cell population is made up of three regions. The most central cells are squamous in appearance and rarely undergo mitosis. The cells in the germinative region, which encircles the central epithelium, are more cuboidal in appearance and undergo mitosis at a slow rate. The lens epithelial cells in the equatorial region elongate into lens fiber cells, lose their nuclei by a process called denucleation, and attach at the anterior and posterior lens sutures. The fiber cells are continually being formed—the newest fiber cells are located peripherally and the oldest become the most centralized and compressed lens fibers. Nearly 80% of glucose metabolism in the lens occurs primarily by glycolysis. The tricarboxylic cycle accounts for 5%, the pentose monophosphate shunt accounts for 15%, and the sorbitol pathway accounts for a negligible portion of glucose metabolism.

Vitreous. The vitreous also refracts light that enters the eye and passes through the lens to focus light on the retina. The vitreous is gel-like and lies posterior to the lens and anterior to the retina. The vitreous is 98% water that is suspended in collagen fibers and glycosaminoglycan matrix. The vitreous body physically holds the retina against the choroid. No continuous turnover of the vitreous occurs.

Sclera. The sclera comprises the posterior 80% of the fibrous tunic. The sclera differs from the cornea in three basic ways. The collagen fibrils of the sclera are irregularly arranged. The scleral epithelium is thicker than the corneal epithelium. It has small basal cells with scanty cytoplasm.[1] Scleral thickness at the entry point of the optic nerve in the sheep is 1.0 to 1.2 mm. It thins at the equator to 0.25 to 0.30 mm and thickens at the corneoscleral junction to 0.4 to 0.5 mm.[1]

Vascular Tunic (Tunica Vasculosa Oculi)

The vascular tunic is comprised of the iris, ciliary body, and choroid. These structures are highly vascularized and usually pigmented.

Iris. The iris is the smallest component of the uvea. It is a muscular diaphragm suspended between the cornea and the lens. It is attached to the sclera at its periphery by the pectinate ligaments and to the ciliary body. The iris divides the space between the cornea and the lens into the anterior and posterior chambers of the anterior segment. Its central aspect has an aperture, the pupil (pupillae), that changes in size to adjust the amount of light entering the eye and reaching the retina. The muscles that regulate pupil size are the sphincter pupillae and the dilator pupillae. The sphincter muscle lies concentrically near the pupillary margin and the dilator muscle has fibers arranged radially from the sphincter to the ciliary border. The pupil is oval in a horizontal plane in sheep and goats and has several round, variably sized black masses at the superior and inferior aspects of the pupillary border called *granula iridica*. The granula iridica are extensions of the posterior pigmented epithelium of the iris. They enhance the effect of pupillary constriction or miosis. In goats the myocytes of the sphincter muscle are occasionally found in the basal portion of the granula iridica.[1]

The iris is grossly divided into two regions divided by the collarette. The central region is the pupillary zone, and the peripheral region is the ciliary zone. The peripheral half of the ciliary zone contains a circumferential artery, the annular major arterial circle. The major arterial circle is an incomplete circle that originates from the dorsal and ventral branches of the medial and lateral LPCAs. The major arterial circle branches into radial arteries that nourish the rest of the iris. Radial vessels provide venous drainage for the iris. They empty directly into the anterior choroidal circulation.

The three cellular layers of the iris are the anterior border layer, the middle stroma (which contains the sphincter muscle), and the posterior epithelial layers. The anterior border layer consists of fibroblasts and melanocytes, and their processes form an incomplete layer across the surface of the iris. No continuous layer of epithelium extends across the iris's anterior surface.[1] The iris stroma is loosely arranged and consists of fibroblasts, fine collagenous fibers, chromatophores, and melanocytes. Iris color depends on the density of the pigmentation in the stroma. The iris sphincter muscle of sheep and goats is probably very similar to that of the horse, another ungulate with an oval pupil in a horizontal direction. In the horse the iris sphincter lies in the main portion of the central stroma and is covered by the granula iridica.[1] It is parasympathetically innervated. The iris dilator muscle is located in the posterior aspect of the iris stroma. It is innervated by sympathetic fibers and is continuous with the pigmented epithelium of the ciliary body. The posterior pigmented epithelium of the iris is continuous with the nonpigmented epithelium of the ciliary body. Both the iris dilator muscle and the posterior pigmented epithelium form the granula iridica in herbivores. The size of the dilator muscle in the sheep and goat is probably similar to that of the horse.[1]

Ciliary body (corpus ciliare). The ciliary body is the middle portion of the uvea that joins the choroid (posterior uvea) to the peripheral iris (anterior uvea). It consists of two sections: the anterior pars plicata (corona ciliaris) and the posterior pars plana. The pars plicata consists of radial folds called *ciliary processes* that are "thick and club-like with shallow valleys in herbivores."[12] The ciliary processes connect the zonular fibers to the lens equator that holds the lens in place. In ungulates the processes have numerous arterioles and veins within the processes' core. The ciliary processes also have well-developed capillary beds that produce the majority of the aqueous humor.[1] The pars plana is the flat portion of the ciliary body that terminates in the pars ciliaris retinae, the junction of the ciliary body and the retina. The pars plana varies in width because the retina extends more anteriorly medially and inferiorly in most species. Aside from the ciliary processes the ciliary muscles comprise the majority of the ciliary body. The ciliary musculature is composed of meridional smooth muscle fibers coursing close to the sclera. This musculature is poorly developed in ungulates, accounting for their poor accommodative ability. Evolution has allowed herbivores to develop large corneas, horizontally oval-shaped pupils, and large anterior chambers for better night vision and good motion detection. However, these evolutionary changes also have led to the loss of ciliary musculature development.

Iridocorneal angle. The iridocorneal angle (ICA) is the most anterior aspect of the ciliary body. The most anterior region of the ICA is the termination of Descemet's membrane.[13] The ICA is bordered by the limbus, the base of the iris, and the ciliary cleft. The ciliary cleft is a triangular region that is the posterolateral extension of the anterior chamber into the ciliary body. Pectinate ligaments are present in the ciliary cleft from the pigmented limbus to the root of the iris.[1] The ICA and ciliary musculature of sheep and goats are similar to those of cattle. The outflow tract has a large ciliary cleft with prominent spaces of Fontana. The large, semi-oval corneoscleral tra-

becular meshwork and the uveal trabecular meshwork form a delineated angular aqueous plexus.[13] The ciliary cleft and pectinate ligaments are smaller in sheep and goats than in cattle and horses because of their smaller globe size. Aqueous humor can take two pathways to exit the eye: the conventional and the unconventional outflow pathway. The majority of aqueous humor exits the eye in most species by the conventional pathway. Specifically, following its production by the ciliary body, aqueous humor passes into the posterior chamber, through the pupil, into the anterior chamber, between the pectinate ligaments, through the trabecular meshwork, into the scleral venous plexus, and then the systemic circulation. Aqueous humor can also exit the eye by a number of ancillary pathways. It can drain anteriorly within the iridal stroma and across the cornea, it can flow posteriorly into the vitreous humor, or it can flow exteroposteriorly along a supraciliary-suprachoroidal space into the adjacent sclera.[1] The uveoscleral (unconventional) pathway is the most prominent of the ancillary routes of aqueous drainage. Aqueous humor is absorbed from the ciliary cleft into the anterior face of the ciliary body and diffuses into the sclera and the systemic venous circulation. The percentage of outflow by the uveoscleral pathway has been determined for many species but not for cattle, sheep, or goats. This outflow pathway is thought to be the major aqueous outflow pathway in the horse and may be a major pathway in other ungulates.

Choroid (choroidea). The choroid is a dense network of blood vessels and pigmented stroma between the retina and the sclera. The choroid supplies nutrition to the posterior layers of the retina. The total choroidal blood supply far exceeds the need for retinal nutrition and it may also serve as a heat exchange mechanism to prevent the retina from overheating. Morphologically the choroid can be divided into four layers: suprachoroidea, large-vessel layer, medium-sized vessel and tapetum layer, and choriocapillaris. The suprachoroidea is the potential space between the choroidal stroma and is attached loosely to the sclera by the lamina fusca. The LPCAs and nerves travel in the suprachoroidea along the horizontal meridian. The large-vessel layer (lamina vasculosa) is the posterior stromal layer. It has large cavernous vessels, primarily veins, that drain the choriocapillaris and some branches of the SPCA. The medium-sized vessel and tapetum layer is the anterior stromal layer of the choroid. It has smaller vessels connecting the choriocapillaris to the large-vessel layer. Within this inner stromal layer lies the tapetum. In ungulates the tapetum is fibrous (tapetum fibrosum) and composed of regularly arranged collagen fibers and occasional fibrocytes. Herbivores are born with mature eyes and well-developed tapeta. Sheep have several hundred layers of well-arranged collagen lamellae.[14] Capillaries penetrate the tapetum at right angles to the collagen lamellae, connecting the choriocapillaris to the medium-sized vessels; when visualized end-on, they are referred to as the "stars of Winslow."[1] The choriocapillaris is the single layer of capillaries between the choroidal stroma and the retinal pigmented epithelium (RPE). These capillaries are fenestrated, and external to their endothelium they have a basement membrane that forms the outermost layer of Bruch's membrane separating the choroid from the RPE.

Neural Tunic

The neural tunic includes the retina and optic nerve, both derivatives of the forebrain. The retina and optic nerve are the only portions of the brain that can be seen on a physical examination and can provide clinical information about an animal's physical status. The retinal vasculature, derivatives of the SPCAs, provides the inner layers of the retina with the majority of its nutrients. The choriocapillaris provides the outer layers of the retina with nutrients, and the vitreous plays a minor role in providing nutrition to the inner layers of the retina. The retinal metabolic rate is one of the highest in the body, and therefore if either the retinal or choroidal vasculature is even marginally compromised, the retina can become ischemic.[1]

The retina has 10 layers, the outermost of which is the RPE; the inner nine layers are known as the *sensory retina*. The five layers of clinical importance (from posterior to anterior) are as follows:

1. RPE
2. The photoreceptors
3. The inner nuclear layer (nuclei of the bipolar cells)
4. The ganglion cell layer
5. The nerve fiber layer (axons of the ganglion cells)

The photoreceptors include the rods and cones. Rods function in dim-light vision. Cones function in bright light and play roles in color recognition and visual acuity. Photoreceptors are composed of inner and outer segments. The outer segments have rhodopsin embedded in their membranes. Bipolar cells synapse with photoreceptors on one side and with ganglion cells on the opposite side. They transfer the electrical potential generated by the photoreceptors to the ganglion cells. The ganglion cells are the innermost cell layer of the retina. Projecting axons run parallel to the retinal surface in the innermost nerve fiber layer and converge at the optic disc. These axons turn posteriorly to form the optic nerve (cranial nerve II). Optic nerve fibers exit the eye through the lamina cribrosa. The density of the ganglion cells has been determined in the area centralis and visual streak of goats. The area centralis is the area of maximal cone density and the visual streak is the area of maximal ganglion cell density. The central retina of sheep is similar to that of other mammals with an area centralis and a single visual streak. Goats have an area centralis and also two

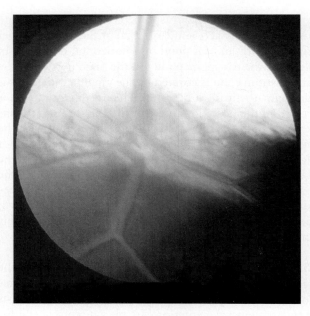

Figure 12-1   Normal fundus of a sheep.

visual streaks—a horizontal streak and a vertical streak.[15] The rod-to-cone ratio for sheep is 30:1 to 40:1.[16] No rod-to-cone ratio has been reported in goats. Both sheep and goats have two types of cones, allowing these animals dichromatic color vision.[17]

The RPE is a single layer of cells between the sensory retina and the choriocapillaris. It is nonpigmented in the dorsal half of the fundus, allowing the tapetum exposure to light. The primary functions of the RPE are metabolism of retinol for phototransduction and phagocytosis of waste products from the sensory retina. The RPE has tight interepithelial junctions that form part of the blood-retinal barrier.

Sheep and goat retinae have a holangiotic vascular pattern. The term *holangiotic* means that all quadrants of the retina are vascularized with vessels extending from the optic nerve to the periphery. Sheep retinae have three or four major venules and numerous branching arterioles. Occasionally the superior arteriole and venule wrap around each other. Goat retinae have five to eight primary venules.

The tapetal fundus is triangular, can be yellow to bluish-purple, and is stippled with the stars of Winslow. The dorsomedial tapetal fundus has more pigment than the other sections. The nontapetal fundus is pigmented because the RPE contains pigment and is located ventral to the tapetal fundus. The tapetal-nontapetal junction separates the two fundi. In sheep the optic nerve is located within the nontapetal fundus just ventral to this junction. Sheep have a kidney bean–shaped optic disc and goats have a rounder optic disc that is often located within the tapetal fundus (Figure 12-1). Goats also have a pigmented ring that surrounds the optic disc (Figure 12-2).[18]

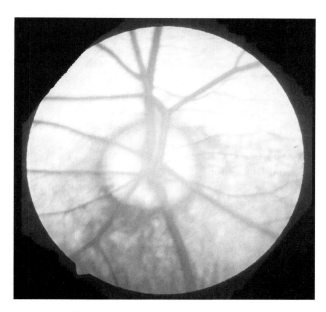

Figure 12-2 Normal fundus of a goat.

The optic nerve is composed of the axons of the retinal ganglion cells. The optic nerve is located ventrolateral to the posterior pole of the globe. It is myelinated in all species; in sheep and goats the myelin is maintained as the fibers enter the globe through the lamina cribrosa. The optic nerve has a small dark central depression called the *physiologic cup* or *pit*. The orbital portion of the optic nerve is enveloped in the thick dura mater and fuses anteriorly with the sclera. Internal to the dura mater is the arachnoid sheath, and within this layer is the pia mater. Herbivores, including sheep and goats, exhibit more than 80% decussation at the optic chiasm to form the optic tracts. Each optic tract is composed of pupillary and visual fibers. The pupillary fibers travel to the pretectal nucleus to control the pupillary light reflex (PLR), whereas the visual fibers travel to the lateral geniculate nucleus and then to the visual cortex for visual perception.

REFERENCES

1. Samuelson DA: Ophthalmic anatomy. In Gelatt KN, editor: *Veterinary ophthalmology,* ed 3, Philadelphia, 1999, Williams & Wilkins.
2. Shively MJ: Integumentary. In Shively MJ, editor: *Veterinary anatomy,* College Station, TX, 1984, Texas A & M University Press.
3. Dyce KM, Sack WO, Wensing CJG: The sense organs. In Dyce KM, Sack WO, Wensing CJG, editors: *Textbook of veterinary anatomy,* ed 2, Philadelphia, 1996, WB Saunders.
4. Sisson S, Grossman JD: The sense organs and common integument. In Grossman JD, editor: *The anatomy of domestic animals,* ed 4, Philadelphia, 1953, WB Saunders.
5. Martin CL, Anderson BG: Ocular anatomy. In Gelatt KN, editor: *Veterinary ophthalmology,* Philadelphia, 1981, Lea and Febiger.
6. Gargiulo AM et al: Ultrastructural study of sheep lacrimal glands, *Vet Res* 30(4):345, 1999.
7. Sinha RD, Calhoun ML: A gross, histologic, and histochemical study of the lacrimal apparatus of sheep and goats, *Am J Vet Res* 27(121):1633, 1966.
8. Brightman AH, Wachsstock RS, Erskine R: Lysozyme concentrations in the tears of cattle, goats and sheep, *Am J Vet Res* 52(1):9, 1991.
9. Whitley RD, Gilger BC: Diseases of the canine cornea and sclera. In Gelatt KN, editor: *Veterinary ophthalmology,* Philadelphia, 1999, Williams & Wilkins.
10. Maurice DM: The structure and transparency of the cornea, *J Physiol* 136:263, 1957.
11. Mir S et al: A comparative histologic study of the fibrillin microfibrillar system in the lens capsule of normal subjects and subjects with Marfan syndrome, *Invest Ophthalmol Vis Sci* 39(1):84, 1998.
12. Duke-Elder S: *The eyes of mammals in the eye of evolution,* St Louis, 1958, Mosby.
13. Samuelson DA: A reevaluation of the comparative anatomy of the eutherian iridocorneal angle and associated ciliary body musculature, *Vet Comp Ophthalmol* 6(3):153, 1996.
14. Bellairs R, Harkness LR, Harkness RD: The structure of the tapetum of the eye of the sheep, *Cell Tissue Res* 157(1):73, 1975.
15. Gonzalez-Soriano J et al: A quantitative study of ganglion cells in the goat retina, *Anat Histol Embryol* 26(1):39, 1997.
16. Braekevelt CR: Retinal photoreceptor fine structure in the domestic sheep, *Acta Anat* 116(3):265, 1983.
17. Jacobs GH, Deegan II JF, Neitz J: Photopigment basis for dichromatic color vision in cows, goats, and sheep, *Vis Neurosci* 15(3):581, 1998.
18. Whittaker CJG, Gelatt KN, Wilkie DA: Food animal ophthalmology. In Gelatt KN, editor: *Veterinary ophthalmology,* ed 3, Philadelphia, 1999, Williams & Wilkins.

OPHTHALMIC EXAMINATION

A thorough ophthalmic history should include a description of signalment, type of environment in which the animal is housed, present and previous diet, ophthalmic complaint, vaccination status, previous medical therapy, and concurrent medical problems. Ophthalmic changes can be clues to an animal's physical status, and therefore questions concerning the animal's ophthalmic problems should be accompanied by inquiries into the animal's physical condition. The examiner should avoid asking questions that may lead the owner to over-interpret the clinical signs they have observed.

After taking the history, the examiner should observe the animal's movements in a small area before beginning the ophthalmic examination. The animal should be encouraged to maneuver around obstacles in bright and dim light. Because sheep and goats have laterally placed eyes, unilateral blindness is less likely to be compensated for by the contralateral eye. An animal often turns its head in an attempt to see in front of it when visual acuity is compromised on one side. If the examiner still harbors doubts concerning vision, he or she can cover each eye individually for better assessment.

The ophthalmic examination can be performed under manual restraint in sheep while they are seated on their rumps; goats can stand for the examination. Before touching the head, the examiner should assess the eyes for symmetry in size and position, note the presence of abnormal ocular discharge, observe the eyelids as they pass over the ocular surface, and record any rubbing, blepharospasm, or other abnormalities. The menace test can be used to evaluate the optic nerve (cranial nerve II) and facial nerve (cranial nerve VII) for presence of vision and ability to blink, respectively. If the palpebral fissures do not close completely, a palpebral reflex test should be performed by touching the skin around the eye. This test assesses the trigeminal nerve (cranial nerves V) and facial nerve (cranial nerve VII). Both pupils should be assessed for size, shape, and symmetry under both light and dark conditions without direct stimulation. Shining a focal bright light source into one eye allows assessment of the PLR. After the response from the stimulated eye is observed, the contralateral eye should be quickly evaluated for the consensual pupillary response. The consensual pupillary response is slower and more incomplete compared with the stimulated eye because of unequal cross-over of the optic nerve fibers at the optic chiasm. The PLR is a subcortical response that requires normal function of the retina, optic nerve (cranial nerve II), midbrain, oculomotor nerve (cranial nerve III), and iris sphincter muscle. Cortically blind animals can have a normal PLR. The dazzle response assesses the visual pathway between the optic nerve and the midbrain. A very bright light source directed toward the eye usually causes a bilateral blink or turning of the head away from the light stimulus. This is a subcortical response that reaches the rostral colliculus and also stimulates the facial nucleus to cause the blink reflex.

Abnormalities of the orbit can be assessed by palpation of the bones of the orbital rim for fractures and asymmetry or by skull radiography. Difficulty in retropulsing the globe (with the eyelids closed) may indicate a retrobulbar space-occupying mass or other orbital disease. Difficulty or pain on opening of the mouth may indicate inflammatory orbital disease. Retrobulbar neoplasia usually does not cause pain on opening of the mouth. The involved orbit or globe should always be compared with the contralateral side. The eyelids should be evaluated for entropion or ectropion, complete closure of the palpebral fissures, increased wetness or ocular discharge on the hair adjacent to the eyelid margins, and distichiasis or trichiasis. The patency of the nasolacrimal apparatus can be assessed by determining whether fluorescein dye passes from the lacrimal lake to the nares after it is placed on the globe and flushed with saline solution. If fluorescein dye is not evident at one or both nares, the examiner can use a 22- or 23-gauge cannula attached to a 6-ml syringe filled with sterile saline solution to flush the nasolacrimal ducts in an orthograde direction. This procedure is performed by first applying topical anesthetic (0.5% proparacaine) to the globe and puncta. The distal blunt end of the cannula is inserted into the superior puncta, and saline solution is injected until fluid is seen to exit the inferior puncta. The cannula is then inserted into the inferior puncta and saline solution is gently injected until fluid is seen exiting the distal naris.

The conjunctiva should not be hyperemic, thickened, or edematous (chemosis). Examination for hemorrhage, foreign bodies (especially beneath the nictitating membrane), and lymphoid follicle hyperplasia should be performed. Samples from the conjunctiva for culture and sensitivity, cytology, immunofluorescent antibody (IFA), and biopsy can be obtained in physically restrained animals after the application of topical anesthetic solution. Fluorescein dye should not be applied before sample collection for IFA because it may result in a false positive result.[1]

The cornea is examined with a focal light source for clarity. A bluish hue is indicative of edema, white opacities may indicate scarring, a yellow-white color is often associated with white blood cell infiltrate, and red is consistent with neovascularization (this condition is generally more prominent at the limbus). Corneal edema can result from injury to the superficial corneal epithelium or corneal endothelium. Corneal ulcers result in focal corneal edema and positive uptake of fluorescein dye. Fluorescein is a hydrophilic dye that binds exposed corneal stroma, but not epithelium or Descemet's membrane. The slit beam on a direct ophthalmoscope can be used to assess the depth of a corneal ulcer by how deeply the beam is projected on the ulcer. If the ulcer is deep and fluorescein dye uptake is not evident, a descemetocele is likely. A perforated corneal ulcer may have aqueous humor draining from the perforation or the iris; fibrin may occlude the perforation. These ulcers should not be manipulated and minimal diagnostics should be performed because surgical intervention is the treatment of choice.

The anterior chamber is evaluated for clarity and depth. Damage to the blood-aqueous barrier allows protein and cells into the aqueous humor, creating turbidity or the Tyndall effect (aqueous flare). The slit beam or the smallest circle on a direct ophthalmoscope can be used to identify aqueous flare. The beam of light is focused directly on the cornea and then observed at 90° to the direction of the beam as it passes through the anterior chamber. There should be no evidence of light absorption within the anterior chamber. Aqueous flare is seen when protein and cells absorb light and the light beam is reflected in the aqueous humor. Iris bombé and intumescent cataracts can cause the anterior chamber depth to appear decreased, and hypermature cataracts can cause the anterior chamber depth to appear increased.[2]

The iris is examined for abnormal shape (dyscoria), color, thickness, miosis, or mydriasis inconsistent with the level of ambient light. Dyscoria can result from lens luxation or subluxation, synechia (adhesions), or a mass caudal to or within the iris. Pupil size should be examined in bright and dim light, and the examiner should determine direct and consensual PLRs. The color and thickness of the iris should be compared with the contralateral side; increased iridal thickness may be obvious in cases of cellular infiltrate and anterior uveitis. The granula iridica should be examined for size and symmetry because severe acute or chronic uveitis can cause them to atrophy.

Intraocular pressure (IOP) in most species is between 15 and 25 mm Hg. The average IOP in sheep and goats has not been established but is likely similar to that of other species. IOP can be measured in small ruminants using a Schiotz tonometer or a TonoPen. The footplate of the Schiotz is curved for use on human corneas and is probably not accurate in sheep or goats. Applanation tonometers such as the TonoPen are more accurate than indentation tonometers and are easier to use in domestic animals because the head does not have to be in a nose-up position, the footplate is only 3.22 mm in diameter, the footplate is not curved, and the reading does not have to be converted.[2] After administering topical anesthesia, the examiner gently taps the cornea with the TonoPen. The instrument takes a number of readings and then provides the average of those readings in mm Hg. A high reading is consistent with glaucoma. Excessive neck restraint should be avoided during the use of either instrument because this elevates the IOP.

The lens, vitreous, and fundus are best evaluated through a dilated pupil. The pupil can be dilated with a short-acting topical parasympatholytic such as 1% tropicamide. Time to effect for tropicamide is 10 to 20 minutes, and the effect lasts between 4 and 8 hours.[2] The lens should be evaluated for position and clarity. Nuclear sclerosis is an aging change that does not preclude evaluation of the fundus but must be differentiated from cataracts.

The fundic examination can be performed by either direct or indirect ophthalmoscopy. Direct ophthalmoscopy is performed at a distance of 2 to 3 cm from the patient's eye. The large circle is used when the pupil is dilated, and the smaller circles are used when the pupil is not dilated. The instrument is set at either 0 or the red 2 to begin the examination. The numbers are sequentially changed to bring a lesion into focus depending on its location. The disadvantages of direct ophthalmoscopy include the small field of view (approximately 2% of the entire fundus) and difficulty in examining the peripheral fundus. The advantages of direct ophthalmoscopy include greater magnification and the ability to alter the dioptric strength of the ophthalmoscope.[2]

Indirect ophthalmoscopy requires a focal light source to be held adjacent to one of the examiner's eyes and an indirect lens (held at arm's length) positioned 2 to 4 cm in front of the patient's eye after the tapetal reflex has been identified. A relatively inexpensive ophthalmic indirect lens ($50 to $75) is effective. The image seen is virtual but is inverted and reversed. The advantages of using indirect ophthalmoscopy include a larger field of view (approximately 40% of the entire fundus depending on the strength of the lens), which allows the peripheral fundus to be examined more completely, and stereopsis (use of both of the examiner's eyes). Disadvantages include the need for a relatively dilated pupil. Examination in a darkened room and use of a dimmed light source and a 28-diopter lens often allow fundic evaluation without dilation in herbivores through their horizontally oval pupils. Another limitation of indirect ophthalmoscopy is that it requires practice for the examiner to become proficient with the technique. When examining the fundus by indirect ophthalmoscopy, the examiner should move his or her head in the direction that is to be visualized within the fundus. The examiner should have a pattern for examining the fundus beginning with the optic nerve, dividing the fundus into quadrants, and examining each one by evaluating the vessels and color of the tapetal and nontapetal fundi.

Auriculopalpebral Nerve Block

The auriculopalpebral nerve is a branch of the facial nerve and provides motor function to the eyelids. Local anesthesia of the auriculopalpebral nerve combined with topical anesthesia (0.5% proparacaine) facilitates removal of foreign bodies and subconjunctival injections. The auriculopalpebral nerve can be palpated along the zygomatic arch near the base of the ear. Using a 25-gauge, 5/8-inch needle, the examiner injects 1 to 2 ml of local anesthetic perineurally to produce akinesia of the eyelids.[3]

SPECIALIZED DIAGNOSTIC TESTS

Corneal and Conjunctival Scrape

Conjunctival scrapings for cytologic examination and aerobic bacterial culture are valuable for the diagnosis of infectious keratoconjunctivitis. Collection of samples for culture should be performed before other diagnostic procedures. Sterile swabs should be moistened with sterile saline or transport media before application. The palpebral margins should not be scraped to reduce the possibility of contamination. Anaerobic bacteria and fungi are rare ocular pathogens in sheep and goats.[4] Fungal cultures are best obtained using a sterile, blunt instrument such as a Kimura spatula or the flat handle end of a scalpel blade. The culture sample should be placed directly onto fungal culture media.[4]

The cornea and conjunctiva should be anesthetized with topical 0.5% proparacaine before the procedure is performed, and a palpebral nerve block may be beneficial. If conjunctival follicles are present, these areas should be avoided to obtain a more representative sample. The sample should be very gently rolled or smeared onto a slide before staining with Diff-Quick or Wright's or Gram's stains.[4-6] Viral, mycoplasmal, or chlamydial organisms are poorly identified by Gram's staining.[4] Healthy conjunctiva is characterized cytologically by numerous epithelial cells, occasional lymphocytes, and rare neutrophils. Melanin granules may be observed in dark-faced breeds and can be mistaken for bacteria. Goblet cells are more common in animals with acute keratoconjunctivitis but also are present in unaffected animals. In acute keratoconjunctivitis, neutrophils become more numerous and plasma cells may be observed. Small numbers of eosinophils in otherwise normal sheep probably indicate a local reaction to environmental irritants.[6]

REFERENCES

1. da Silva-Curieal JMA et al: Topical fluorescein dye: effects on immunofluorescent antibody test for feline herpesvirus keratoconjunctivitis, *Prog Vet Comp Ophthalmol* 1(2):99, 1991.
2. Strubbe DT, Gelatt KN: Ophthalmic examination and diagnostic procedures. In Gelatt KN, editor: *Veterinary ophthalmology*, ed 3, Philadelphia, 1999, Williams & Wilkins.
3. Skarda RT: Local and regional anesthetic techniques: ruminants and swine. In Thurmon JC, Tranquilli WJ, Benson GJ, editors: *Veterinary anesthesia*, ed 3, Baltimore, 1996, Williams & Wilkins.
4. Ramsey DT: Surface ocular microbiology in food and fiber-producing animals. In Howard JL, Smith RA, editors: *Current veterinary therapy, food animal practice*, ed 4, Philadelphia, 1999, WB Saunders.
5. Pickett JP: Ophthalmic examination techniques for food animals. In Howard JL, Smith RA, editors: *Current veterinary therapy, food animal practice*, ed 4, Philadelphia, 1999, WB Saunders.
6. Dagnall GJR: Use of exfoliative cytology in the diagnosis of ovine keratoconjunctivitis, *Vet Rec* 135(6):127, 1994.

PATHOLOGY OF THE EYELIDS AND NASOLACRIMAL DUCTS

Entropion

Entropion is an inward deviation or rolling of the eyelid that causes a contact irritation of the cornea and conjunctiva by the eyelashes and periocular hair. Entropion has been reported to be the most common ocular disease of neonatal lambs.[1] If entropion is congenital (or primary), which is common, usually only the lower eyelid is affected and the condition is bilateral.[2-4] Secondary (or acquired) entropion may result from trauma, severe dehydration, loss of retrobulbar fat because of emaciation, old age, microphthalmia, phthisis bulbi, or painful ocular conditions that cause contraction of the retractor bulbi muscle and blepharospasm.

Clinical signs. Clinical signs are ordinarily observed in lambs during the first few days to weeks of life and may include blepharospasm, photophobia, eye rubbing, and

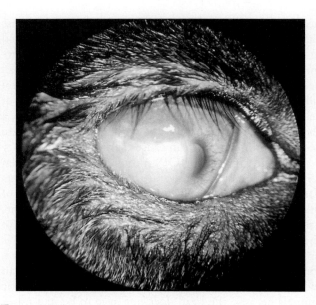

Figure 12-3 Entropion of the lower eyelid and secondary keratitis in a goat. Dorsal corneal neovascularization and central corneal edema with a superficial corneal ulcer also are present. (Courtesy Dr. Mary B. Glaze, Baton Rouge, Louisiana.)

keratoconjunctivitis. Initially epiphora may be present, but ocular discharge becomes mucopurulent as secondary bacterial keratoconjunctivitis develops (Figure 12-3).[1-4] Secondary entropion is usually unilateral and may affect either the upper or lower eyelid. Animals of any age may be affected.[3,4]

Treatment. Initial treatment of entropion is generally conservative and involves the administration of topical antibiotic ointments and attempts to evert the affected eyelid(s). Antibiotic ointments should be applied at least every 8 to 12 hours; more severe cases may require more frequent administration. Topical 1% atropine is indicated in animals with severe ocular pain and ciliary spasm. Atropine is administered every 8 to 12 hours until the pupil is dilated, after which the frequency of administration may be reduced.[3]

Nonsurgical eversion of the affected eyelid may be attempted using a variety of methods. Subcutaneous palpebral injection of benzathine or procaine penicillin immediately corrects entropion and acts as a local irritant that often causes sufficient fibrosis to correct the problem. Approximately 1 to 2 ml of penicillin (sufficient to evert the eyelid) is injected in a linear fashion just parallel to the affected eyelid margin.[1-3,5,6] The skin of the affected eyelid may be clamped with a mosquito hemostat to create swelling and resultant fibrosis that may permanently correct the entropion. The hemostat is applied just below and parallel with the eyelid margin and left in place for 30 seconds.[1,3,4,7] Another method involves the placement of two or three vertical mattress sutures, skin staples, or Michel wound clips to evert the eyelid.[1-7] In most cases entropion is effectively treated with these techniques, and surgical correction should be considered only when temporary eversion techniques have not been successful.[6] Some authors suggest that surgical procedures should be performed only on older animals (at least 4 to 6 months of age).[6]

Surgical correction of entropion is best undertaken with the animal anesthetized and placed in lateral recumbency (see Chapter 16). A crescent-shaped flap of skin is removed from the affected eyelid using a #15 scalpel blade and sharp dissection. The flap of skin to be removed is incised 1 to 2 mm distal to the eyelid margin and 3 to 4 mm wider than the affected area. The underlying section of the orbicularis oculi muscle also should be excised. Placement of a sterile tongue depressor, Jaeger lid plate, or scalpel handle underneath the eyelid in the conjunctival fornix facilitates incision and dissection of the eyelid. The skin is closed in one layer with a simple interrupted pattern. Closure should begin in the middle of the incision and proceed to the edges to ensure even skin tension across the suture line. Soft (silk or monofilament nylon), fine (3-0 to 4-0) suture material is suggested. The clinician should take care to tie knots away from the cornea to prevent irritation. Sutures should be removed in 10 to 14 days. Topical antibiotics should be continued for several days after surgery or until any corneal ulcers have healed.

Prevention. Congenital entropion is suspected to be a heritable trait, and affected animals should not be used for breeding purposes.[2,3,6,7] The genetic factors resulting in congenital entropion are unknown, but the trait is believed to be multifactorial and caused by more than a simple, autosomal recessive inheritance.[2,4,8] Dusty or windy conditions may contribute to the development of entropion in genetically predisposed animals.[6] From 4% to 80% of a flock may be affected with congenital entropion, and usually several lambs are affected in the new lamb crop.[9] In contrast, secondary entropion (e.g., that resulting from dehydration) normally affects only single animals.[4]

Ectropion

The most common etiologies of ectropion include iatrogenic overcorrection of entropion and trauma.[1,3,4] Ectropion is relatively rare in sheep and goats.[3,4]

Clinical signs. Clinical signs of ectropion include drooping of the affected eyelid, epiphora, and exposure keratoconjunctivitis.[4] Some sheep have mild drooping of the eyelids as a normal conformational variation. Mildly affected animals may be predisposed to conjunctivitis but most have no clinical signs of ocular disease.[1]

Treatment. If surgical correction is necessary, a V to Y blepharoplasty or eyelid shortening procedure is rec-

ommended, using techniques as described for other species.[1,3]

Viral Blepharitis

Blepharitis has numerous etiologies, and several of these are systemic diseases that are likely to affect other body systems. Viral causes of blepharitis include cutaneous ecthyma (orf), ulcerative dermatosis, and bluetongue.[3,4]

Clinical signs. Lesions of contagious ecthyma are characterized by vesicles or pustules that rapidly progress to proliferative, scab-like crusts.[10] Owners and clinicians should wear gloves when treating animals with clinical signs of cutaneous ecthyma virus because of its zoonotic potential. Similarly, ulcerative dermatosis virus causes encrusted ulcerations of the eyelids of sheep. Clinical signs of bluetongue virus infections are more likely to be observed in sheep than goats and include blepharitis, blepharospasm, and conjunctivitis.[3,4] Other ocular lesions of bluetongue include hyperemia and eczema of the adnexal skin and retinal dysplasia.[3]

Treatment. Treatment of viral blepharitis is largely symptomatic and may involve the administration of antiinflammatory agents and topical ophthalmic antibiotics to prevent secondary bacterial infections.[3] Affected animals should be isolated, and contamination of ointment tubes must be avoided.[3]

Bacterial Blepharitis

Bacterial blepharitis may be caused by *Dermatophilus congolensis*, *Actinobacillus lignieresii*, and *Clostridium novyi*.[3,4] *A. lignieresii* infections are characterized by pyogranulomatous nodules with draining tracts. Impression smears of exudate reveal clumps of filamentous gram-negative bacteria and inflammatory cells.[3] Bighead (*C. novyi* infection) usually occurs in rams as a sequela to head trauma during fighting and butting. Affected animals have extensive facial and cervical swelling that may affect the eyelids.[3,4] Blepharoedema may be severe enough to obliterate the palpebral fissure and blind the animal or cause exposure keratitis because of an inability to close the eyelids fully.[4]

Treatment. Treatment of *C. novyi* infection requires intensive therapy with systemic antiinflammatory therapy, antimicrobial agents (e.g., penicillin, florfenicol), and topical antibiotic ointments.[4]

Fungal Blepharitis

Clinical signs. Clinical signs of dermatophytosis include facial alopecia and crusting that may affect the eyelids. Young goats are most commonly affected, and cases are most likely to occur during late winter and early spring.[3] Diagnosis may be based on fungal culture, fungal growth on dermatophyte test media, and microscopic examination of affected hairs after application of potassium hydroxide (KOH). Dermatophytes are potentially zoonotic and people should wear gloves when treating infected animals.

Treatment. Fungal blepharitis is usually self-limiting, and most animals recover in the spring with improved pasture conditions and increased dietary vitamin A concentrations. Symptomatic therapy may involve the administration of topical antifungal ointments or shampoos.[3]

Parasitic Blepharitis

A variety of external parasite infestations can cause blepharitis. Blepharitis may be caused by the parasites directly or may result from rubbing or scratching in pruritic animals. *Psoroptes, Psorergates,* and *Chorioptes* infestations may cause intense itching and rarely involve only the facial area.[3] Diagnosis is based on clinical signs and confirmed by microscopic examination of skin scrapings.

Treatment. Other external parasites that may cause blepharitis include sheep keds, lice, and ticks.[3,4] Mite infestations are treated by ivermectin administration, dipping in insecticides, and local application of insecticides as necessary.[3]

Elaeophoriasis (Sorehead)

Elaeophora schneideri (sorehead) may aberrantly infect sheep and goats. Sorehead occurs in the high mountain regions of the western United States where small ruminants are pastured near deer.[1,6] Clinical signs of *E. schneideri* infection in small ruminants and elk include facial swelling, blepharospasm, keratoconjunctivitis, alopecia, ulceration, and encrusted lesions of the face.[1,6] Sorehead most commonly affects adult sheep during the fall and winter.[1,6] Diagnosis is based on consistent clinical signs in small ruminants in endemic areas and the demonstration of *E. schneideri* microfilaria in skin or conjunctival biopsies.

Treatment. Reported effective treatments include piperazine (50 mg/kg by mouth [PO]) and diethylcarbamazine (100 mg/kg PO). The efficacy of ivermectin against the parasite is unknown.[6]

Other causes of blepharitis and blepharoedema include photosensitization, solar dermatitis, contact hypersensitivity dermatitis, and cutaneous myiasis.[3,5]

Neoplasia

Neoplasms reported to affect the eyelids of sheep and goats include squamous cell carcinoma, fibroma, fibrosarcoma, and melanoma.[3,5] Papilloma virus infection causes eyelid warts.[3,5] In immunocompetent animals, warts are generally fairly benign and self-limiting. Papillomas that interfere with eyelid function or irritate the cornea should be removed.[3]

Treatment. Treatment of eyelid neoplasms is determined by the invasiveness of the tumor but may involve surgical removal, cryotherapy (possible complications include eyelid fibrosis and corneal damage), CO_2 laser excision, or local hyperthermia therapy. Topical antibiotic ointments should be administered for several days after surgery.

Facial Nerve Paralysis

Locoweed (*Astragalus* and *Oxytropis* species) produces paralysis of the palpebral nerve and secondary exposure keratoconjunctivitis sicca (KCS).[6] Locoweed toxicity also causes marked cytoplasmic vacuolization of the lacrimal gland secretory epithelium. The resultant decrease in tear production further contributes to KCS and may cause animals to have a "dull-eyed" appearance.[11] Listeriosis should be ruled out as a possible cause of cranial nerve abnormalities, especially in animals with unilateral deficits.

Nictitating Membrane

Abnormalities of the nictitating membrane are uncommon. Lymphoid follicles of the third eyelid may be very prominent in cases of infectious conjunctivitis, especially if the condition is caused by chlamydial organisms. Carcinomas and adenocarcinomas affecting the third eyelid may be treated by local excision or preferably by removal of the entire nictitating membrane.[3]

Nasolacrimal Duct Disease

Disease of the nasolacrimal duct of sheep is most commonly caused by larvae of the nasal bot (*Oestrus ovis*). Normally the larvae of the nasal bot fly mature in the frontal and nasal sinuses until they are sneezed out to complete their life cycle. Occasionally, larvae may aberrantly migrate into the nasolacrimal duct or ocular mucous membranes. Clinical signs of ocular or nasolacrimal infection include epiphora and conjunctivitis. Affected animals also may exhibit frenzied behavior to avoid adult botflies, stomp, sneeze, and may have a nasal discharge.

Treatment. Treatment involves removal of visible larvae, flushing of the nasolacrimal ducts, and administration of ivermectin (200 μg/kg PO). Nasal bot infections are most effectively treated in the fall when larvae are smaller.[3,6]

REFERENCES

1. Moore CP, Wallace LM: Selected eye diseases of sheep and goats. In Howard JL, editor: *Current veterinary therapy, food animal practice,* ed 3, Philadelphia, 1993, WB Saunders.
2. Miller TR, Gelatt KN: Food animal ophthalmology. In Gelatt KN, editor: *Veterinary ophthalmology,* ed 2, Philadelphia, 1991, Lea and Febiger.
3. Moore CP, Whitley RD: Ophthalmic diseases of small domestic ruminants, *Vet Clin North Am Large Anim Pract* 6(3):641, 1984.
4. Wyman M: Eye diseases of sheep and goats, *Vet Clin North Am Large Anim Pract* 5(3):657, 1983.
5. Lavach JD: Disorders of the eyelids, conjunctivae, and nasolacrimal system. In: *Large animal ophthalmology,* St Louis, 1990, Mosby.
6. Pickett JP: Selected eye diseases of food and fiber-producing animals. In Howard JL, Smith RA, editors: *Current veterinary therapy, food animal practice,* ed 4, Philadelphia, 1999, WB Saunders.
7. Rook JS, Cortese V: Repair of entropion in the lamb, *Vet Med Small Anim Clin* 76(4):571, 1981.
8. Taylor M, Catchpole J: Incidence of entropion in lambs from two ewe flocks put to the same rams, *Vet Rec* 118(13):361, 1986.
9. Gelatt KN: Congenital entropion in a Hampshire lamb, *Vet Med Small Anim Clin* 65(8):761, 1970.
10. Smith MC, Sherman DM: Skin. In Smith MC, Sherman DM, editors: *Goat medicine,* Philadelphia, 1994, Lea and Febiger.
11. Van Kampen KR, James LF: Ophthalmic lesions in locoweed poisoning of cattle, sheep, and horses, *Am J Vet Res* 32(8):1293, 1971.

PATHOLOGY OF THE CONJUNCTIVA AND CORNEA

Conjunctival Trauma

Goats and sheep have large, prominent eyes that may be traumatized by fencing, feeders, and coarse forage during browsing. Dusty or windy conditions also may cause an irritant conjunctivitis.

Clinical signs. Animals with conjunctival trauma often have conjunctival hemorrhage and swelling. If the globe appears soft (decreased IOP) or the anterior chamber is shallow or flat, a scleral or corneal laceration is likely. Subconjunctival hemorrhage is often an incidental finding in neonates and is caused by minor trauma during parturition.

Treatment. Uncomplicated cases of conjunctival irritation and minor trauma can be treated with topical broad-spectrum antibiotic ointments (e.g., triple antibiotic) to prevent secondary bacterial infections and to provide corneal lubrication.[1]

Corneal Trauma

Corneal trauma may be caused by penetrating foreign bodies, lacerations, and abrasions causing ulcerative keratitis. The most common ocular foreign bodies are small particles of plant material that become embedded in the conjunctiva or corneal stroma.

Treatment. Removal of small, superficial foreign bodies is often accomplished with topical anesthesia using 0.5% proparacaine and manual restraint. Foreign bodies are usually easily removed using cotton-tipped applicators or ophthalmic forceps. After foreign body removal, topical antibiotics should be administered every 6 to 8 hours for several days. Nonpenetrating corneal lacerations may be treated as simple corneal ulcers with topical antibiotics and 1% atropine.[1] Chemical injuries to the cornea and conjunctiva are caused by insecticide dips or sprays, shampoos, and disinfectants. In the case of chemical injuries, immediate lavage with large volumes of isotonic saline or ordinary tap water is essential to flush the conjunctival sac and dilute the offending agent. After lavage the affected eyes should be treated with topical antibiotics and atropine. Topical anticollagenase preparations such as acetylcysteine may be beneficial to reduce ongoing corneal degeneration. Systemic antiinflammatory agents are indicated to control secondary uveitis.[1]

Infectious Conjunctivitis

Reports describing the normal conjunctival flora of sheep and goats are scarce. In clinically normal sheep, 60% of eye swabs were negative for bacterial growth.[2] In sheep the most commonly isolated bacteria were similar to *Branhamella (Neisseria) ovis* and were recovered in low numbers. Other frequently isolated organisms were *Micrococcus* and *Streptococcus* species. Less commonly isolated bacteria were of the genera *Corynebacterium, Achromobacter, Bacillus, Neisseria* (other than *N. ovis*), *Staphylococcus, Pseudomonas, Moraxella,* and *Escherichia coli.*[2,3] *Moraxella bovis* is not a cause of infectious keratoconjunctivitis in goats.[3] However, conflicting reports indicate the possible pathogenicity of *Moraxella* in ovine keratoconjunctivitis.[4,5] Other known ocular pathogens, including *Mycoplasma conjunctivae* and *Chlamydia psittaci,* can be cultured from the eyes of sheep and goats after resolution of keratoconjunctivitis and in clinically normal animals.[3,6-10]

Mycoplasma Conjunctivitis

Mycoplasma species are important and frequent pathogens causing keratoconjunctivitis in sheep and goats. Reported mycoplasmal pathogens include *M. conjunctivae, M. mycoides* subsp. *mycoides, M. capricolum, M. agalactiae,* and *M. arginini.*

Clinical signs. Clinical signs of ocular mycoplasmal infections are hyperemia of the conjunctival blood vessels, photophobia, blepharospasm, and epiphora that may become mucopurulent (Figure 12-4).[8-15] Corneal neovascularization and opacity beginning at the limbus and progressing centrally may occur in some cases (Figure 12-5).[8,10-12,14,15] Severely affected animals may develop iridocyclitis, corneal ulcers, or blindness because of intense corneal opacity.[3,9-13] Some authors state that clinical signs are more common and severe in adult sheep than in lambs.[8,12]

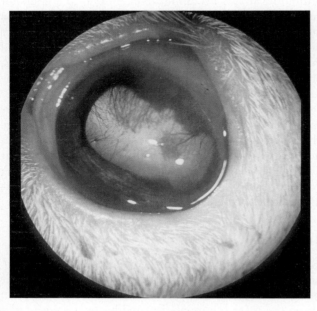

Figure 12-4 Keratoconjunctivitis with conjunctival hyperemia, chemosis, epiphora, and corneal neovascularization. (Courtesy Dr. Ron Ofri, Rehovot, Israel.)

Diagnosis. Diagnosis of mycoplasmal infection is based on clinical signs, IFA staining of conjunctival scrapings, and positive culture of lacrimal secretions, blood, or milk.[8,11] Conjunctival scrapings stained with Giemsa-type stains may reveal basophilic, coccobacillary organisms within the cytoplasm of the epithelial cells.[8,11,12] Conjunctival neutrophils, lymphocytes, and plasma cells, as well as necrotic epithelium also may be observed (Figure 12-6).[11] Culture and cytology results are more likely to be positive when obtained soon after the onset of clinical signs.[12]

Treatment. Many cases of mycoplasmal keratoconjunctivitis are self-limiting and resolve completely within a few weeks without treatment.[10,13,15] Both systemic and topical antibiotic therapy have been recommended, and antibiotics may speed the recovery of affected animals.[15,16] Systemic tylosin, oxytetracycline (10 to 20 mg/kg intramuscularly [IM] or subcutaneously [SC]), chlortetracycline (80 mg/head/day in the feed), and streptomycin have been found to be effective in vitro against isolates taken from sheep.[16] Topical tetracycline alone[12] or combined with polymyxin B[15] also is reported to be effective. The prophylactic use of long-acting oxytetracycline (20 mg/kg every 48 to 72 hours IM or SC) may prevent the appearance of clinical signs in other members of the herd or flock.[12]

Prevention. Affected animals should be isolated to prevent the spread of disease.[11] Carrier animals and apparently uninfected animals are an important source of infection because *M. conjunctivae* may persist for months

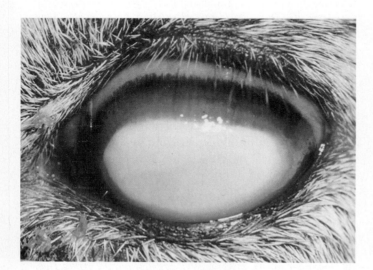

Figure 12-5 Keratoconjunctivitis in a goat. Periocular swelling, epiphora, and generalized corneal edema with circumlimbal deep neovascularization also are present. (Courtesy Dr. M.A. Salisbury, Sarasota, Florida.)

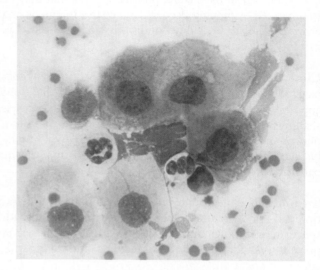

Figure 12-6 Photomicrograph of a conjunctival scraping from the goat in Figure 12-5. Neutrophils, erythrocytes, and conjunctival epithelial cells with basophilic coccobacillary pleomorphic bodies within the cytoplasm are present, consistent with *Mycoplasma* infection. Wright's stain, 250× magnification. (Courtesy Dr. M.A. Salisbury, Sarasota, Florida.)

in the conjunctival sac and nares after recovery.[8] Recently affected herds or flocks often have a history of introduction of new members that were inapparent carriers of *M. conjunctivae*.[3,8,12,15] The infection is spread by direct contact with infective ocular secretions, fomites, and face flies.[3,11,12] Some authors recommend isolation and prophylactic treatment of new animals before they are added to the herd or flock[11] (see Chapter 5).

Chlamydia psittaci Conjunctivitis

Ocular *C. psittaci* infections in sheep and goats cannot be distinguished from *M. conjunctivae* infections based on clinical signs alone because they appear similar clinically.[3] Two strains of *C. psittaci* exist and are characterized by their ability to cause keratoconjunctivitis alone or as part of a systemic disease process such as pyrexia, polyarthritis, respiratory tract infection, and abortion.[3,11] Keratoconjunctivitis in lambs caused by *C. psittaci* is more likely to be bilateral than *M. conjunctivae* infection.[3]

Clinical signs.   As many as 80% of lambs are affected bilaterally, but lesions may be asymmetric.[3,11,17,18] In one report,[17] all affected lambs with polyarthritis also had some degree of conjunctivitis. Clinical signs are generally more severe in lambs than adult sheep and as many as 90% of lambs may become infected.[3,11] Initial clinical signs of ocular *C. psittaci* infection include conjunctival petechiae and hyperemia, corneal edema, neovascularization, and ocular discharge that may vary from serous to mucoid or purulent. As the condition progresses, severe conjunctival hyperemia, neovascularization, and corneal ulceration occur, along with a neutrophilic corneal infiltrate (Figure 12-7).[3,11,17-20] A characteristic clinical sign of chlamydial keratoconjunctivitis is the formation of conjunctival lymphoid follicles. Lymphoid follicles begin as small, discrete, pale, elevated areas in the conjunctiva that gradually enlarge and coalesce to form pink to red folds in the lower conjunctival fornix. The follicles can protrude as much as 8 to 10 mm to fill the conjunctival fornix and become confluent with the follicles on the surface of the nictitating membrane.[18]

Diagnosis.   Diagnostic tests for *C. psittaci* keratoconjunctivitis include culture of blood or ocular secretions, serology using complement fixation tests, and specific IFA staining or microscopic examination of conjunctival smears.[3,8,11,12,17-19] A four-fold or greater rise between acute and convalescent serum samples (taken 2 weeks apart) using the complement fixation test may confirm the diagnosis.[8] Organisms are more likely to be found using culture or cytologic methods early in the disease process.[12,20] Conjunctival scrapings reveal numerous neutrophils with some lymphocytes and plasma cells.[18] In chlamydial infections, conjunctival epithelial cells are shed singly or in groups of two or three, whereas in unaf-

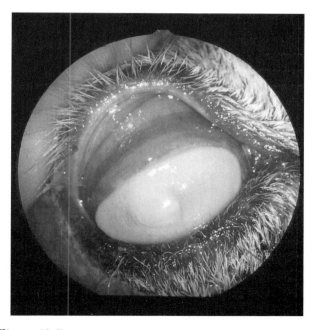

Figure 12-7   *Corneal stromal abscess in a sheep. Corneal cellular infiltrate, deep neovascularization, and severe conjunctival hyperemia also are present. (Courtesy Dr. P. Lybaert, Brussels, Belgium.)*

fected animals these cells are found in sheets of several cells.[18] Chlamydial inclusions are usually juxtanuclear[17] and may be found in approximately 50% of conjunctival scrapings if Giemsa stain is used.[8,11]

Treatment and prevention.   Treatment of *C. psittaci* infection is as described for mycoplasmal infections. Systemic and topical tetracycline is reportedly effective.[3,11] In uncomplicated cases the disease is usually self-limiting and recovery can be expected within 2 to 3 weeks.[11,18,20] Transmission of *C. psittaci* occurs by infective secretions, direct contact, and insects.[11,18] Recovered animals may shed *C. psittaci* in tears and nasal secretions for several months after the resolution of clinical signs.[11] In 8- to 10-month-old lambs a degree of resistance appears to develop.[18] Although some authors[12,20] state that some sheep are carriers for *C. psittaci*, others report that chlamydial organisms cannot be cultured from the eyes of clinically normal animals[3] (see Chapter 5).

Colesiota conjunctivae Conjunctivitis

Colesiota conjunctivae is a member of the family Chlamydiaceae, and similar to *C. psittaci* it also can cause conjunctivitis in sheep. Previously *C. conjunctivae* was presumed to be a Rickettsia-like organism based on its morphologic appearance.[11,20,21] However, this classification was probably based on misidentification of epithelial inclusions of *C. psittaci* as rickettsial organisms.[11,20] The bacterium has not been cultured and has only been identified from conjunctival scrapings.[11]

Branhamella ovis Conjunctivitis

Branhamella (Neisseria) ovis may cause conjunctivitis, epiphora, injected scleral blood vessels, photophobia, and corneal neovascularization in sheep and goats.[11,22] Only a small number of affected sheep develop keratitis.[11] The role of B. ovis as a primary pathogen is unclear and the bacteria may be primarily opportunistic with infections by other organisms such as M. conjunctivae and C. psittaci.[3,8,11,12] Diagnosis of B. ovis infection is based on bacterial culture results and Gram's staining of conjunctival scrapings, which reveals a predominance of gram-negative diplococci.[22]

Treatment. Successful treatment of B. ovis infection in goats involves parenteral tylosin for 5 days combined with topical application of bacitracin-neomycin-polymyxin B ointment. Animals without any corneal involvement recover within 48 hours.[22] B. ovis may be cultured from the eyes of both diseased and unaffected sheep and goats[3,6,8,10-12] but has been isolated more frequently from the eyes of affected sheep.[10,12]

Acholeplasma oculi Conjunctivitis

Clinical signs of Acholeplasma oculi (or A. oculusi) infection in sheep and goats include conjunctivitis, keratitis, blepharospasm, epiphora, and pannus.[23,24]

Treatment. Treatment of A. oculi infection in ewes is successful with subconjunctival injections of oxytetracycline; a second treatment is necessary in only a few animals.[23]

Listeria monocytogenes Conjunctivitis

In sheep, Listeria monocytogenes may cause conjunctivitis as well as encephalitic disease.[25] Infections tend to be unilateral and are characterized by blepharospasm, apparent blindness, hypopyon, corneal edema, and catarrhal conjunctivitis. Clinical signs may resolve within 2 weeks without corneal scarring. Animals may be infected by feeding on contaminated silage.

Treatment. Response to antibiotics, including topical oxytetracycline and systemic ampicillin, appears to be poor.

Viral Keratoconjunctivitis

Severe conjunctivitis, keratoconus, corneal opacity, and blindness has been reported in two goats naturally affected with infectious bovine rhinotracheitis virus.[26] The virus was isolated from the nasal secretions of both goats. The goats had clinical signs of respiratory tract disease before ocular involvement was noted, and both recovered. Bluetongue virus infection may cause conjunctivitis, blepharitis, and blepharoedema.[27]

Mycotic Keratitis

Mycotic keratitis is rare in ruminants.[27] If fungal elements are cultured or observed in conjunctival scrapings, their presence as possible contaminants should be carefully considered. Saprophytic fungi such as Aspergillus and Mucor species have been isolated from both diseased and unaffected eyes in sheep and goats.[15,18]

Treatment. Treatment involves the application of topical antifungal agents, including natamycin, miconazole, itraconazole/dimethyl sulfoxide (DMSO), or ketoconazole. Topical miconazole is usually the most cost-effective therapy and should be administered every 4 to 6 hours. Superficial keratectomy can be used for both therapeutic and diagnostic purposes. Keratectomy removes diseased corneal material, providing tissue for fungal culture and cytology while increasing the penetration of topical medications.

Parasitic Keratitis

Thelazia rhodesii, the eye worm, causes widespread infection in North America. However, clinical disease is uncommon.[28,29] Eye worm infections may cause conjunctivitis, conjunctival cysts, and keratitis. In severe cases, corneal edema, ulceration, and neovascularization may occur.[29] Face flies and other Musca species are intermediate hosts for the parasite, and therefore fly control is essential for reducing infections.

Treatment. Therapy can involve manual removal of worms after the application of topical anesthetics[29,30] or organophosphate (echothiophate iodide, phospholine iodide)[31] and irrigation of the conjunctival sac. In cattle, both ivermectin (200 μg/kg SC)[30] and doramectin (200 μg/kg SC)[32] have greater than 99% efficacy against eye worms. Levamisole (5 mg/kg PO) also may be efficacious.[31]

O. ovis larvae can aberrantly migrate into the conjunctiva or nasolacrimal duct of sheep, causing epiphora and conjunctivitis.[28] Keratoconjunctivitis, blepharospasm, and blepharoedema may occur in small ruminants as sequelae to E. schneideri infection.[28] Treatment of O. ovis and E. schneideri infection is described in the section on pathology of the eyelid.

Conjunctivitis Therapy

Most of the bacterial ocular pathogens of sheep and goats are susceptible to tetracycline. Combination therapy with long-acting injectable (20 mg/kg IM or SC) and topical tetracycline (every 6 to 8 hours) is usually effective for most bacterial infections.[33] Topical ophthalmic ointments are generally preferred over solutions because of their prolonged contact time and because less drug is likely to be lost in ocular secretions. For these same reasons, ointments are administered less frequently than solutions. However, ointments should be avoided if a perforating corneal ulcer is suspected because they are very irritating to intraocular structures. Powdered preparations are not recommended for topical ophthalmic use because they are extremely irritating and have low drug bioavailability. Topical administration of therapeutic agents provides higher drug levels in the cornea, conjunctiva, aqueous humor, iris, and ciliary body.[33]

Another method to achieve high local concentrations of therapeutic agents is subconjunctival injection. Before injection an auriculopalpebral nerve block and sedation may be necessary. The conjunctiva should be anesthetized with 0.5% proparacaine. In sheep and goats a maximum volume of 0.5 ml may be administered in the dorsal conjunctival fornix with a 25-gauge needle. Subconjunctival injection of antibiotics may be used to achieve initial high concentrations of antibiotics but should not be administered in place of topical antibiotics.[33]

Third eyelid flaps. Third eyelid flaps may be used in some cases of ulcerative keratitis as a temporary ophthalmic bandage. The clinician applies a topical anesthetic to the eye and performs a line block over the dorsal aspect of the upper eyelid. The third eyelid is sutured to the dorsal fornix of the upper eyelid with two or three simple interrupted horizontal mattress sutures using monofilament suture (00) material. The sutures are placed using a curved cutting needle directed through the skin of the upper eyelid 1 cm from the palpebral margin; the needle is then passed into the third eyelid 2 to 3 mm from its edge on the palpebral side before being passed parallel to the eyelid margin into the fibrous tissue of the third eyelid to obtain a 3- to 4-mm piece of tissue. The clinician next passes the needle through the palpebral conjunctiva and skin and ties it off to complete the suture. The suture should not penetrate the bulbar mucosa of the third eyelid, and the nictitating membrane should be seated as deeply as possible in the dorsal conjunctival cul-de-sac to avoid corneal injury by the sutures. If absorbable suture material such as chromic gut is used, sutures usually dissolve in 2 or 3 weeks. Nonabsorbable sutures should be removed as soon as ocular disease has resolved.[31] One large disadvantage of third eyelid flaps is that the cornea and intraocular structures cannot be examined. Third eyelid flaps should be avoided in cases of melting corneal ulcers, ulcers deeper than three quarters of the corneal stromal thickness, and infected ulcers.

Prevention of Conjunctivitis

In epizootic cases of suspected bacterial keratoconjunctivitis, several control measures have been suggested to reduce the spread of disease.[31] Infected animals and animals in direct contact with them should be isolated. Exposure to environmental irritants such as flies, dust, pollen, and wind should be avoided. Pastures should be mowed to eliminate long-stemmed or rough weeds and grasses. Contaminated stall bedding should be removed, and water troughs and feeders should be cleaned and disinfected. Affected animals may have visual deficits and should be either confined or kept near readily accessible feed and water sources.

Miscellaneous

Dermoids (choristoma) are ectopic patches of epidermal tissue and can be found on the conjunctiva, limbus, and cornea. They rarely occur in sheep and goats.[28] Dermoids affecting the conjunctiva or palpebral mucosae are often easily removed with sharp dissection under topical or regional anesthesia. Corneal dermoids are removed by superficial lamellar keratectomy. Regeneration can occur if the entire lesion is not removed.[34]

REFERENCES

1. Whitley RD: Ocular trauma. In Smith BP, editor: *Large animal internal medicine*, ed 2, St Louis, 1996, Mosby.
2. Spradbrow PB: The bacterial flora of the ovine conjunctival sac, *Aust Vet J* 44(3):117, 1968.
3. Ramsey DT: Surface ocular microbiology in food and fiber-producing animals. In Howard JL, Smith RA, editors: *Current veterinary therapy, food animal practice*, ed 4, Philadelphia, 1999, WB Saunders.
4. Baker JR, Faull WB, Ward WR: Conjunctivitis and keratitis in sheep associated with *Moraxella (Haemophilus)* organisms, *Vet Rec* 77(14):402, 1965.
5. Wood DR, Watson WA, Hunter D: Conjunctivitis in sheep, *Vet Rec* 77(19):551, 1965.
6. Dagnall GJR: Use of exfoliative cytology in the diagnosis of ovine keratoconjunctivitis, *Vet Rec* 135(6):127, 1994.
7. Trotter SL et al: Epidemic caprine keratoconjunctivitis: experimentally induced disease with a pure culture of *Mycoplasma conjunctivae*, *Infect Immun* 18(3):816, 1977.
8. Hosie BO: Infectious keratoconjunctivitis in sheep and goats, *Vet Ann* 29:93, 1989.
9. Jones GE et al: Mycoplasmas and ovine keratoconjunctivitis, *Vet Rec* 99(8):137, 1976.
10. Egwu GO et al: Ovine infectious keratoconjunctivitis: a microbiological study of clinically unaffected and affected sheep's eyes with special reference to *Mycoplasma conjunctivae*, *Vet Rec* 125(10):253, 1989.
11. Moore CP, Wallace LM: Selected eye diseases of sheep and goats. In Howard JL, editor: *Current veterinary therapy, food animal practice*, ed 3, Philadelphia, 1993, WB Saunders.
12. Greig A: Ovine keratoconjunctivitis, *In Practice* 11(3):110, 1989.
13. McCauley EH, Surman PG, Anderson DR: Isolation of *Mycoplasma* from goats during an epizootic of keratoconjunctivitis, *Am J Vet Res* 32(6):861, 1971.
14. Dagnall GJR: Experimental infection of the conjunctival sac of lambs with *Mycoplasma conjunctivae*, *Br Vet J* 149(5):429, 1993.
15. Baas EJ et al: Epidemic caprine keratoconjunctivitis: recovery of *Mycoplasma conjunctivae* and its possible role in pathogenesis, *Infect Immun* 18(3):806, 1977.
16. Egwu GO: In vitro antibiotic sensitivity of *Mycoplasma conjunctivae* and some bacterial species causing ovine infectious keratoconjunctivitis, *Small Rumin Res* 7(1):85, 1992.

17. Stephenson EH, Storz J, Hopkins JB: Properties and frequency of isolation of chlamydiae from eyes of lambs with conjunctivitis and polyarthritis, *Am J Vet Res* 35(2):177, 1974.

18. Hopkins JB et al: Conjunctivitis associated with chlamydial polyarthritis in lambs, *J Am Vet Med Assoc* 163(10):1157, 1973.

19. Wilsmore AJ, Dagnall GJR, Woodland RM: Experimental conjunctival infection of lambs with a strain of *Chlamydia psittaci* isolated from the eyes of a sheep naturally affected with keratoconjunctivitis, *Vet Rec* 127(9):229, 1990.

20. Cello RM: Ocular infections in animals with PLT *(Bedsonia)* group agents, *Am J Ophthalmol* 63(5):1270, 1967.

21. König CDW: Keratoconjunctivitis infectious ovis (KIO), "pink eye" or "zere oogjes" (a survey), *Vet Q* 5(3):127, 1983.

22. Bulgin MS, Dubose DA: Pinkeye associated with *Branhamella ovis* infection in dairy goats, *Vet Med Small Anim Clin* 77(12):1791, 1982.

23. Arbuckle JBR, Bonson MD: The isolation of *Acholeplasma oculi* from an outbreak of ovine keratoconjunctivitis, *Vet Rec* 106(1):15, 1979.

24. Al-Aubaidi JM et al: Identification and characterization of *Acholeplasma oculi* spec. nov. from the eyes of goats with keratoconjunctivitis, *Cornell Vet* 63(1):117, 1973.

25. Walker JK, Morgan JH: Ovine ophthalmitis associated with *Listeria monocytogenes*, *Vet Rec* 132(25):636, 1993.

26. Mohanty SB et al: Natural infection with infectious bovine rhinotracheitis virus in goats, *J Am Vet Med Assoc* 160(6):879, 1972.

27. Wyman M: Eye diseases of sheep and goats, *Vet Clin North Am Large Anim Pract* 5(3):657, 1983.

28. Pickett JP: Selected eye diseases of food and fiber-producing animals. In Howard JL, Smith RA, editors: *Current veterinary therapy, food animal practice,* ed 4, Philadelphia, 1999, WB Saunders.

29. English RV, Nasisse MP: Ocular parasites. In Smith BP, editor: *Large animal internal medicine,* ed 2, St Louis, 1996, Mosby.

30. Soll MD et al: The efficacy of ivermectin against *Thelazia rhodesii* (Desmarest, 1828) in the eyes of cattle, *Vet Parasitol* 42(1-2):67, 1992.

31. Moore CP, Whitley RD: Ophthalmic diseases of small domestic ruminants, *Vet Clin North Am Large Anim Pract* 6(3):641, 1984.

32. Kennedy MJ, Phillips FE: Efficacy of doramectin against eyeworms *(Thelazia* spp.) in naturally and experimentally infected cattle, *Vet Parasitol* 49(1):61, 1993.

33. Ramsey DT: Ophthalmic therapeutics. In Howard JL, Smith RA, editors: *Current veterinary therapy, food animal practice,* ed 4, Philadelphia, 1999, WB Saunders.

34. Miller TR, Gelatt KN: Food animal ophthalmology. In Gelatt KN, editor: *Veterinary ophthalmology,* ed 2, Philadelphia, 1991, WB Saunders.

PATHOLOGY OF THE UVEAL TRACT AND LENS

Uveitis

Clinical signs. Clinical signs of uveitis may include miosis, photophobia, iris hyperemia, aqueous flare, hypopyon, hyphema, blindness, and fibrin deposition within the anterior chamber.[1-5] Uveitis is a frequent clinical sign of septicemia and is often observed in neonates with failure of passive transfer. *Mycoplasma* species often cause septicemia and systemic disease in both neonates and adult animals. In addition to ocular disease, clinical signs of mycoplasmal infections include polyarthritis, mastitis, and agalactia.[1,2,4] Animals infected with mycoplasmal organisms should be isolated because bacteria are transmitted by direct contact with infected animals, infective secretions, and fomites.[1]

L. monocytogenes infections can result in septicemia in 4- to 6-month-old feedlot lambs fed silage-based rations. Lambs may have clinical signs of uveitis, conjunctivitis, and endophthalmitis, as well as cranial nerve deficits.[2,5,6]

Toxoplasma gondii is an uncommon cause of anterior uveitis in sheep and goats.[6] In sheep, ocular toxoplasmosis most frequently involves the iris, ciliary body, and retina, and a nonsuppurative iridocyclitis is often present.[7]

Diagnosis and treatment. Antibiotic and antiinflammatory therapy are indicated for treatment of anterior uveitis. In septicemic neonates, blood culture and sensitivity results are valuable to determine appropriate antimicrobial agents. Culture of ocular secretions or blood may identify pathogenic *Mycoplasma* species. Both topical and systemic antibiotics should be administered for bacterial septicemia and secondary uveitis. Topical 1% atropine ointment is indicated to promote pupillary dilation, relieve iris and ciliary muscle spasm, and thereby decrease intraocular pain.[1,3,5] If corneal ulceration is not present, topical, subconjunctival, or parenteral corticosteroids may be administered for their antiinflammatory effects.[1,3,5] Nonsteroidal antiinflammatory drugs (NSAIDs) are often beneficial to reduce the intraocular inflammatory response and provide analgesia. *Mycoplasma* species are usually susceptible to tetracycline, erythromycin, and tylosin.[1,5] Penicillin or tetracycline[5] is generally effective against *L. monocytogenes*. Systemic pyrimethamine and sulfadiazine in combination with topical 10% sulfacetamide, atropine, and steroid ointments have been recommended for treatment of ocular toxoplasmosis.[5]

Cataracts

Cataracts are the most common lens abnormality of sheep and goats. The majority of cataracts are congenitally acquired.[6] Any opacity in the lens is a cataract, except nuclear sclerosis, which is an aging change that results from compression of the oldest lens material. Cataracts are described by their appearance, location, and size. The smallest cataracts (less than 5% of the total lens) are incipient. Immature cataracts can be subdivided into early immature (6% to 50% lens coverage) and late immature (51% to 99% lens coverage). Mature cataracts involve the entire lens (Figure 12-8). Hypermature cataracts are characterized by lens fiber liquefaction, wrinkling of the lens capsule, and the development of dense plaques on

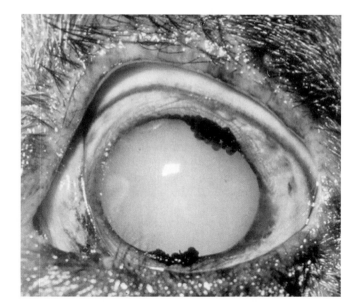

Figure 12-8 Mature cataract in a sheep. In this animal, cataracts were bilateral and caused by an unknown etiology. (Courtesy Dr. Brad Nadelstein, Chesapeake, Virginia.)

the anterior and posterior lens capsules.[8] Cataracts with an autosomal dominant inheritance have been described in New Zealand Romney sheep.[9] These cataracts were bilateral and the majority of them developed in animals between 2 to 4 months of age; however, some lambs were affected at birth. Congenital, nonprogressive nuclear cataracts that do not interfere with vision have been observed in sheep and goats.[3] Incipient cataracts and confirmed diabetes mellitus have been reported in twin male lambs.[10] Cataracts also may occur as sequelae to ocular trauma and severe uveitis.[3,6] Any uveitis can potentially cause cataracts. Septicemic infection such as that caused by *Mycoplasma agalactiae* can result in uveitis-induced cataracts.[6] Intraocular *E. schneideri* infection may cause posterior synechia and cataract formation.[11]

Miscellaneous

Persistence of the hyaloid artery may be an incidental finding during ophthalmoscopic examination of sheep and goats.[12] In the embryo the hyaloid artery supplies blood to the lens and normally atrophies after birth. However, as many as 30% of sheep between 1 and 3 years of age and approximately 40% of goats may have unilateral or bilateral persistent hyaloid arteries. The remnant of the hyaloid artery appears as a tight linear structure extending from the posterior lens capsule to the optic disc.

Persistent pupillary membranes have been reported in sheep.[3] The remnants of the embryonic pupillary membrane appear as pigmented strands of iris tissue extending from the iris collarette to the anterior lens capsule or corneal endothelium. Mild cases may appear only as small

pigmented foci over the anterior lens capsule. Focal opacities may be present in the cornea or on the anterior lens capsule in areas where the persistent pupillary membranes adhere. An essential iris atrophy has been reported in Shropshire sheep.[13] Affected sheep are born normal but develop ocular lesions by 1 to 1½ years of age. Lesions are bilateral but not symmetric and include partial- or full-thickness holes in the iris stroma and an absent or a rudimentary corpora nigra. Pupils are pear-shaped and respond poorly to both light and the administration of topical tropicamide.

References

1. Moore CP, Wallace LM: Selected eye diseases of sheep and goats. In Howard JL, editor: *Current veterinary therapy, food animal practice*, ed 3, Philadelphia, 1993, WB Saunders.
2. Moore CP, Whitley RD: Ophthalmic diseases of small domestic ruminants, *Vet Clin North Am Large Anim Pract* 6(3):641, 1984.
3. Lavach JD: Lens, uvea, and glaucoma. In: *Large animal ophthalmology*, St Louis, 1990, Mosby.
4. Whitley RD, Albert RA: Clinical uveitis and polyarthritis associated with *Mycoplasma* species in a young goat, *Vet Rec* 115(9):217, 1984.
5. Wyman M: Eye diseases of sheep and goats, *Vet Clin North Am Large Anim Pract* 5(3):657, 1983.
6. Pickett JP: Selected eye diseases of food and fiber-producing animals. In Howard JL, Smith RA, editors: *Current veterinary therapy, food animal practice*, ed 4, Philadelphia, 1999, WB Saunders.
7. Piper RC, Cole CR, Shadduck JA: Natural and experimental ocular toxoplasmosis in animals, *Am J Ophthalmol* 69(4):662, 1970.
8. Colitz CMH et al: Histologic and immunohistochemical characterization of lens capsular plaques in dogs with cataracts, *Am J Vet Res* 61(2):139, 1999.
9. Brooks HV et al: An inherited cataract in New Zealand Romney sheep, *N Z Vet J* 30(2):113, 1982.
10. Mattheeuws D et al: Diabetes mellitus in two twin male lambs, *Vet Q* 4(3):135, 1982.
11. Abdelbaki YZ, Davis RW: Ophthalmoscopic findings in elaeophorosis of domestic sheep, *Vet Med Small Anim Clin* 67(1):69, 1972.
12. Rubin LF: Fundus of ox, sheep, and other ruminants and pig. In: *Atlas of veterinary ophthalmoscopy*, Philadelphia, 1974, Lea and Febiger.
13. Aguirre G, Greene B, Gross S: Essential iris atrophy in sheep, *Proc Am Coll Vet Ophthalmol* 12:84, 1981.

PATHOLOGY OF THE RETINA

Many infectious organisms and septicemic conditions can cause retinitis or retinal changes. Septic neonates and feedlot lambs with listeriosis may develop chorioretinitis.[1] In sheep, toxoplasmosis frequently causes focal retinal necrosis and cyclitis or iridocyclitis.[2]

E. schneideri infections in sheep can result in retinal disease. An ophthalmoscopic examination can greatly aid in the identification of this parasite.[3] Reported ophthalmoscopic changes include chorioretinal atrophy with proliferation of tapetal pigment, attenuation of retinal vasculature, and optic nerve atrophy.[3] The optic discs of affected animals may have a hazy outline and appear edematous and pale gray. In contrast to elk, affected sheep do not become blind.[3]

A necrotizing retinopathy and retinal dysplasia occurs in lambs if their dams are naturally infected with bluetongue virus or a modified live vaccine is administered during the first half of gestation.[4] Lambs born to infected or vaccinated ewes have visual impairment and central nervous system defects.[1] Goats are more resistant to bluetongue virus than sheep.[5] Modified live bluetongue vaccine should not be administered to pregnant ewes, particularly during the first half of gestation.[6]

Scrapie has been shown to be a rare cause of blindness.[7] In one report[7] affected sheep lacked a menace reflex and walked into objects, although they maintained a PLR to bright light. Ophthalmoscopy revealed several oval-shaped, blister-like lesions scattered throughout the tapetum lucidum; these lesions ranged from one to three quarters of the size of the optic disc. Histologically the lesions were caused by an accumulation of lipid pigment between the RPE and photoreceptors in the retina.

Plant Toxicity

If it is chronically grazed, bracken fern *(Pteridium aquilinum)* causes a progressive retinal degeneration in sheep colloquially called *bright blindness*.[8-10] The majority of affected sheep are noticed to be blind between September and November,[8] several months after they begin to graze bracken fern.[10] Most sheep are affected between 3 and 4 years of age.[8] The earliest detectable clinical sign of bright blindness is an increased hyperreflectivity from the tapetum lucidum.[8] Affected sheep are permanently blind and very alert. The pupils are dilated and rounded and the PLR is poor.[8,10] Ophthalmoscopic examination may reveal attenuated retinal vessels that appear more widely separated than normal. In advanced cases the nontapetal fundus is pale with small cracks and gray foci. The optic disc may appear pale or gray-pink in color.[8,10] Choroidal vessels may be visible in some areas of the fundus.[10] The exact toxin responsible for bright blindness remains unknown, but retinal lactate dehydrogenase activity in experimentally affected sheep is significantly lower than in controls.[9] Platelet and leukocyte counts also are significantly lower in affected sheep.[9] Microscopic lesions are limited to the retina and are characterized by a complete destruction of the outer nuclear layer and photoreceptors.[8]

Locoweed *(Astragalus* and *Oxytropis* species) toxicity causes marked cytoplasmic vacuolization of the retinal ganglion and bipolar cells, which may result in visual deficits.[11]

Inherited Retinal Degeneration

Ceroid lipofuscinosis (Batten's disease) is an inherited lysosomal storage disease that causes blindness, ataxia, and tremors in South Hampshire sheep.[12] Blindness occurs by two mechanisms. Early loss of vision results from atrophy of the cerebral cortex. A concurrent retinal dystrophy also occurs in the rod and cone outer segments as the retinal cells accumulate ceroid lipofuscin pigment.[13,14] Affected animals have abnormal electroretinograms.[13,14] Retinal degeneration characterized as a rod-cone dysplasia has been reported in a 4-month-old Toggenburg doe.[15] Clinical signs of blindness became apparent after weaning and included bumping into objects, decreased weight gain, horizontal nystagmus, and poor PLRs.

Vitamin A Deficiency

The retina requires a constant supply of vitamin A to maintain vision. Phototransduction depends on vitamin A and progressive retinal degeneration results from a dietary deficiency.[16] Rhodopsin initiates the cascade of phototransduction and is made up of opsin (a protein that determines the wavelength of the photon the pigment will absorb) and retinol (a vitamin A derivative).[16] After light stimulation, rhodopsin undergoes a series of conformational changes and activates transducing activating phosphodiesterase, which results in hyperpolarization in the outer segments of the photoreceptors.[16] Ruminants are efficient in converting dietary beta-carotene into vitamin A if they have access to good-quality green forage sources. Vitamin A is stored in the liver, and hepatic stores may prevent vitamin A deficiency disease for many months if dietary deficiency occurs.

Clinical signs. Clinical signs of vitamin A deficiency may not become apparent for at least 3 months in goats[17] and 200 days in sheep[18] if they have previously been grazing good-quality pasture. Under the same conditions of dietary vitamin A deficiency, male animals are apparently more susceptible to developing clinical signs of deficiency than females.[19] Nyctalopia (night blindness) is a consistent clinical sign of vitamin A deficiency in sheep and goats, along with anorexia and poor body condition.[20,21] Severely affected animals may be completely blind and lack a PLR.[19,21] Ophthalmoscopy reveals papilledema, papillary and peripapillary retinal hemorrhages, and depigmentation of the nontapetal retina.[19,22] In young animals, vitamin A deficiency induces bony remodeling, narrowing of the optic canal, and thickening of the dura mater, which in turn causes an ischemic necrosis of the optic nerves.[19,23] Remodeling of the optic canal does not occur in skeletally mature animals and blindness is likely caused by retinal degeneration.[19,23]

Treatment. Nyctalopia is reversible with vitamin A replacement. However, completely blind animals probably will not respond to therapy.[19,22] Allowing free access to green forages or parenterally administering a commercially available vitamin A product is usually preventive in areas in which dry, brown hay is fed for extended periods and the inclusion of vitamin A in a feed or mineral supplement is required.

References

1. Pickett JP: Selected eye diseases of food and fiber-producing animals. In Howard JL, Smith RA, editors: *Current veterinary therapy, food animal practice,* ed 4, Philadelphia, 1999, WB Saunders.
2. Piper RC, Cole CR, Shadduck JA: Natural and experimental ocular toxoplasmosis in animals, *Am J Ophthalmol* 69(4):662, 1970.
3. Abdelbaki YZ, Davis RW: Ophthalmoscopic findings in elaeophorosis of domestic sheep, *Vet Med Small Anim Clin* 67(1):69, 1972.
4. Silverstein AM et al: An experimental, virus-induced retinal dysplasia in the fetal lamb, *Am J Ophthalmol* 72(1):22, 1971.
5. Wyman M: Eye diseases of sheep and goats, *Vet Clin North Am Large Anim Pract* 5(3):657, 1983.
6. Moore CP, Wallace LM: Selected eye diseases of sheep and goats. In Howard JL, editor: *Current veterinary therapy, food animal practice,* ed 3, Philadelphia, 1993, WB Saunders.
7. Barnett KC, Palmer AC: Retinopathy in sheep affected with natural scrapie, *Res Vet Sci* 12(4):383, 1971.
8. Watson WA, Barnett KC, Terlecki S: Progressive retinal degeneration (bright blindness) in sheep: a review, *Vet Rec* 91(27):665, 1972.
9. Watson WA et al: Experimentally produced progressive retinal degeneration (bright blindness) in sheep, *Br Vet J* 128(9):457, 1972.
10. Watson WA, Barlow RM, Barnett KC: Bright blindness—a condition prevalent in Yorkshire hill sheep, *Vet Rec* 77(37):1060, 1965.
11. Van Kampen KR, James LF: Ophthalmic lesions in locoweed poisoning of cattle, sheep, and horses, *Am J Vet Res* 32(8):1293, 1971.
12. Jolly RD, West DM: Blindness in South Hampshire sheep: a neuronal ceroid-lipofuscinosis, *N Z Vet J* 24(6):123, 1976.
13. Mayhew IG et al: Ceroid-lipofuscinosis (Batten's disease): pathogenesis of blindness in the ovine model, *Neuropathol Appl Neurobiol* 11(4):273, 1985.
14. Graydon RJ, Jolly RD: Ceroid-lipofuscinosis (Batten's disease) sequential electrophysiologic and pathologic changes in the retina of the ovine model, *Invest Ophthalmol Vis Sci* 25(3):294, 1984.
15. Buyukmichi N: Retinal degeneration in a goat, *J Am Vet Med Assoc* 177(4):351, 1980.
16. Ofri R: Optics and physiology of vision. In Gelatt KN, editor: *Veterinary ophthalmology,* ed 3, Philadelphia, 1999, Williams & Wilkins.
17. National Research Council: Nutrient requirements. In National Research Council, editor: *Nutrient requirements of goats: Angora, dairy, and meat goats in temperate and tropical countries,* Washington, DC, 1981, National Academy Press.
18. National Research Council: Nutrient requirements and signs of deficiency. In National Research Council, editor: *Nutrient requirements of sheep,* ed 6, Washington, DC, 1985, National Academy Press.
19. Paulsen ME et al: Blindness and sexual dimorphism associated with vitamin A deficiency in feedlot cattle, *J Am Vet Med Assoc* 194(7):933, 1989.
20. Schmidt H: Vitamin A deficiencies in ruminants, *Am J Vet Res* 2(5):373, 1941.
21. Eveleth DF, Bolin DW, Goldsby AI: Experimental avitaminosis A in sheep, *Am J Vet Res* 10(36):250, 1949.
22. Divers TJ et al: Blindness and convulsions associated with vitamin A deficiency in feedlot steers, *J Am Vet Med Assoc* 189(12):1579, 1986.
23. Hayes KC, Nielsen SW, Eaton HD: Pathogenesis of the optic nerve lesion in vitamin A–deficient calves, *Arch Ophthalmol* 80(6):777, 1968.

BLINDNESS

Severely ill or septicemic animals may appear blind as a result of depression or systemic disease. Evaluation of vision is difficult in neonatal animals because they normally lack a menace reflex for several days after birth. Blindness can be caused by neurologic diseases such as hydrocephalus, intracranial neoplasia, and any encephalitis, including caprine arthritis-encephalitis, scrapie, toxoplasmosis, cerebral abscesses, and aberrant parasite migration *(Parelaphostrongylus tenuis).*[1-3] *L. monocytogenes* infections may cause blindness as a sequela to septicemia, which generally causes severe endophthalmitis and hypopyon or (less commonly) meningoencephalitis.[3,4] Other clinical signs of listeriosis are optic neuritis, amaurosis, decreased PLRs, head tilt, and unilateral cranial nerve deficits.[3] Pituitary abscesses or neoplasia may lead to blindness if the optic chiasm is compressed. Pregnancy toxemia and ketosis may produce clinical signs of blindness because of cerebral energy deprivation and swelling.[5] Lightning strike, trauma, and improper use of debudding irons may damage the cerebral cortex and cause secondary blindness.[2,4,6]

Central blindness is a clinical syndrome characterized by ophthalmoscopically normal eyes, absence of the menace reflex, absent dazzle response, and a normal PLR.[2] Etiologies of central blindness in sheep and goats include polioencephalomalacia, lead poisoning, and sodium toxicosis and water deprivation (see Chapter 11).

References

1. Lavach JD: Ophthalmoscopic anatomy and disorders of the optic nerve, retina, and choroid. In: *Large animal ophthalmology,* St Louis, 1990, Mosby.
2. Collins BK: Neuro-ophthalmology in food animals. In Howard JL, editor: *Current veterinary therapy, food animal practice,* ed 3, Philadelphia, 1993, WB Saunders.
3. Miller PE: Neurogenic vision loss. In Howard JL, Smith RA, editors: *Current veterinary therapy, food animal practice,* ed 4, Philadelphia, 1999, WB Saunders.
4. Moore CP, Whitley RD: Ophthalmic diseases of small domestic ruminants, *Vet Clin North Am Large Anim Pract* 6(3):641, 1984.

5. Smith MC: Polioencephalomalacia in goats, *J Am Vet Med Assoc* 174(12):1328, 1979.
6. Smith MC, Sherman DM: Ocular system. In Smith MC, Sherman DM, editors: *Goat medicine*, Philadelphia, 1994, Lea and Febiger.

PATHOLOGY OF THE ORBIT

Glaucoma

Glaucoma in sheep and goats usually results from ocular inflammatory conditions such as severe keratoconjunctivitis, corneal ulcers, anterior uveitis, ocular trauma, and septicemia.[1,2] Glaucoma develops from a decreased outflow of aqueous humor, which may result from extensive anterior synechia or filtration angle obstruction with inflammatory cells or fibrin.[1]

Clinical signs.   Clinical signs of glaucoma include congestion of conjunctival and episcleral blood vessels, corneal edema, buphthalmos, blindness, exposure keratitis, lens luxation, and cataracts.[2]

Treatment.   Buphthalmic eyes should be enucleated, especially if exposure keratitis is present.[1,2] A silicone intraorbital prosthesis may be implanted in some cases if a cosmetic appearance is desired and the animal is unilaterally affected.[1] If the animal retains vision in the affected eye, diode laser cycloablation can be performed to destroy some of the ciliary body epithelial cells, which decreases aqueous humor production. Medical therapy of glaucoma may be attempted and is similar to that used in horses.[3]

Exophthalmos

Exophthalmos can be caused by retrobulbar abscesses or neoplasia, especially lymphoma and squamous cell carcinoma. Orbital cellulitis is rare but may result from periocular puncture wounds, plant awns migrating from the oral cavity, and caseous lymphadenitis abscesses.[4]

Cyclopia

Cyclopia in fetal lambs, a developmental anomaly characterized by the presence of only one orbit, has been associated with the consumption of *Veratrum californicum* (skunk cabbage, corn lily, or false hellebore) by ewes on the fourteenth day of gestation.[5,6] The plant grows in the mountain ranges of the western United States. Other congenital defects attributed to grazing *V. californicum* include anophthalmia, shortening or absence of the maxillary and nasal bones, cebocephalus (monkey face), hydrocephalus, and harelip (Figure 12-9).[5,6] The incidence of congenital deformities may range from 1% to 25% of lambs in flocks grazing pastures contaminated with

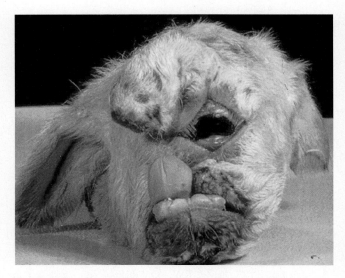

Figure 12-9   Cyclopia and facial malformations in a lamb. (Courtesy Dr. Robert Poppenga, Kennett Square, Pennsylvania, and the University of Pennsylvania Poisonous Plants Home Page, http://cal.nbc.upenn.edu/poison/)

skunk cabbage.[6] Occasionally only one lamb of twins is affected.[5,6]

Miscellaneous Ophthalmic Problems

Congenital microphthalmia, along with other ocular defects such as aphasia, aniridia, and optic nerve hypoplasia, may be inherited as an autosomal recessive trait in Texel sheep.[7] Several ocular abnormalities may occur in lambs born to ewes grazing seleniferous pastures.[8] Microphthalmia, conjunctival cysts, aphasia or displacement of the lens, aniridia or rudimentary iris, and a lack of a division between the cornea and sclera have been reported. Some 75% of affected lambs died at birth.

REFERENCES

1. Moore CP, Whitley RD: Ophthalmic diseases of small domestic ruminants, *Vet Clin North Am Large Anim Pract* 6(3):641, 1984.
2. Lavach JD: Lens, uvea, and glaucoma. In: *Large animal ophthalmology*, St Louis, 1990, Mosby.
3. Lavach JD: Glaucoma. In: *Large animal ophthalmology*, St Louis, 1990, Mosby.
4. Pickett JP: Selected eye diseases of food and fiber-producing animals. In Howard JL, Smith RA, editors: *Current veterinary therapy, food animal practice*, ed 4, Philadelphia, 1999, WB Saunders.
5. Binns W et al: Chronologic evaluation of teratogenicity in sheep fed *Veratrum californicum*, *J Am Vet Med Assoc* 147(8):839, 1965.
6. Binns W et al: A congenital cyclopian-type malformation in lambs induced by maternal ingestion of a range plant, *Veratrum californicum*, *Am J Vet Res* 24(103):1164, 1963.
7. Moore CP, Wallace LM: Selected eye diseases of sheep and goats. In Howard JL, editor: *Current veterinary therapy, food animal practice*, ed 3, Philadelphia, 1993, WB Saunders.
8. Rosenfeld I, Beath OA: Congenital malformations of eyes of sheep, *J Agri Res* 75(3):93, 1947.

ENUCLEATION

Enucleation is indicated for removal of eyes damaged by severe keratitis, perforating injury, glaucoma, and intraocular neoplasia. Exenteration may be necessary in cases of severe ocular infections or neoplasia; this procedure involves removal of the entire globe, extraocular muscles, and adnexa. The contralateral eye should be carefully evaluated to ensure normal vision before enucleation or exenteration is performed. If keratitis or endophthalmitis is present, systemic and topical antibiotics should be administered preoperatively.

Retrobulbar Anesthesia

General anesthesia or sedation (see Chapter 16) with local retrobulbar anesthesia may be used for enucleation in sheep and goats.[1] In small ruminants a 3.75-cm, 22-gauge, slightly curved needle may be used for retrobulbar anesthesia. A four-site retrobulbar injection technique desensitizes the optic nerve, extraocular muscles, and sensory portions of the eye and adnexa. Landmarks for the injections are the dorsal, ventral, medial, and lateral edges of the bony orbit. Topical ophthalmic anesthetic (0.5% proparacaine) should be applied before injection to desensitize the cornea and conjunctiva. The surgeon's index finger should be used to deflect the globe and protect it from the needle as each injection is administered. The clinician palpates the wall of the bony orbit and inserts the needle from the conjunctival fornix until it encounters the apex of the orbit. Approximately 1 to 2 ml of local anesthetic (2% lidocaine) or mepivacaine is injected at each site as the needle is advanced.

Surgery

Enucleation may be performed using the subconjunctival or transpalpebral technique. The subconjunctival approach removes only the globe and usually causes less hemorrhage. If a prosthesis is to be placed for a more cosmetic result, the subconjunctival approach should be used. The transpalpebral approach is indicated in cases of ocular infection or neoplasia; it involves removal of the entire globe, conjunctiva, extraocular muscles, and nictitating membrane. Because enucleation is often performed to remove severely infected and ruptured globes, the transpalpebral approach is most often indicated to reduce surgical contamination. After induction of general anesthesia or sedation and retrobulbar anesthesia, the patient is placed into lateral recumbency with the eye to be enucleated toward the surgeon. The affected orbit should be lavaged with a 1:50 dilution of povidone iodine solution and isotonic saline. Before clipping and aseptic preparation of the surgical field, the affected eyelids should be sutured closed using a monofilament, nonabsorbable suture material in a simple continuous pattern. A tail of suture should be left at each end of the incision to facilitate manipulation of the eye during surgery. The palpebral skin is incised 3 to 4 mm from the eyelid margins using a #15 or #10 scalpel blade. Blunt dissection is then performed circumferentially, using curved scissors and proceeding deeply into the eyelids and external to the extraocular muscles. The optic nerve and vessels should be clamped with a curved hemostat, then ligated and transected. The bony orbit should be gently lavaged several times with sterile saline solution containing a broad-spectrum antibiotic. Closure of the remaining soft tissues may be attempted to reduce postoperative sinking of the eyelids; however, this is often difficult in small ruminants because of their rather deep and wide bony orbit. The subcutaneous tissues are closed using absorbable suture (2-0 to 3-0) in a simple continuous or subcuticular pattern. The skin is closed using nonabsorbable suture (2-0) in a simple interrupted pattern. Systemic antibiotics and antiinflammatory drugs should be continued for several days after surgery. Some surgeons place a modified head bandage for a few days to compress the enucleated orbit and decrease postoperative swelling. All enucleated eyes should be submitted for histopathologic examination to determine the exact cause of ocular disease.

REFERENCE

1. Skarda RT: Local and regional anesthetic techniques: ruminants and swine. In Thurmon JC, Tranquilli WJ, Benson GJ, editors: *Veterinary anesthesia*, ed 3, Baltimore, 1996, Williams & Wilkins.

Chapter 13

*D*iseases of the Mammary Gland

DAVID E. ANDERSON, BRUCE L. HULL, AND D.G. PUGH

Diseases of the teats and udders of sheep and goats are less extensively discussed in the veterinary literature than those of dairy cattle. However, these diseases are no less important or significant to the dairy or meat goat or sheep farmer. Mastitis is a significant problem for the goat and sheep dairy industries and can result in poor milk production and low weaning weights among meat breeds. Problems of the teat and udder that require surgery seem to be much less common in small ruminants than in cattle. This is especially true in sheep, where the most common teat and udder surgeries include udder amputation following a gangrenous mastitis and removal of large, fibrotic udders so that the genetic potential of the animal is preserved. Indications for teat surgery may change as the dairy sheep industry grows in the United States.

ANATOMY

The mammary system of sheep and goats includes two glands, each of which have one teat.[1,2] The principal support for the udder is the medial and lateral suspensory ligaments. The medial suspensory ligament is elastic in nature; each half of the udder has a medial suspensory ligament, and they adhere tightly to each other. The medial laminae are composed of elastic sheets of tissue arising from the ventral abdominal wall and dividing the udder into two halves. The lateral suspensory ligament arises from the pelvic symphysis, subpelvic tendon, and prepubic tendon. Secondary laminae arise from the medial and lateral laminae to support lobes of the udder. The indentation formed between the two halves of the udder is associated with the medial laminae and is referred to as the *intermammary groove.*

The two halves of the udder are distinct and are supplied by separate arteries, veins, and nerves. The main ar-

terial blood supply to the udder is provided by the external pudendal artery. Blood from this artery courses through the inguinal ring after originating from the abdominal aorta and traveling through the external iliac artery, deep femoral artery, and pudendal epigastric trunk. The venous blood from the udder is drained by the external pudendal veins, the caudal superficial epigastric veins, and the perineal veins. The iliohypogastric and ilioinguinal nerves innervate the cranial udder. The genitofemoral nerve innervates the caudal udder.

The teat wall is composed of five layers. The innermost layer is very thin and is made up of epithelium and mucosal tissue. A layer of connective tissue, rich in blood supply, surrounds the inner layers. External to the connective tissue layer is the muscular layer, which is composed of both circular and longitudinal muscle fibers. Externally the teat is covered by stratified squamous epithelium. The teat mucosa surrounds a teat cistern (teat sinus, lactiferous sinus) that is filled with milk during lactation. The teat cistern is continuous proximally with the gland cistern but is demarcated from it by a distinct annular ring. This annular ring contains a large vein that encircles the base of the teat and is occasionally referred to as *Furstenberg's venous ring.* Located at the distal end of the teat and connecting the teat cistern to the outside is the streak canal (teat canal, papillary duct). This structure is lined by longitudinal folds of stratified squamous epithelia that produce keratin plugs. At the junction of the teat cistern and the streak canal is the rosette of Furstenberg. This rosette is created when the epithelium of the teat cistern meets the stratified squamous epithelium of the streak canal. The circular teat sphincter muscle lies directly beneath the rosette of Furstenberg at the proximal end of the streak canal. The streak canal varies from 0.5 to 1.0 cm in length and ends externally at the teat orifice.

MILK PRODUCTION

Much of the emphasis on milk and milk production has traditionally dealt with feeding meat and fiber sheep and goats for optimal milk production to maximize weaning weights. Chapter 2 addresses some of the feeding concerns in this area with dairy goats and sheep. Other production concerns include the length of lactation and the amount of milk produced, the effects of machine milking, and production-related diseases. Dairy goats that kid annually lactate for 305 days of the year. Similar to sheep, dairy goats experience peak milk production at 6 to 8 weeks after giving birth.[3] As with their dairy cow counterparts, they usually "dry off" 60 days before giving birth. Goats allowed a shorter dry period may experience depressed production in the following lactation.[3] The lactation curve of meat goats and sheep is much steeper than that of dairy goats.[3]

As a general rule, feeding the dairy goat (and to some extent the dairy sheep) is similar to feeding dairy cows. Similar to cows, high-producing dairy goats are in a negative balance for energy and some other nutrients during early lactation.[4] As production begins to taper off, they begin to replete their body stores. As with dairy cows, the three basic problems limiting productivity of dairy goats and sheep are nutrition, reproduction, and mastitis (see Chapters 2 and 6).

Inflammation of the mammary gland can result from trauma, infective organisms (viruses, bacteria, fungi), and environmental insults (freezing temperatures, irritating substances). When treating a doe or ewe with a mammary disease, unless an emergency situation such as excessive hemorrhage exists, the clinician should gather a complete history and perform a thorough physical examination.

The gland should be uniformly soft and symmetric. It should have a similar temperature to the rest of the body and be free of swelling, edema, and pain. The superficial inguinal (supramammary lymph) node should be barely palpable, not excessively hot, and pain-free on light palpation. Careful palpation alone is an excellent diagnostic tool; teats should be thin, uniform, and normal in appearance. Milk should be easily expressed or stripped out without overt signs of pain. If the female is lactating, the examiner should express some milk into a black plate or strip cup to evaluate it for abnormal color, consistency, and clots or flakes. Other diagnostic tests to augment the assessment of the mammary gland include the California mastitis test (CMT).

ULTRASOUND

Real-time ultrasonography may be useful for identifying tumors, abscesses, granulomas, and excessive fibrosis. Many practitioners only have access to 5 MHz linear array ultrasound equipment, but this equipment can be successfully employed. A sector scanning machine usually provides a wider view of the udder, and a 3.5 MHz transducer allows for deeper udder visualization. Obviously, all types of equipment have their limitations. On ultrasound examination, the normal udder displays a uniform mixture of hyperechogenic and hypoechogenic material. Abscesses, tumors, and fibrotic tissue are hyperechogenic, and milk is hypoechogenic. If the clinician is in doubt about the status of a female's udder, comparing the results with ultrasound images of a normal female's udder can greatly aid in assessment. The anatomy of the gland, annual ligament, and teat cistern can all be evaluated.

BIOPSY

Mammary biopsies are not commonly performed. In rare cases in which mammary tumors are suspected, a clinician can sedate the animal, anesthetize and aseptically scrub the skin over the area, insert a biopsy instrument (14 gauge) through the skin, and collect the tissue. The area to be biopsied should be carefully palpated for proper placement of the biopsy needle. This procedure is enhanced by first measuring the depth of the abnormality with real-time ultrasound equipment or using ultrasound to help guide the operator in collecting the biopsy. If a seepage of milk occurs, the biopsy site was located too close to a superficial duct or cistern. In this case a purse-string suture should be applied around the biopsy site after the biopsy has been taken. However, these rare milk leaks usually heal without intervention.

MILK CULTURE AND ANTIBIOTIC SENSITIVITY

Whenever milk is encountered that is abnormal in color, consistency, or odor or comes from a hot and inflamed udder, it should be collected from the affected half for microbial culture and antibiotic sensitivity patterns. After a standard washing and drying of the teat, the teat end should be scrubbed with an alcohol swab or pad (70% ethanol), the teat should be expressed and "first n fore" milk should be discarded, and then several milliliters of milk should be aseptically collected into a sterile milk culture tube or container. The sample should be refrigerated (4° C or 39° F) if it is not immediately cultured, but it should be swabbed onto a blood agar plate within 24 hours. Samples should be frozen if more than 24 hours will elapse before submission to the laboratory. *Mycoplasma* may be a cause of mastitis, and when it is suspected *Mycoplasma*-specific culture media may be employed.

SOMATIC CELL CULTURE

Cells in the milk are somatic cells and can be assessed with somatic cell culture (SCC). Infection that results in an increase in inflammatory cells increases the cells noted on SCC. SCCs in goats are less reflective of subclinical intramammary infection than an SCC of cow's milk.[3] The cytoplasmic droplets produced by the goat's apocrine secretion of milk result in an artificially elevated SCC if electronic counting methods are used. Methods of determining the SCC that measure deoxyribonucleic acid (DNA) or involve direct microscopy are more applicable for the goat. Still, an increased SCC may be used to indicate an inflammatory response in the goat.

CALIFORNIA MASTITIS TEST

The CMT is a commonly used method of estimating the cellularity of milk in cows, sheep, and goats. Milk (2 to 3 ml) is stripped into the CMT paddle, an equal volume of reagent is added, and the changes in viscosity of the mixture of milk and CMT reagent is graded a negative, trace, +1, +2, and +3. The greater the degree of viscosity (or the higher the number), the more cellular the milk and possibly the greater the degree of inflammation. This test is a good screen to predict the potential for infection and to compare the two halves.[3]

DISEASES

Supernumerary Teats

Accessory teats or supernumerary teats may be separate and not connected to the primary mammary gland, or they may be connected to the primary teat or gland. However, usually they are separate and have a functionally separate mammary gland.[1,2] Small supernumerary teats that are completely separate from the main teats are rarely observed in goats. When seen, supernumerary teats are generally located caudal to the main teats and are usually much smaller. When supernumerary teats are found in rams and bucks, these teats are usually located cranial to the scrotum. A distinction must be made between supernumerary and bifid teats (see the next section).

Treatment.   Supernumerary teats are usually removed with serrated scissors when the kid or lamb is young. Teats should always be removed so the resultant cut is craniocaudal and the scar blends with the normal folds of the udder. If supernumerary teats are not removed until the animal is older, they should be dissected and sutured after tranquilization and local anesthesia.

After tranquilization and the administration of local anesthesia, the supernumerary teat should be dissected with an elliptic incision in a cranial-to-caudal orientation. This dissection provides visualization of the glandular epithelium and mucosa from which the supernumerary teat arose. This tissue is closed with a simple continuous suture of fine (3-0 or 4-0) absorbable monofilament material. The adjacent connective tissue should also be closed with a continuous suture of fine absorbable material. The skin should then be closed with interrupted sutures of nonabsorbable material (polymerized caprolactam, polypropylene). An alternate method is to crush the teat base with a Burdizzo emasculatome and cauterize the base with silver nitrate.

Bifid Teats

Bifid teats (fused teats, forked teat) may be fused for a variable distance but always have two teat sphincters and two teat orifices (Figure 13-1). They are considered to be

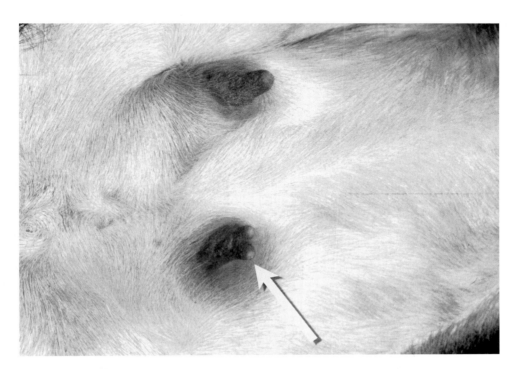

Figure 13-1   Bifid teat in a goat. Note the presence of two orifices.

an inherited defect, and surgical correction of them is considered unethical. Therefore unless an extra teat is clearly a separate and distinct teat the kid or lamb should not be used as a dairy or meat replacement animal. These abnormalities appear to be more common among pygmy goats and other non-dairy goat breeds.[2]

Weeping Teats

Weeping teats (Figure 13-2) are probably a variation of what is called a *web teat* in dairy cattle. In goats these small masses of secretory tissue, which are usually numerous, are commonly located on the teat near its base, but may be located on the udder near the base of the teat.[2] These masses of secretory tissue usually communicate to the outside through small pores in the side of the teat. Ultrasound examination (real-time, B-mode) is useful to confirm the diagnosis (Figure 13-3). These tissues become obvious in early lactation because of contamination of the teat skin with the secretions. Occasionally one or two of these small masses of secretory tissue does not have an opening and accumulates milk to form a milk cyst in the wall of the teat (usually near its base). In rare cases, gland development may be extensive with a true web teat formation (see Figure 13-3).

Although chemical cauterization using silver nitrate has been suggested to treat these cystic structures, this treatment is often not satisfactory because of the widespread nature of the extraneous secretory tissue.[2] A hereditary component of this defect must be considered, although no breeding studies have been done to date.

Poor Suspensory Ligament Support

The suspensory ligaments of the udder may become prematurely disrupted or may be congenitally malformed, resulting in abnormal udder conformation. The base of the udder is abnormally low, the teats may be splayed (angled laterally), and the walls of the teats may expand (balloon teat) if connective tissue damage includes the teats. Abnormalities of udder conformation are undesirable, and affected animals and their offspring should not be selected for use as replacement stock.

Uneven (Asymmetric) Udders

An asymmetric udder is seen occasionally in goats, but rarely in sheep. This abnormality should not be the sole reason to cull an affected animal. Goats seem to be more prone to this type of udder problem than other domestic species. Asymmetric udder abnormality may occur at freshening, in which the udder is more developed on one side than the other (Figure 13-4). This is more common in primiparous animals, but affected animals may have normal udder conformation in subsequent lactations. The abnormality may be caused by unsynchronized or uneven udder development.

Precocious Udder

Udder development in non-pregnant goats is not uncommon[2] (see Figure 13-5). Examination of precocious udder development should be aimed at differentiating between udder enlargement because of fat deposition, high estrogen concentrations in feeds (e.g., moldy corn,

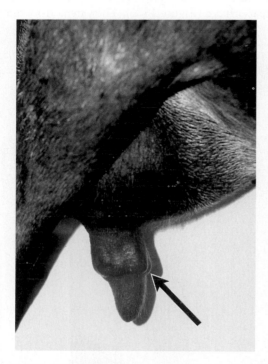

Figure 13-2 Weeping teat in a goat. Note the presence of cystlike structures at the base of the teat.

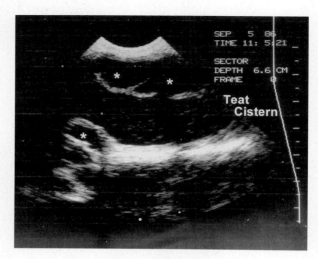

Figure 13-3 An ultrasound image of the teat in Figure 13-2. Note the presence of cysts (*) in the wall of the base of the teat.

clover), intersex, and true milk production associated with persistent corpus luteum or natural prolactin-like substances. Response to empirical treatment with prostaglandin $F_{2\alpha}$ (5 mg intramuscularly [IM]) suggests the influence of a persistent corpus luteum. These goats should not be milked because they are at an increased risk of mastitis. If milking is required to relieve pain, infusion of an intramammary product may be advisable to guard against the development of mastitis. Also, feeding management to attempt "dry off" should be done. This may include eliminating grain sources and feeding poor-quality roughage but should not include water deprivation. In rare cases the precocious udder may become pendulous, self-traumatized, or mastitic or may suffer teat damage severe enough to warrant udder amputation (see Chapter 7).

Udder Edema

Udder edema occurs sporadically in dairy breeds of sheep and goats. It can be diagnosed by finding pitting edema around the external aspect of the mammary glands, especially cranial to the udder. Affected animals do not exhibit hot udders or changes in milk quality. Udder edema may be present before or can develop after parturition.[4] If prepartum udder edema is present, the glands should not be milked out. Prepartum milking increases the risk of hypocalcemia and mastitis, which may contribute to the failure of passive transfer of colostral antibodies to lambs or kids. Udder edema is most common in primiparous females and may be associated with inadequate development of venous and lymphatic drainage from the udder. Inadequate drainage may be caused by rapid engorgement of the udder in the final stages of gestation without venous and lymphatic adaptation. Occasionally blood is seen in the milk and is presumed to

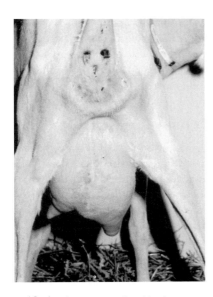

Figure 13-4　An asymmetric udder in a young goat.

result from the vascular fragility associated with hydrostatic congestion.

Treatment.　Udder edema usually resolves with time, but treatment is occasionally warranted. When needed, treatment may involve the administration of antiinflammatory drugs (flunixin meglumine 1 to 2 mg/kg intravenously [IV] or IM), diuretics (furosemide 2 to 10 mg/kg IV or IM), steroids (dexamethasone 0.1 to 1 mg/kg IV or IM), as well as more frequent milking and possibly hydrotherapy. If edema recurs in subsequent lactations, viral involvement (ovine progressive pneumonia virus [OPPV] or caprine arthritis-encephalitis [CAE] virus) or genetic influences should be suspected.[4] These animals should be selected for culling when possible.

Gynecomastia

Some male goats from heavy milk-producing lines of certain breeds (e.g., Saanen, Alpine) can experience udder development, lactate, and on occasion develop mastitis. Excessive udder development in these males more commonly occurs in the summer months. Energy and protein intake in these males should be reduced during times of the year when they are prone to lactate (spring and summer) or when these animals begin to lactate. Affected males appear to be of normal fertility. A mastectomy, when necessary, can be performed as described for females.

Skin Diseases

Diseases affecting the skin of the udder are discussed in Chapter 7.

OBSTRUCTION TO MILK FLOW

Blind Half

Rarely, "blind" mammary glands may be observed when females begin their first lactation. Blind glands usually occur on one side only and may be caused by congenital defects of the mammary gland or by granulomatous or viral mastitis early in the development of the udder. A Saanen goat was determined to have a congenitally blind udder because the milk ducts failed to unite with the gland cistern.[5]

Hard Milker

"Hard milkers," as seen in the cow, are rarely encountered in sheep or goats. However, when they are observed they may be treated in a similar manner as affected cattle. A hard milker in a sheep or goat may be caused by trauma to the teat end or may just be due to a congenitally small (tight) teat sphincter. When trauma occurs it is usually in the form of a crushing injury and is often self-inflicted. Animals occasionally crush their teat between their leg and the floor when trying to rise. Obviously, because of their small udder size this injury is extremely rare in sheep. Other causes for this type of trauma are poor milking machine function (delivering excess vacuum to the teat end) and frostbite of the teat end. Frostbite is obviously a seasonal event. Any traumatic insult to the area of the teat sphincter causes the formation of scar tissue in this area, which may lead to a small stream of milk and slow milking. This type of injury is therefore often self-perpetuating. The typical history is that one half of the udder takes a lot longer to milk out than the other half in dairy breeds or that one half of the udder is never milked out in meat breeds. This longer milking effort increases the trauma to the end of the teat and may in time increase the amount of scar tissue and make the animal even more difficult to milk. The trauma to the teat end coupled with incomplete milking may lead to mastitis.

Treatment. If surgery is indicated to increase the size of the milk stream, the use of a small teat knife is preferable to other methods of opening a hard milker because most other instruments (designed for cattle) open the sphincter too far and create permanent leakage. Surgery for a stenotic teat sphincter should be performed before the morning milking so that surgical response can be monitored and proper aftercare can be initiated throughout the day. After aseptic preparation of the teat skin and end, the surgeon inserts a teat knife through the streak canal, taking care to avoid cutting the entire length of the streak canal. The surgeon angles the knife at 45 degrees and makes a cut at the rosette of Furstenberg (area of the sphincter muscle) before gently removing the knife from the teat. The teat is forcefully milked to assess progress. If necessary the teat sphincter is cut 180 degrees from the first cut. These cuts can be repeated at 90 degrees separation if necessary. Milk flow should be evaluated after each cut. Evidence of the correct amount of cut is provided by the teat dripping a fine stream of milk for a minute or two after a forceful stream of milk is expelled from the teat.

After surgery the quarter should have several streams of milk expressed every 15 minutes for the next 2 or 3 hours and then once every hour until the next milking. This stripping must be forceful because the goal is to prevent closure of the incisions. The owner or clinician can help break down any fibrinous adhesions that may start to form between the cut edges by rolling the end of the teat between the thumb and finger.

Overzealous treatment of the hard milker may cause permanent leakage and increase the risk of mastitis. An enlarged teat orifice is very difficult to treat. Treatment may be attempted by injecting 0.1 ml of Lugol's iodine at four places around the teat end (each at 90 degrees' separation). The solution is injected using a tuberculin (TB) syringe and a 27-gauge needle. The goal of this procedure is to tighten the teat sphincter by stimulating scar tissue development. Unfortunately, this is often unrewarding. The owner should be warned that injecting Lugol's might result in sloughing of the tissues because goats' teats seem to be even more sensitive than those of cattle.

Teat "Spider" and Lactoliths (Milk Stones)

The term *teat spider* is usually used to describe scar tissue from the wall of the teat that hinders complete and rapid milking. As such, teat spiders seldom occur in small ruminants. However, small ruminants are somewhat prone to small floating pieces of scar tissue that have broken off from within the secretory tissue of the udder as a sequela to mastitis. Goats also occasionally get lactoliths, which are small, mineralized deposits. Lactoliths, or milk stones, are concretions formed within the teat cistern. These concretions are most likely caused by incomplete milking and may be formed by precipitation of debris and mineral composites contained in the milk. In either case these small floating objects may occlude the streak canal and obstruct milk flow.

Treatment. If the offending mass is small it may be manually massaged out of the streak canal with a combination of hydrostatic pressure (forceful milking) and manipulation of the teat end. If this is not possible and the mass is small or pliable it can be extracted with an alligator forceps inserted into the teat cistern through the streak canal.

If neither procedure works, the teat must be opened (thelotomy) to remove the offending foreign object. Elective thelotomy does not carry the high risk of incision failure that is commonly observed after laceration suturing. The success of thelotomy results from its minimal tissue damage, limited contamination, and the short time interval between incision and closure. The teat should be opened along its long axis. At this point the teat cistern can be explored and the offending foreign body or scar tissue removed. The teat is then closed as described for teat lacerations in the following section.

Teat Lacerations

Teat lacerations in sheep and goats appear to be less common than teat lacerations in cattle, but they can be just as devastating if left untreated. If repair of teat lacerations is to be attempted, the clinician should tranquilize the animal and use ring block of a local anesthetic (2% lidocaine hydrochloride); general anesthesia may be preferable in some cases. The prognosis for teat laceration treatment depends on several factors and can vary from good to hopeless.[6-11] Needless to say, full-thickness lacerations (into the teat cistern) have a much poorer prognosis than partial-thickness lacerations. The fresher a laceration is, the better it heals. The prognosis is poorer for lacerations that are more than 4 hours old, and after about 12 hours the prognosis is extremely poor. Because of the nature of the blood supply of the teat, vertical (longitudinal) lacerations heal far better than horizontal lacerations and lacerations near the base of the teat (its attachment to the udder) heal better than lacerations of the distal teat. Lacerations that involve the teat sphincter and streak canal have a much poorer prognosis than those that do not involve these structures because anatomic repair and return to complete function are more difficult to achieve in this area.

Treatment. Before attempting repair the clinician must clean and thoroughly evaluate the laceration for any small, deep holes that may be covered by fibrin clots. Even small fistulas change the method of repair and the prognosis. If the clinician is to attempt repair of a laceration of unknown duration or a laceration known to be more than 4 hours old, extensive débridement may be necessary. Any tissue that is infected, necrotic, or devitalized must be completely removed. Often, however, very little "extra" tissue is available and delicate dissection is necessary to remove desiccated tissue while preserving all the normal tissue possible. Débridement should continue until fresh bleeding tissue is uncovered.

After anesthesia and débridement have been accomplished, suturing with fine (4-0 or smaller) absorbable suture increases the chance of success. If full-thickness lacerations are not sutured but rather left to granulate, the majority will heal by second intention with fistula formation. The lining tissue should be sutured with a simple continuous pattern using fine (4-0 or 5-0) absorbable suture material with a swaged-on atraumatic needle. The tissue must be sutured carefully to obtain a milk-tight seal. After completely closing the tissue the clinician may wish to insert a teat cannula through the teat sphincter and gently probe the suture line to check for holes or weak areas. If the inner lining is not sutured, granulation tissue may proliferate into the lumen of the teat cistern and obstruct milk flow. When suturing full thickness in the mucosal surface the clinician is more certain to seal the mucosa completely and prevent milk fistulas. Because this inner surface tissue is very thin and delicate it should be supported by another simple continuous layer of fine absorbable suture placed in the submucosa. The submucosa of a teat is not a distinct layer, but rather the tissue directly adjacent to the mucosa and epithelial lining. The remainder of the teat wall should be closed with vertical mattress sutures of a non-capillary material. A *deep* "bite" of the vertical mattress suture is placed adjacent to the submucosal suture line to give it support. If the animal is being machine milked she can be put back on the machine at the next scheduled milking. Research in cattle suggests that one quarter can be rested for 7 days and still return to function if daily palpation of the gland for mas-

titis detection is performed. If she is being hand milked the owner or clinician may choose to prepare the teat carefully with alcohol and drain the milk with a teat tube for 4 or 5 days before resuming hand milking.

If a horizontal laceration that is not full thickness results in a ventrally based skin flap, the blood supply should be carefully evaluated. If the blood supply is inadequate, the flap should be trimmed to healthy tissue. The remaining wound may be closed in some cases or left to granulate if the remaining tissue is inadequate for closure.

Any full-thickness teat laceration or laceration that damages the teat end should be treated as though it were a case of mastitis. Culture and sensitivity tests are probably indicated and certainly appropriate antibiotics (both intramammary and systemic) should be employed. However, the clinician should be careful during intramammary infusion to avoid damaging the repair. Because the teat has an excellent blood supply the skin sutures can usually be removed in 10 days.

Teat Fistula

Teat fistulas are rare in sheep and goats and usually result from the unsuccessful repair of a teat laceration or from a laceration in which no repair was attempted.

Treatment. If the initial repair fails, the laceration should be allowed to granulate until the swelling and infection subside. During this period the wound should be cleaned daily and mastitis prevention measures instituted for 2 to 4 weeks.

After the wound has granulated to an end-stage fistula, surgery should be performed to correct it.[6-11] After preparation and administration of a ring block, the entire fistulous tract is dissected out of the surrounding tissue. This may be accomplished with an elliptic incision (around the fistula) parallel to the long axis of the teat. This dissection must be performed all the way to the teat cistern. After the dissection has been completed, the defect is closed as described for teat lacerations (three-layer closure).

Dissection of teat fistulas is extremely difficult if not impossible in sheep or goats with small teats. In these cases, teat size precludes surgery because insufficient teat tissue is available to dissect the fistula and close the wound adequately.

Udder Amputation

Udder amputation is perhaps the most common mammary surgery in small ruminants. This surgical procedure is performed when an owner wishes to keep the animal (either for genetic potential or as a pet) after the udder has become too pendulous for normal function. In sheep of exceptional value the udder may be amputated after long-term chronic mastitis has left a non-secretory

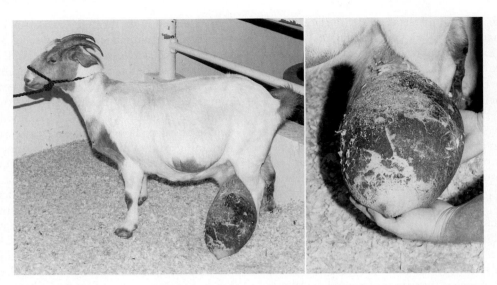

Figure 13-5 Large udders are a common finding in goats. These illustrations show an enlarged injured udder of a pregnant 6-year-old Boer-cross goat. She had been grazing and doing well (body condition score 3) until the owner noticed her dragging something behind her.

fibrotic mass for an udder. In these cases the animal is often a "poor doer" because of the chronic infection. In goats, udders may be amputated because of chronic fibrotic mammary tissue (as with sheep) or excessive size (Figure 13-5) resulting from inappropriate lactation syndrome (see Chapter 7). Goats are more prone to precocious milking than any other domestic species. Although many medical therapies have been attempted to cease this milking, they are seldom successful. Often these are pet animals that the owner does not wish to milk. In other cases the owner gets tired of milking the animal on a continual basis. Regardless, without milking the udder in some cases increases in size over time until it grows large enough to become uncomfortable for the animal and unsightly for the owner. At this point the owner of a pet sheep or goat often elects udder amputation.

Udder amputation is not a procedure to be undertaken lightly because the animal is often in poor physical condition and/or anemic as a result of the chronic nature of the infectious process.[12] Additionally, the clinician must consider the mass of the udder to be removed and the potential for serious hemorrhage. The owner should be made aware of these potentially serious consequences. General anesthesia, although not an absolute necessity, is certainly preferable.

A blood donor should be available or blood should be drawn and banked in case a blood transfusion is needed. Most of the time, udder amputation is an elective procedure. Therefore the animal should be fasted for 24 to 48 hours, and broad-spectrum antibiotics should be administered up to 4 hours before surgery. Although this surgery can be attempted on a heavily sedated animal with lumbosacral epidural anesthesia, general anesthesia is usually required (see Chapter 16). If possible the

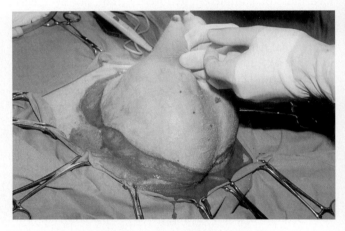

Figure 13-6 Circumferential incision made around the base of the udder.

animal should be positioned in dorsal recumbency to facilitate working on both sides of the udder. If dorsal recumbency is not possible the animal will need to be rolled from one side to the other during surgery and the appropriate preparations should be made. The ventral abdomen is clipped and aseptically prepared for surgery.

The external pudendal artery should be ligated before any of the venous system is occluded. This allows the blood contained by the udder to drain back into the circulation before the udder is removed. The surgeon makes a skin incision parallel to the base of the udder and about 3 to 5 cm ventral to the dorsal edge of the mammary tissue (Figure 13-6). Eventually this incision will extend completely around the udder in an elliptic manner. Hemorrhage can be controlled by either cautery or ligation. After incising the skin, the surgeon carefully extends the incision through the lateral suspensory ligament of the udder. Care should be taken at this point because the external pudendal artery and vein lie directly beneath the lateral suspensory ligament. The external pudendal artery and vein course from the inguinal ring in a tortuous manner. They should be ligated separately where they exit the inguinal ring. The clinician should exercise extreme caution during this procedure. If separation is difficult, the artery and vein can be ligated or double-ligated together. This raises the possibility of an arteriovenous shunt, but this rarely occurs. After the artery and vein have been ligated on one side, the procedure should be repeated on the opposite side unless only half of the udder is being amputated.

At this point the clinician extends the incisions (each side) cranially and ligates the subcutaneous abdominal veins. Traditionally reports have suggested that there is one subcutaneous abdominal vein for each half of the udder, more commonly these veins have numerous branches as they approach the udder. Each branch must be individually ligated or double-ligated. After the subcutaneous abdominal veins have been ligated, the skin incisions are extended caudally and the perineal veins are ligated. There should be one perineal vein on each side, although this is somewhat variable.

After ligating all the major vessels, the clinician cuts the median suspensory ligament near the body wall. Ideally, about 1 to 2 cm of medial suspensory ligament should remain on the body to provide a place to anchor the skin and help obliterate dead space during closure. If only half of the udder is being amputated, the right and left half of the median suspensory ligament can be separated, with the half of the median suspensory involved with the amputated half being severed.

After amputating the udder, the clinician closes the skin, obliterating the dead space if possible. This usually includes placing some of the sutures into the median suspensory ligament while closing the skin. The surgeon may choose to place a drain in the dead space for several days after surgery.

After surgery first intention healing is desired, but second intention healing seems to be more common. Although umbilical tape has been traditionally used as the ligature of choice, postoperative infection is much less of a problem with absorbable ligatures. If absorbable sutures are used, the clinician should be aware of the large vessels that are being ligated and employ appropriately sized sutures. Antibiotics should be continued as needed, and any postoperative pain should be managed.

Mastitis

Mastitis is common among all dairy and meat production livestock. Cold or wet environments and climatic conditions, muddy areas, and nutritional stress all may predispose to mastitis by reducing the blood flow to the udder and/or suppressing local immune function (secondary to increased stress-related cortisol output).[13] Grazing improved pastures and implementing feeding practices that favor excessive milk production may predispose to mastitis.[13] Surveys of goat dairy herds indicate that mastitis may occur in 13% to 20% of lactating does.[14,15] Sheep, goats, and cattle share many pathophysiologic processes, and diagnostic and treatment principles established for cattle can easily be adapted to use on sheep and goats.

Replacement livestock and animals with mastitis should be examined for predisposing factors, including teat fistula, accessory teats, trauma, pendulous udder, and udder edema. Dairy animals are most susceptible to mammary infections at parturition but may be infected through lactation or even after drying off. Brood ewes and does most commonly develop mastitis between parturition and weaning. Ewes have the same risk factors as goats, but after their lambs are 4 to 6 weeks of age, if milk needs (such as those of twins) exceed production, teat trauma can result from hungry lamb bites, particularly in poor producers.[3] With mastitis the udder becomes hot, swollen, and painful; however, affected animals also may display few or no outward signs. Nevertheless, meat and fiber animals suffering from mastitis and referred for treatment are usually sick, anorexic, and febrile and are often toxic. Animals affected with subclinical mastitis often fail to produce enough milk to raise their young or wean smaller young and have increased scar tissue on some areas of the udder. Whenever possible, owners or clinicians should palpate udders before purchase, before breeding, and at parturition. Herd problems from mastitis or increased somatic cell counts should be thoroughly investigated. With dairy animals, milking technique, milking hygiene, milking machine function (proper vacuum pressure), environmental risk factors, and personnel should all be evaluated.[16]

Agalactia

Agalactia has many causes in sheep and goats, including age of the female, poor prepartum gestation, genetics, and some diseases. Some infectious causes include CAE and ovine progressive pneumonia (OPP); previous bouts of mastitis that destroyed mammary tissue also can predispose to agalactia. Whenever agalactia is encountered females should undergo a complete physical examination and be tested for these diseases. Affected animals should be quarantined or, if genetics is the probable cause, culled.

Acute Mastitis

Acute mastitis may be recognized by the presence of heat, redness, pain, swelling of the udder, and/or lameness or stiff walking. Palpation of the udder may reveal edema, firmness of the gland, and enlargement of the supramammary lymph nodes. Milk stripped from the gland may have an abnormal color, contain flakes or clots (garget), and be thinner (serous) or thicker than normal. Bacteria such as *Escherichia coli* and *Mycoplasma* species also may cause septicemia or toxemia in the affected animal. This may be recognized by increased rectal temperature, elevated heart rate, decreased appetite, and marked reduction in milk production.[14]

Coliform Mastitis

Coliform mastitis seems to be less common among small ruminants when compared with cattle. *E. coli* and *Klebsiella* species are the most common coliform bacteria implicated in mastitis.[2,5] Coliform mastitis is more common in the post-parturient period and is associated with severe systemic disease. It can be either a persistent or transient infection.[3]

Clinical signs. Affected animals may have fever, anorexia, apparent depression, lethargy, and high heart rate; shock and death may ensue if the infection is not treated. Milk changes to a small volume of a watery serosanguineous secretion. Palpation of the gland reveals heat, swelling, edema, and pain. Endotoxin and inflammation may cause vascular thrombosis and gangrene, which can appear clinically similar to bluebag.

Treatment. Treatment should include antiinflammatory drugs (e.g., flunixin meglumine, 1 to 2 mg/kg IV), systemic antibiotics (oxytetracycline 10 mg/kg IV), and IV fluid therapy (see Appendix II) as needed. Use of aminoglycoside antibiotics should be avoided in food-producing animals because of prolonged and unpredictable drug elimination times. Intravenous administration of 5% hypertonic saline solution (HSS) (dosed at 5 ml/kg body weight over 5 minutes) is useful as a form of shock therapy to improve cardiac output.

Prevention. Coliform bacteria are environmental pathogens. Therefore control measures should be aimed at proper hygiene. Bedding should be kept clean and dry. Other prevention measures include milking clean, dry teats; providing teat dips (0.25 0 0.5 iodine) before and after milking; wiping teats with a towel (used only on that animal); and maintaining optimal milking machine function to avoid teat end injury.[3] Post-milking dips should contain ingredients that are effective but do not result in milk residues. Vaccination against gram-negative "core proteins" may be beneficial.

Bluebag

The bluebag form of mastitis is an infectious disease that is only rarely contagious.[15] It is a common concern for sheep and goat farmers (Figure 13-7). Its name comes

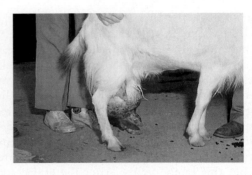

Figure 13-7 A goat with gangrene mastitis. Note the dark color of the distal portion of the left (far) gland. (Courtesy Dr. Tom Powe, Auburn, Alabama.)

from an alteration in mammary blood flow during the disease process that causes a change in udder color. The most common pathogens isolated from affected udders are *Staphylococcus aureus* and *Pasteurella haemolytica*.[18] *S. aureus* is most commonly associated with the gangrenous form of the disease. *P. haemolytica* may be more common among range ewes. Mastitis can occur as an acute, a subacute, or a chronic infection. The disease may progress rapidly and be severe enough to result in the death of affected animals. The incidence of this infection increases with age and the number of lactations and is most common during lactation.

S. aureus is a non-motile, non-encapsulated, non-spore-forming, gram-positive, coagulase-positive, coccoid, aerobic bacterium. Milk cytology reveals bacteria as singles, pairs, or chains of cocci. This bacterium is common on the skin and mucous membranes of normal sheep and goats. It can be destroyed by heat (60° to 80° C for 30 minutes) and some antiseptic agents (1% phenol for 35 minutes contact time; 0.5% mercuric chloride for 60 minutes; 10% formalin for 10 minutes).[18]

P. haemolytica is a non-motile, non–spore-forming, encapsulated, gram-negative, bipolar, pleomorphic, aerobic rod bacterium. It is found in the upper respiratory tract of normal sheep and goats. This bacterium is more easily destroyed than *S. aureus* and is susceptible to heat (60° C for 10 minutes) and antiseptic chemicals (0.5% phenol for 15 minutes). *P. haemolytica* can survive for weeks in a favorable environment. This infection is more common in sheep than in goats, but outbreaks of *P. haemolytica* have been documented in goats.[19] In sheep, *P. haemolytica* often results from lamb-induced teat injuries, but some ewes may be chronic carriers.

These bacteria are most likely inoculated onto the teat end by flies, excessive or aggressive nursing that causes teat end damage, poor milking machine hygiene, or contaminated bedding and pastures. Infection is followed rapidly by a severe inflammatory response. Pain and inflammation cause a marked decrease in milk production. *S. aureus* toxins cause vascular thrombosis and subsequent gangrene and tissue sloughing. *P. haemolytica* infection may lead to abscess formation; these abscesses may rupture through the skin of the udder.

Clinical signs. The acute form of bluebag produces the clinical signs of fever (41° to 42° C), decreased feed intake, refusal to lay down, and lameness because of udder pain. Animals infected by *P. haemolytica* may exhibit lameness of the rear legs early in the course of the disease. Typically only half of the udder is infected. The skin is initially erythematous and hot, but becomes cyanotic (hence the name *bluebag*) and cold as the infection progresses.[17] The udder may become very edematous. Animals that survive may slough the udder or the affected half. Milk decreases in volume and becomes a serous and watery or bloody and brown secretion with fibrinous debris. In cases of mastitis caused by *P. haemolytica*, concurrent lamb pneumonia may be encountered. In sheep flocks, 5% of sheep may be infected. Mortality rates approach 50% for *P. haemolytica* and 80% for *S. aureus* infection if no treatment is provided. Toxemia and shock may cause death in either case. The affected gland usually does not return to complete milk production in surviving sheep and goats.

Treatment. Antimicrobial drug therapy should be based on culture and sensitivity results, but empirical selection of β-lactam or tetracycline antibiotics based on historical susceptibility patterns is justified. In cases of *S. aureus* infection, antibiotics do not appear to reach the organism and are therefore of limited value. Toxemia may be treated with fluid therapy (see Appendix II) and nonsteroidal antiinflammatory drugs (NSAIDs; flunixin meglumine 1 to 2 mg/kg IV or IM). However, in most cases therapy is unrewarding. Affected animals that survive should be culled. In severe cases of gangrenous mastitis, udder amputation may be the treatment of choice. If a chronic problem exists in a flock, the production and use of an autogenous bacterium should be considered.

Miscellaneous Bacterial Mastitis

Pseudomonas species have been associated with mastitis and are usually spread by a contaminated water supply or teat dips.[3] Mastitis may be severe enough to cause systemic clinical signs, including septicemia and hemorrhagic milk. *P. aeruginosa* and *P. pseudomallei* have been isolated from animals with clinical cases of mastitis. In one study, *P. aeruginosa* was associated with purulent mastitis that progressed to gangrene and death in some goats.[5] Experimental inoculation with the isolated bacteria caused hemorrhagic mastitis in some goats and a watery greenish secretion in others; severe inflammation in the udder, fever up to 41° C (106° F), and decreased milk production also were observed.

Treatment. Response to therapy is often poor, but if treatment is instituted it should be based on culture and sensitivity results.

Arcanobacterium pyogenes may cause infection in non-lactating animals. Development and rupture of udder abscesses are typical of this infection. Milk becomes purulent and has a foul odor. Although susceptible to a variety of antibiotics, infection with this bacterium is difficult or impossible to cure because of the formation of udder abscesses. Therefore these animals serve as carriers of infection in the herd. Affected animals should be culled to prevent continued contamination of the milking equipment and/or herd mates. Affected halves in genetically superior animals may be treated to cease milk production by the infusion of some caustic solutions (60 to 120 ml of a 2% chlorhexidine solution twice a day for 2 to 3 days).

Streptococcal mastitis is caused by a variety of *Streptococcus* species. Streptococci may cause individual or herd outbreaks of mastitis. Some streptococci (e.g., *S. zooepidemicus*) may cause udder abscesses, atrophy, and chronic mastitis. *S. agalactiae* causes mastitis sporadically in goats. Infection with this bacterium may result in fibrosis and loss of milk production but is often not associated with systemic signs. *S. dysgalactiae* and *S. uberis* are more common causes of mastitis. These bacteria are spread by poor milking machine or personnel hygiene.

Bacillus cereus and other *Bacillus* species cause mild to severe (gangrenous) mastitis in goats. This organism is a soil and water contaminant.[3] Other pathogens rarely reported in sheep include *Clostridium perfringens* and *Leptospira hardjo*. *C. perfringens* is associated with an acute gangrenous mastitis, whereas *L. hardjo* may result in a sudden depression in milk output.

Clinical signs. Acute mastitis produces udder swelling, pain, decreased milk production, and abnormal milk.

Treatment. Treatment includes a combination of systemic and intramammary antibiotics based on culture and sensitivity tests. Empirical systemic antibiotic therapy may be instituted with trimethoprim-sulfadimethoxine, and intramammary treatment may be instituted with cephalosporin-based products.

Subclinical Mastitis

Subclinical mastitis is one of the most common causes of culling animals from the flock. As the name implies, it is a form of mastitis or inflammation of the mammary gland that insidiously drains the animal's productive ability. Subclinical mastitis in sheep and goats is caused by a variety of bacteria, including *Bacillus* species, *Staphylococcus epidermidis*, *E. coli*, *P. aeruginosa*, *A. (Actinomyces, Corynebacterium) pyogenes*, *A. pseudotuberculosis*,

BOX 13-1

Pathogens Isolated from Mastitic Milk Samples in Goats

SUBCLINICAL MASTITIS (FREQUENCY %)	MASTITIS (FREQUENCY %)	CHRONIC MASTITIS (FREQUENCY %)
Staphylococcus species (59.1%; 12 species):	*Staphylococcus epidermidis* (24.6%)	Culture positive (66.7%)
S. aureus (17.2%)	*Escherichia coli* (11%)	*Staphylococcus aureus*
S. epidermidis (14.2%)	*Pseudomonas aeruginosa* (8%)	Beta-hemolytic *Streptococcus*
S. capitis (12.8%)	*Staphylococcus aureus* (7%)	*Streptococcus agalactia*
Bacillus species (29.9%)	*Arcanobacterium pyogenes* (3%)	Coagulase negative
Coliforms (4.3%)	*Arcanobacterium pyogenes* (3%)	*Staphylococcus*
Micrococcus species (2.6%)	*Enterobacter cloacae* (3%)	*Arcanobacterium pyogenes*
Streptococcus species (1.9%)	*Streptococcus* species (3%)	*Pseudomonas* species
Corynebacterium,	*Pseudomonas putida* (1%)	*Pasteurella* species
Arcanobacterium (1.5%)	*Bacillus* species (1%)	No growth (33.3%)
Pseudomonas species (0.7%)	*Klebsiella pneumoniae* (1%)	
	Gram-positive rods (1%)	
	No growth (35.6%)	

From Turner CW, Berousek ER: Blind halves in a goat's udder, *J Dairy Sci* 25:549, 1942; Kalogridou-Vassiliadou D: Mastitis-related pathogens in goat milk, *Small Rumin Res* 4:203, 1991; Lerondelle C, Richard Y, Issartial J: Factors affecting somatic cell counts in goat milk, *Small Rumin Res* 8:129, 1992; Chineme CN, Addo PB: Chronic caprine mastitis: clinical, microbiological and pathological findings in spontaneously occurring cases in Nigerian goats, *Intl Goat and Sheep Res* 3:266, 1984; Rowe JD: Milk quality and mastitis, *Proceedings of the 1998 Symposium on the Health and Disease of Small Ruminants Western Veterinary Conference,* 1998, Las Vegas, NV; Van Tonder EM: Notes on some disease problems of Angora goats in South Africa, *Vet Med Rev* 1:109, 1975.

Klebsiella species, and other environmental pathogens (Box 13-1).[21,22]

Clinical signs. Subclinical mastitis may be recognized by poor lamb or kid growth, neonatal malnutrition, and neonatal death caused by starvation in meat breeds. In dairy breeds, low daily milk production is the most common finding. Occasionally, udder abscesses are recognized by swelling, edema, or rupture and subsequent purulent exudate.

Diagnosis. Diagnosis of subclinical mastitis is by palpation of the udder and/or milk culture. Other tests helpful for identifying animals with subclinical mastitis are SCCs and CMTs. Herd managers should be encouraged to perform routine udder palpation and milk tests when animals freshen and at appropriate intervals according to the management system. Differentiation of various types of pathogenic bacteria has become easier and may be performed in a general practice without submitting samples to commercial laboratories (Table 13-1). However, accurate identification of species of bacteria may require the use of a commercial microbiology laboratory. Whenever culturing halves, the clinician should communicate to the diagnostic laboratory that non-hemolytic *Staphylococcus* may be a cause of subclinical mastitis and should be included in any findings. The CMT is based on pH and the

presence of DNA-containing cells. The test solution lyses cells to release DNA, which then coagulates to a visible gelatin- or mucus-like material. The pH detector turns dark purple in alkaline milk and tan to yellow in acidic milk. The CMT is not interpreted as stringently in sheep and goat milk because these species typically have higher somatic cell counts; a CMT of trace or 1+ should be considered within normal limits for this test (Table 13-2). Sheep and goat milk contains relatively higher somatic cell counts compared with that of cattle. A typical somatic cell count range for sheep and goats is 0 to 500,000 cells/ml (see Table 13-2). Mild inflammation increases the count to the 500,000 to 2,000,000 cells/ml range. The somatic cell count is inversely related to milk production. As milk production decreases in late lactation, the somatic cell count increases because a similar number of cells are diluted in a lesser volume of milk.[23] The count approaches 5,000,000 cells/ml in normal goats near the end of lactation. A more useful application of CMT and SCC is to compare results between udder halves. In one study, udder halves infected with coagulase-negative *Staphylococcus* had a mean somatic cell count of 932,000 cells/ml, udder halves infected with other major pathogens had a mean somatic cell count of 2,443,000 cells/ml, and uninfected udder halves had a mean somatic cell count of 272,000 cells/ml. If milk from one half of the udder scores markedly higher on the

TABLE 13-1

DIFFERENTIATION OF BACTERIAL CULTURE ISOLATES

GRAM-POSITIVE ORGANISMS				GRAM-NEGATIVE ORGANISMS		
Cocci		Rods		Yeast Uncommon	Rods	Cocci Rare
Catalase		Catalase			Oxidase	
Positive	Negative	Positive	Negative		Positive	Negative
Staphylococcus	*Streptococcus*	*Bacillus*	*Actinomyces*		*Pasteurella*	*Escherichia coli*
		Corynebacterium	*pyogenes*		*Pseudomonas*	*Klebsiella*
		Pseudotuberculosis				*Enterobacter*
						Serratia
						Proteus

From Smith MC, Sherman DM: Mammary gland and milk production. In Smith MC, Sherman DM, editors: *Goat Medicine*, Baltimore, 1994, Williams & Wilkins.

TABLE 13-2

MILK TESTS AND INTERPRETATION

CALIFORNIA MASTITIS TEST RESULT	SOMATIC CELL CULTURE (CELLS/ML)	INTERPRETATION
Negative	0 to 480,000	Normal
Trace	0 to 640,000	Normal
1+	240,000 to 1,440,000	Normal
2+	1,080,000 to 5,850,000	Mastitis
3+	More than 10,000,000	Mastitis

From Smith MC, Sherman DM: Mammary gland and milk production. In Smith MC, Sherman DM, editors: *Goat medicine*, Baltimore, 1994, Williams & Wilkins.

CMT or SCC compared with the contralateral gland, a diagnosis of subclinical mastitis is justified and culture should be performed. Research investigating improved diagnostic tests for mastitis continues. Some recent techniques include measuring electrical conductivity, antitrypsin, *N*-acetyl-β-*D*-glucosaminidase (NAGase), fat, and protein content.[15,22-25]

S. epidermidis is commonly associated with mastitis in dairy goats and may be the most common bacterium implicated in chronic progressive mastitis.[3] This bacteria is spread from the skin of goats or milking personnel and may cause acute mastitis.

Prevention. Preventive measures include keeping all housing and dry lots clean and avoiding muddy areas. When "drying off" or at weaning, the owner or clinician may choose to infuse halves with a "dry cow" infusion. If halves were treated during lactation, a different class of antibiotics should be used for "dry off" infusion.

Treatment and Prevention of Bacterial Mastitis

A variety of regimens have been used to treat mastitis in sheep and goats. Response to therapy varies with the type of pathogen causing the disease. Difficulties with parenteral treatment of mastitis during lactation are discussed by Pyorala et al.[26] In this study, 452 dairy cows were treated with either parenteral procaine penicillin G, spiramycin, or enrofloxacin; 35 cows were treated with supportive care only (all 35 had *E. coli* infection). The cure rate was 34% for *S. aureus*, 76% for coagulase-negative *Staphylococcus*, and 65% for *Streptococcus*. Heifers experiencing their first lactation had higher cure rates than older cows. Mastitis caused by *E. coli* was cured in 74% of cows receiving procaine penicillin G and 71% of cows receiving supportive care only. Cows affected with mastitis early in the course of lactation suffered more severe clinical signs when infected with coagulase-negative *Staphylococcus* or *E. coli*. The authors of the study concluded that penicillin therapy may be beneficial in heifers in their first lactation, but not in older cows and not for coliform mastitis.[26] The results of this study appear to be applicable to sheep and goats.

In cases of toxic or gangrenous mastitis, treatment consists of hydration maintenance with either IV or oral fluids (see Appendix II) or hypertonic saline (4 ml/kg IV), administering NSAIDs (flunixin meglumine 1 to 2 mg/kg), and milking out every 2 to 3 hours.[27] Oxytocin administered at each milk-out may aid in milk removal. The use of antibiotics is controversial. Still, many owners and clinicians include broad-spectrum antibiotics in their treatment protocols. If the mastitis is not associated with systemic signs, stripping the affected half out every 2 to 3 hours may be all that is required.[27] If the animal survives and the udder does not slough, a partial mastectomy (previously discussed) can be performed. An alternative procedure to surgery is the infusion of the udder with Lugol's iodine or chlorhexidine solution. Infusion with either of these results in drying and "killing" the half.[28]

Intramammary infusions are an accepted practice at dry-off in dairy cattle and may be of some value in sheep and goats.[26-28] In one study, 49 does with bacterial mastitis (coagulase-negative *Staphylococcus*, *C. bovis*, *S. uberis*) had the infected udder half treated at dry-off with cephapirin benzathine intramammary infusion.[29] Udder halves were monitored for treatment success or the development of new infection. Also, antibiotic residues were determined at freshening. At the time of freshening, 78.9% of infected quarters had been cured. All treatment failures occurred in udder halves infected with coagulase-negative *Staphylococcus* (8 of 40 were not cured). Fewer than 7% of udder halves not infected at dry-off were found to be infected at the time of freshening. This study emphasized the possibility of selective treatment of udder halves at dry-off rather than the standard practice of dry treatment of all udders (current recommendations for dairy cows include the use of nonselective dry cow infusion). Antibiotic residues were detected in only one goat, suggesting that prolonged antibiotic residues may remain when bovine intramammary preparations are used in goats. Another study evaluated the effect of intramammary infusions on bacterial infection and somatic cell count in goats. Treatments included infusion of a combination product after the last milking (penicillin, nafcillin, dihydrostreptomycin) and no infusion at dry-off.[30] Only 19.8% of control goat udder halves were culture-negative 2 weeks after freshening, compared with 71% of udder halves treated by intramammary infusion. One study[31] evaluated the effect of intramammary infusion of ewes that were infused at the time of lamb weaning and cultured again 1 to 3 weeks after freshening. Untreated control ewes were 2.6 times more likely to develop new intramammary infections compared with treated ewes. Interestingly, the presence of one infected udder half was associated with a higher risk of the other half of the udder becoming infected.[31] In a Canadian study,[32] tilmicosin given parenterally to multiparous ewes 1 month before lambing was shown to improve the growth of their lambs compared with lambs from untreated control ewes. Lambs from tilmicosin-treated ewes were 0.52 kg heavier at 50 days of age, compared with lambs from untreated ewes. The tilmicosin treatment resulted in a 43% decrease in palpable udder abnormalities compared with the controls. However, no difference in the incidence of clinical mastitis was noted between the two groups. Therefore a management protocol of giving tilmicosin (10 mg/kg IM) at the time of prelambing vaccination may improve lamb weaning weights by decreasing the incidence of subclinical mastitis.[32] Tilmicosin is not approved for use in sheep in the United States, but it is approved in Canada. Its use should be avoided in goats (see Appendix I).

Where possible, identification (by milk culture or CMT) and culling of all affected animals should be carried out because these animals may serve as sources of continuing flock infection. As previously stated, milking technique, milking machine function, and diet should all be carefully evaluated. Ewes or does that are thin (body condition score less than 2.5) should be fed enough to ensure adequate milk output. This may help minimize teat and udder trauma from hungry lambs or kids. Lambs or kids whose dams are poor milkers should be identified and fed a supplement. Hungry lambs and kids may transmit infection if they are "bumming" or nursing milk from numerous ewes and does. This may be more of a problem in lambs infected with bacterial respiratory disease (*Pasteurella* species) (see Chapter 5). Contagious ecthyma should be prevented because it may predispose to bacterial or fungal mastitis. Providing proper shelter; clean, non-muddy paddocks; and clean, uncontaminated bedding are all paramount in preventing both clinical and nonclinical mastitis. All handling, lounging, or feeding areas should be well drained. Dry ewe or doe teat infusion and possibly post-infusion teat dipping at weaning or drying off also can reduce flock infection rates.[13,20,28] If teat or udder infusion with antibiotics is used, good aseptic technique should be emphasized. The drastic practice of withholding feed and/or water 24 to 48 hours before weaning is probably of only marginal value. Still, decreasing feed intake to meet but not exceed maintenance at or just before weaning may be of some value in decreasing milk output and reducing mastitis cases. All ewes and does should be closely monitored for signs of mastitis for the first 2 weeks after weaning.

Mycoplasma Mastitis

Mycoplasma species are increasingly recognized as significant pathogens in the udder.[33-41] *Mycoplasma*-induced mastitis should be suspected when clinical signs support a diagnosis of mastitis but repeated attempts to culture bacteria fail to identify a significant pathogen. Diagnostic laboratory techniques have improved greatly in recent years, and identification of *Mycoplasma* species pathogens is performed more readily. *Mycoplasma*-infected milk may be a significant source of infection for young animals, which then develop arthritis and keratoconjunctivitis. Feeding of mastitic milk to young kids and lambs is discouraged because it may result in lifelong infection (see Chapters 5 and 9).

M. agalactiae (the causative organism of contagious agalactia) may produce acute or chronic mastitis in sheep and goats.[2] This pleomorphic gram-negative bacterium is hemolytic on blood agar. Contagious agalactia is most common in European and Middle Eastern countries and rare in the United States; it is a federally reportable disease. Infective organisms contaminate the environment through milk, urine, nasal and ocular secretions, exudate from joints, and secretions from the reproductive tract.

Clinical signs.   Clinical cases are observed most often during spring months. Often infection of the udder occurs during the final trimester of gestation. After being ingested, *M. agalactiae* invades the intestinal wall, where it multiplies and then gains entry into the bloodstream, causing a sustained septicemia. During the septicemic period the animal's temperature may rise to 41° or 42° C (105° to 107° F) and the affected animal becomes anorectic. Foci of infection may become established in the udder, uterus, eyes, and joints. Clinical signs may be observed as soon as 5 to 7 days after inoculation of infective organisms or as late as 60 days after ingestion of infective organisms from the environment. Interstitial mastitis causes fibrosis and reduced milk production. Milk from infected udders is more alkaline than normal, has a yellow color, segregates into layers on standing with a green-yellow supernatant, and exhibits granular sedimentation in the bottom of the receptacle. As the disease progresses, the udder atrophies and milk production is severely decreased.

M. arginini, although considered non-pathogenic, has been associated with mastitis in goats.[39,40] Affected goats suffer marked decreases in milk production and exhibit purulent exudate and large numbers of leukocytes in the milk.

M. putrefaciens has been isolated from cases of acute and subclinical mastitis. Acute mastitis caused by this organism may be associated with agalactia, abortion, and arthritis. However, glandular fibrosis is not a common finding despite the marked leukocyte increases in milk.

M. mycoides subspecies *capri,* *M. mycoides* subspecies *mycoides,* and *M. capricolum* have been associated with mastitis in goats.[2,41] Mastitis caused by these pathogens is characterized by purulent exudate in the milk, thickening of the milk, markedly decreased milk production, enlarged supramammary lymph nodes, and systemic diseases such as arthritis, pneumonia, and conjunctivitis. A 6-year-old French Alpine goat exhibited decreased appetite and milk production, fever (41° C), an auricular abscess, and mastitis.[41] In this case the milk was watery and yellow. Serology confirmed a diagnosis of *M. mycoides* subspecies *mycoides.*[37]

Agalactia caused by *Mycoplasma* species infection is followed by udder atrophy. However, resolution of the udder may be followed by normal lactation after the next parturition because glandular fibrosis is not common with *Mycoplasma*-induced mastitis.

Treatment.   Although treatment for mastitis caused by *Mycoplasma* may be attempted with tiamulin, tylosin (20 mg/kg IM twice a day [BID]), erythromycin (3 to 5 mg/kg IM BID), or tetracycline (10 mg/kg IV once a day [SID] to BID or 20 mg/kg every 48 hours), success rates are variable, prognosis is poor, and a carrier state may persist.

Prevention.   Because udder damage is considered permanent, culling of infected sheep and goats is advised. Carrier animals may remain clinically normal and shed organisms for months or years during times of stress (e.g., parturition, relocation). Herd control measures may include serologic testing (if available for the specific strain identified), intermittent bulk tank cultures to detect dairy animals with subclinical disease, culture of colostrum at freshening, pasteurization of milk before feeding to young stock, isolation or culling of clinically affected animals, use of individual towels for each udder when cleaning in the dairy parlor, and close attention to hygiene by personnel. Vaccination with strain-specific vaccines may be useful, but concerns about the persistence of carrier animals in the herd remain (see Chapter 5).

Because milk is the major route for infection for *Mycoplasma* in kids, many of the same protocols for prevention of CAE are useful in preventing *Mycoplasma* mastitis.[37] Removing kids from dams at birth and feeding them heat-treated colostrum (60 minutes at 56° C) helps prevent this disease. Identifying carrier animals through culture testing, removing them from the herd or flock, and implementing proper milking hygiene practices also are crucial to preventing *Mycoplasma* mastitis.[37,38]

ZOONOTIC PATHOGENS

Raw milk consumption poses certain risks for the transmission of zoonotic disease (Box 13-2). *Listeria monocytogenes* rarely causes interstitial mastitis. However, this bac-

---

BOX 13-2

Zoonotic Pathogens Potentially Contaminating Raw Sheep or Goat Milk

SECRETED INTO MILK	CONTAMINANTS
Brucellosis	*Campylobacter*
Corynebacterium	*Escherichia coli*
pseudotuberculosis	*Listeria monocytogenes*
Leptospirosis	*Listeria monocytogenes*
Salmonella	
Coxiella burnetii	
Mycobacterium bovis	
Mycobacterium avium	
subsp. *paratuberculosis*	

From Smith MC, Sherman DM: Mammary gland and milk production. In Smith MC, Sherman DM, editors: *Goat medicine,* Baltimore, 1994, Williams & Wilkins.

terium is occasionally isolated from milk cultures. The zoonotic potential of this pathogen is of great concern and affected animals should either be treated until proven free of disease or culled from the herd. However, the owner and clinician should bear in mind that proving an animal free of disease is difficult. *Mycobacterium bovis, M. tuberculosis,* and *M. avium* may cause subacute or chronic mastitis. Palpation of the udder reveals hard nodules in the parenchyma. Infection is confirmed by an intradermal tuberculin skin test, and affected animals are culled under federal supervision.

Fungal Mastitis

Fungal infection of the udder is infrequently diagnosed. Most often, fungal infection is associated with prolonged or repeated administration of antimicrobial drugs into the udder by intramammary infusion. A variety of infective fungi have been identified, including *Candida albicans, Aspergillus fumigatus, A. terreus, Cryptococcus albidus, C. neoformans, Yersinia pseudotuberculosis, Nocardia* species, *Rhodotorula glutinis,* and *Geotrichum candidum.* Treatment of fungal mastitis is not generally recommended because it requires the administration of drugs not approved for use in food-producing animals.

VIRAL MASTITIS

Chronic Indurative Mastitis of Sheep

Sheep flocks infected with OPPV suffer high morbidity but low mortality.[2] The udder appears full but has a firm texture on palpation. Milk production is markedly reduced and the teats fail to fill up with milk.[38] Although the disease may be present at first lactation, the incidence is highest among ewes older than 3 years. Milk color and content appear normal. This viral infection causes periductal lymphoid proliferation and lymphoid follicle formation, which results in alveolar atrophy. Milk flow is inhibited; fibrosis of the parenchyma results in firmness on palpation. Clinical signs among meat breeds include poor lamb or kid growth. Dairy breeds suffer decreased milk production. Diagnosis is made by virus isolation or serology (see Chapters 6 and 14).

Hard Udder of Goats

Hard udder is a chronic fibrosing mastitis of goats caused by the CAE virus, which is nearly identical to OPPV in sheep.[2,18,42] This viral infection causes an interstitial mastitis characterized by periductal lymphocytic infiltration and subsequent fibrosis. Although the udder is extremely firm on palpation and little milk can be expressed, udder edema, erythema, and heat are not evident. Superficial inguinal lymph nodes may become enlarged. This form of mastitis is seen in some animals at puberty.[43] Milk production may increase as the lactation cycle con-

tinues, but total production levels are generally depressed. Milk production was evaluated in a herd of Alpine goats infected with CAE.[44] Approximately 36% of the herd was seropositive to CAE by agar gel immunodiffusion (AGID). Production parameters were higher for seronegative goats (696 kg milk, 24 kg butterfat, and 21 kg of nonfat solids) than for seropositive goats (656 kg milk, 20 kg butterfat, 20 kg nonfat solids). Diagnosis is by thorough palpation of the udder, failure to yield *Mycoplasma* species or other bacteria on culture, observation of mononuclear infiltrates on histology, and positive serology or immunofluorescent antibody tests. Affected goats should be culled because treatment response is poor. Kids born to affected does should be removed immediately from the doe and given colostrum and milk free of CAE virus and *Mycoplasma* species (see Chapters 6, 9, and 14).

Prevention of Mastitis

Prevention of mastitis is best accomplished by close attention to hygiene, milking equipment maintenance, optimal nutrition, and proper animal care and housing.[37] Various guidelines have been established for the prevention of mastitis (Table 13-3). Maintaining clean, dry bedding and properly cleaning lambing jugs helps prevent the spread of some organisms (e.g., *P. haemolytica*). If milking machines are used on sheep or goat dairies, careful monitoring and maintenance of equipment is required.[5] Post-milking teat dipping, dry doe or ewe treatment, and identification of all infected animals (by culture testing) are paramount in control of the more contagious pathogens (*S. aureus* and *Mycoplasma* species).[3] Dry doe or ewe teat infusion can be based on culture and antibiotic sensitivity testing, but broad-spectrum infusions without culture and sensitivity testing are commonly administered with good response. When *Mycoplasma* infection is suspected, removing kids at birth and feeding them only pasteurized colostrum are good preventive techniques. Clipping or burning udder hair, cleaning the teats before and after milking (using a separate towel for each animal), and dipping before and after milking are good procedures in problem herds.[3] Performing CMTs, identifying infected animals, maintaining them in a separate area from uninfected animals, and milking them last helps minimize the spread of disease. Ewes and does that are marginal milk producers near weaning should be provided a palatable creep feed for their young (see Chapter 2) to help minimize udder trauma caused by aggressive nursing. Whenever chronic mastitis occurs or chronically high somatic cell counts are encountered, the dietary adequacy of energy, protein, water, macronutrients, and micronutrients should be investigated. Adequate dietary selenium (0.2 to 0.3 ppm), copper (7 to 11 ppm in sheep; 10 to 15 ppm in goats), zinc (more than 25 ppm), molybdenum (a copper-to-molybdenum ratio of 6:1), and vitamin E should be made available.

TABLE 13-3

TECHNIQUES USED TO PREVENT MASTITIS IN DAIRY ANIMALS

RISK FACTOR	INTERVENTION
Pathogen exposure	Provide clean, dry bedding
	Eliminate overcrowding
Bedding material	Provide sand or crushed limestone for bedding material
	Avoid wood shavings and straw unless excellent management is available
Milking procedures	Maintain a clean, stress-free parlor
	Check foremilk, California mastitis test (CMT), black plate, strip cup, and milk
	Identify affected animals (CMT, culture, somatic cell culture testing) and milk them last or with a separate claw
	Wash teats and udder
	Strip milk
	Dry teats with single-use towels
	Pre-dip teats (optional)
	Dry teats again with single-use towels
	Attach teat cup as soon as teats are full of milk
	Adjust and monitor milking unit
	Vacuum off before removing teat cups
	Dip teats after milking
	Disinfect teat cups between animals
	Check milking machine vacuum and function periodically
Herd health	Provide teat infusion for the doe or ewe using appropriate antibiotics at "dry off"

Adapted from Turner CW, Berousek ER: Blind halves in a goat's udder, *J Dairy Sci* 25:549, 1942; Sharma SP, Iyer PKR: Pathology of chronic lesions in the mammary glands of goats *(Capra hircus)*. 2: Fibrocystic disease and intraductal carcinomas, *Ind J Anim Sci* 44:474, 1974; Nickerson SC: Mastitis management: strategies to combat mastitis, *Agri-Pract* 16:17, 1995.

Neoplasia

Neoplastic conditions of the udders of sheep and goats are rare. Skin tumors are most common and include squamous cell carcinoma and papilloma. Saanen goats have a breed-specific predisposition to udder papillomatosis.[6] This condition also is associated with white udder skin color. One selection criterion for replacement dairy goats should be darker skin color (tan versus white). Teat and udder papillomas may progress to squamous cell carcinoma or erode into the teat cistern and cause mastitis and permanent loss of the affected udder half. The most common mammary neoplasia reported in goats is intraductal carcinoma, but the prevalence of this neoplasm is very rare (0.08% in two studies).[45,46] Mammary adenocarcinoma also has been diagnosed in a goat.[47] Both adenocarcinoma and fibroepithelial hyperplasia have been diagnosed in goats.[43]

Drug Residue Avoidance

Preservation of a wholesome milk product that is free of contaminants is paramount to the dairy sheep and goat industry. Nearly all treatments for mastitis and udder diseases are performed in an extra-label manner because relatively few drugs are approved for use in either sheep or goats. Veterinarians must work diligently with dairy industry personnel to achieve milk quality assurance.

Treatment recommendations should respect guidelines described in the Animal Medicinal Drug Use Clarification Act (AMDUCA) to avoid residue contamination of meat and milk. Sheep and goats differ from cattle in many drug dosages and drug elimination times. Therefore, whenever possible, drug withdrawal times should be drawn from research performed specifically on sheep or goats. One author has recommended doubling the withdrawal times established for cattle when applying the same products in goats.[2] The main component in avoidance of drug resistance is proper record-keeping and identification of treated animals.

REFERENCES

1. Pasquini C, Spurgeon T: *Anatomy of domestic animals,* ed 5, Pilot Point, TX, 1989, Sudz Publishing.
2. Smith MC, Sherman DM: Mammary gland and milk production. In Smith MC, Sherman DM, editors: *Goat medicine,* Baltimore, 1994, Williams & Wilkins.
3. Rowe JD: Milk quality and mastitis, *Proceedings of the 1998 Symposium on the Health and Disease of Small Ruminants Western Veterinary Conference,* 1998, Las Vegas, NV.
4. East NE, Birnie EF: Diseases of the udder, *Vet Clin North Am Food Anim Pract* 5:591, 1983.

5. Turner CW, Berousek ER: Blind halves in a goat's udder, *J Dairy Sci* 25:549, 1942.

6. Arighi M et al: Invasive teat surgery in dairy cattle II. Long-term follow-up and complications, *Can Vet J* 28:763, 1987.

7. Bristol DG: Teat and udder surgery in dairy cattle—Part I, *Comp Cont Ed Pract Vet* 11:868, 1989.

8. Bristol DG: Teat and udder surgery in dairy cattle—Part II, *Comp Cont Ed Pract Vet* 11:983, 1989.

9. Ducharme NG et al: Invasive teat surgery in dairy cattle I. Surgical procedures and classification of lesions, *Can Vet J* 28:757, 1987.

10. Modransky P, Welker B: Management of teat lacerations and fistula, *Vet Med* 88:995, 1993.

11. Trent AM: Teat surgery, *Agri-Pract* 14:6, 1993.

12. Kerr HJ, Wallace CE: Mastectomy in a goat, *Vet Med* 72:1177, 1978.

13. Bruere AN, West DM: *The sheep: health, disease and production*, Palmerston North, New Zealand, 1993, Massey University Press.

14. Lewter MM et al: Mastitis in goats, *Comp Cont Ed Vet Pract* 6:S417, 1984.

15. Vihan VS: Determination of NA-Gase activity in milk for diagnosis of subclinical caprine mastitis, *Small Rumin Res* 2:359, 1989.

16. Kalogridou-Vassiliadou D, Manolkidis K, Hatziminaoglou J: Changes in mastitis pathogens in goat milk throughout lactation, *Small Rumin Res* 4:197, 1991.

17. Kimberling CV: Diseases of ewes. In Kimberling CV, editor: *Jensen and Swift's diseases of sheep, ed 3*, Philadelphia, 1988, Lea & Febiger.

18. Van Tonder EM: Notes on some disease problems of Angora goats in South Africa, *Vet Med Rev* 1:109, 1975.

19. Chineme CN, Addo PB: Chronic caprine mastitis: clinical, microbiological and pathological findings in spontaneously occurring cases in Nigerian goats, *Intl Goat and Sheep Res* 3:266, 1984.

20. Clarkson MJ, Winter AC: *A handbook for the sheep clinician, ed 5*, Liverpool, UK, 1997, Liverpool University Press.

21. Kalogridou-Vassiliadou D: Mastitis-related pathogens in goat milk, *Small Rumin Res* 4:203, 1991.

22. Lerondelle C, Richard Y, Issartial J: Factors affecting somatic cell counts in goat milk, *Small Rumin Res* 8:129, 1992.

23. Park YW: Interrelationships between somatic cell counts, electrical conductivity, bacteria counts, percent fat and protein in goat milk, *Small Rumin Res* 5:367, 1991.

24. Maisi P: Analysis of physiological changes in caprine milk with CMT, NAGase, and antitrypsin, *Small Rumin Res* 3:485, 1990.

25. Maisi P: Milk NAGase, CMT, and antitrypsin as indicators of caprine subclinical mastitis infections, *Small Rumin Res* 3:493, 1990.

26. Pyorala SHK, Pyorala EO: Efficacy of parenteral administration of three antimicrobial agents in treatment of clinical mastitis in lactating cows: 487 cases (1989-1995), *J Am Vet Med Assoc* 212:407, 1998.

27. Gessert ME: Flock health, Part II. Nutritional and infectious diseases, *Proceedings of the 1998 Symposium on the Health and Disease of Small Ruminants Western Veterinary Conference*, 1998, Las Vegas, NV.

28. Matthews JG: *Outline of clinical diagnosis in the goat*, London, 1996, Wright Publishing.

29. Fox LK, Hancock DD, Horner SD: Selective intramammary antibiotic therapy during the nonlactating period in goats, *Small Rumin Res* 9:313, 1992.

30. Poutrel B et al: Control of intramammary infections in goats: impact on somatic cell counts, *J Anim Sci* 75:566, 1997.

31. Hueston WD, Boner GJ, Baertsche SL: Intramammary antibiotic treatment at the end of lactation for prophylaxis and treatment of intramammary infections in ewes, *J Am Vet Med Assoc* 194:1041, 1989.

32. Croft A et al: The effect of tilmicosin administered to ewes prior to lambing on incidence of clinical mastitis and subsequent lamb performance, *Can Vet J* 41(4):306, 2000.

33. DaMassa AJ: Recovery of *Mycoplasma agalactiae* from mastitic goat milk, *J Am Vet Med Assoc* 183:548, 1983.

34. DaMassa AJ et al: Caprine mycoplasmosis: acute pulmonary disease in newborn kids given *Mycoplasma capricolum* orally, *Aust Vet J* 60:125, 1983.

35. DaMassa AJ, Brooks DL, Holmberg CA: Induction of mycoplasmosis in goat kids by oral inoculation with *Mycoplasma mycoides* subsp. *mycoides*, *Am J Vet Res* 47:2084, 1986.

36. DaMassa AJ, Wakenell PS, Brooks DL: Mycoplasmas of goats and sheep, *J Vet Diagn Invest* 4:101, 1992.

37. East NE: *Mycoplasma mycoides* polyarthritis of goats. In Smith BP, editor: *Large animal internal medicine, ed 2*, St Louis, 1996, Mosby.

38. East NE et al: Milkborne outbreak of *Mycoplasma mycoides* subspecies *mycoides* infection in a commercial goat dairy, *J Am Vet Med Assoc* 182:1338, 1983.

39. Prasad LN, Gupta PP, Singh N: Isolation of mycoplasmas from goat mastitis, *Ind J Anim Sci* 54:1172, 1984.

40. Prasad LN, Gupta PP, Singh N: Experimental *Mycoplasma arginine* mastitis in goats, *Aust Vet J* 62:341, 1985.

41. Blikslager AT, Anderson KL: *Mycoplasma mycoides* subspecies *mycoides* as the cause of a subcuticular abscess and mastitis in a goat, *J Am Vet Med Assoc* 201:1404, 1992.

42. Bulgin MS: Ovine progressive pneumonia, caprine arthritis-encephalitis, and related lentiviral diseases of sheep and goats, *Vet Clin North Am Food Anim Pract* 6:691, 1990.

43. Dawson M: Caprine arthritis encephalitis. In Boden E, editor: *Sheep and goat practice*, London, 1991, Bailliere Tindall.

44. Smith MC, Cutlip R: Effects of infection with caprine arthritis-encephalitis virus on milk production in goats, *J Am Vet Med Assoc* 193:63, 1998.

45. Sharma SP, Iyer PKR: Pathology of chronic lesions in the mammary glands of goats *(Capra hircus)*. 2: Fibrocystic disease and intraductal carcinomas, *Ind J Anim Sci* 44:474, 1974.

46. Singh B, Iyer PKR: Mammary intraductal carcinoma in goats *(Capra hircus)*, *Vet Path* 9:441, 1972.

47. Anderasen CB, Huber MJ, Mattoon JS: Unilateral fibroepithelial hyperplasia of the mammary gland in a goat, *J Am Vet Med Assoc* 202:1279, 1993.

Chapter 14

Diseases of the Hematologic, Immunologic, and Lymphatic Systems (Multisystem Diseases)

CHRISTOPHER CEBRA AND MARGARET CEBRA

BASIC HEMATOLOGY

An adequate volume of blood for hematologic and bio-chemical analysis is best obtained from the jugular vein of sheep and goats. The animal should be restrained in a standing position (goats or sheep) or tipped up (sheep only) with the head turned away from the jugular vein to be used. Ideally the animal should be restrained by someone other than the blood collector, although the same person may be able to both restrain a sheep and collect blood if the animal is tipped up or a halter is used (Figure 14-1). The animal should be at rest, with minimal excitement. The collector parts or clips the wool or hair to visualize the jugular vein and then uses the hand not holding the needle to apply digital pressure proximally just above the thoracic inlet to block blood movement through the vein. The vessel may take a second or more to distend after pressure is applied. The collector may then use the needle-bearing hand to "strum" the vessel and cause the blood to oscillate. If in doubt about whether the distended vessel is the jugular vein, the collector can release the hand placing pressure on the vessel and observe whether the distended vessel disappears; if it does, the distended vessel was probably the jugular vein. The collector should avoid vessels that pulsate because these are likely the carotid arteries. The area should be cleaned with alcohol or other disinfectant, water, or a clean, dry gauze sponge. An 18- or 20-gauge, 1- to 1.5-inch needle is usually adequate to collect blood from an adult sheep or goat, whereas a 22-gauge needle may be used in a neonate. The skin of adults or males may be thicker and more difficult to penetrate with the needle. A syringe or evacuated tube attached to a Vacutainer (Becton Dickinson Inc., Rutherford, NJ) can be used to collect blood. The needle should be plunged through the skin into the vein at an approximate 30-degree angle. The blood should not come out of the vessel in pulsatile waves; this is suggestive of an arterial stick. After aseptically obtaining an adequate volume of blood, the collector removes the needle and releases the pressure on the vessel near the thoracic inlet. Pressure should be applied to the site of puncture for a minute or more to prevent extravascular leakage of blood and hematoma formation. The blood should be carefully transferred to a vial containing the appropriate anticoagulant to prevent red blood cell (RBC) rupture. Goat erythrocytes are small and particularly prone to hemolysis. To minimize this problem, goat blood should be collected with a needle and syringe, not a Vacutainer. White blood cell (WBC) differential distribution, individual blood cell staining characteristics, and morphology may be assessed by microscopic examination of a stained blood film. The differential distribution provides more information than total WBC count because inflammatory conditions in sheep and goats often result in a shift in neutrophil populations toward more degenerate, toxic, or immature forms without changing the overall WBC count.[1] The preferred anticoagulant for a complete blood count (CBC) is ethylenediaminetetraacetate (EDTA), and tubes should be filled to capacity to ensure the proper blood-to-anticoagulant ratio. Blood samples should be processed as soon as possible after collection. If a delay is anticipated, the blood sample should be refrigerated (4° C) and an air-dried blood smear should be made because prolonged contact of blood with EDTA causes changes in WBC morphology and the separation of some RBC parasites. Blood can be refrigerated for 24 hours and still yield an accurate CBC.

A reference range for hematologic data for sheep and goats is provided in Table 14-1. Goats tend to have a low

TABLE 14-1

NORMAL HEMATOLOGIC PARAMETERS FOR SHEEP AND GOATS

PARAMETER (UNITS)	ADULT SHEEP	ADULT GOAT
Hematocrit (%)	27 to 45	22 to 36
Hemoglobin (g/dl)	9 to 15.8	8 to 12
Red blood cell count ($\times 10^6/\mu$l)	9 to 17.5	8 to 17
Mean corpuscular volume (fL)	28 to 40	15 to 26
Mean corpuscular hemoglobin concentration (g/dl)	31 to 34	29 to 35
Platelet count ($\times 10^5/\mu$l)	2.4 to 7.0	2.8 to 6.4
Total white blood cell count (/μl)	4000 to 12,000	4000 to 13,000
Segmented neutrophils (/μl)	1500 to 9000	1400 to 8000
Band neutrophils (/μl)	0	0
Lymphocytes (/μl)	2000 to 9000	2000 to 9000
Monocytes (/μl)	0 to 600	0 to 500
Eosinophils (/μl)	0 to 1000	0 to 900
Basophils (/μl)	0 to 300	0 to 100
Total plasma protein (g/dl)	6.2 to 7.5	6.0 to 7.5
Fibrinogen (mg/dl)	100 to 600	100 to 500

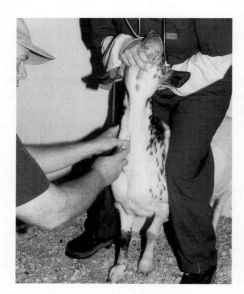

Figure 14-1 Placement of a needle into the jugular vein to attain a blood sample.

mean corpuscular volume (MCV) because of their small erythrocytes. Small ruminants younger than 6 months old tend to have lower hematocrit, RBC count, hemoglobin, and plasma protein concentrations, as well as a higher total WBC count. Neonates often have a high hematocrit at birth that decreases with colostral ingestion. Lactating animals may have decreased hematocrits, RBC counts, and hemoglobin concentrations. Animals grazing at high altitude (mountain goats and Bighorn sheep) tend to have increased RBC counts, hematocrits, and hemoglobin concentrations.

BONE MARROW

Bone marrow aspirates and core biopsy samples taken from sites of active erythropoiesis can be useful to evaluate erythrocyte production and determine the cause of anemia and other hemogram abnormalities. The sites of biopsy in sheep and goats include the sternebra, femur, and ileum. The procedure should be done under chemical sedation or anesthesia. The area over the biopsy site is clipped and surgically prepared; the sampler should wear sterile gloves to maintain asepsis. Aspirates can be obtained by inserting a sterile needle attached to a 3- or 6-cc syringe containing one or two drops of EDTA through the bone and into the bone marrow. Drawing back on the syringe plunger several times may aid in the procurement of an acceptable sample; such a sample may consist of as little as 0.5 ml of bone marrow. If the sample is going to be processed immediately, no anticoagulant is required. Core biopsies are obtained using a Jamshidi or Westerman-Jensen biopsy needle. The skin is incised with a scalpel and the biopsy needle is inserted into the bone and turned several times to obtain a core sample. More than one site may be used. The sampler then closes the skin with sutures or staples. Biopsy samples are preserved by placing them in 10% neutral buffered formalin solution. Impression smears can be made from these samples by gently rolling them on a clean glass slide before placing them in the formalin solution (Figure 14-2). Information obtained from bone marrow samples includes subjective data regarding cell density, megakaryocyte numbers, abnormal cells, maturation patterns of RBCs and WBCs, and the ratio of erythroid to myeloid cells. Prussian blue stain can be used on bone marrow to

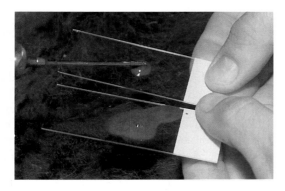

Figure 14-2   After collection of the bone marrow aspirate, a few drops are placed on clean slides for cytologic evaluation.

demonstrate iron stores. Bone marrow aspirates and biopsies are painful and invasive procedures. Therefore animals should be placed on antibiotics and antiinflammatory drugs prophylactically.

BLOOD CULTURES

Blood cultures can be useful in diagnosing bacteremia in an intermittently or persistently febrile sheep or goat or an animal with numerous sites of organ infection. Ideally the clinician should obtain the sample before instituting antimicrobial therapy. However, if this is impossible, antimicrobial therapy should be discontinued 48 to 72 hours before sampling. Samples should be taken before and during febrile episodes. The jugular vein is most commonly used to attain a blood culture. As described previously, the skin over the jugular vein should be clipped and surgically prepared. The person collecting the blood sample should wear sterile gloves and use a sterile needle and syringe. Blood samples should be placed immediately in a blood culture flask. The chances of attaining a positive culture from bacteremic animals increases with the size of the sample up to about 30 ml, but adding more than the recommended amount to any one culture vial may overwhelm the capacity of the specialized antibiotic-absorbing resins within the flasks. The clinician should change the needle on the sample syringe after collecting the blood and before putting the sample in the culture medium. Samples should be refrigerated until they can be sent to a diagnostic laboratory, where aerobic and sometimes anaerobic cultures are made.

CHANGES IN THE HEMOGRAM

The most common and significant abnormality of the hemogram is anemia. In sheep and goats, anemia occurs most commonly after blood loss, hemolysis, and chronic disease. Blood loss is usually covert and commonly caused by gastrointestinal or external parasites. Overt blood loss is usually caused by major trauma such as that caused by

dog bites, severe lacerations, and complications of castration or dehorning. CBC values appear normal immediately after acute blood loss. However, after a few hours of fluid redistribution, anemia and hypoproteinemia are evident. Evidence of red cell regeneration (macrocytosis, reticulocytosis, nucleated red cells) should appear within a day or two of the blood loss.

Hemolysis occurs most commonly after ingestion of toxic plants, RBC parasitism, intravenous (IV) injection of hypotonic or hypertonic agents, contact with bacterial toxins, water intoxication, or immune-mediated destruction of opsonized erythrocytes. Ingested toxins include sulfur compounds from onions and *Brassica* plants (kale, canola), nitrates, nitrites, and copper. Except for that caused by copper, hemolysis usually occurs within a day or two after ingestion. Copper toxicosis can occur after acute overingestion but more commonly is seen in animals that are chronically overfed copper and suffer some stressful event. Goats are more tolerant of excess copper than sheep, and certain breeds of sheep, particularly the Suffolk, are highly sensitive to copper toxicosis (see Chapters 2, 4, and 10).

Hemolytic bacterial toxins include those from *Clostridium perfringens* type A, *C. haemolyticum* and *Leptospira interrogans*. Intraerythrocytic parasites include *Anaplasma* species, *Eperythrozoon ovis*, and *Babesia* species. Immune-mediated RBC destruction is very uncommon except with parasitemia, the administration of certain drugs (penicillin), or bovine colostrum to small ruminant neonates. Rapid reduction of plasma osmolality can lead to osmotic lysis of erythrocytes. This can occur locally as a sequela to rapid IV injection of hypotonic substances or after ingestion of a large quantity of water following a period of water deprivation and dehydration (water intoxication).

Parasite infestation, opsonization, and ingestion of toxic plants typically cause extravascular hemolysis. In these cases damaged erythrocytes are removed by cells of the reticuloendothelial system, resulting in anemia, pallor, weakness, depression, icterus, and dark urine. Bacterial toxins, changes in plasma osmolality, and copper toxicosis cause intravascular hemolysis, resulting in the additional signs of hemoglobinemia and hemoglobinuria. Other signs such as fever, neurologic symptoms, and sudden death may be seen with specific diseases. Signs of regeneration should be seen on the hemogram 1 to 2 days after the onset of hemolysis.

Anemia that is not related to the loss or destruction of erythrocytes usually results from a lack of production. By definition, these anemias are nonregenerative. Although mild forms may exist in pregnant sheep and goats and those deficient in vital minerals (e.g., iron, selenium, copper, zinc), the most common cause of nonregenerative anemia is chronic disease. Under these conditions, iron is sequestered in an unusable form in the bone marrow; staining a marrow sample with Prussian blue stain reveals large iron stores, differentiating this disease from iron-deficiency anemia. The causes of anemia of chronic disease are numerous and include infectious conditions (e.g., pneumonia, footrot, caseous lymphadenitis), malnutrition, and environmental stressors.[1]

TREATMENT OF ANEMIA

Most anemia does not require treatment. Unless loss of RBC volume is rapid and severe, the animal is usually able to compensate to the decreased oxygen-carrying capacity by decreasing activity. It is important to remember in this regard that anemia often first becomes apparent to the manager of a sheep or goat flock when animals appear overly stressed or die during movement or handling.

If possible, the cause of the anemia should be addressed. This can involve trying to control internal and external parasites, changing the diet, and treating infectious diseases. Maintaining adequate hydration is essential in animals with intravascular hemolysis to avoid hemoglobin-induced renal tubular damage. Specialty compounds such as molybdenum salts for copper toxicosis and methylene blue for nitrate toxicity are usually too expensive or difficult to be used on a flock-wide basis, but may be useful in valuable individual animals.

Animals with severe acute blood loss or hemolysis may benefit from a whole blood transfusion. Because transfusion reactions are rare and strong erythrocyte antigens have not been identified in sheep and goats, almost any donor of the same species is acceptable for a first transfusion. Cross-matching can be done to ensure compatibility, which becomes more important if the animal receives more than one transfusion. Blood should be withdrawn aseptically from the donor and collected by a bleeding trocar into an open flask or by a catheter into a special collection bag. Blood should be mixed at a 4:1 ratio with acid-citrate dextrose, sodium citrate, or another suitable anticoagulant and administered through a filtered blood administration set. If the jugular vein is not accessible, blood may be infused into the peritoneal cavity, but the slower absorption from that site makes it less effective for treating acute blood loss. The first 15 to 30 minutes of administration should be slow. If no reaction is seen (fever, tenesmus, tachypnea, tachycardia, shaking), the rate may be increased. Transfused erythrocytes may only survive a few days, and therefore the original cause of the anemia must be addressed.[1]

CHANGES IN THE LEUKOGRAM

Peripheral WBCs include granulocytes (neutrophils, eosinophils, and basophils) and mononuclear cells (lymphocytes and monocytes). Immature forms of neutrophils and lymphocytes may be seen during severe inflammatory diseases. Abnormalities of the neutrophil line are usually the best cellular evidence of inflammation in small rumi-

nants, and inflammation is almost always a sequela of infection. An increase in neutrophil numbers and their proportional contribution to the total WBC count is usually seen in mild gram-positive, subacute, or chronic bacterial infections. Animals with more severe disease may exhibit high or normal counts, but a greater proportion of the neutrophils will have toxic changes or be immature forms (band cells, metamyelocytes, or myelocytes). In severe, acute inflammation and many diseases caused by gram-negative bacteria, a temporary reduction in neutrophil numbers is observed, often with a concurrent shift toward more toxic or immature forms. If the animal survives the peracute disease, neutropenia should resolve over 3 to 4 days, first through an increase in immature cells, and later through a mature neutrophilic response. The most important cause of increased total and relative neutrophil counts is stress (or glucocorticoid administration), which inhibits neutrophil margination and extravasation and thereby increases the number of these cells in the midstream blood.

Increases in eosinophil counts are usually related to exposure to eukaryotic parasites. Decreases are rarely of clinical significance and may be seen as part of the stress response. Idiopathic allergic-type reactions also are indicators of pathology but are very rare. Increases in basophils are rarely clinically significant.

Increases in lymphocyte counts often reflect chronic inflammatory disease such as that seen with internal abscesses. In rare cases, lymphocytosis may consist of abnormal, blast-type cells and indicate a lymphoproliferative neoplasm. Lymphopenia is an important part of the stress response; nevertheless, the clinician must keep in mind that many diseases stimulate a stress response. Therefore lymphopenia and neutrophilia may represent either stress or inflammation, and an examination of neutrophil morphology and plasma fibrinogen concentrations may be useful in distinguishing the two situations. A high fibrinogen concentration, toxic changes, and high counts of immature neutrophils indicate inflammation under those circumstances. Blood monocyte counts also may indicate stress or chronic inflammation. The difficulties in interpreting individual cell count abnormalities highlight the importance of obtaining a differential WBC count and description of cellular morphology in assessing sick sheep and goats.

Leukogram abnormalities are rarely given specific treatment. It is far more common and useful to use the information from the leukogram to develop a plan to treat the disease responsible for the abnormality.

ASSESSMENT OF THE LYMPHATIC SYSTEM

Palpation of external lymph nodes is part of the thorough physical examination. Lymph nodes that can be found in normal sheep and goats include the submandibular, prescapular, and prefemoral nodes. None of these should be prominent or painful on palpation. Additional nodes that may be palpated occasionally in normal animals include the parotid, retropharyngeal, supramammary, perirectal, and popliteal nodes. Internal lymph nodes that may be identified during specialized diagnostic procedures include the mediastinal, mesenteric, and other abdominal nodes.

Enlargement of lymph nodes may be focal, multifocal, or generalized. Identification of a single enlarged superficial node does not always rule out a multifocal or generalized disorder because the status of the internal nodes often cannot be determined. Enlargement generally indicates either inflammation or neoplasia. Inflammatory enlargement is generally related to an associated disease with an infectious component. Small ruminants are particularly sensitive to lymph node–based infections (e.g., caseous lymphadenitis), so the search often does not extend beyond aspirating or draining the lymph node itself. Neoplastic enlargement almost always results from lymphosarcoma.

DISEASE OF THE LYMPHATIC SYSTEM

Lymphosarcoma

Pathogenesis. Neoplastic transformation of a member of the lymphocyte cell line leads to unregulated clonal expansion of that cell. The cause of transformation is usually unknown; in rare cases, especially in flock outbreaks in sheep, it can be linked to exposure to the bovine leukemia virus, which has occurred experimentally and as a result of the administration of whole blood *Anaplasma* vaccines. Whether the bovine leukemia virus can induce lymphosarcoma in goats is still unclear. Proliferation of lymphocytes leads to mass lesions and infiltration of viscera. These cause physical obstruction (to breathing, blood flow, urination, defecation), ulceration of mucosal surfaces (blood loss, bacterial invasion), immune system dysfunction, organ failure, and generalized malaise and cachexia. Tissues masses may be internal or visible on external examination.

Clinical signs. Signs vary according to the site of the masses. Slowly progressive weight loss is the most common finding. In some cases, expansile masses are noted; at first they usually are presumed to be caseous lymphadenitis abscesses. Most masses form at the sites of internal or external lymph nodes. Leukemia is rare. The most common abnormalities are those of chronic disease and cachexia, and include nonregenerative anemia and hypoalbuminemia. Bone marrow examination may reveal clonal expansion of lymphoid precursor cells.

Diagnosis. Postmortem lesions include homogeneous white to tan masses that bulge on the cut surface. They may be small or large. Less commonly, diffuse paleness of the reticuloendothelial organs is noted. Microscopic examination of these tissues reveals infiltrates of abnormal cells of the lymphocyte line.

Prevention. Avoiding exposure to the bovine leukemia virus and avoiding the use of instruments contaminated with blood on more than one animal may help prevent the spread of lymphosarcoma. However, most animals appear to develop this neoplasm spontaneously.

Failure of Passive Transfer

Pathogenesis. Lambs and kids are born with functional lymphocytes that are capable of producing endogenous immunoglobulin. These cells develop the ability to respond to foreign antigens in the fetus at approximately 80 days of gestation. However, because of a lack of in utero exposure, basal concentrations of immunoglobulin are low at birth. Therefore these cells respond too sluggishly to new challenges to provide an adequate defense against acute infection for approximately the first 6 weeks of life. Additionally, as with other ruminants, no transplacental passage of immunoglobulin to fetal sheep and goats occurs. Lambs and kids depend on intestinal absorption of ingested colostral antibodies to provide a ready supply of immunoglobulin and allow opsonization of pathogens for the first months of life.

Adequate passive transfer requires delivery of a sufficient quantity of good-quality colostrum into the gastrointestinal tract as well as adequate absorption of antibodies from the colostrum into the blood. In general, this is left to chance: the quality of the colostrum, amount ingested, and adequacy of absorption are rarely monitored. Problems in colostral quality can arise from young, sick, undernourished, and poorly vaccinated dams. Problems in availability can arise from prepartum leakage or nursing by another lamb or kid. Problems in ingestion can arise from weak or sick neonates, competition with other lambs or kids, and separation of the neonate from the dam. Problems in absorption can arise from weakness, sickness, hypothermia, hypoxemia, dehydration, previous exposure of the gut to protein, delay in ingestion, and other factors that affect gut function in the neonate. Sheep and goats are especially prone to many of these causes of failure of passive transfer because of their tendency to have numerous offspring; the earliest-nursing, most vigorous offspring may ingest more than their share of colostrum.

Extrapolating from equine research, a finding of 800 mg/dl of immunoglobulin in the plasma of a 1-day-old lamb or kid is considered indicative of adequate passive transfer. No research has been done to show that this particular concentration is significantly protective in small ruminants, and it is probably more important that immunoglobulin against specific opportunistic and primary pathogens be absorbed than any bulk amount. Moreover, this amount should be considered minimally acceptable—most healthy small ruminant neonates achieve immunoglobulin concentrations that are 50% to 200% higher.

In addition to immunoglobulin, colostrum also contains large quantities of fat-soluble vitamins that do not cross the placenta. The most important of these are vitamins A, D, and E, which are important in bone development and the immune or inflammatory response. Neonates that have not ingested enough colostrum are likely to be deficient in these vitamins.

Diagnosis. A diagnosis of failure of passive transfer can be deduced from the history if the neonate is known not to have ingested colostrum in the first day of life or the dam is known not to have had colostrum. Owners occasionally pick a lamb or kid up, hold it at ear level while carefully cradling the head and neck, and shake the abdomen in order to hear milk in the abomasum. A presumptive diagnosis can be made if the neonate shows signs of undernourishment or sepsis in the first few days after birth. A definitive diagnosis can be made by direct laboratory measurement (radioimmunoassay) of immunoglobulin concentrations. Numerous semi-quantitative methods of estimating immunoglobulin exist, including various agglutination (glutaraldehyde) and precipitate assays (sodium sulfate) and measurement of blood protein fractions. The use of a hand-held refractometer to measure total protein in a well-hydrated animal may be used as a quick screen. A total protein of 5.5 to 6 mg/dl or greater is usually suggestive of successful transfer of colostral antibodies in a normally hydrated neonate. These methods may be relied on to give an overall flock assessment of adequacy of passive transfer, but they are rarely accurate enough to provide definitive information on individual animals (see Chapter 6).[2]

Treatment. Failure of passive transfer is not by itself a disease, but it greatly increases the neonate's susceptibility to infectious diseases. The amount of colostrum absorbed across the gut decreases with time, especially in animals that have been ingesting other proteins (e.g., the casein in milk); it also decreases with illnesses that decrease gastrointestinal function. Sufficient immunoglobulin likely cannot be absorbed more than 24 hours after birth. Therefore oral colostrum is the best treatment in the immediate postpartum treatment in still-healthy neonates. Same-species colostrum is best: hemolysis has been reported in lambs receiving cattle colostrum. To make up for complete failure, approximately 5% of the neonate's body weight by volume of colostrum (or about 1.25 g of immunoglobulin per kg of body weight) should be administered on two separate occasions, 4 to 12 hours apart.

Colostral substitutes generated from slaughterhouse blood are becoming available, but their absorption and efficacy remains largely untested. After the window for immunoglobulin absorption has closed, plasma administered intravenously or intraperitoneally is the best way to raise the neonate's blood immunoglobulin concentrations. Adult donor plasma contains approximately 2.5 to 3.5 g of immunoglobulin per dl, so a volume equivalent to 10% of body weight is necessary to achieve similar concentrations as with normal passive transfer. If plasma is used instead of colostrum, administration of vitamins A, D, and E also may be beneficial.

If colostrum and plasma are unavailable or cost prohibitive, "closing" the gut as quickly as possible with milk, maintaining high standards of hygiene, and possibly administering prophylactic antibiotics offer the greatest prospects for preventing infectious disease. Vaccination of the neonate or the administration of antitoxin hyperimmune serum should not be considered protective, but may be of value.

Prevention. Ensuring colostral quality is best done through good nutrition, health care, and vaccination of dam (see Chapter 2). Administration of vaccines 6 weeks prepartum, followed in 2 weeks with a booster, provide the highest quantity of protective immunoglobulin in the colostrum. Prepartum leakage is rarely the problem in small ruminants that it is in horses and cattle. However, in a flock or hard environment, still-pregnant dams may steal babies from other sheep or goats. To prevent theft and the resultant loss of colostrum by the "adopted" neonate, owners may choose to keep pregnant stock separate from those that have already delivered. If complete separation is not possible, the dam and her offspring should be allowed to bond to each other in a private pen ("jug" or "crate") for at least 24 hours before being placed back with the flock. Clipping excessive wool or mohair from around the perineal area and udder before lambing or kidding, expressing the teats to ensure they are not plugged, and having extra colostrum when placing pregnant females in jugs or crates are other good preventive measures.

Neonatal Sepsis

Pathogenesis. Sepsis is the condition resulting from systemic bacterial infections or toxemia. Most systemic bacterial infections are caused by opportunistic infections in immunocompromised animals or the overwhelming of a competent immune system with massive challenge. Rarely, small numbers of aggressive primary pathogens are the cause. The most common cause of immune dysfunction in neonates is failure of passive transfer. Less common causes include nutritional deficiencies (notably in selenium, copper, or vitamin E), stress, and other illnesses.

Bacteria enter the body through the gastrointestinal or respiratory tracts or through a break in the skin (e.g., umbilicus, castration site, docked tail, wound). The role of the umbilicus is usually overemphasized over the other, more common routes. Bacteria proliferate locally and either enter the circulation or produce toxins that enter the circulation. After entering the bloodstream, bacteria seed various body sites, including the lungs, kidneys, liver, central nervous system, joints, umbilicus, lymphoid tissue, and body cavities. Toxins tend to damage blood cells, vascular endothelium, and various organ tissues. Overwhelming bacteremia or toxemia is usually fatal; less severe disease is associated with localization of the bacteria to one or more sites of chronic infection such as the umbilicus, lymph nodes, organ abscesses, and joints. The greater the immune responsiveness of the animal, the more likely it is to prevent invasion and clear the infection.

The major opportunistic causes of neonatal sepsis include most *Escherichia coli*, *Streptococcus*, *Actinomyces* (Arcanobacter), and other organisms (often gram-negative enteric bacteria). Most of these organisms are normal inhabitants of the ruminant gastrointestinal tract or soil and therefore are likely to be found in the highest concentrations around areas with the poorest hygiene. The major primary causes of neonatal sepsis include some *E. coli*, *Salmonella dublin* or *S. typhimurium*, and *Erysipelothrix rhusiopathiae*. These organisms may be associated with illness in adults and outbreaks in neonates in spite of good nutrition, hygiene, and adequate passive transfer.

Clinical signs.   The clinical signs of acute sepsis are the same as those of shock. Fever is present in the most acute phase but is transient, and the absence of fever should not be taken as evidence against bacterial infection. Hypothermia is often present in advanced cases. Other common clinical signs include obtundation; anorexia with a weak suckle reflex; cold extremities; dry or tacky mucous membranes with purple-blue discoloration (buccal) or enlarged, engorged blood vessels (sclera); tachycardia; tenting skin; and poor filling of the jugular veins. Diarrhea, swollen joints, tachypnea, and specific neurologic signs may be present if the pertinent organs are affected.

Diagnosis.   A presumptive diagnosis can be made on finding a neonate with the previously described clinical signs. Other disorders that can produce these signs include hypothermia, hypoxemia, congenital cardiovascular or nervous system anomalies, and starvation. These other disorders often coexist with sepsis as predisposing factors or complications of the infectious disorder. Clinical pathology data that support a diagnosis of sepsis include evidence of failure of passive transfer, hyperfibrinogenemia, and left shift of the leukogram, particularly when neutropenia, toxic changes to neutrophils, or myelocytes and metamyelocytes are present. Serum bio-

chemical analysis may be helpful in assessing overall condition.[2] Definitive diagnosis of sepsis is achieved by isolating the bacteria. Blood culture or postmortem internal organ culture are the best diagnostic tools for acute, untreated bacteremia. Aspirates of abscesses or infected joints are more accurate if sepsis is long-standing, particularly if the animal has been treated with antibiotics.

Treatment.   Treatment for neonatal sepsis is most rewarding when initiated early in the infection. Although cost and residues are always a concern when treating young food animals, their small size and long time interval until slaughter or milk production gives the clinician greater leeway in choosing appropriate antimicrobial agents. Because both gram-positive and gram-negative infections are possible, broad-spectrum coverage through single antibiotics or combinations of them is preferred (ceftiofur 1 to 2.2 mg/kg intramuscularly [IM] once a day [SID] to twice a day [BID]). Treatment should be continued for at least 5 days to ensure clearance of the infection. Nonsteroidal antiinflammatory drugs (NSAIDs) also are beneficial in their antipyretic, antiinflammatory, and antiendotoxic roles (flunixin meglumine 1 to 2 mg/kg IV or IM).

If the neonate is severely dehydrated or obtunded, fluid treatment should be initiated. Because septic neonates are often deficient in immunoglobulin as a result of failure of passive transfer or consumption of milk, plasma transfusions are often beneficial. Plasma should come from the same species; whole blood can be used in an emergency situation. Adverse reactions are rare.

Prevention.   Methods to improve colostral quality and passive transfer are helpful in preventing sepsis. Decreasing overcrowding, separating neonates from most adult stock (except their dams), and decreasing fecal and soil contamination of facilities decrease the amount of bacterial challenge. Sanitizing common equipment and minimizing contamination of tail docking and castration sites also are important. Dipping the umbilicus is of questionable importance and is probably unnecessary in well-managed, clean flocks. However, the procedure is harmless and provides an opportunity to examine the newborn, so current recommendations include dipping the umbilicus with dilute iodine or chlorhexidine solutions.[2]

Neonatal Uncomplicated Diarrhea

Pathogenesis.   Uncomplicated diarrhea may be caused by viral, bacterial, and protozoan pathogens. They differ from the causative agents of complicated diarrhea in that they do not invade beyond the gut wall or result in systemic toxemia (see Chapter 4).

The net result of such an infection is that a large volume of isotonic intestinal fluid is lost into the bowel with the unabsorbed ingesta. If enough fluid and electrolytes are lost, dehydration and metabolic acidosis induce systemic clinical signs similar to those seen in complicated diarrhea. This disease in kids is one component of "floppy kid syndrome."

Clinical signs. Profuse, watery diarrhea without fever is the hallmark clinical sign. With severe dehydration or acidosis, affected lambs and kids become weak and dull and lack appetite. Mucous membranes become tacky, and skin tenting becomes prolonged. Shock signs may develop. Physical assessment often has to take the place of clinical pathology analysis in lambs and kids.

Mild, nonclinical uncomplicated diarrhea is characterized by profuse diarrhea with minimal systemic signs. The animal is bright and alert. Minimal skin tenting is evident. The animal is able to stand and eat readily and has a strong suckle reflex. The animal is less than 5% dehydrated, with a blood pH of 7.35 to 7.50 and a bicarbonate deficit of 0 mEq/L.

Moderate uncomplicated diarrhea is characterized by profuse diarrhea in a dull but responsive animal. Skin tenting is prolonged, but eye luster is normal. The sheep or goat is able to stand and eat, but eats slowly and has a weak suckle reflex. The animal holds its head down. It is 5% to 7% dehydrated, with a blood pH of 7.10 to 7.25 and a bicarbonate deficit of 5 mEq/L.

Severe uncomplicated diarrhea is characterized by profuse diarrhea. The sheep or goat is dull and minimally responsive with a very long skin tent and dull, sunken eyes. It can only stand with assistance and prefers to stay in sternal recumbency with its head up. The animal eats very slowly, if at all, and has a minimal suckle reflex. It is 8% to 10% dehydrated, with a blood pH of 6.90 to 7.10 and a bicarbonate deficit of 10 mEq/L.

Very severe uncomplicated diarrhea is characterized by profuse diarrhea and profound weakness. The animal's skin remains tented for more than a minute and its eyes are very sunken and dull. It is nonresponsive with no suckle response. It is unable to maintain sternal recumbency (lateral). The animal is 10% to 12% dehydrated, with a blood pH of 6.8 to 7.0 and a bicarbonate deficiency of 15 to 20 mEq/L.

Clinical pathology. The leukogram should be normal or have abnormalities compatible with stress. Serum biochemical or blood gas analysis may reveal evidence of intestinal electrolyte loss (hyponatremia, hypochloremia, metabolic acidosis) and dehydration (hyperalbuminemia, azotemia).

Diagnosis. A presumptive diagnosis may be based on the characteristic clinical signs and exclusion of causes of complicated diarrhea ("scours"). Response to conservative treatment also is supportive of this diagnosis. Identification of the specific causative agent is less important than proper treatment of infected animals. To identify the causative agent, feces should be examined by electron microscopy to identify the viruses, by culture to determine a bacterial cause, by light or fluorescent microscopy after sugar flotation, acid-fasting, auramine, or fluorescent antibody staining for *C. parvum*.

Treatment. The immediate goals of treatment are rehydration, replacement of lost electrolytes, and restoration of acid-base balance. Less immediate goals are provision of nutrition and replacement of ongoing losses. The aggressiveness of treatment is dictated by the severity of the condition as well as economic considerations[3]:

1. Rehydration: Calculate the percentage of dehydration. Example: 10% dehydration in a 3-kg lamb: $0.1 \times 3 \text{ kg} \times 1 \text{ kg/L} = 0.3 \text{ L}$, or 300 ml
2. Replace lost electrolytes—Sodium, chloride, bicarbonate, and potassium are lost roughly in proportion to extracellular fluid; replace in roughly the same proportions (except provide more bicarbonate and less chloride; see next step). Replace with fluid that is similar in composition to extracellular fluid.
3. Restore the acid-base balance—Estimate bicarbonate deficit by blood gas analysis (24, measured) or physical assessment. Then calculate the whole-body deficit. Example: Assessment suggests a deficit of 16 mEq/L bicarbonate in a 3-kg, comatose lamb with prolonged skin tenting (0.5 is the multiplier for extracellular fluid in a neonate)—$0.5 \times (16 \text{ mEq/L}) \times 3 \text{ kg} \times 1 \text{ kg/L} = 24 \text{ mEq}$ bicarbonate

Therefore the immediate goal is to provide 300 ml of fluid and 24 mEq of bicarbonate to this lamb in a fluid that resembles normal extracellular fluid (ECF). Fluids can be given by various routes:

Oral
- Advantages: Oral fluids are inexpensive (non-sterile) and easy to give. They are less likely to cause fatal arrhythmias or neurologic disease than IV fluids.
- Disadvantages: An animal receives a maximum of its gastric volume (5% of body weight) and good gastric motility is required. Oral fluids may not be well absorbed by a damaged gut. Absorption also is slow.

Intravenous
- Advantage: This method allows rapid correction of all deficits, even in moribund animals.
- Disadvantages: It is expensive (sterile), requires venous access, and can rapidly lead to overcorrection.

Subcutaneous
- Advantages: This method does not require venous access or good gut motility.

- Disadvantages: It is expensive (sterile) and the fluids may not be well absorbed in very dehydrated animals. Absorption is not as quick as by IV administration. Animals should only be given hypotonic or isotonic fluids.

Intraperitoneal
- Advantages: This method does not require venous access or gut motility. Fluids are absorbed quickly by this route.
- Disadvantages: It is expensive (sterile) and can cause peritonitis. Isotonic fluids are best used in this route. Only a limited volume can be given.

In general, lambs and kids with good appetites (especially those being fed by bottle) and those that have recently lost their appetites (including those being fed by tube or working the bottle) may be treated with oral fluids, but those that have a lack of appetite coupled with severe dehydration should be treated with IV or subcutaneous (SC) fluids. SC fluids are most useful as an adjunct: the owner or clinician can give a few hundred ml to a neonate treated with an IV bolus to provide a prolonged effect. If oral fluids have not produced an improvement within 2 to 4 hours, IV treatment should be strongly considered.

Many good commercial oral fluids are available. These contain electrolytes (sodium similar to plasma), an alkalinizing agent (bicarbonate, propionate, acetate, citrate; most good ones have about 80 mEq/L of base), and glucose or glycine to slow gastric emptying and aid in sodium absorption. The amount of carbohydrates varies; it is higher in "high-energy" solutions. Less carbohydrate is needed in less severely affected animals because they are less likely to have severe hyponatremia. Fluids to be avoided include medicated milk replacers and unbuffered saline solutions.

IV treatment should be provided with a sterile commercial product. These typically contain 25 to 30 mEq/L of base. Additional sodium bicarbonate solution or powder can be added (12 mEq of bicarbonate per g of powder, or 1 mEq/ml of 8.4% solution) to replace the base deficit. The bicarbonate deficit should be replaced over 4 hours to avoid the development of neurologic signs.

After deficits are replaced, the following continued treatments and adjuncts may be considered:

1. Continued administration of fluids (oral rather than IV if possible) to replace ongoing losses (see Appendix II):

   - A volume equal to 5% of the body weight can be given orally at a time; feedings can be increased from two (normal) to three to six feedings a day. After 24 hours, less hypertonic fluids can be used.
   - IV fluids can be continued at twice the maintenance fluid rate until appetite is restored.
   - More bicarbonate may be necessary.

2. Consideration of the addition of milk to the treatment regimen:

   - Milk has more energy but fewer electrolytes per unit of fluid.
   - Milk can be used for up to half of the feedings: Lambs fed milk lose less weight with scours. Free water helps prevent hypernatremia.
   - Milk should not be mixed with electrolytes because they inhibit curd formation (although acetate is allegedly safe).
   - Milk may exacerbate diarrhea in the early stage: Large intestine fermentation leads to osmotic diarrhea and further fluid loss. Withholding milk for 24 hours may help, but longer delays lead to cachexia.
   - Milk is a good potassium source.

Other Causes of Weakness and Depression in Neonates

Ruling out infectious causes of depression and weakness is difficult, and clinicians often do well to assume that an infectious disease is contributing to clinical signs when making treatment decisions. However, a number of noninfectious systemic disturbances also can depress neurologic and muscular function. Successful treatment often requires identification and correction of each of these disturbances. Among the more common abnormalities leading to depression in neonates are hypoxemia, metabolic or respiratory acidosis, hypothermia, hyperthermia, hypoglycemia, dehydration, azotemia, and imbalances in some electrolytes.

Hypothermia and hyperthermia can easily be diagnosed with a rectal thermometer. Hypothermia is far more common and can result from weakness, shock, and environmental stress. Cold, windy weather or tube feeding with cold milk replacer or fluids can lead to a rapid drop in core body temperature, especially in neonates that are small or weak or have been inadequately licked off or rejected by their dams. Strong, vigorous neonates usually are protected by heat produced during muscular activity and are able to seek food and shelter. Clinical signs begin when the rectal temperature drops to 98° F or below. Protection from wind and cold such as an individual ewe jug or pen, heat lamps (positioned far enough away so as not to burn the neonate), hot water bottles, blankets, and warm fluids are helpful in treating and preventing hypothermia. Shearing the ewe before lambing is of value because it forces the ewe to seek shelter. If this management technique is used, care should be taken to avoid inducing severe hypothermia in the dam.

Environmental hyperthermia is much less common than fever in neonates. Therefore treatment for infectious diseases in young animals with high temperatures is usually warranted. Providing cool shelter with good ventilation, minimizing stressful events, ensuring adequate fluid intake, and shearing the adults are the best defenses against environmental heat stress.

Hypoglycemia also is easy to diagnose with the aid of an inexpensive, portable glucose meter. Lambs and kids typically develop hypoglycemia under the same circumstances as hypothermia. Administering 50 ml/kg of dextrose (approximately 3.5 fl oz/lb, or 5% of body weight) in warm milk replacer or 1 ml/kg of 50% dextrose IV or by mouth (PO, diluted to 5% dextrose) should provide ample energy to correct hypoglycemia. IV treatment may be necessary if gut motility is absent. Follow-up treatment may be necessary if the neonate does not regain its appetite.

Except during severe conditions, normal lambs and kids should be able to maintain normal body core temperature. Therefore they should be examined for an underlying disorder if they exhibit signs of hypothermia or hyperthermia. Clinicians and owners should not assume that warming and feeding a cold, weak neonate will always correct its condition.

Hypoxemia is much more difficult to diagnose. Portable blood gas meters for arterial analysis and radiography units for thoracic imaging are available but still uncommon in small ruminant practice. For those reasons, hypoxemia is usually under-diagnosed. Hypoxemia can result from prematurity or dysmaturity, infection, depression or weakness (decreased ventilation), meconium aspiration, bullous emphysema, hernias, and other thoracic fluid or tissue masses. It is likely to be a contributing factor to illness and death in most weak neonates younger than 3 days old. Such animals benefit from the provision of supplemental oxygen, either through a nasal insufflation tube or oxygen tent. In addition to its direct effect on attitude, hypoxemia at birth leads to poor gut function and subsequent poor colostral absorption. Many animals that exhibit failure of passive transfer and subsequent sepsis had a previous bout of hypoxemia.

Azotemia, metabolic acidosis, and electrolyte imbalances are difficult to diagnose without clinical pathology analysis. Therefore they are best treated in animals showing signs of dehydration with the administration of a balanced, physiologic electrolyte solution. Metabolic acidosis is usually accompanied by either obvious evidence of bicarbonate loss (diarrhea) or severe dehydration. However, neither of these conditions is present with floppy kid syndrome. This descriptive title is applied to muscle weakness, anorexia, and depression in kids in the first 2 weeks of life. By its strictest definition, *floppy kid syndrome* refers to metabolic acidosis with a high anion gap without dehydration or any known cause in young kids that were normal at birth. A variety of etiologies have been proposed for metabolic acidosis without dehydration, including intestinal fermentation of milk in well-fed kids with subsequent absorption of volatile fatty acids, transient neonatal renal tubular acidosis, and lactic acidosis following toxic impairment of cardiovascular function. Overgrowth of *C. perfringens* type A is often suggested as a source of the toxin. Because of the high anion gap, a pathologic condition that leads to overproduction of an organic acid should be considered more likely than one that leads to bicarbonate loss. The disease can occur in individuals or in outbreaks; although parity of the dam and number of offspring have not been associated with the disease, aggressively feeding kids are more likely to suffer from milk fermentation or clostridial overgrowth. An infectious etiology appears more likely in herds that have an increased incidence as the kidding season progresses. The disease also is reported to be more common in meat goats than dairy goats. Incidence can vary tremendously from year to year in a single flock or region. A similar disease has been reported in calves and llama crias, and lambs also are likely to be susceptible under the right conditions.

Because blood gas analysis and exclusion of other diseases often are impractical, the term *floppy kid syndrome* frequently is used by owners to refer to any kid that is weak and does not have an overt, organ specific sign (e.g., diarrhea). Different pathologic processes are grouped together by their common clinical endpoint (as with "thin ewe syndrome"), and the veterinarian is charged with determining the etiology in a specific flock. Most possible causes are found in the previously provided list of conditions that cause weakness and depression in neonates. Sepsis and hypoxemia are the most important items on that list and therefore also must be considered important causes of possible floppy kid syndrome. Treatment and prevention of floppy kid syndrome currently follow the same lines as the treatment and prevention of neonatal sepsis or enteritis. Spontaneous recovery of animals with floppy kid syndrome may occur. However, in valuable kids, quick assessment of blood chemistry and base deficits allows correction of electrolyte and blood pH abnormalities with 1.3% sodium bicarbonate.[4]

References

1. Morris DD: Anemia. In Smith BP, editor: *Large animal internal medicine,* ed 2, St Louis, 1996, Mosby.
2. Koterba AM, House JK: Neonatal infection. In Smith BP, editor: *Large animal internal medicine,* ed 2, St Louis, 1996, Mosby.
3. Naylor JM: Neonatal ruminant diarrhea. In Smith BP, editor: *Large animal internal medicine,* ed 2, St Louis, 1996, Mosby.
4. Rowe JD, East NE: Floppy kid syndrome (metabolic acidosis without dehydration in kids), *Proceedings of the 1998 Symposium on the Health and Disease of Small Ruminants Western Veterinary Conference,* 1998, Las Vegas, NV.

Tissue-Invading *Clostridia*

Tissue-invading *Clostridia* are large, straight, gram-positive rods that are 3 to 10 μm in length. *C. perfringens* and *C. haemolytica* are smaller bacteria and *C. novyi, C. chauvoei,* and *C. septicum* are larger. The bacteria grow best under anaerobic conditions and produce waste gases. *Clostridia* bear spores that may be the only viable form in soil. Identification of these spores within bacteria on microscopic examination is useful to identify *Clostridia.* Spores in *C. perfringens* are central and do not affect the shape, whereas most other species have the spore toward one end and appear slightly club-shaped.

Clostridia cause infectious, noncontagious disease. The bacteria inhabit the intestinal tract and are present in the feces of many healthy animals. Small numbers of organisms in their dormant spore form also may reside in tissues such as the liver and skeletal muscle. They can be isolated from soil, where most are thought to have short life spans. Soil concentrations are highest in locations recently contaminated with ruminant feces, especially crowded, overused facilities such as feedlots and lambing sheds. Environmental contamination also appears highest during cool, damp times of the year such as late winter and spring.

The concentration of organisms and their toxins found in the feces, gut contents, and internal organs of most adult ruminants is usually small. Competition and peristalsis prevent overgrowth in the gut and aerobic conditions prevent overgrowth in other tissues in live animals. However, rapid overgrowth and tissue invasion occur after death, making rapid postmortem examination essential to ascertain whether clostridial organisms are responsible for the death.

Pathogenic clostridial organisms all produce heat-labile protein exotoxins. Most make a variety of toxins, and the relative contribution of each toxin to the disease state is not known. The major exotoxins of *C. perfringens* are alpha, a phospholipase that lyses mammalian cells; beta, a trypsin-labile necrotizing toxin; epsilon, a trypsin-activated necrotizing toxin; and iota, another trypsin-activated necrotizing toxin. Toxin production is used to classify *C. perfringens* organisms according to type. All five types of *C. perfringens* make alpha toxin. Types B and C also make beta toxin (with B making epsilon toxin as well), Type D makes epsilon toxin, and Type E makes iota toxin. Because the necrotizing toxins cause more prominent lesions than alpha toxin, they are used to characterize diseases caused by *C. perfringens* infection with types other than A. Other tissue-invasive clostridial organisms make toxins similar to those produced by *C. perfringens* in addition to various other necrotizing and hemolyzing toxins. In many cases these toxins can be chemically altered to produce antigenic toxoids.[1-4]

Enteric Infections

Pathogenesis.   Enteric clostridial organisms are thought to proliferate under conditions of decreased peristalsis and poor ruminal and abomasal function. Weather and handling stresses, feed changes, and an overabundance of high-energy feeds are thought to promote overgrowth. Milk, bakery products, and cereal grains are the most common high-energy feeds associated with outbreaks. Toxin production occurs with overgrowth and precipitates disease. Other enteric infections that disrupt the mucosal border may increase systemic absorption of toxins.

C. perfringens type A occurs worldwide and is the most common type of this species isolated from soil. It causes "yellow lamb disease" in younger animals, a condition reported much more commonly in sheep than in goats. Risk factors for infection have not been established. This disease occurs most commonly in lambs 2 to 6 months old. Under favorable conditions the organisms proliferate and cause a corresponding increase in alpha toxin production. The alpha toxin causes minor gastrointestinal lesions and is absorbed across the gut wall to cause hemolysis and vasculitis. The clinical course is usually less than 24 hours (see Chapter 4).

Clinical signs.   The clinical signs include weakness, depression, fever, icterus, anemia, hemoglobinuria, tachypnea, and terminal recumbency. Laboratory evaluation reveals evidence of intravascular hemolysis. Necropsy reveals evidence of hemolysis, hyperemic intestines, and multifocal internal petechial hemorrhages. Positive diagnosis is based on identification of the alpha toxin and the absence of other toxins by newer enzyme-linked immunospecific assay (ELISA) tests or older live-animal assays. Morbidity in a flock is lower than for many of the other enteric clostridial diseases, but the mortality rate is very high.

Adult animals also are susceptible to hemolytic disease and vasculitis caused by *C. perfringens* type A infection. The organism has been isolated from sites distant from the infection, including muscle and the mammary gland. Fatal abomasitis and rumenitis in neonates and juveniles also has been blamed on *C. perfringens* type A, but the rapid postmortem proliferation of the organism makes substantiation of this claim difficult.

Clinical pathology.   The most characteristic change is neutrophilic leukocytosis with a left shift. Other evidence of systemic toxemia (metabolic acidosis, azotemia, increases in liver and muscle enzymes) also may be seen.

Treatment.   Administration of antibiotics such as penicillin and *Clostridium* antitoxin are the mainstays of treatment, although animals may die acutely before treatment can be instituted.

Prevention.   A toxoid against the clostridial alpha toxin is available in some countries, but not in the United States. Prevention efforts should focus on environmental hygiene and avoiding favorable gut conditions for proliferation of the organism. Because this type appears to survive better in soil than other types, preventing ingestion of soil may be important in preventing disease.

C. perfringens types B and C cause very similar diseases called *lamb dysentery* and *hemorrhagic enterotoxemia*, respectively. Both lambs and kids can be affected. With both diseases the beta toxin is important, and inactivation of this toxin after maturation of pancreatic trypsinogen secretion effectively limits the susceptible population to neonatal animals. Older animals may become susceptible as a result of overwhelming infection or trypsin inhibition by some soy and sweet potato products. The reported geographic range of both neonatal diseases appears to be limited (type B to the United Kingdom and South Africa and type C to the United Kingdom and North America), even though infection with *C. perfringens* type C appears to occur worldwide.

The diseases initially affect lambs and kids less than 3 days old, with illness occasionally occurring in older lambs. Because of the age of the animals, fecal contamination of teats, hands, and equipment that enter the mouths of the neonates (orogastric tubes, nipples) is a major cause of infection. Severely affected animals or those at the beginning of an outbreak are usually found dead. Less acutely affected animals display yellow, fluid feces that may contain brown flecks of blood; splinting of the abdomen, especially when handled; colic signs; and feed refusal. The clinical course is usually short, and the disease is almost always fatal. Terminal convulsions and coma are occasionally noted, especially with the disease in the United States. Postmortem examination reveals small hemorrhagic ulcers in the small intestine with type B infection and diffuse reddening with hemorrhage and necrosis of the abomasum and the entire intestine with type C infection. Animals that die very rapidly may have minimal or no gross abnormalities of the intestine.

C. perfringens type C in older sheep causes "struck." Temporary suppression of pancreatic trypsin production may be important in the development of this disease. Affected animals are usually found dead or with signs of toxemia. Specific antemortem signs of gastrointestinal disease are rare. Postmortem changes include neutrophilic leukocytosis with a left shift. Other evidence of systemic toxemia (metabolic acidosis, azotemia, increases in liver and muscle enzymes) also may be seen.

Diagnosis. Diagnosis of these diseases is made by identification of characteristic lesions and positive toxin assays. Because the beta toxin is very labile, negative toxin assays are less significant than negative assays with other tissue-invading *Clostridia*.

Treatment. If identified early in the disease course, antibiotics such as penicillin products and *Clostridium* antitoxin may be beneficial. Fluids and antiinflammatory

agents may be indicated as well. Usually the condition is not recognized until the animal is dead or dying.

Prevention. A beta toxoid is available in the United States and other countries. It is usually packaged with an epsilon toxoid. The best protection is achieved by vaccinating pregnant dams twice, with the second dose administered approximately 3 to 4 weeks before lambing or kidding. Juveniles also should be vaccinated twice, starting around weaning time. Adults should receive an annual booster.

C. perfringens type D produces epsilon toxin, which is responsible for increasing gut permeability and widespread tissue damage. The organism proliferates best and produces the most toxin in the duodenum under conditions of excess fermentable starch, such as occurs after over-ingestion of high-energy feeds (milk, grain, lush pasture). Overindulgence can be a primary condition or reflect failure of the ruminal flora to adjust to an abrupt feed change such as increasing the grain portion of the ration or moving a flock onto an ungrazed, lush pasture. In addition to providing substrate for the organisms, these rapidly fermentable diets may decrease peristalsis, allowing the toxin to accumulate. Because of the need for trypsin cleavage of the protoxin, animals less than 2 weeks of age are rarely affected. The disease occurs worldwide.

Natural disease caused by *C. perfringens* type D differs between sheep and goats, possibly because of a difference in relative local and systemic action of the toxin, although experimental models have demonstrated that both species develop similar lesions. Sheep tend to develop enterotoxemia. Peracutely affected sheep may die before or shortly after illness is noted and may have no postmortem lesions. Acutely affected sheep develop tachypnea, tachycardia, fever, colic signs such as lateral recumbency and splinting of the abdomen, anorexia, and neurologic signs that begin as dullness and progress to seizures or coma. Yellow, watery diarrhea may be evident terminally and is a more prominent sign in subacutely or chronically affected lambs. Postmortem lesions include subendocardial hemorrhage around the mitral valve and pericardial effusion. The disease is more common in ewe lambs; in single, rapidly growing lambs 3 to 8 weeks of age; and in feedlot lambs 2 to 3 weeks after they enter the lot. Tail docking, castration, and other forms of intervention are thought to decrease the incidence of this disease by temporarily decreasing appetite. The disease also affects unvaccinated adult sheep, even without any history of stressors or feed changes.

Goats tend to develop more severe enteritis but fewer neurologic and systemic signs. Postmortem findings include pseudomembranous enterocolitis with mucosal ulceration, as well as fibrin, blood clots, and watery contents in the bowel lumen. Evidence of systemic toxemia, including multifocal petechial and ecchymotic hemorrhage, proteinaceous exudates in body cavities, pulmonary edema, and cerebral malacia with perivascular cuffing, is seen after both natural and experimental infections but is less common and less pronounced than lesions seen in sheep.

Clinical pathology.   Characteristic changes include neutrophilic leukocytosis with a left shift. Other evidence of systemic toxemia (metabolic acidosis, azotemia, increases in liver and muscle enzymes) also may be seen.

Treatment.   If identified early in the disease course, antibiotics such as penicillin products and *Clostridium* antitoxin may be beneficial. Fluids and antiinflammatory agents may be indicated as well. Usually the condition is not recognized until the animal is dead or dying.

Prevention.   Vaccination of pregnant ewes with two doses of toxoid, with the second dose coming 3 to 4 weeks before lambing, and adequate ingestion of colostrum are the best methods of protecting newborn lambs. Vaccination of the lamb itself before it is 6 weeks old provides minimal protection. Lambs should be vaccinated twice around weaning or at entrance to a feedlot. Males and adult females that are not part of the breeding program may be vaccinated annually. Vaccination has been shown to protect goats from experimental disease, but clinical evidence suggests that well-vaccinated goats are still susceptible to developing clostridial enteritis. The toxoids may not protect against local action of the toxins in the goat, which appears to play a greater role in their disease than it does in sheep[1-4] (see Chapter 4).

NON-ENTERIC CLOSTRIDIAL INFECTIONS

C. novyi (black disease, necrotic hepatitis, bighead) is found worldwide in the soil, feces, and gastrointestinal tracts of healthy ruminants. The organism also can be found in the liver of some healthy ruminants. It is a very large, straight, rod-shaped organism with terminal oval spores. Two types exist: type A secretes alpha, gamma, and epsilon toxins and is one of the organisms responsible for bighead and a minor contributor to malignant edema (see the later section on *C. septicum*); type B secretes alpha and beta toxins and is responsible for black disease. The temporal and geographic distributions of black disease resemble those of fascioliasis, with the greatest incidence of disease occurring in milder, moister months in many countries. Black disease is less common in sheep than in cattle, and also is rare in goats.[5,6]

Bighead

Pathogenesis and clinical signs.   Fecal and soil contamination of wounds received during head-butting leads to proliferation of *C. novyi* type A in damaged head and neck tissues. Secreted toxins lead to swelling, edema,

serohemorrhagic exudates, and local tissue necrosis. Wounds appear and smell gangrenous. Systemic toxemia may affect internal organs, leading to the death of the animal. *C. sordelli* causes identical disease.

Diagnosis.   Laboratory analysis may reveal an increase in enzymes of muscle or liver origin as well as neutrophilic leukocytosis with many immature and toxic neutrophils. Postmortem findings include local necrosis around the injury site. Diagnosis is usually made by identifying characteristic lesions.

Treatment.   Wound management (disinfection, débridement) and administration of antibiotic products (penicillin G sodium 20,000 IU/kg IV every 6 hours) are important treatment considerations.

Prevention.   Ram management may aid in prevention of head-butting wounds. Annual vaccination with multivalent clostridial toxoids also may be helpful. In flocks with a high prevalence of this disorder, a booster vaccine given to rams 1 month before the breeding season may provide additional protection.[6]

Black Disease

Pathogenesis.   Sporulated organisms within Kupffer's cells and spores of the organism present in the liver are thought to proliferate and begin secreting toxins when migrating fluke larvae create adequate anaerobic conditions. Infective organisms also may be brought into the liver by the flukes. Necrotizing toxins cause local hepatic necrosis and systemic toxemia.

Clinical signs.   Affected sheep are debilitated, fail to keep up with the flock, and exhibit weakness, recumbency, separation, and anorexia. Tachypnea and tachycardia may be seen; fever occurs early in the disease. The patches of subcutaneous hemorrhagic edema that give this disease its name are less likely to develop in sheep than in cattle, and therefore are rarely noted before the animal dies. The clinical course usually lasts less than 1 day, and the disease is uniformly fatal. The short course often prevents producers from noticing any abnormalities before the death of the animal.

Diagnosis.   The most characteristic clinical pathology changes are neutrophilic leukocytosis with a left shift. Other evidence of systemic toxemia (metabolic acidosis, azotemia, increases in liver and muscle enzymes) also may be seen. Postmortem findings include multifocal hepatic necrosis, straw-colored body cavity exudates, and patches of subcutaneous hemorrhagic edema.

Treatment and prevention.   Although black disease is rarely identified before the animal dies, it is best treated with flukicides (clorsulon 7 mg/kg PO) and antibiotics (penicillin G sodium 20,000 to 40,000 IU/kg IV every 6 hours). Supportive care, including nutritional support, fluids, and stress reduction, may be beneficial. Efforts to control fluke infestation are the most effective way to prevent this disease. Annual administration of multivalent clostridial vaccines also may be helpful. In flocks at high risk for developing this disorder, a booster vaccine given 1 month before fluke exposure may provide additional protection.[5,6]

Malignant Edema and Braxy

C. septicum is the most important cause of malignant edema. However, other tissue-invasive *Clostridia* can cause this disease, and mixed infections are common. The pathogenesis of infection is often similar to that seen with bighead and blackleg: soil or fecal *Clostridia* invasion of a contaminated wound. Activation of dormant bacteria in damaged tissue similar to that seen in clostridial necrotic hepatitis also occurs. In both cases, bacterial toxins lead to local tissue necrosis and systemic toxemia. The alpha, beta, gamma, and delta toxins are lecithinase, deoxyribonuclease, hyaluronidase, and hemolysin, respectively. Commonly affected sites include castration, dehorning, and injection sites; the umbilicus; and the postpartum uterus. Invasion through the lining of the abomasum causes braxy. Factors that promote braxy have not been identified, although ingestion of frozen feedstuffs in yearlings has been implicated. Both forms of the disease have worldwide distribution and are described more commonly in sheep than goats.

Clinical signs. Malignant edema is characterized by local or regional pain, edematous swelling, fever, and signs of shock. Evidence of subcutaneous gas production is less common in this infection than in blackleg. Uterine infections may cause a fetid vaginal discharge. Death occurs within hours to a few days after the onset of signs. Braxy usually causes death before any abnormalities are noted. On rare occasions, signs of depression, weakness, and colic may be seen.

Diagnosis. Characteristic clinical pathology changes include neutrophilic leukocytosis with a left shift. A decrease in WBC and RBC counts also is possible because of the leukocidal and hemolytic effects of the toxins. Other evidence of systemic toxemia (metabolic acidosis, azotemia, increases in liver and muscle enzymes) also may be seen. Postmortem changes with malignant edema include dark red, swollen muscle filled with hemorrhagic, proteinaceous exudate and little or no gas. With braxy the abomasal wall is hemorrhagic and necrotic. Both diseases cause rapid postmortem decomposition of the carcass.

Treatment and prevention. Wound management and antibiotics are important in treating braxy. Ancillary treatments such as fluids, antiinflammatory agents (flunixin meglumine 2 mg/kg IV), nutritional support, and blood transfusions may be necessary. Hygiene during invasive procedures such as castration, obstetric manipulation, shearing, tail docking, and administering injections is helpful in preventing malignant edema. Multivalent clostridial toxoids may provide some protection and should be given annually to animals at risk.[7,8]

Blackleg

C. chauvoei is the most important cause of blackleg. However, other tissue-invasive *Clostridia* can cause this disease, and mixed infections are common. The pathogenesis of infection is often similar to that seen with bighead and malignant edema: soil or fecal *Clostridia* invasion of a contaminated wound. Tail-docking, castration, and shearing wounds appear to be especially important sites of infection in sheep. Activation of dormant bacteria in damaged tissue, similar to that seen in clostridial necrotic hepatitis, also occurs, and the original cause of tissue damage such as a wound is not always evident. In some cases, bacterial proliferation appears to occur in a site distant from the original wound (fetal infections after shearing of a ewe). Bacterial toxins lead to local tissue necrosis and systemic toxemia. This bacterium produces similar toxins to those produced by *C. septicum*, and the disease is seen worldwide. *C. chauvoei* also causes severe gangrenous mastitis in postparturient ewes.

Clinical signs. Blackleg is characterized by local to regional painful, edematous swelling; fever; and signs of shock. Focal signs such as lameness, udder swelling, and subcutaneous swelling are more commonly seen with this disease than with malignant edema. Evidence of subcutaneous gas production is common. Uterine and mammary infections may cause a fetid vaginal or mammary discharge. Death often occurs within hours to a few days after the onset of signs, but the focal nature of this disorder gives affected animals a better prognosis than those affected by other nonintestinal clostridial disorders.

Diagnosis. Characteristic clinical pathology changes include neutrophilic leukocytosis with a left shift. A decrease in WBC and RBC counts also is possible because of the leukocidal and hemolytic effects of the toxins. Other evidence of systemic toxemia (metabolic acidosis, azotemia, increases in liver and muscle enzymes) also may be seen. Postmortem changes with blackleg most commonly consist of focal, crepitant, red, brown, or black areas of myonecrosis. Other regions such as the fetus, tail head, or mammary gland also may be affected. Degenerative changes can occur in internal organs, especially if postmortem evaluation is delayed. Diagnosis is made by isolating the organism. Fluorescent antibody tests are available to differentiate *C. chauvoei* from *C. septicum*.

Treatment and prevention.   Wound management, administration of antibiotics (penicillin G sodium 20,000 to 40,000 IU/kg IV every 6 hours), and supportive care (nutritional support, fluids, antiinflammatory agents) are important. Hygiene during invasive procedures such as castration, obstetric manipulation, shearing, tail docking, and administering injections is helpful in preventing blackleg. Multivalent clostridial toxoids may provide some protection and should be given annually to animals at risk[7] (see Chapter 9).

Red Water Disease

C. haemolyticum is the etiologic agent associated with red water disease. The organism appears to be related closely to *C. novyi* and may be referred to as type D of that species. The major difference between the two organisms is that *C. novyi* type B produces a phage-associated alpha toxin in addition to the beta toxin produced by both species. *C. haemolyticum* has a similar life cycle to other *Clostridia* and appears to thrive on alkaline pastures with standing water. It colonizes the livers of healthy animals and proliferates after liver damage, including damage caused by migrating flukes or liver biopsies. The beta toxin causes intravascular hemolysis and damages the capillary endothelium. Anemia, hepatic infarction, hemorrhagic enteritis, and hemoglobin-induced tubular nephritis are the primary results. The disease is seen worldwide and is more commonly reported in sheep than in goats. Seasonality varies with the life cycle of the flukes.

Clinical signs.   Affected animals appear weak and depressed and produce red urine and feces. Heart and respiratory rates are high and become much higher with any sort of effort or stress. Fever and icterus are seen early and late, respectively, in the course of the disease. Death occurs within hours to a few days after the onset of signs.

Diagnosis.   Hematologic evaluation reveals evidence of intravascular hemolysis, including severe anemia, hemoglobinemia, and hemoglobinuria. Mature neutrophilia with a degenerative left shift (immature forms of neutrophils and toxic changes) is often present. Serum biochemical evaluation may reveal evidence of organ failure and shock. The most characteristic postmortem finding is a large pale center of necrosis in the liver that results from bacterial proliferation and regional infarction of the portal vein. Microscopic evaluation reveals numerous *Clostridia*-like organisms within the necrotic region. Hemorrhagic polyserositis with blood-tinged body cavity exudates also are common. A presumptive diagnosis can be made based on the lesions. Positive diagnosis is made by isolating the organism.

Treatment and prevention.   Treatment includes the administration of antibiotics (penicillin G sodium 20,000 to 40,000 IU/kg IV every 6 hours) and flukicides (clorsulon 7 mg/kg PO) and the provision of supportive care (nutritional support and administration of antiinflammatory agents, blood transfusions, and fluids). Efforts to control liver flukes and prevent other causes of liver damage are most important. Polyvalent clostridial toxoids may provide some protection. In addition to the annual booster, a second or biyearly booster vaccination given 1 month before fluke exposure may provide additional protection to flocks at high risk for developing this disorder.[9]

Noninvasive *Clostridia*

Both tetanus and botulism are important diseases in small ruminant medicine. These two diseases are covered in Chapter 11.

References

1. Hagan WA, Bruner DW, Timoney JF: *Clostridium perfringens.* In Hagan WA, Bruner DW, Timoney JF, editors: *Hagan and Bruner's microbiology and infectious diseases of domestic animals,* ed 8, Ithaca, NY, 1988, Comstock Publishing.
2. Blackwell TE: Clinical signs, treatments, and postmortem lesions in dairy goats with enterotoxemia: 13 cases (1979-1982), *J Am Vet Med Assoc* 200:214, 1992.
3. Uzal FA, Kelly FA: Enterotoxemia in goats, *Vet Res Comm* 20:481, 1996.
4. Uzal FA, Kelly FA: Experimental *Clostridium perfringens* type D enterotoxemia in goats, *Vet Pathol* 35:142, 1998.
5. Hagan WA, Bruner DW, Timoney JF: *Clostridium novyi.* In Hagan WA, Bruner DW, Timoney JF, editors: *Hagan and Bruner's microbiology and infectious diseases of domestic animals,* ed 8, Ithaca, NY, 1988, Comstock Publishing.
6. Hamid ME et al: First report of infectious necrotic hepatitis (black disease) among Nubian goats in Sudan, *Rev Elev Med Vet Pays Trop* 44:273, 1991.
7. Hagan WA, Bruner DW, Timoney JF: *Clostridium septicum.* In Hagan WA, Bruner DW, Timoney JF, editors: *Hagan and Bruner's microbiology and infectious diseases of domestic animals,* ed 8, Ithaca, NY, 1988, Comstock Publishing.
8. Eustis SL, Bergeland ME: Suppurative abomasitis associated with *Clostridium septicum* infection, *J Am Vet Med Assoc* 178:732, 1981.
9. Hagan WA, Bruner DW, Timoney JF: *Clostridium haemolyticum.* In Hagan WA, Bruner DW, Timoney JF, editors: *Hagan and Bruner's microbiology and infectious diseases of domestic animals,* ed 8, Ithaca, NY, 1988, Comstock Publishing.

Juvenile and Adult Sepsis

Pathophysiology.   Older animals are generally more resistant to sepsis than neonates because they have larger amounts of circulating antibodies. However, this resistance can be overwhelmed by aggressive bacteria, or loss of immune function can allow invasion by opportunistic bacteria. Malnutrition, parasitism, transport, overcrowding, other diseases, extreme weather conditions, and other stressors are the major causes of immune suppression.

Clinical signs. Sepsis may produce peracute, acute, or chronic disease signs. Peracute signs include fever, injected mucous membranes (including the sclera), tachycardia, tachypnea, dyspnea, swollen joints, lameness, splinting of the abdomen, weakness, depression, anorexia, recumbency, seizures, coma, and sudden death. Acute signs are similar, except that they persist for a longer period and therefore are more likely to be noticed. Chronic signs usually result from the partial clearance of infection after an acute episode, which may be clinical or inapparent.

IMPORTANT BACTERIAL CAUSES OF SEPSIS

Actinobacillus seminis is a gram-negative bacillus or coccobacillus that primarily affects the male and female reproductive tracts. Infection causes posthitis, epididymitis, and orchitis in rams and metritis and abortion in ewes. Other sites of infection, including rare occurrences of chronic sepsis, also are possible. Serologic tests are much more useful for identifying infected flocks than infected individuals within flocks. Definitive diagnosis depends on bacteriologic culture of the organism and differentiation of it from *Brucella ovis*. The bacillus is common in sheep in some parts of the world but is uncommon in North American sheep and goats.[1]

Arcanobacterium (Actinomyces) pyogenes is best known as an abscess-forming bacterium because of the thick pus formed in response to infection by it and the fibrinous response it elicits. It occasionally also causes sepsis. Its association with chronic sepsis lends credence to the belief that *Arcanobacterium* is often a secondary invader that colonizes tissues damaged by another bacterium (see Chapter 8).

Bacillus anthracis is a large, gram-positive, anaerobic bacillus that causes anthrax. It forms spores under aerobic conditions (such as on culture plates) but rarely does so when oxygen tensions are low, as in carcasses. The organism affects most mammals, with herbivores being most susceptible. It is usually carried from one area to another by shedding or dying animals and also can multiply in alkaline, nitrogenous soils. Periods of heat and intermittent flooding promote overgrowth of the organism. *B. anthracis* spores may be inhaled or ingested; in rare cases the bacillus itself may be spread by biting flies. After local replication the organism gains access to the blood, where it multiples readily. Large numbers of the organisms colonize the spleen. *B. anthracis* secretes a holotoxin made of edema factor (EF), protective antigen (PA), and lethal factor (LF). This toxin impairs phagocytosis, increases capillary permeability, and inhibits clotting. Splenic engorgement, generalized edema, circulatory shock, and bleeding diathesis are the most common lesions and signs of anthrax. Generalized infection should be considered uniformly fatal. Death may occur before or within hours of initial recognition that the animal is sick. Prophylactic antibiotic treatment of healthy animals (oxytetracycline 10 mg/kg IV SID) may decrease spread and mortality during outbreaks. The disease is reportable in many areas. Local forms of anthrax also occur, most commonly after transmission through a skin wound or fly bite. Local heat, pain, swelling, and necrosis are seen first, and the generalized syndrome often follows.[2]

Borrelia burgdorferi is thought to spread to ruminants from its mouse host by *Ixodes* ticks. The condition is zoonotic, causing Lyme disease in humans. The organism is thought to be responsible for fever, weight loss, and chronic septic arthritis in some ruminants, based on the finding that these animals are seropositive and occasionally respond to tetracycline antibiotics. Abundant evidence for this is lacking, and it is likely that some of those animals have mycoplasmal or other infections. A similar organism, possibly *Borrelia theileri*, is responsible for rare cases of bacteremia and fever[3] (see Chapter 9).

ZOONOTIC INFECTIONS

Brucella melitensis is more common in goats than sheep. Swine, cattle, and other ruminants are common hosts. The disease is zoonotic. Infection usually causes inapparent mammary infection and abortions. Diagnosis is made by serology, culture, or agglutination tests[4] (see Chapter 6).

Chlamydia psittaci has a life cycle that is not particularly well understood. It is an obligate intracellular parasite that spreads from cell to cell in the form of elementary bodies. It colonizes epithelial membranes, including the intestinal mucosa, where it may persist within a flock. Transmission between animals may occur through direct contact (ocular secretions, abortions), fecal-oral passage of infective elementary bodies, and possibly through insect bites, birds, and breeding (venereal spread). Polyarthritis, conjunctivitis, pneumonia, orchitis, epididymitis, and middle- to late-pregnancy abortion are the most common disease manifestations; the different manifestations may be caused by different strains. Chlamydial diseases are more commonly reported in sheep than in goats. Diagnosis of chlamydial disease is often difficult. Elementary bodies may be seen on histopathologic examination of affected tissues, including the placenta. Serologic and cytopathologic assays also exist. Vaccines are available to prevent chlamydial abortion in sheep[5] (see Chapters 6 and 12).

Coxiella burnetii is a rickettsial organism that is an important cause of abortion in sheep and goats and also causes zoonotic disease. It is spread between animals by ticks and also possibly by inhalation of aerosolized particles or contaminated dust. In addition to abortion, newly infected sheep and goats occasionally have mild, transient fevers. *C. burnetii* is far more important as the cause of Q fever in humans, who become infected after inhaling particles, handling contaminated animals, or coming into contact with contaminated body fluids (uterine fluid, milk) from infected animals. Results of vaccination trials in animals have been equivocal both at preventing abortion and limiting shedding of the organism. Currently no vaccine is available in the United States[6] (see Chapter 6).

More common in sheep than goats, *E. rhusiopathiae* has many hosts (including domestic swine and wild rodents). It appears to be plentiful in some environments and is zoonotic by wound infection. The organism appears to enter through skin breaks such as tail docking, castration, and shearing wounds. Chronic septic arthritis is the most common manifestation. Diagnosis is by culture.[7]

Francisella (Pasteurella) tularensis is more common in sheep than goats. The organism has many hosts, of which the most important are wild rabbits and rodents. It can contaminate water sources. It is zoonotic, causing tularemia, or rabbit fever. Transmission to sheep is usually through biting arthropods (ticks, flies) that have previously fed on an infected wild mammal. Acute or chronic sepsis may be seen, with more widespread and severe disease occurring in sheep with poor immune function. Healthy sheep are thought to be resistant to infection. Granulomatous splenitis and hepatitis are seen at necropsy[8] (see Chapter 5).

Leptospira interrogans

Pathogenesis. *Leptospires* are spirochete bacteria that live in moist environments. Their survival time outside of hosts is usually short, so their most important reservoirs are the kidneys of infected animals, especially rodents. Infected animals shed the organisms through urine and most other body fluids. Organisms enter new hosts through mucous membranes and skin breaks and cause bacteremia. Signs of sepsis range from severe, especially in neonates, to inapparent. Intravascular hemolysis may result from the action of hemolytic toxins or agglutinating antibodies. Animals that survive the acute stage localize the infection in sites such as the kidneys, eyes, and fetoplacental unit. Abortion may occur a month or more after acute signs first become evident; renal shedding may occur for several months. Leptospirosis is zoonotic, causing flulike signs and encephalitis. Because sheep and goats are not commonly infected, they are less likely to be sources of infection than other domestic and wild species.

Clinical signs. Acute leptospirosis causes signs of sepsis, including fever, depression, dyspnea, exercise intolerance, weakness, and death. Additionally, many affected animals show signs of intravascular hemolysis such as anemia, icterus, and hemoglobinuria.

Diagnosis. Evidence of intravascular hemolysis such as anemia, hyperbilirubinemia, hemoglobinuria, and hemoglobinemia is specific to this disease. In chronic infection nonspecific inflammatory changes and azotemia may be seen. Animals dying in the acute hemolytic stage are likely to have dark, discolored urine, bladder, and kidneys. Spirochetes can be identified on dark-field microscopy of fresh urine or plasma from infected animals and may be cultured with special techniques. In animals with less severe infection, a rise in antibody titers can be used to support a diagnosis of leptospirosis.

Prevention. Numerous vaccines are available for sheep. Because protection is serotype-specific, it is important to vaccinate against common serotypes in the area. *L. pomona* is the most consistent isolate from sheep and goats. Vaccination immunity is thought to be short lived; boosters should be given at least twice a year in endemic areas[10] (see Chapter 6).

Listeria monocytogenes

Pathogenesis. *L. monocytogenes* causes disease with similar frequency in sheep and goats. The organism is a common soil and fecal contaminant, especially if pH is greater than 5.0. It also proliferates in silage that is not properly acidified and in rotting, woody debris. Risk of exposure depends on the feed and environment of the animals. Environmental and fecal contamination are more common sources than silage in small ruminants overall because most sheep and goats throughout the world are never fed silage. Infection almost always results from ingestion.

Listeria may invade the body through the gastrointestinal tract. The most common form of listerial infection is sepsis, especially in animals younger than 1 year old. The organism appears to be cleared quickly from the blood but causes persistent problems resulting from localized infections. Hepatitis, abortion, and nervous system disease are the most common manifestations. *Listeria* may have a predilection for the central nervous system because many affected animals have clinical signs and necropsy lesions compatible with diffuse meningoencephalitis or spinal myelitis. Animals with the latter lesions appear bright but have hindlimb paresis or tetraparesis. A better known form of listeriosis in ruminants is a specialized brainstem disease.

Clinical signs. The most common signs are those of sepsis, with the majority of affected animals also exhibiting neurologic signs. Animals with the brainstem form of the disease display signs that differ according to the nerve nuclei affected.

Diagnosis. Diagnosis is made by isolating the organism from lesions, body fluids, or feeds (silage). A presumptive diagnosis of the brainstem form of the disease can be made by histopathologic identification of the microabscesses.

Prevention. No vaccine is available, so efforts to avoid infection include providing adequate passive transfer of immunoglobulin to neonates, properly fermenting silage, and removing rotting, woody vegetation from pastures[11] (see Chapters 6 and 11).

Mycoplasmal Diseases

Pathogenesis. *Mycoplasma* are very small, simple bacteria that parasitize cells of higher species. They are common inhabitants of mucous membranes and can have either a commensal or pathogenic relationship with the host. Transmission between animals is most likely through direct or indirect contact with infected body fluids from infected animals, inhalation of respiratory droplets, and arthropod vectors. Common sites for superficial infection include the ocular membranes, lung, mammary gland, and female reproductive tract. The organisms can also enter the blood and cause septicemia, abortion, pleuritis, and polyarthritis. Flare-ups often occur during times of crowding and during lambing or kidding, when neonates can spread the organisms from the mother's mouth to her udder and in turn become infected by ingesting contaminated milk.

The most important *Mycoplasma* species in sheep and goats in the United States are *M. conjunctivae*, *M. capricolum*, and the less pathogenic *M. ovipneumoniae.* They are most commonly associated with keratoconjunctivitis (Figure 14-3), acute or chronic sepsis, and pneumonia, respectively. *M. conjunctivae* and *C. psittaci* are the most common causes of pinkeye in North American small ruminants. *Mycoplasma* are thought to inhibit tracheal ciliary function and thus have a role similar to viruses in "shipping fever pneumonia" in facilitating lower respiratory tract invasion by *Pasteurella* and *Mannheimia*. Many of the major pathogenic serotypes found in other countries (some of which cause severe pleuropneumonia without the participation of another bacteria), including *M. mycoides* subsp. *mycoides, M. mycoides* subsp. *capri, M. agalactiae,* and strain F38, are not found in or have been eradicated from North America.

Clinical signs. Keratoconjunctivitis, mastitis, exudative vulvovaginitis, fever, cough, dyspnea, exercise intolerance, abortion, lameness, swollen joints, neonatal death, and depression may all be seen with *Mycoplasma* infections.

Diagnosis. No specific clinical pathologic findings occur with these diseases. *Mycoplasma* infection should be suspected in sheep and goats with severe exudative pleuropneumonia in some parts of the world. *Mycoplasma* can be identified by bacteriologic culture or staining of exudates. Examiners must take care in interpreting positive cultures from body surfaces because nonpathogenic *Mycoplasma* are common.

Prevention. Vaccines against mycoplasmal infections are available in some parts of the world, but not in the United States. Providing fly control, preventing stress and overcrowding, and isolating sick animals from healthy ones may help prevent the spread of disease[12] (see Chapters 5, 12, and 13).

Fusobacterium Infections

Fusobacterium necrophorum causes or is associated with a variety of diseases in sheep and is likely to cause many similar diseases in goats. It is best known as a cause of footrot and hepatic abscesses and also appears to be important in lip-leg ulceration. It is an enteric gram-negative anaerobe and as such can cause gram-negative sepsis after entrance of the bacteria or its toxins into the circulation.

F. necrophorum has a poor ability to invade healthy tissue. However, it readily colonizes regions damaged by trauma, persistent moisture, and infection. In addition to endotoxin the bacterium produces leukocidal and cytolytic toxins that form zones of necrosis around bacterial colonies. This tissue necrosis as well as the foul-smelling waste gases produced by the bacteria are characteristic of necrobacillosis, or *F. necrophorum* infection. Clinical signs include necrotic, fetid lesions, usually of the mouth or feet, that can cause ingestion or lameness problems. Efforts to maintain good hygiene are helpful in preventing fecal contamination. Additionally, preventing trauma to foot and mouth tissues through good surface choices and proper pasture drainage is important[9] (see Chapter 9).

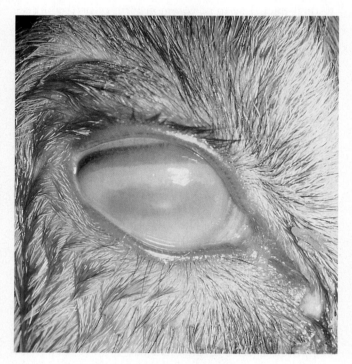

Figure 14-3 Keratoconjunctivitis in a goat caused by *Mycoplasma* species. (Courtesy Drs. Tom Powe and D.G. Pugh, Auburn University, Alabama.)

PASTEURELLA AND PASTEURELLA-LIKE INFECTIONS

Pasteurella multocida

Pathogenesis. *P. multocida* is a small, gram-negative, bipolar, ovoid rod that inhabits the pharynx of healthy ruminants, similar to other *Pasteurella* species and *Mannheimia haemolytica*. It can survive in soil and water for varying amounts of time after contamination with ruminant nasal secretions. Healthy ruminants shed *P. multocida* much more frequently than *M. haemolytica*. Disease occurs when bacteria colonize the lower respiratory tract or enter the blood. Risk factors for pulmonary and systemic infection include viral or mycoplasmal respiratory diseases, temperature extremes, respiratory tract irritants, transport, overcrowding, changes to higher-energy feeds, and handling stress. These factors are thought both to increase bacterial replication in the airway and suppress mechanisms to clear the infection. Pasteurellosis is a major problem in feedlot sheep but less common in small breeding or hobby flocks. Pasteurellosis also is a significant disease in certain wild small ruminants such as Bighorn sheep.

Direct spread of the organism between animals occurs with nasal contact, and indirect spread occurs after contact with infected nasal secretions. The organism persists in the environment for longer periods during warm, moist weather. *Pasteurella* produces a polysaccharide capsule that inhibits phagocytosis and an endotoxin that contributes to clinical signs. Unlike *M. haemolytica*, *P. multocida* does not appear to produce a leukotoxin that has a direct lytic effect on host cells and leads to extensive secondary damage resulting from the release of proteolytic enzymes from lysed neutrophils. The major disease caused by *P. multocida* is pneumonia. However, *Pasteurella* species also are capable of entering the blood to cause septicemia in neonates and hemorrhagic septicemia in adults. Occasionally focal infections such as septic arthritis and mastitis are found.

Clinical signs. Clinical signs of pneumonic and septicemic pasteurellosis include bilateral purulent nasal discharge, coughing, diarrhea, anorexia, and high fever. The disease course can be short with septicemic pasteurellosis and is usually more insidious with *P. multocida* pneumonia. *Pasteurella* mastitis is characterized by the bluebag condition or gangrene of the udder.

Diagnosis. Inflammatory changes in the leukogram and hyperfibrinogenemia are the most frequent abnormalities. With severe disease and in the septicemic form, immature neutrophils may predominate over mature cells. Inflammation of the intestine and abomasum also may be seen. Hemorrhage and fibrin are usually absent or less prominent than in pneumonia caused by *M. haemolytica*. Samples for bacteriologic culture are usually obtained postmortem. Blood or tracheal fluid may be obtained before death if the value of the animal warrants it.

Prevention. Vaccines are available for control of pneumonic pasteurellosis, although they are of questionable efficacy in controlling that infection[13] (see Chapters 5 and 6).

Pasteurella haemolytica

M. haemolytica (*P. haemolytica* biotype A) is a gram-negative rod that is a common commensal inhabitant of the tonsils of young animals. It is gradually replaced by *P. trehalosi* in older animals. Disease is much more frequently described in sheep than in goats and occurs when the organism gains access to the lower respiratory tract.

Clinical signs and diagnosis. The most common syndrome is enzootic pneumonia, which is seen in young lambs and their dams. Hemorrhagic bronchopneumonia is the major lesion and respiratory signs predominate. Gangrenous mastitis (bluebag) is seen in some of the dams, presumably after they have been nursed by infected offspring. Factors that promote respiratory disease, including viral infections, airborne irritants, high stocking density, and stress, are thought to promote invasion of the lower airway by these bacteria.

Prevention. Vaccines are available for control of pneumonic pasteurellosis, but they are of questionable efficacy in controlling that infection[14] (see Chapters 5 and 6).

Pasteurella trehalosi

P. trehalosi (*P. haemolytica* biotype T) is a gram-negative rod that gradually replaces *M. haemolytica* as the major commensal inhabitant of the tonsils. Disease is much more frequently described in sheep than in goats and occurs when the organism gains access to the lung or blood. Replication occurs in the lung and systemic toxemia or bacteremia result. Hemorrhagic pneumonia, necrotic hepatitis, erosions of the tonsils and gastrointestinal tract, and hemorrhagic serositis are seen. The case fatality rate is high. Studies have not determined whether vaccines against *M. haemolytica* provide any protection against *P. trehalosi* infection[14] (see Chapter 6).

Yersiniosis

Pathogenesis. *Yersinia* are gram-negative bacteria. *Y. enterocolitica* and *Y. pseudotuberculosis* both have many mammalian and avian hosts, including humans, and cause clostridial enteritis–like disease in goats. Rodent and bird hosts may be important reservoir populations for infections in domestic animals. Kids younger than 6 months old develop enteritis, bacteremia, and diarrhea that is watery but not bloody. Severe toxemia and sudden death can occur. Older kids and flocks with chronic exposure tend to have less severe acute disease. Instead, chronic diarrhea and weight loss are seen, usually in association with gut wall and abdominal abscesses. Sheep are rarely affected.

Clinical signs. Signs of enteritis or sepsis predominate in acute disease, whereas signs of wasting are more common in chronic disease.

Diagnosis. Evidence of acute or chronic inflammation is provided by blood work. Characteristic necropsy lesions include numerous microabscesses in the gut wall and mesenteric lymph nodes, as well as other evidence of enteritis or sepsis. Culture of lesions and demonstration of a rising antibody titer are diagnostic.

Prevention. Avoiding exposure to sources and maintaining overall flock health are helpful in preventing losses caused by yersiniosis.

Gram-Negative Sepsis

Pathogenesis. Gram-negative bacteria and their toxins gain access to the blood from a site of proliferation or destruction. The most important toxin is endotoxin, a group of lipopolysaccharide molecules that reside within the wall of the bacteria. Bacteria or endotoxins incite a systemic inflammatory response, chiefly through activation of host macrophages and stimulation of host cytokine release. These cytokines cause inflammation, produce leukocyte recruitment, increase capillary permeability, induce fever through stimulation of the hypothalamus, and have regional or diffuse vasomotor effects.

Because the ruminant gut has a plentiful population of gram-negative bacteria, it is implicated as the source of most cases of gram-negative sepsis. Grain overload causes a die-off of the normal gram-negative ruminal flora, ulcerative enteric disease allows invasion of bacteria or absorption of their toxins, and ingestion of pathogens provides a suitable place for proliferation and route for invasion of the body. Gram-negative sepsis caused by opportunistic organisms is best recognized in the immunocompromised neonate but also can be seen in stressed or immunocompromised sheep or goats of all ages. In those cases a predisposing cause or source of overwhelming challenge should be sought. *E. coli* is commonly found in fecal material, *Klebsiella pneumoniae* is found in feces and wood products, *F. necrophorum* lives in the gastrointestinal tract and in soil and invades through compromised gastric mucosa or footrot lesions, and *Pseudomonas aeruginosa* is found in water and wash solutions.

Primary pathogens are relatively more common in adults. Although some coliform bacteria may fit into this category, by far the most important genus is *Salmonella*. Sources of *Salmonella* infection are numerous and include carrier animals of the same species, cattle, rodents, birds, other animals, and possibly feedstuffs. Only one serotype of *Salmonella* is specifically adapted to sheep *(S. abortus ovis)*, and it is not found in North America. No strain is known to be host-adapted to goats. Therefore all infections in sheep and goats have the potential to spread to and from other species, including humans. Serotypes of *Salmonella* that have caused important infections in sheep or goats include *S. typhimurium, S. dublin,* and *S. montevideo.* Most of these infections lead to bacteremia with mild systemic signs, followed by abortion. *S. dublin* and *S. typhimurium* tend to cause more illness in adults because of fibrinonecrotic enteritis.

Clinical signs. Affected animals can exhibit anything from mild depression with a low-grade fever to shock. Common signs include fever, tachycardia, tachypnea, depression with slow or absent eating and drinking, weakness or recumbency, and injection or cyanosis of mucous membranes. Organ-specific signs may betray the source or at least the primary location of the infection. Fetid discharge may be seen with metritis or abortion; dyspnea and abnormal lung sounds may be seen with pulmonary infection; and bloat, ruminal atony, abdominal distention, and diarrhea may be seen with gastrointestinal infections.

Diagnosis. The most common abnormality identified on a CBC with peracute gram-negative sepsis is panleukopenia. Over the course of several days this condition may resolve, first through an increase in immature neutrophils and later through an increase in mature neutrophils and restoration of lymphocyte counts. Very immature cells, severe toxic changes, and persistence of neutropenia suggest a poor prognosis. Serum biochemical changes often reflect the severity of the condition; that is, the more normal the blood work, the less severe the disease. The greater the evidence of shock or tissue damage, the worse the prognosis. Metabolic acidosis with a large anion gap and azotemia suggest advanced disease. Necropsy findings include diffuse evidence of inflammation, including pulmonary congestion, and polyserositis with body cavity exudates. Hemorrhagic pneumonia or fibrinonecrotic enteritis may be seen and reflect the source of bacterial invasion. In all cases, diagnosis is best confirmed by bacteriologic culture of body tissues or fluids. In the live animal, culture of blood, feces, or tracheal fluid yields the best results. When numerous animals are infected, environmental samples (including feed, water, and bedding) should be tested for the presence of the bacteria. However, bacteriologic culture of aborted fetuses or placentas frequently yields heavy growth of the organism.

Prevention. Maintaining overall good health and hygiene is the best means of preventing gram-negative sepsis. Anti-endotoxin bacterins are available for cattle in the United States, but their use in small ruminants has been too limited to assess their efficacy.[15] During a flock outbreak, the use of autogenous bacterin may help prevent the spread of disease on a farm (see Chapter 6).

TREATMENT FOR SEPSIS (ADULT AND JUVENILE)

Bacterial organisms are rarely identified before important treatment decisions must be made. Therefore treatment should follow general principles and have a wide spectrum of efficacy. Antimicrobial drugs are the cornerstone of treatment. In meat- or milk-producing small ruminants the veterinarian must be careful to use drugs within label directions or have a rational plan for extra-label drug use (see Appendix I). The issue of extra-label drug use is especially important in goats, because very few pharmaceutical products have been licensed for them in North America. Cost and convenience of treatment also may dictate the drugs to be used.

Unless the clinician strongly suspects a particular organism (as with clostridiosis or anaplasmosis), he or she should use a single antibiotic or combination of antimicrobial drugs to provide a broad spectrum of coverage. Penicillins, macrolides, tetracyclines, and cephalosporins all provide reasonably effective coverage against gram-positive pathogens, but of these drugs only the newer cephalosporins are reasonably effective against many systemic and enteric gram-negative pathogens. The gram-negative pathogens of the respiratory tract are often sensitive to other classes of antibiotics. Macrolides and tetracyclines also are effective against *Mycoplasma* species and rickettsial organisms (see Appendix I).

NSAIDs almost always are beneficial in severe infectious conditions because of their antiinflammatory, antipyretic, and antiendotoxic effects. They are likely to be more effective than corticosteroids because they provide benefits without suppressing the immune response. All such drug use should be considered extra-label and instituted accordingly (see Appendix I). Specific antisera are available for some of the clostridial diseases and may be beneficial if given before widespread tissue necrosis has occurred. Severely compromised animals should be treated with fluids for shock (see Appendix II).

OTHER CAUSES OF DISEASE

Common Abscess-Forming Bacteria

Pathophysiology.   Abscess-forming bacteria are usually able to survive phagocytosis and thereby avoid destruction by cells of the immune system. Alternatively, they invoke such an inflammatory response that the host body "walls off" the entire region with fibrous tissue. Abscesses may occur locally, frequently after a wound infection, or at numerous or distant sites from the point of infection. For abscesses to occur at the latter sites, the organism must travel to either by way of the blood or within leukocytes. Therefore disease characterized by multifocal or internal abscesses usually results from a low-grade, transient event of bacteremia.

The best known and most important abscess-forming bacterium in small ruminants is *Corynebacterium pseudotuberculosis,* the gram-positive, facultative anaerobic coccobacillus that causes caseous lymphadenitis. Infection is usually maintained in a flock by infected animals that spread the organism to others through purulent material draining from open abscesses. The organism is very hardy, so infection can occur through direct contact or indirect contact with contaminated common instruments and facilities. Infection is usually introduced into a flock through acquisition of an infected animal, although it also can occur when a naive flock is moved into a contaminated area. Horses, cattle, and humans also are minor hosts. Infection is thought to occur after ingestion, inhalation, or wound contamination. Except for lower respiratory tract invasion, a surface break is thought to be necessary. Contaminated shears, tail-docking knives, and emasculators readily spread the organisms through a flock. Abscesses can form at the site of invasion or more commonly at the site of the local lymph node.

Clinical signs.   Clinical signs of external abscesses include surface swellings and draining lesions. Drainage may be intermittent and usually consists of thick, yellow-white purulent material. Internal abscesses are more difficult to diagnose. Thoracic masses may cause inspiratory dyspnea or occlude venous return to the heart. Abdominal lesions may cause tenesmus, stranguria, and occasionally colic. The most common sign of internal abscesses is weight loss with or without intermittent fever. Common external sites include the submandibular or retromandibular space, preinguinal, prefemoral, and supramammary nodes. Head and neck lesions are more common in goats, whereas sheep have a more even distribution of cranial and caudal lesions, presumably as a result of shearing wounds. External infections rarely cause clinical illness beyond the draining abscess, although some degree of cachexia may be present. More important are internal infections.

Diagnosis.   Diagnosis is often made by the characteristic lesions with their thick, non-malodorous pus. Bacteriologic culture provides a more specific answer, which may be important for flock management. Serologic tests have been developed to identify carrier animals and may be useful if the manager wishes to eliminate infection from the flock.

Treatment.   Treatment is often unrewarding: antibiotic sensitivity profiles do not reflect the degree of protection afforded the organisms within the abscesses. Long-term treatment with antibiotics and drainage of any compromising masses may lead to some degree of resolution, but internal abscesses are likely to persist.

Prevention. Prevention through the use of vaccines has been attempted. Vaccines appear to reduce the severity of the disease, but do not completely prevent infection. Moreover, live attenuated bacterins lead to de facto infection of all vaccinated animals, and therefore should not be used in naive flocks[16] (see Chapter 8).

Other abscess-forming bacteria are most important as differential diagnoses for caseous lymphadenitis. *Arcanobacterium (Actinomyces, Corynebacterium) pyogenes* is another wound contaminant that affects focal areas or regional external lymph nodes. It also commonly colonizes damaged internal tissues such as post-pneumonic lungs, post-acidotic livers, and damaged feet and heart valves. It is thought to be ubiquitous and poorly invasive in ruminants, and therefore does not have the same flock significance as *C. pseudotuberculosis.* Flocks with outbreaks of this infection often have suboptimal management. *F. necrophorum* causes similar disease and often co-infects with *A. pyogenes.* It is generally more necrotizing and leads to greater systemic signs of acute illness, including death. *F. necrophorum* also produces fetid pus, whereas *A. pyogenes* usually does not. *Rhodococcus equi* is a rare cause of pulmonary abscesses in sheep.

Numerous small, coalescent, nodular skin abscesses may result from *Pseudomonas pseudomallei* infection (melioidosis). Infection usually occurs after the sheep or goat is bitten by an insect that previously fed on an infected rodent. This organism is found in many subtropical regions, including the Caribbean, but is not reported in North America.

Mycobacteria

Pathogenesis. *Mycobacteria* are small, aerobic, straight or curved pleomorphic rods with thick lipid cell walls. They can be stained with acid-fast stains and are usually gram-positive. The bacteria live within infected animals of many mammalian species and survive for several years in warm, moist environments. Infection occurs after ingestion or inhalation. An identifying characteristic of the mechanism of infection by *Mycobacteria* is the bacteria's ability to survive within macrophages by preventing fusion of phagosomes and lysosomes. The organisms are carried to local lymphatic vessels or lymph nodes, where they form granulomas. As they enlarge, granulomas may develop necrotic or mineralized centers surrounded by macrophages and giant cells. Disease can be local, regional, or generalized, depending on the distance the organism is carried from the original site of infection. Granulomatous pneumonia, enterocolitis, and lymphadenitis are the most common local and regional forms of the disease.

Organisms from ruptured granulomas may be spread in contaminated respiratory secretions and feces. Mycobacterial infections of all types are uncommon in North American sheep and goats, and these species are considered to be relatively resistant to infection. *M. bovis* is the most common organism associated with ovine tuberculosis in other countries, but *M. avium* is more common in the United States. The most common mycobacterial infection is Johne's disease (paratuberculosis), whose causative organism has been reclassified recently as *M. avium* subsp. *paratuberculosis. M. tuberculosis* is rare in the United States (see Chapter 4).

Mycobacterial infections are reportable in most parts of the United States. Some debate is ongoing about human susceptibility to *M. avium* subsp. *paratuberculosis;* the other organisms are known to be pathogenic in people.

Clinical signs. The most common clinical sign is emaciation. Diarrhea may be seen terminally in both tuberculosis and paratuberculosis. The disease is insidious, with signs becoming more apparent over several weeks to months. Respiratory signs may be seen, especially with infection by *M. bovis* or *M. avium.*

Diagnosis. Reports of clinicopathologic abnormalities are rare. Hypoalbuminemia and hypoproteinemia are likely to be common with chronic enterocolitis caused by either tuberculosis or paratuberculosis. The most common necropsy lesions seen in tuberculosis are nodular lesions of the lung, liver, lymph nodes, spleen, and intestines. Histologic evaluation reveals the nodules to be granulomas with giant cells and acid-fast organisms. Frequently the center of the lesion is necrotic and mineralized. Intestinal lesions appear to be more common than pulmonary lesions in goats. The lesions of paratuberculosis are centered around the ileocecocolic junction and the adjacent mesentery. The regions may appear normal or be notably thickened. Postmortem diagnosis is made by identifying characteristic lesions and culturing the organisms. Antemortem diagnosis of tuberculosis is best achieved by observing the reaction to intradermal injection of tuberculin with or without comparative injection of purified protein derivatives of *M. bovis* and *M. avium.* All tuberculosis testing should be done in accordance with local regulations. Antemortem diagnosis of Johne's disease can be achieved by fecal culture of the organism, but this test takes several weeks to months to complete. Newer serologic tests (e.g., ELISA) are available and appear to be sensitive and specific for Johne's disease.

Prevention. Tuberculosis should not be endemic in flocks in the United States because positive animals are quarantined or destroyed. Therefore preventing exposure to wild ruminants and other possible sources is crucial. Except in goat flocks raised for the production of milk that is to be sold unpasteurized, testing is uncommon, so animals are usually not identified until they develop overt disease.

Paratuberculosis is much more common and may be maintained in flocks by carrier animals. No effective treatment is available for either disease, nor should any be encouraged because efforts should be concentrated on eliminating infection from the flock or herd[17] (see Chapter 4).

REFERENCES

1. Hagan WA, Bruner DW, Timoney JF: *Actinobacillus seminis.* In Hagan WA, Bruner DW, Timoney JF, editors: *Hagan and Bruner's microbiology and infectious diseases of domestic animals,* ed 8, Ithaca, NY, 1988, Comstock Publishing.
2. Hagan WA, Bruner DW, Timoney JF: *Bacillus anthracis.* In Hagan WA, Bruner DW, Timoney JF, editors: *Hagan and Bruner's microbiology and infectious diseases of domestic animals,* ed 8, Ithaca, NY, 1988, Comstock Publishing.
3. Hagan WA, Bruner DW, Timoney JF: *Borrelia burgdorferi.* In Hagan WA, Bruner DW, Timoney JF, editors: *Hagan and Bruner's microbiology and infectious diseases of domestic animals,* ed 8, Ithaca, NY, 1988, Comstock Publishing.
4. Hagan WA, Bruner DW, Timoney JF: *Brucella melitensis.* In Hagan WA, Bruner DW, Timoney JF, editors: *Hagan and Bruner's microbiology and infectious diseases of domestic animals,* ed 8, Ithaca, NY, 1988, Comstock Publishing.
5. Hagan WA, Bruner DW, Timoney JF: *Chlamydia psittaci.* In Hagan WA, Bruner DW, Timoney JF, editors: *Hagan and Bruner's microbiology and infectious diseases of domestic animals,* ed 8, Ithaca, NY, 1988, Comstock Publishing.
6. Hagan WA, Bruner DW, Timoney JF: *Coxiella burnetii.* In Hagan WA, Bruner DW, Timoney JF, editors: *Hagan and Bruner's microbiology and infectious diseases of domestic animals,* ed 8, Ithaca, NY, 1988, Comstock Publishing.
7. Hagan WA, Bruner DW, Timoney JF: *Erysipelas rhusiopathiae.* In Hagan WA, Bruner DW, Timoney JF, editors: *Hagan and Bruner's microbiology and infectious diseases of domestic animals,* ed 8, Ithaca, NY, 1988, Comstock Publishing.
8. Hagan WA, Bruner DW, Timoney JF: *Francisella tularensis.* In Hagan WA, Bruner DW, Timoney JF, editors: *Hagan and Bruner's microbiology and infectious diseases of domestic animals,* ed 8, Ithaca, NY, 1988, Comstock Publishing.
9. Hagan WA, Bruner DW, Timoney JF: *Fusobacterium necrophorum.* In Hagan WA, Bruner DW, Timoney JF, editors: *Hagan and Bruner's microbiology and infectious diseases of domestic animals,* ed 8, Ithaca, NY, 1988, Comstock Publishing.
10. Hagan WA, Bruner DW, Timoney JF: *Leptospira interrogans.* In Hagan WA, Bruner DW, Timoney JF, editors: *Hagan and Bruner's microbiology and infectious diseases of domestic animals,* ed 8, Ithaca, NY, 1988, Comstock Publishing.
11. Hagan WA, Bruner DW, Timoney JF: *Listeria monocytogenes.* In Hagan WA, Bruner DW, Timoney JF, editors: *Hagan and Bruner's microbiology and infectious diseases of domestic animals,* ed 8, Ithaca, NY, 1988, Comstock Publishing.
12. Hagan WA, Bruner DW, Timoney JF: The genera *Mycoplasma* and *Ureaplasma.* In Hagan WA, Bruner DW, Timoney JF, editors: *Hagan and Bruner's microbiology and infectious diseases of domestic animals,* ed 8, Ithaca, NY, 1988, Comstock Publishing.
13. Hagan WA, Bruner DW, Timoney JF: *Pasteurella multocida.* In Hagan WA, Bruner DW, Timoney JF, editors: *Hagan and Bruner's microbiology and infectious diseases of domestic animals,* ed 8, Ithaca, NY, 1988, Comstock Publishing.
14. Hagan WA, Bruner DW, Timoney JF: *Pasteurella haemolytica.* In Hagan WA, Bruner DW, Timoney JF, editors: *Hagan and Bruner's microbiology and infectious diseases of domestic animals,* ed 8, Ithaca, NY, 1988, Comstock Publishing.
15. Hagan WA, Bruner DW, Timoney JF: The genus *Salmonella.* In Hagan WA, Bruner DW, Timoney JF, editors: *Hagan and Bruner's microbiology and infectious diseases of domestic animals,* ed 8, Ithaca, NY, 1988, Comstock Publishing.
16. Hagan WA, Bruner DW, Timoney JF: *Corynebacterium pseudotuberculosis.* In Hagan WA, Bruner DW, Timoney JF, editors: *Hagan and Bruner's microbiology and infectious diseases of domestic animals,* ed 8, Ithaca, NY, 1988, Comstock Publishing.
17. Hagan WA, Bruner DW, Timoney JF: The genus *Mycobacterium.* In Hagan WA, Bruner DW, Timoney JF, editors: *Hagan and Bruner's microbiology and infectious diseases of domestic animals,* ed 8, Ithaca, NY, 1988, Comstock Publishing.

BLOOD AND TISSUE PARASITES

Anaplasma ovis, Eperythrozoon ovis, and *Babesia* Species

Pathogenesis. *A. ovis* and *E. ovis* are small bacteria that lack cells walls and parasitize erythrocytes. They were initially classified as rickettsial bacteria, although work in recent years suggests a close relationship between *Eperythrozoon* and *Mycoplasma.* The organisms are spread from animal to animal by insect or mechanical vectors. Known arthropod vectors for *A. ovis* include ticks and horseflies; other biting flies may be more important with *E. ovis* infection. Hypodermic needles and equipment used for tail-docking, castrating, or disbudding animals may be important in iatrogenic transmission. After being introduced into a naive host, the organisms proliferate and the number of red cells infected increases rapidly until an effective immune response begins 1 to 2 weeks later. A similar proliferation of organisms may occur in chronically infected animals after temporary immune suppression. The humoral and cellular immune responses against *A. ovis* lead to opsonization of parasitized erythrocytes and their removal by cells of the reticuloendothelial system; *Eperythrozoon* infection is thought to cause more intravascular hemolysis. The result in both cases is hemolytic anemia.

The protozoon parasites *Babesia ovis* and *B. motasi* have similar life cycles and cause similar diseases, but they have been eradicated and are reportable in the United States. *Babesia* affecting small ruminants are generally less pathogenic than their bovine counterparts.

Animals that survive the acute hemolytic crisis reduce the parasites to low numbers but rarely clear the infection completely; they serve as sources of infection for other animals. Sheep and goats are susceptible to infection by either organism; goats generally appear to be more resistant to the development of severe parasitemia and clinical signs.

Clinical signs. Animals may have fever after acute infection and during the hemolytic period. Other signs present during the hemolytic crisis may include weakness, mucous membrane pallor, and dark urine. Urine discoloration results from increased amounts of bilirubin in most cases, although hemoglobinuria may be seen in some sheep with eperythrozoonosis. Icterus is usually present only after the acute hemolytic crisis. Clinical signs are exacerbated during times of stress, and infection is often first noted when the animals are moved or handled. Chronically infected animals may appear clinically normal, may have recrudescence of infection after stress, or may display signs of ill-thrift such as poor body condition and fleece (Figure 14-4). Babesiosis occasionally causes concurrent central neurologic signs.

Diagnosis. The major clinical laboratory finding is regenerative anemia with detection of the intraerythrocytic bodies. Chronically infected sheep often have high counts of nucleated erythrocytes. Because *Eperythrozoon* consumes glucose, hypoglycemia and metabolic acidosis may be detected, especially in blood samples that are not processed immediately. Diagnosis is by identification of the organisms on blood smears. Special stains are available to make the organisms more visible. Postmortem lesions include pallor or icterus of membranes and splenomegaly. Some evidence of vasculitis, including edema or exudates in body tissues or cavities, may be seen with *E. ovis* infection.

Treatment. *Eperythrozoon* and *Anaplasma* are sensitive to tetracycline antibiotics (oxytetracycline 10 mg/kg IV SID). *Babesia* is more difficult to treat. Drugs effective against it include diminazene, pentamidine, and imidocarb dipropionate (1.2 mg/kg IM, repeat in 10 days). Supportive care for all blood parasite infections includes whole blood transfusions, nutritional support, and administration of fluids.

Prevention. Prevention in most cases involves maintaining low levels of parasites rather than eliminating them entirely. This method ensures continual stimulation of the immune response, whereas eradication often leaves the animal susceptible to another bout of acute infection. Vector control also is important.[1,2]

Ehrlichia Infections

Pathogenesis. *Ehrlichia* infections of WBCs cause fever, immune suppression, and some organ damage. Their major importance lies in the fact that they cause abortion if infection occurs during late pregnancy and that they act as facilitators of other infectious diseases. *Ehrlichia (Cytoecetes) phagocytophilia* is spread by *Ixodes* ticks and causes tick-borne or pasture fever. The incidence of disease is seasonal with the life cycle of the tick. The organism infects granulocytes and some monocytes, leading to severe persistent neutropenia and acute lymphopenia. Fever occurs 1 to 2 weeks after infection, lasts as long as 2 weeks, and has occasional relapses. Chronic infection is common. Spleen, lung, liver, and kidney tissue may show some damage because of immune destruction of infected cells, but organ-specific signs are usually the result of secondary infection. Establishing ehrlichiosis as a contributor to flock illness often requires looking beyond the obvious clinical signs.

Diagnosis. *E. ovis* causes fever (benign ehrlichiosis) 1 to 2 weeks after infection. Because of this organism's predilection for mononuclear cells, the degree of immune suppression and subsequent importance of this disease are much less than for *E. phagocytophilia* infection. Specific diagnosis is best made by identifying darkly stained bodies at the periphery of granulocytic cells, as well as occasional large bodies deep within the cytoplasm of some cells. Stained bodies also can be seen on the periphery of mononuclear cells from a blood smear during the acute febrile stage or in tissues during chronic infection. Lymphadenopathy and splenomegaly may be seen.

Both of these infections affect sheep and goats (*E. phagocytophilia* also affects many other ruminants), but neither has been reported in North America. *E. phagocytophilia* is found in northwestern Europe, including the United Kingdom, Scandinavia, and India, and *E. ovis* is found mainly in the countries bordering the Indian Ocean.

Treatment and prevention. Treatment and prevention efforts should focus on reducing vectors and bacterial counts during vector season.[3,4]

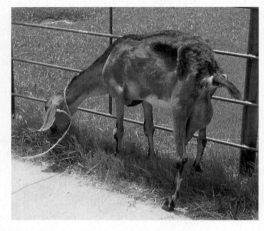

Figure 14-4 Chronic weight loss in a goat as a sequela to anaplasmosis. (Courtesy Drs. Tom Powe and D.G. Pugh, Auburn University, Alabama.)

Sarcocystis Species and *Neospora caninum*

Pathogenesis. *Sarcocystis* is a protozoon parasite that has a two-host life cycle. Sexual reproduction occurs in the bowel of a carnivore (mainly dogs and wild canids) after the carnivore ingests cysts in the muscles of sheep or goats. Sporocysts are passed in the carnivore's feces and later ingested by a sheep or goat. The sporocysts hatch in the ruminant gut and invade the vascular endothelium during three phases of asexual reproduction. After the third phase (approximately 8 to 10 weeks after ingestion), merozoites enter the ruminant's muscle tissue and encyst. Clinical signs are uncommon but can occur during the stages of reproduction and muscle invasion of the host. *Neospora caninum* has a similar life cycle and causes similar disease, except that it appears more likely to cause abortion and affect the central nervous system.

Clinical signs. Most infections are asymptomatic. However, if a large number of sporocysts are ingested, tissue damage may occur during the intestinal, vascular, and muscle stages of the *Sarcocystis* life cycle. Fever, lameness or a stiff gait, reluctance to move, and diarrhea may be seen. Central neurologic signs (blindness, changes in mentation, seizures) may occur if the organisms invade the brain or interrupt blood flow to it. Abortion can occur as early as 4 weeks after ingestion. With severe chronic infections, emaciation and anorexia are seen.

Diagnosis. The most characteristic abnormality is an increase in muscle enzyme activity (creatine kinase [CK], aspartate aminotransferase [AST]) in the blood. Anemia is common and may result from extravascular hemolysis. Cerebrospinal fluid may show mild mononuclear pleocytosis or may appear normal. On necropsy, muscles may display pale streaks or macroscopic cysts throughout. Other evidence of vasculitis includes hemorrhagic serosal surfaces, body cavity fluids, and lymphadenopathy. Microscopic or ultrastructural examination of affected tissues should reveal the presence of organisms. Specific antibody tests are available and do not cross-react with *Toxoplasma gondii* antibodies. Blood antibody titers often peak around the onset of clinical signs and should be markedly higher than baseline values. Antibody preparations also are available for identification of organisms in tissue preparations.

Treatment. Sheep infected with *Sarcocystis* species can be treated with salinomycin (200 ppm in complete feed), monensin (0.5 to 1 mg/kg PO), or amprolium (25 to 40 mg/kg PO). Drugs such as sulfadiazine or trimethoprim (25 to 44 mg/kg IM SID), pyrimethamine (0.5 to 1 mg/kg PO SID), and clindamycin have shown some success in treating *Neospora* infections.

Prevention. Preventing contamination of feedstuffs with the feces of infected carnivores and preventing ingestion of raw meat by carnivores are most important, but these measures may not be possible in flocks handled with dogs or those living on range land. Anticoccidial drugs appear to decrease the chance of clinical disease.[5]

Toxoplasma gondii

Pathogenesis. *T. gondii* is a protozoon parasite with a life cycle very similar to *Sarcocystis,* except that the definitive host is the cat and that a wider range of mammalian and avian species, including humans, appear to be capable of acting as intermediate hosts. Sporocysts are infective a few days after passage in cat feces, and most ruminants are infected by eating feed contaminated with cat feces. People can become infected by ingesting raw meat or milk from infected animals.

Abortion, stillbirth, and neonatal death are the most common forms of clinical disease in sheep and goats, and *Toxoplasma* should be considered one of the most common causes of perinatal losses in small ruminants. Abortion usually occurs during the final month of pregnancy. Fever, vasculitis-induced disease, and neurologic disease are less common manifestations.

Clinical signs. Beyond abortion, clinical disease is rare in adults and resembles systemic sarcocystosis. Clinical signs include fever, dyspnea, depression, and anorexia. Neurologic signs are more common than with *Sarcocystis* infection, especially in lambs and kids infected in utero.

Diagnosis. No specific laboratory abnormalities are associated with toxoplasmosis. Nodular lesions similar to sarcocysts may be seen in various tissues, including the brain. Aborted or stillborn fetuses may appear normal except for histologic lesions in the brain, liver, or lung, but more commonly fetuses are macerated. The placenta is usually abnormal with gross and microscopic evidence of necrosis of the cotyledons. Microscopic identification of the organism in body tissues is the most common means of diagnosis. Serologic tests also are available.

Treatment and prevention. Drugs similar to those used to treat *Neospora* are effective against *Toxoplasma*. Preventing contamination of feeds with cat feces and preventing ingestion of dead animals by cats are the most important ways of stemming the spread of this organism. Both methods are likely to be difficult in most flocks. Direct spread from one sheep or goat to another is rare. Anticoccidial drugs may have some prophylactic effect[6] (see Chapter 6).

References

1. Hagan WA, Bruner DW, Timoney JF: *Anaplasma ovis.* In Hagan WA, Bruner DW, Timoney JF, editors: *Hagan and Bruner's microbiology and infectious diseases of domestic animals,* ed 8, Ithaca, NY, 1988, Comstock Publishing.
2. Hagan WA, Bruner DW, Timoney JF: *Eperythrozoon ovis.* In Hagan WA, Bruner DW, Timoney JF, editors: *Hagan and Bruner's microbiology and infectious diseases of domestic animals,* ed 8, Ithaca, NY, 1988, Comstock Publishing.

3. Hagan WA, Bruner DW, Timoney JF: *Ehrlichia phagocytophilia*. In Hagan WA, Bruner DW, Timoney JF, editors: *Hagan and Bruner's microbiology and infectious diseases of domestic animals*, ed 8, Ithaca, NY, 1988, Comstock Publishing.
4. Lepidi H et al: Comparative pathology, and immunohistology associated with clinical illness after *Ehrlichia phagocytophilia*–group infections, *Am J Trop Med Hyg* 62:29, 2000.
5. Dubey JP: Sarcocystosis. In Howard JL, editor: *Current veterinary therapy*, ed 3, Philadelphia, 1993, WB Saunders.
6. Dubey JP: Toxoplasmosis. In Howard JL, editor: *Current veterinary therapy*, ed 3, Philadelphia, 1993, WB Saunders.

ACUTE VIRAL DISEASES

Bluetongue

Bluetongue is an acute viral disease of domestic and wild ruminants caused by a ribonucleic acid (RNA) virus in the genus *Orbivirus* and family *Reovirus;* it is transmitted by the insect vector *Culicoides varipennis* (gnat)[1,2] (see Chapters 3, 6, and 8).

Clinical signs. Bluetongue disease has two different manifestations—reproductive problems and vasculitis of several organ systems. A spiked fever often leads to depression, anorexia, and rapid weight loss. Leukopenia is present. Affected animals may develop edema of the lips, tongue, throat, ears, and brisket. Other signs include excessive salivation and hyperemia or cyanosis of the oral mucosa, including the tongue (hence the name *bluetongue*). Affected sheep often produce profuse serous nasal discharge that soon becomes mucopurulent and produces crusts and excoriations around the nose and muzzle. Oral lesions progress to petechial hemorrhages, erosions, and ulcers. Pulmonary edema is often severe and pneumonia may develop. Skin lesions can progress to localized dermatitis. Affected sheep may exhibit stiffness or lameness because of muscular changes and laminitis. Cyanosis or hemorrhagic changes of the skin of the coronet can extend into the horny tissue. After recovery a definite ridge in the horn of the hoof may be present for many months. Mortality varies widely. In Africa the virus is much more virulent than in the United States and mortality ranges from 2% to 30%.

The reproductive or teratogenic form of the disease varies greatly with strain, host, and environmental factors. Teratogenic effects include abortions, stillbirths, and weak, live "dummy lambs." Congenital defects may include hydranencephaly.

Diagnosis. In parts of the world in which the disease is common, the diagnosis is usually based on clinical signs alone. The virus can be isolated from blood, semen, or tissues (spleen and brain from aborted fetuses). Viral isolation from blood obtained during the viremic, febrile state is the most definitive means of diagnosis. Serologic evaluation involves two types of viral antigen groups called *P7* and *P2*. The former is found in all bluetongue viruses, and the latter determines the serotype. Sera are commonly tested with complement fixation, agar gel immunodiffusion (AGID), or one of several ELISA tests. A competitive ELISA is considered the best serologic test for detecting group antibodies to bluetongue virus. A direct fluorescent antibody test is available. Polymerase chain reaction– (PCR-) based tests for bluetongue have recently become available and are extremely sensitive and specific.

Other clinicopathologic signs that aid in diagnosis include leukopenia during the early febrile stage of the disease and an increase in serum CK corresponding to the latter phase of muscle stiffness and lameness.

Treatment. Treatment is nonspecific and consists of nursing care. Because of the reluctance of animals to eat, they should be fed a gruel of alfalfa pellets by stomach tube or encouraged to eat soft feeds and green grass. Broad-spectrum antimicrobials (oxytetracycline 5 mg/kg IM SID to BID) are often used to treat secondary pneumonia and dermatitis. Animals should be kept on soft bedding with good footing. Water and shade should be readily available. NSAIDs (flunixin meglumine 1.1 to 2 mg/kg IV) are commonly used.

Prevention. The *Culicoides* vector is difficult to eliminate, so animals should be kept indoors during periods of peak gnat activity (dusk and early evening). Owners should attempt to eliminate gnat breeding grounds such as overflowing watering troughs and shallow septic systems and should limit exposure of sheep to gnats with the use of repellent sprays.

Modified live vaccines based on local strains and serotypes are available in some parts of the world. Some cross-protection among serotypes does occur. The vaccine should be administered at least 2 weeks before breeding season to prevent teratogenic effects. Vaccinated breeding rams may have a slight risk of decreased fertility. Lambs can be vaccinated in the face of an outbreak. Pregnant animals cannot be vaccinated with modified live vaccines.

Sheep that have recovered from an attack of bluetongue are solidly resistant for months to infection by the same viral strain and to some other viral types. Active immunity in sheep requires both humoral and cellular immunity.[1,2]

Peste des Petits Ruminants (Pseudorinderpest)

Etiology. Peste des petits ruminants (PPR) is an acute or peracute, febrile, often fatal disease of ruminants caused by a virus in the family *Paramyxoviridae* and genus *Morbillivirus*. Sheep are less susceptible than goats and white-tailed deer. Cattle are only subclinically infected. The virus is serologically related to the virus that causes rinderpest.

Pathogenesis. The route of infection is respiratory and is spread by airborne droplets. All secretions and excretions of infected animals are contagious throughout the course of the disease, but no carrier state exists. The virus targets lymphoid tissue. Lymphocytes are destroyed in germinal centers in lymph nodes, Peyer's patches, tonsils, splenic corpuscles, and cecal lymphoid tissue. Immunosuppression results from lymphoid destruction. Lymphocytes are partially replaced by plasma cells, macrophages, an eosinophilic acellular matrix, and occasionally neutrophils. The epithelial lining of the mouth and digestive tract is highly vulnerable to the PPR virus. With the loss of the alimentary tract mucosa, weight loss and diarrhea become severe. The incubation period is usually 2 to 6 days.

Clinical signs. The clinical disease produced by PPR virus in sheep and goats closely resembles that of rinderpest, but the course is much more rapid. With the acute form, sheep and goats typically display an abrupt rise in temperature to 104° to 106° F (40° to 41° C). Within a few days infected animals develop nasal and lacrimal discharge, depression, thirst, anorexia, and leukopenia. Congestion of the conjunctival and other mucous membranes occurs, followed by serous and mucopurulent exudates. Sheep and goats develop oral erosions with necrotic foci, which results in excessive salivation. Diarrhea that may be profuse but is rarely hemorrhagic develops later (within 2 to 3 days) and is accompanied by abdominal pain, tachypnea, emaciation, and severe dehydration. Bronchopneumonia, particularly that caused by *Pasteurella* species, may be a terminal sequela. Death usually occurs 5 to 10 days after the onset of fever. Pregnant sheep or goats with PPR may abort.

Diagnosis. A presumptive diagnosis of PPR can be made on the basis of clinical, pathologic, and epizootiologic findings. The diagnosis can be confirmed by isolating the virus from blood or tissues, including lymph nodes, tonsils, spleen, and lung. Serologic tests (complement fixation or AGID) cannot differentiate between PPR and rinderpest. Characteristic postmortem findings include necrotic stomatitis that is generally confined to the inside of the lower lip and adjacent gum, the cheeks near the commissures, and the ventral surface of the free portion of the tongue. Abomasal erosions are often present. In the small intestine, Peyer's patches are markedly affected particularly in the first portion of the duodenum and terminal ileum. The large intestine may be severely affected. Lesions occurring near the ileocecal valve, at the cecocolic junction, and in the rectum are often described as *zebra stripes* that indicate areas of congestion along the folds of the mucosa.

Treatment and prevention. PPR virus infection has no specific treatment. Mortality can be reduced by supportive care, including the administration of antimicrobial and antiinflammatory agents, as well as nutritional support. In the United States, state and federal veterinarians should be notified if PPR virus is suspected. Methods used to eradicate rinderpest are useful in the eradication and control of PPR. All sick sheep and goats and those exposed should be slaughtered and disposed of by burning, burying, or rendering. The premises should be decontaminated and the area quarantined. Sheep and goats can be protected against PPR by immunization with rinderpest vaccines or by the simultaneous administration of PPR hyperimmune bovine serum and virulent PPR virus.[3,4]

Louping Ill

Pathogenesis. Louping ill is caused by a togavirus related to the other arthropod-borne encephalitis viruses. It mainly affects lambs; occasionally also affects grouse, goats, and cattle; and infrequently affects pigs, deer, rodents, and humans. Currently, it is thought to occur only in and near Scotland and Ireland, although a second focus in Eastern Europe is suspected. Transmission is most common during tick season, and *Ixodes ricinus* is thought to be the most important infective host. Coinfection of sheep with *Cytoecetes (Ehrlichia) phagocytophilia* is common and may contribute to central nervous system infection.

Many sheep clear the infection after a few days of fever and viremia, but others develop severe, fatal viral encephalitis. The virus is shed in many secretions, including milk, which is an important source of infection for other animals (and humans). The severity of the disease depends on herd immunity because previous exposure gives long-lasting immunity. Colostrum from immune females is protective for the neonate. High antibody titers also appear to shorten the duration and level of viremia and thereby prevent invasion of the central nervous system. Naive flocks may have fatality rates as high as 60%.

Clinical signs. High biphasic fever, anorexia, and depression are seen in most infected sheep. Lambs may die quickly before illness is noted. Some sheep also develop central neurologic signs, including hyperexcitability, muscle tremors, and rigidity. Abnormal coordination and muscle activity may cause sheep to move with a bounding gait (hence the name *louping ill*).

Diagnosis. The condition has no characteristic gross lesions. Microscopic examination of animals with neurologic signs reveals evidence of viral meningoencephalitis. Diagnosis is made by history (based on location, signs, and time of year), the identification of characteristic lesions, virus isolation, or fluorescent antibody staining of fresh brain tissue. A demonstrated increase in specific antibody titers in survivors strongly suggests the presence of this infection.

Prevention. Vaccines are available in endemic areas to control infection. Vector control during tick season also is important. Lambing season should also be timed so that lambs have high colostral antibody protection at the time of exposure to ticks.[5,6]

Foot-and-Mouth Disease and Vesicular Stomatitis

Pathogenesis. Foot-and-mouth disease is caused by a highly contagious picornavirus and has been eradicated from the United States. Vesicular stomatitis is caused by a rhabdovirus and is intermittently eradicated from the United States. Both diseases are zoonotic, nearly indistinguishable from each other, and reportable. Foot-and-mouth disease has a broad host range that includes most hoof stock (including pigs but not horses) and several other mammalian species. Vesicular stomatitis also affects many species of hoof stock, including both pigs and horses. Small ruminants are relatively less susceptible than cattle, particularly to vesicular stomatitis.

The viruses are spread by aerosol and mechanical vectors and primarily colonize skin or mucous membranes. Milking machines, flies, birds, and humans all may be important mechanical vectors. Vesicular stomatitis tends to remain at the site of infection, and colonization is facilitated by damage to the skin. Oral mucous membranes, coronary bands and interdigital skin, and teat-end skin are common sites of lesions. Vesicular stomatitis outbreaks in the United States tend to occur in the summer or fall and end with the first killing frost.

Viremia plays more of a role with foot-and-mouth disease. The virus is present in most body tissues and fluids in infected animals and can be transmitted through milk, meat, bone, and hide products; semen; equipment that pierces the skin; and biting arthropods. It also tends to spread through the circulation from the site of infection to other susceptible tissues, including the sites of vesicular stomatitis, as well as to the nasal cavity, mammary glandular epithelium, and ruminal pillars. A rare "malignant" form of foot-and-mouth disease also causes fatal myocarditis.

The basic lesion for both diseases is the vesicle that forms and quickly ruptures approximately 2 to 14 days after infection. Ruptured vesicles leave deep erosions on the skin or mucous membranes and appear to cause pain. Tissue damage and inflammation are often compounded by secondary bacterial infection, which can cause greater morbidity and mortality than the original viral infection. Morbidity is related to feed refusal, increased recumbency, and secondary infections of the mouth, udder, and feet.

Clinical signs. Vesicles, erosions, and ulcers are seen at target sites. They may appear mildly inflamed and erythematous; if they are infected, they may appear severely inflamed with hemorrhage and necrosis. Other signs vary according to the location and severity of the lesions. Lingual and buccal lesions cause salivation, dysphagia, and feed refusal. Foot lesions cause lameness and recumbency. Teat lesions cause reluctance to be milked or nursed and a drop in production. Fever also may be seen early in the disease, when vesicles are most apparent. The fever then usually abates and vesicles are replaced by erosions or ulcers. Abortion may occur, especially with foot-and-mouth disease, and is probably related to the fever rather than to fetal infection. Except for the malignant form of foot-and-mouth disease and infection complicated by severe secondary infection, the disease is usually self-limiting; most animals recover within 2 to 3 weeks. Shedding of the virus causing vesicular stomatitis is thought to subside soon after healing of lesions. Foot-and-mouth disease virus may be shed for as long as 6 months and all body secretions and tissues should be considered contagious, including milk, semen, meat, and offal. Both viruses have zoonotic potential and cause a disease in humans that resembles mild influenza. The diseases are self-limiting, but people can shed the viruses in sufficient quantities to infect other animals.

Diagnosis. No characteristic clinicopathologic changes are reported for either virus. Gross lesions resemble those seen before death and include vesicular, erosive, and ulcerative lesions of the mouth, feet, and teat ends; foot-and-mouth disease also causes lesions of the mammary gland and ruminal epithelium. Microscopic findings include hydropic degeneration of cells of the stratum spinosum of the epidermis without inclusion bodies. Secondary bacterial infection may lead to deeper ulcers and complicate identification of the viral etiology of these lesions. "Tiger-heart" striping of the myocardium may be seen with the malignant form of foot-and-mouth disease.

A presumptive diagnosis may be made by identifying characteristic lesions during a season and in an area at risk for one of these infections. In North America, bluetongue should be considered as an important differential diagnosis for ulcerative oral lesions in sheep. A confirmed diagnosis of foot-and-mouth disease is achieved by a combination of virus isolation (from vesicles), immunohistochemistry, and serology. Identifying the source of infection also is very important. Diagnosis of vesicular stomatitis is achieved by complement fixation or fluorescent antibody staining of virus in vesicular fluid or detection of a rise in antibody titers. Flocks with either of these diseases in the United States are subject to quarantine and possible destruction (especially for foot-and-mouth disease).

Prevention. Meticulous personal hygiene and avoidance of contact with new animals are important during outbreaks to prevent spread between flocks. Vaccines against foot-and-mouth disease are available in many parts of the world, but not in the United States. Most nations slaughter or quarantine affected animals. Vaccines against vesicular stomatitis are available and are most commonly used if the risk of outbreak is high, but vaccination does not prevent infection or shedding. Good hoof and teat care and soft feeds may help prevent spread of the virus by providing a healthy, intact barrier against invasion.[7-9]

Contagious Ecthyma (Orf, Sore Mouth)

Contagious ecthyma is caused by a parapoxvirus that has zoonotic potential. All ages can be affected, but it generally only causes clinical disease in young nursing animals. Papules or pustules on the lips, nose, and udder may last 2 to 4 weeks (see Chapters 3 and 10).

Sheep and Goat Pox

Pathogenesis.   Sheep and goat pox are caused by two closely related poxviruses. Some strains are infective to both sheep and goats; most are species-specific. They are maintained in populations by infected animals, and transmission occurs by aerosol or direct or indirect contact. Flies may play an important role as mechanical vectors in some flocks. Viruses remain infective in the environment for as long as 6 months.

After infection, viremia and inflammation of the oral, nasal, and ocular mucous membranes occur. Erythematous papular pox lesions appear a few days later. Mild infections are characterized by lesions concentrated in the non-wooled or hairless regions of the skin. Severe infections produce lesions throughout the oral cavity, respiratory tract, and peritoneal cavity. Secondary infection is common with the severe form and mortality is high. Severity varies according to strain pathogenicity, breed susceptibility, and immune status. If the animal survives, lesions heal in 3 to 4 weeks. Both diseases have been eradicated from the United States and are reportable. People can develop mild disease on exposure to these viruses.

Clinical signs.   Fever, inappetence, conjunctivitis, and upper respiratory signs are seen in the initial stages. Pox lesions are visible shortly thereafter. Secondary infection can lead to a variety of more serious signs indicative of respiratory disease, sepsis, and shock.

Diagnosis.   Characteristic pox lesions are highly suggestive of this disease. Microscopic analysis reveals eosinophilic intracytoplasmic inclusion bodies, acantholysis, and pustule formation within the epidermis and occasionally the dermis. Viral particles may be seen on ultrastructural examination.

Gross and microscopic lesions are characteristic with the severe form, but mild disease may produce mild

lesions that are difficult to differentiate from other viral diseases that cause oral proliferative or ulcerative lesions. Virus can be isolated from blood or tissues (mainly skin) during the acute viremic stage and identified by antibody staining of more chronic lesions. Serologic tests are available to detect rising titers in convalescent animals.

Treatment and prevention.   No specific treatment is available for sheep or goat pox. Antibacterial drugs may be useful to treat secondary infection. Judicious use of insecticides and confinement of affected animals may prevent spread. Vaccines are available in some countries, but not in the United States. Infected flocks are placed under quarantine or destroyed in regions where the diseases are not endemic. These viruses are difficult to eradicate from flocks because of their environmental persistence and the constant supply of susceptible hosts.[10,11]

References

1. Hagan WA, Bruner DW, Timoney JF: Bluetongue. In Hagan WA, Bruner DW, Timoney JF, editors: *Hagan and Bruner's microbiology and infectious diseases of domestic animals,* ed 8, Ithaca, NY, 1988, Comstock Publishing.

2. Walton TE: Bluetongue in sheep. In Howard JL, editor: *Current veterinary therapy,* ed 3, Philadelphia, 1993, WB Saunders.

3. Hagan WA, Bruner DW, Timoney JF: Peste des petits ruminants. In Hagan WA, Bruner DW, Timoney JF, editors: *Hagan and Bruner's microbiology and infectious diseases of domestic animals,* ed 8, Ithaca, NY, 1988, Comstock Publishing.

4. Commission on Foreign Animal Disease: Pest of small ruminants. In Commission on Foreign Animal Disease, editor: *Foreign animal diseases,* Richmond, VA, 1984, US Animal Health Association.

5. Hagan WA, Bruner DW, Timoney JF: Louping ill. In Hagan WA, Bruner DW, Timoney JF, editors: *Hagan and Bruner's microbiology and infectious diseases of domestic animals,* ed 8, Ithaca, NY, 1988, Comstock Publishing.

6. Commission on Foreign Animal Disease: Louping ill of sheep. In Commission on Foreign Animal Disease, editor: *Foreign animal diseases,* Richmond, VA, 1984, US Animal Health Association.

7. Hagan WA, Bruner DW, Timoney JF: Foot and mouth disease. In Hagan WA, Bruner DW, Timoney JF, editors: *Hagan and Bruner's microbiology and infectious diseases of domestic animals,* ed 8, Ithaca, NY, 1988, Comstock Publishing.

8. Hagan WA, Bruner DW, Timoney JF: Vesicular stomatitis. In Hagan WA, Bruner DW, Timoney JF, editors: *Hagan and Bruner's microbiology and infectious diseases of domestic animals,* ed 8, Ithaca, NY, 1988, Comstock Publishing.

9. Commission on Foreign Animal Disease: Foot and mouth disease. In Commission on Foreign Animal Disease, editor: *Foreign animal diseases,* Richmond, VA, 1984, US Animal Health Association.

10. Hagan WA, Bruner DW, Timoney JF: The genus *Capripoxvirus.* In Hagan WA, Bruner DW, Timoney JF, editors: *Hagan and Bruner's microbiology and infectious diseases of domestic animals,* ed 8, Ithaca, NY, 1988, Comstock Publishing.

11. Commission on Foreign Animal Disease: Sheep and goat pox. In Commission on Foreign Animal Disease, editor: *Foreign animal diseases,* Richmond, VA, 1984, US Animal Health Association.

CHRONIC VIRAL DISEASES

Caprine Arthritis-Encephalitis Virus Infection

Caprine arthritis-encephalitis virus (CAEV) is an enveloped, single-stranded RNA virus in the subfamily *Lentivirinae.* Similar to other retroviruses, CAEV integrates into the host chromosomal deoxyribonucleic acid (DNA) before replicating. The virus is able to remain latent or undergo sporadic bouts of productive viral replication.

Clinical signs. Clinical disease may be evident in only 10% of goats from a CAEV- infected herd at any given time. As many as 85% of seropositive goats may be clinically normal. CAEV produces four clinical syndromes: encephalomyelitis, arthritis (Figure 14-5), interstitial pneumonia, and indurative mastitis. The pattern of disease usually varies with age. Arthritis is generally seen in sexually mature goats, whereas encephalomyelitis is generally seen in kids 2 to 4 months old. Interstitial pneumonia and indurative mastitis are more common in adult goats. Some goats suffer from a wasting disorder characterized by poor body condition and rough hair coat.

Diagnosis. A presumptive diagnosis of CAEV can be made on the basis of history and clinical signs suggestive of one or more of the syndromes. In general, ELISA tests are better for detecting disease in an individual animal because the sensitivity of the test is higher than that of the AGID, whereas the AGID is better for herd screening that requires high specificity. With the AGID test, false negatives may occur in goats that have not yet seroconverted to recent infection. Individual goats may take months or years to seroconvert or may never do so. Parturition or advanced stages of disease also may contribute to a false negative result. False positives may occur in goats younger than 90 days old that have colostral antibodies.

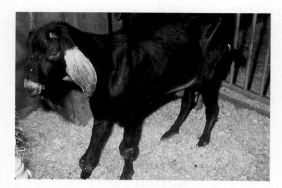

Figure 14-5 This Nubian goat tested positive for CAEV. Note the large, round carpal joints. This goat appeared to be in a great deal of pain and preferred to eat while on its knees. (Courtesy Drs. Tom Powe and D.G. Pugh, Auburn University, Alabama.)

For this reason it is often suggested that kids be at least 6 months old before they are first tested. PCR testing has a high specificity and sensitivity and can detect infection within a day of exposure. Other less commonly used tests include a Western blot to detect antibodies and a Northern blot to look for mitochondrial RNA (mRNA). Because of the limitations in interpreting serologic results, CAEV-induced disease can only be definitively diagnosed by identification of characteristic lesions from examination of biopsy specimens or postmortem viral isolation.

Treatment. No specific treatments are available for any of the syndromes associated with CAEV, although chemotherapeutics currently used for acquired immunodeficiency syndrome (AIDS) may be useful (zidovudine [AZT], interferon α and γ, interleukin-2, and antiviral agents). Young goats suffering from encephalomyelitis may benefit from physical therapy if they are recumbent, and bottle feeding may help maintain hydration and caloric intake. Antibiotics may be beneficial to goats affected with interstitial pneumonia or mastitis if secondary bacterial infection is present. Generally the prognosis is poor for the encephalitic form and guarded for the other forms.

Prevention. Prevention of CAEV is crucial because infection is lifelong. Infected colostrum and milk are the most important sources of infection. Newborn kids should be prevented from ingesting colostrum from infected does and should instead be fed pasteurized goat's milk (heated to 56° C for 60 minutes) or milk from CAEV-negative goats. All goats in a herd should undergo serologic testing twice yearly; seropositive goats should be segregated or culled to prevent direct contact between infected and uninfected animals. When no seropositive animals remain after two successive testing periods, the herd is considered free of CAEV.[1,2]

Ovine Progressive Pneumonia Virus Infection

Ovine progressive pneumonia (OPP) is an ultimately fatal retroviral disease that causes chronic, progressive, debilitating inflammatory conditions of the lungs (United States) and central nervous system (other parts of the world). It also is called *maedi-* (Icelandic for "shortness of breath") *visna* (meaning "wasting"). The virus is a member of the *Lentivirinae* subfamily of retroviruses and is closely related to CAEV. The disease has a long incubation period and protracted clinical course.

Pathogenesis. Only sheep older than 2 years are affected by ovine progressive pneumonia virus (OPPV). The virus is spread by direct contact, probably in respiratory and salivary secretions, and by excretion in the milk.

Transplacental transfer is of minor importance. Infection is established in the monocyte and macrophage cell line and spread by these cells to the lungs, lymph nodes, choroid plexus, spleen, bone marrow, mammary gland, and kidneys. Similar to CAEV, OPPV evades the cellular and humoral immune system of the host by incorporation of its provirus in host DNA, low-grade replication of virus only when monocytes differentiate into macrophages (restricted replication), and production of antigenic variants that are not neutralized by existing antibodies. Continual antigenic stimulation of the host by low-grade replication of OPPV results in chronic inflammation and resultant lymphoid proliferation in various target tissues. The virus may prevent B lymphocytes from differentiating into plasma cells in lymph nodes and may thereby impair immunoregulation. Seroconversion occurs within 2 to 3 weeks after infection.

Clinical signs. In the United States serologic surveys reveal infection rates of between 30% and 67%, but rarely is more than 5% of a flock lost to OPPV. Icelandic, Texel, Border Leicester, and Finnish Landrace appear to be susceptible sheep breeds. Goats also are susceptible. Resistant sheep breeds include Rambouillet and Columbia.

Various clinical syndromes are associated with OPPV and include wasting (thin ewe syndrome), pneumonia, mastitis ("hard bag"), posterior paresis, arthritis, and vasculitis. In North America, pneumonia and indurative aseptic mastitis are common sequelae of infection.

Diagnosis. A presumptive diagnosis can be made on the basis of clinical signs, poor response to treatment, characteristic postmortem findings, and serologic testing. Definitive diagnosis requires isolation of the virus from WBCs (buffy coat of whole blood sample) or tissues. Less expensive and faster serologic tests include AGID, ELISA, and an indirect immunofluorescence test. The AGID test is frequently used as a flock screening test, but the ELISA is more sensitive on an individual basis and can detect antibodies earlier in the course of the disease. As with CAEV, false negatives and false positives are possible (see the section on CAEV, which discusses instances in which each occur).

Treatment. No effective treatment is available for OPPV. Supportive therapy that includes appropriate husbandry and control of secondary infection with antibiotics may prolong life for a few weeks or months but ultimately the disease is fatal. Because of the poor prognosis and risk of exposure of naive animals to clinical disease, long-term treatment is not recommended.

Prevention. The only known method of preventing OPPV infection in a flock is to prevent exposure to the virus. Management practices that help decrease the incidence of horizontal transmission include disinfection of milking equipment, dehorning instruments, and tail docking and castration tools before use and between animals. Contaminated feed and water also are potential routes of infection and should not be shared among infected and uninfected animals. Serologic testing and separation or culling of seropositive animals may help reduce infection. Although OPPV can readily be isolated from ewe colostrum, colostral transmission of OPPV has not be definitively established. However, many prevention guidelines recommend that offspring from infected dams be separated from the dam before they nurse and then be fed cow colostrum and artificially reared. Quarantine and serologic testing of flock additions before placing them with the current flock and purchase of sheep only from OPPV-free flocks are important to prevent the introduction of new infections. Serologic testing should be performed at least annually in a flock until two consecutive negative test results are obtained.[3,4]

Scrapie

Another member of the slow infection group of diseases of small ruminants is scrapie (see Chapter 11). It is an afebrile, chronic, progressive degenerative disorder of the central nervous system of sheep and occasionally of goats. The causative agent is poorly characterized and is postulated to consist of protein fibrils (scrapie-associated fibrils).

Sheep (and goats to a lesser degree) are the natural hosts for scrapie. Clinical signs often do not appear until animals are 2 years old and animals as old as 5 years may exhibit clinical disease. Both vertical and horizontal transmission have been demonstrated experimentally in sheep and goats.

Clinical signs. The onset of scrapie is insidious. Initially, sheep show subtle changes in behavior such as mild apprehension, staring or fixed gaze, failure to respond to herding dogs, and boldness around humans. Several months later, the animals become intolerant of exercise and develop a clumsy, unsteady gait and floppy ears. Later the sheep develop itchy skin that causes them to rub themselves excessively against firm, immobile objects (origin of the name *scrapie*). This leads to excoriations and wool damage.

Diagnosis. Histologically the only consistent lesions are degenerative changes in the central nervous system consisting of bilaterally symmetric vacuolation of the neurons in the brainstem and spinal cord with accompanying spongy degeneration.[5]

Border Disease Virus

Border disease virus (BDV) is very similar to the bovine viral diarrhea virus (BVD) and hog cholera virus. The virus is a helical, enveloped, noncytopathic RNA virus that is a member of the *Togavirus* family and *Pestivirus* genus. It rarely causes disease in adults and is most important as a cause of in utero infection of lambs and kids. The condition gets its name from the fact that it was first reported in sheep along the Welsh border of the United Kingdom. Sheep also are susceptible to BDV.

Pathogenesis. Horizontal transmission of border disease virus occurs through contact with secretions and excretions of body fluids and tissues from infected animals. The virus crosses intact mucous membranes and can spread rapidly through a flock. The major reservoir is the persistently infected sheep or goat. These reservoirs are asymptomatic, congenitally infected, and often seronegative animals that shed large quantities of virus.

If a pregnant animal is infected, the virus may be transmitted vertically to the embryo or fetus. Depending on the stage of gestation, embryonic or fetal infection may have different outcomes ranging from embryonic reabsorption to normal birth. These infections are the most important aspect of border disease.

The major organ system targeted by BDV is the fetal central nervous system. The hallmark lesion is hypomyelination, or degeneration of oligodendroglial cells. Three factors contribute to this lesion. The first is direct viral damage. The second is viral-induced inhibition of the thyroid gland that causes decreased secretion of thyroid hormones. In the absence of these hormones, a resultant lowered concentration of a specific nucleotide in the central nervous system also contributes to the hypomyelination. The third factor is altered immune function. The virus causes the host to produce a virus-specific delayed hypersensitivity reaction that causes inflammation in the central nervous system. It also causes immunosuppression. Death often results from opportunistic conditions such as parasitism, diarrhea, and bronchopneumonia.

Clinical signs. Clinical signs depend on the time during gestation when the fetus or embryo is exposed to the virus. Clinical signs also may vary in severity from animal to animal because different fetuses develop competent immune systems at different times. If the fetus or embryo is exposed to the virus within 45 days of conception, it dies and is resorbed or aborted. These losses are not usually noticed by the flock manager. The principal manifestation in the flock is a large number of open ewes and a small lamb crop. Infection of the fetus between days 45 and 80 of gestation causes damage to rapidly growing systems such as the skin and nervous, lymphoid, thyroid, and skeletal systems. Congenital malformations are seen at birth. Lambs have abnormal fleece (hairy rather than woolly in consistency), small stature, domed heads, shortened legs, and dark pigmentation of the skin, particularly on the dorsal aspect of the neck. The lamb may exhibit

tonic-clonic tremors when awake, which may prevent standing or suckling. Most of these lambs die within a few days of birth. If they survive, the hair changes disappear in 9 to 12 weeks and the central nervous system signs resolve by 20 weeks. Goats infected at this time have similar symptoms except that they rarely exhibit hair coat changes. If lambs are infected before day 80 of gestation and are still viable, they may become persistently infected and immunologically compromised. They are small at birth and generally weak.

Typical outbreaks of border disease cause abortions and birth of weak lambs in the first year as the virus rapidly spreads throughout a susceptible flock, and then insignificant losses in the succeeding years as adult sheep develop immunity.

Diagnosis. Border disease viral antigens can be demonstrated in abomasum, pancreas, kidney, thyroid, skin, and testicle tissues from aborted fetuses and persistently infected animals using fluorescent antibody tests. The virus can be isolated from serum, heparinized whole blood, and tissue taken from brain, spinal cord, spleen, and bone marrow from affected lambs. Whole blood is better than serum if colostral antibodies are likely to be high; serum is an adequate sample in neonates and juveniles that have not suckled.

Antibodies to the virus may be quantified by serum neutralization, AGID, and complement fixation with hyperimmune BVD antiserum. Serologic tests are useful to detect exposure in late-gestation (after day 80) neonates and unvaccinated animals, but may be confounded by colostral antibodies in suckling neonates, previous exposure, and vaccination in older animals. Any titer in a presuckling neonate indicates in utero exposure, whereas a serum neutralization titer of 1:20 to 1:320 suggests infection in adults. The presence of specific antibodies in the cerebral spinal fluid suggests border disease virus infection. Negative presuckling serologic tests do not rule out exposure because persistently infected lambs tend to be immunotolerant to the border disease virus and therefore are born without an antibody titer. These animals may subsequently develop a titer that is indistinguishable from that of a normal animal. Although persistently infected animals do not respond immunologically to the strain of the virus they carry, they may respond to other strains of the virus, including vaccine strains.

Gross postmortem findings include hydranencephaly, porencephaly, microcephaly, cerebellar hypoplasia, abnormal rib curvature, brachygnathia, doming of the frontal bones of the skull, narrowing of the distance between the orbits, shortening the crown-to-rump length, shortening of the diaphyseal length, retention of secondary hair fibers, and abnormal skin pigmentation. The major histopathologic changes include hypomyelination and hypercellularity of the white matter. Glial cells appear normal.

Treatment. No treatment is available for border disease infection. Supportive care may include assistance in nursing and standing for affected lambs, provision of good bedding and solid footing, and treatment of secondary opportunistic infection.

Prevention. Control is primarily achieved by eliminating persistently infected carrier animals from the flock and preventing the addition of new carrier animals. This is easiest in a closed flock but especially difficult in small ruminant flocks because of the frequent desire to import new genetics. To identify carriers, virus isolation must be performed on every animal in the flock; carrier animals must be culled. Additionally, all unborn animals must be considered potential carriers and should be tested at birth. After two lamb or kid crops are born without any positive animals, the flock is likely to be free of border disease. An alternative solution in hobby flocks is to arrest breeding activity until all animals have been shown to be free of infection. New animals should be quarantined and tested before admission to the flock. Herd screening with the ear skin biopsy test using fluorescent antibody staining to detect virus is less expensive and more convenient than the whole blood virus isolation test.

The role of vaccination in preventing infection is still unclear. No vaccine against border disease virus is available, but some reports suggest that BVD vaccines (inactivated or killed products) for cattle may be helpful for sheep at risk. However, these vaccines have proven to be more effective at preventing clinical disease in vaccinated animals than in preventing in utero infection because they do not prevent transient viremia. Vaccination decreases viremia and fetal infection, but does not eliminate them. Therefore vaccines play a role in decreasing economic loss but do not replace culling of carrier animals as the major method of control. [6,7]

REFERENCES

1. Hagan WA, Bruner DW, Timoney JF: Caprine arthritis-encephalitis. In Hagan WA, Bruner DW, Timoney JF, editors: *Hagan and Bruner's microbiology and infectious diseases of domestic animals,* ed 8, Ithaca, NY, 1988, Comstock Publishing.
2. Phelps SL, Smith MC: Caprine arthritis-encephalitis virus infection, *J Am Vet Med Assoc* 203:1663, 1993.
3. Hagan WA, Bruner DW, Timoney JF: Maedi-visna. In Hagan WA, Bruner DW, Timoney JF, editors: *Hagan and Bruner's microbiology and infectious diseases of domestic animals,* ed 8, Ithaca, NY, 1988, Comstock Publishing.
4. Cutlip RC: Maedi-visna. In Howard JL, editor: *Current veterinary therapy,* ed 3, Philadelphia, 1993, WB Saunders.
5. Hagan WA, Bruner DW, Timoney JF: Scrapie. In Hagan WA, Bruner DW, Timoney JF, editors: *Hagan and Bruner's microbiology and infectious diseases of domestic animals,* ed 8, Ithaca, NY, 1988, Comstock Publishing.
6. George LW: Diseases of the nervous system. In Smith BP, editor: *Large animal internal medicine,* ed 2, St Louis, 1996, Mosby.
7. Radostits OM, Gay CC, Blood DC: *Veterinary medicine,* ed 9, Philadelphia, 2000, WB Saunders.

Chapter 15

Diseases of the Cardiovascular System

CHRISTOPHER CEBRA AND MARGARET CEBRA

EXAMINATION OF THE CARDIOVASCULAR SYSTEM

Auscultation of the Heart

The most basic method of assessing cardiac health is thoracic auscultation. The clinician places a stethoscope against the chest wall in the axillary region and then assesses heart rate, rhythm, and strength and listens for any abnormal sounds. The axillary region, the ventral third of the chest between the second and fourth or fifth rib, has relatively little fleece or hair cover, allowing good contact between the bell of the stethoscope and the skin. The clinician should listen to the heart from both sides of the chest at two or three intercostal spaces on each side. He or she must take care to push the bell under the elbow to assess the cranial aspects of the heart and not to push the bell too ventral, where it overlies the sternum and not the thorax.

Normal heart rate varies with the age of the sheep or goat. Neonatal lambs and kids frequently have rates of 120 to 140 beats per minute, whereas adults of both species often have rates between 66 and 80 beats per minute. Juveniles typically attain an adult rate by 3 months of age. Rates can be increased in stressed or excited animals; such animals should be given time to acclimate to restraint before the clinician assesses their heart rate. Other reasons for tachycardia include anxiety, hypovolemia, venous pooling of blood, arterial hypotension, tachyarrhythmia, and poor cardiac function. Causes of bradycardia include lesions affecting the vagus nerve, bradyarrhythmia, and the late stage of shock.

Normal heart rhythm is regular. The most common rhythm anomaly is sinus arrhythmia, in which the heart rate speeds with inspiration and slows with expiration. Descriptions of other dysrhythmias in sheep and goats are uncommon, but a reasonable presumption is that atrial and ventricular fibrillation, varying degrees of atrioventricular block, premature and escape beats, and pathologic tachyarrhythmias occur under similar conditions as in other species.

Assessment of the strength of cardiac contractions is often subjective. Sounds are louder on the left side than the right side and vary inversely in strength with the body condition of the animal. Both S_1 (closure of the atrioventricular valves; onset of ventricular systole) and S_2 (closure of the semilunar valves; onset of ventricular diastole) should be audible.[1]

Peripheral Pulses

Assessment of peripheral pulse strength and synchronicity with cardiac contractions is the simplest way of evaluating the effectiveness of cardiac output. Peripheral arteries can be difficult to find in sheep and goats, especially in adults. The largest include the femoral artery (medial thigh) and brachial artery (proximal medial foreleg). The facial artery (ventrolateral mandible) and carotid artery (ventrolateral neck) also can be used for pulse assessment in some animals. Weak or absent pulses are consistent with hypotension and poor cardiac output. Exuberant pulses are consistent with hyperdynamic shock or regurgitation of blood from the aorta into the heart (aortic valve insufficiency) or lung (patent ductus arteriosus with left-to-right shunting). Pulses are usually assessed manually because of the difficulty of placing any sort of manometric device on a conscious sheep or goat.[1]

Venous Filling, Pulses, and Pressures

Monitoring jugular vein filling and pulses allows the operator to assess right heart function and blood volume. Sheep and goats with hypovolemia may have small jugular veins that are not visible or palpable even after manual occlusion for several minutes. In contrast, sheep and goats with right heart failure or restrictive pericardial disease may have large jugular veins that are visible or palpable without being occluded and have positive pressures. Pulses in the jugular vein result from backflow of blood during right atrial or ventricular systole. No valve is present to prevent regurgitation during right atrial systole; slight pulses that disappear when the head is elevated or do not extend above the level of the heart base are common and nonpathologic. Pulses that extend further up the neck even when the head is elevated most commonly result from tricuspid valve insufficiency. Such pulses coincide with right ventricular systole and are caused by regurgitation of ventricular blood through the incompetent valve. Tricuspid insufficiency can occur with right heart failure (and jugular distention) or as a separate entity.

Monitoring venous pressures requires a manometer. The most common form of monitoring involves inserting a fluid-filled line into the jugular vein. The line is attached to a pressure transducer and measuring instrument. Many electrocardiographs also have the capability of measuring pressures. The venous line may be left in the jugular vein or advanced into the central veins and heart. The jugular and central veins usually have pressures that are negative to as high as 5 cm H_2O. Positive pressures result from hypervolemia (caused by excess fluid administration or renal dysfunction), restrictive pericardial disease, and cardiac dysfunction. If venous hypertension becomes severe, especially over a long period, edema develops.[1]

Mucous Membranes

Mucous membranes can be assessed for color, appearance of vessels, hydration, and capillary refill time. The most common membranes evaluated are the buccal, conjunctival, scleral, and vaginal membranes. Normal membranes are pale pink to pale red, although the high frequency of dark-pigmented membranes in some breeds of sheep and goats sometimes makes this assessment difficult. Overly pale membranes can be attributed to anemia or hypoperfusion; however, the clinician should keep in mind that ruminant membranes tend to be paler than many monogastric species because of their smaller erythrocytes and keratinized membranes. Abnormal ruminant membranes are often white, not pale pink, and scleral vessels become very small. In some animals, anemia can be differentiated from hypoperfusion by observing capillary refill time after slight digital pressure is applied to the buccal or vaginal membranes. In normal animals, color returns in 1.5 to 2 seconds. A shorter refill time is seen in hyperdynamic shock (which is often accompanied by a reddening of the membranes) and a longer time is seen in hypoperfusion.

Change of the normal membrane color toward a purple or blue hue is indicative of cyanosis. Cyanosis results from poorly oxygenated hemoglobin and can be seen with poor central oxygenation (right-to-left cardiac shunting, pulmonary disease), nonfunctional hemoglobin (methemoglobinemia or sulfhemoglobinemia), and local vascular stasis (hypodynamic shock, poor cardiac output, hypothermia). Poor central oxygenation is characterized by purple-blue discoloration of all mucous membranes and possibly of nonpigmented skin, whereas vascular stasis may only affect certain areas such as the gingival margins. Scleral vessels often become engorged, tortuous, and purple during vascular stasis. Approximately one third to one half of blood hemoglobin must be deoxygenated for membranes to become cyanotic; therefore cyanosis usually only occurs when blood oxygen pressures (local or central) are already very low.

Accumulation of bilirubin leads to yellow discoloration of the mucous membranes (jaundice or icterus). Icterus can develop as a result of intravascular or extravascular hemolysis, decreased hepatic uptake of bilirubin, and decreased biliary excretion; the hemolytic causes are most common in sheep and goats.

Hydration can be estimated by the moistness or tackiness of the mucous membranes. This is a subjective determination that is improved by practice on normal animals. A loss of body water suggests that fluids should be part of the treatment protocol. However, dehydration only becomes clinically apparent when body fluid loss exceeds 5% of total body weight (see Appendix II).

Blood Gases

Analysis of blood gases can provide valuable information about animals with hypoperfusion. Metabolic acidosis in sheep and goats without diarrhea, ketonemia, or grain overload often results from lactic acid production by underperfused tissues. The clinician can collect venous blood for analysis from any accessible peripheral vein; the blood should be collected anaerobically and stored in a heparinized container. A determination of whether underperfusion is attributable to inadequate blood oxygen content (pulmonary gas exchange) or inadequate tissue blood flow (blood volume and pressure) requires arterial blood gas analysis. Arterial blood is most commonly collected from the brachial and femoral arteries, but these arteries are poorly accessible in vigorous animals. Clinicians must avoid unnecessary stress when restraining sick animals for blood collection. The auricular arteries and peripheral limb arteries can be used in anesthetized patients. Inadequate arterial blood oxygen content suggests right-to-left cardiac shunting (right-to-left patent ductus arterious or septal defect with or without abnormalities of the great vessels) or pulmonary disease. Differentiation of the causes of inadequate arterial blood oxygen content requires an extensive cardiopulmonary examination.[1]

Electrocardiogram

Electrocardiographic evaluation is most useful for sheep and goats with cardiac dysrhythmias. The most common technique uses the base-apex lead: the positive electrode

(LA) is placed over the cardiac apex in the left fifth intercostal space at the level of the elbow, the negative electrode (RA) is placed in the right jugular furrow at the height of the base of the heart, and the ground (LL) is placed on the dorsal spine or another site distant from the heart. Topical application of alcohol improves skin contact and clipping of fleece may be necessary if the complexes are small (Figure 15-1). Panting behavior and muscle tremors often lead to baseline interference in adult sheep.

The electrocardiogram (ECG) should reveal a distinct P wave (atrial depolarization), QRS complex (ventricular depolarization), and T wave (ventricular repolarization). The R component (negative deflection after a positive deflection) of the QRS complex is usually the most prominent and the Q component (negative deflection before the first positive deflection) is usually absent. The T wave can be either positive or negative and may vary on a single strip (Figure 15-2).

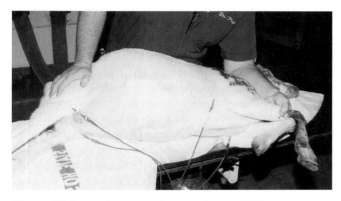

Figure 15-1 Performing an electrocardiogram (ECG) on a goat. The leads are attached to the front two legs and the back two legs. (Courtesy Drs. Hui-Chu Lin and D.G. Pugh, Auburn University, Alabama.)

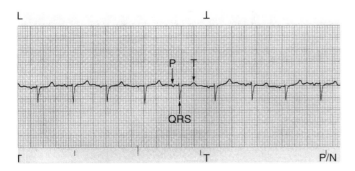

Figure 15-2 Normal ECG complex recorded from a conscious goat using standard limb lead II. The P wave indicates atrial depolarization, whereas the QRS complex and T wave represent ventricular depolarization and repolarization, respectively. (The paper speed is 25 mm/sec.) The magnitude and duration of these waveforms depend on many factors, including the age of the goat, lead examined, size of the cardiac chambers, and method of electrical activation. ECG can be used to monitor cardiac rhythm and detect cardiac diseases. (Courtesy Dr. Hui-Chu Lin, Auburn University, Alabama.)

The ECG should be evaluated for regular appearance of P waves and QRS complexes, regular P-P, R-R, and P-R intervals, appearance of P waves and QRS complexes that are identical in appearance, and appearance of T waves of normal amplitude. The Q-T interval varies inversely with heart rate. An absence of P waves indicates atrial fibrillation or ascension of a ventricular or supraventricular pacemaker. The absence of QRS complexes indicates atrioventricular block.[1]

Echocardiography

Echocardiography is a diagnostic modality that is safe, noninvasive, and convenient to perform in a standing animal; however, it is seldom used in small ruminants because of expense. Nevertheless, it is extremely useful in sheep and goats to confirm intracardiac and pericardial diseases, including valvular endocarditis, pericarditis and pericardial effusions, cardiomyopathy, congestive heart failure, and congenital heart defects. Echocardiography can be used to assess heart chamber size, valve motion, wall thicknesses, blood flow, and intracardiac hemodynamics.

Echocardiography has three basic types:

1. M-mode echocardiography is used to evaluate wall thickness, heart chamber diameters, and valve motion.
2. Dimensional echocardiography is used to evaluate anatomic relationships between cardiac structures and define their movement relative to each other.
3. Doppler echocardiography is used to evaluate blood flow direction, turbulence, and velocity.

Pressure gradients can be estimated within the heart and great vessels such as the pulmonary artery and aorta. Pulse wave Doppler and continuous wave Doppler echocardiography also can be employed. Color flow Doppler converts the Doppler signals to an arbitrarily chosen color scale to semi-quantitatively depict the direction, velocity, and turbulence of blood. The use of color flow Doppler is mainly restricted to specialty practices and referral institutions because significant expertise and experience are required to interpret the image and the equipment is cost-prohibitive for many practices.

Echocardiography can be performed on a standing or laterally recumbent small ruminant. The best location for placement of the transducer is the right third intercostal space at the level of the elbow; the examiner should use a high-frequency transducer that fits well in the intercostal space. The same spot on the left side can be used if the entire heart cannot be visualized from the right side. The examiner may choose to clip the fleece of a sheep or the hair of a goat to improve resolution of the image before applying the coupling gel.

Performing echocardiography involves systematically examining chamber size, myocardial function, valve appearance and motion, and aorta and pulmonary artery blood flow and noting the presence of abnormal structures within or around the heart. Both long- and short-axis views of all cardiac structures should be imaged.[1]

Other Imaging Modalities

Thoracic radiographs are used diagnostically by many private practitioners with access to portable radiographic equipment or a stationary small animal x-ray machine. Most sheep and goats can be treated with the same radiographic techniques used for large dogs. Radiographic studies are most helpful if the practitioner suspects that heart failure, valvular lesions, or abnormal extracardiac or intracardiac communication may be causing chamber or great vessel enlargement or dilatation. Some pulmonary disorders also can be visualized.

Lateral thoracic radiographs are easiest to obtain in sheep and goats and may be performed with physical restraint only. Ventrodorsal (VD) views may require sedation and are of limited usefulness in deep-chested small ruminants. Dirt and foreign bodies in the fleece of sheep can create artifacts on the radiographic film, so the fiber should be examined before the radiograph is taken.[1]

GENERAL CARDIAC DISEASE

Congenital Cardiac Disease

Congenital cardiac defects are abnormalities of cardiac structure or function that are present at birth. Proposed causes include maternal viral infections leading to fetal infection or metabolic dysfunction, fetal anoxia from placental insufficiency, use of pharmacologic agents in pregnant dams, exposure to toxins, nutritional deficiencies in early pregnancy, and heredity. The most common defect in sheep and goats is a ventricular septal defect (VSD). Other reported defects include atrial hypoplasia, cardiomegaly, and cardiac anomalies such as patent ductus arteriosus (PDA), atrial septal defect, and tetralogy of Fallot.

Pathogenesis. A VSD is an opening, primarily in the membranous portion of the ventricular septum, that separates the right and left ventricles. The defect is suspected to occur as a result of failure of the ventricular septum to fuse during gestation. Blood flows through the hole from the left ventricle to the right ventricle and right ventricular outflow tract after birth. This shunting increases the blood flow to the pulmonary circulation and the venous return to the left atrium and ventricle, causing volume overloading the left heart. Eventually left heart failure may lead to the backup of blood through the lung into the right heart and cause subsequent right heart failure. If the defect is large and a great deal of the blood is shunted, right-sided congestive heart failure may occur first. This defect is thought to be inherited as a simple autosomal re-

cessive trait in Southdown sheep and as a sporadic occurrence in other breeds.

Rarely a large VSD may cause such severe right ventricular hypertrophy that deoxygenated blood is pumped into the left side of the heart and out the aorta. This "reverse VSD" or "Eisenmenger syndrome" results in hypoxemia.

Tetralogy of Fallot is a more complex abnormality that includes a VSD, as well as pulmonic stenosis, an overriding aorta, and right ventricular hypertrophy. The result is an increase in deoxygenated blood entering the systemic circulation, which severely decreases the oxygen content of arterial blood.

PDA and atrial septal defects are uncommon and often transient. Both result in recirculation of oxygenated blood through the lung, without diminishment of the oxygen content of arterial blood. Unless a large volume of blood is recirculated, these lesions often do not cause clinical disease. Both may be detected in some neonates and then resolve spontaneously over the first months of life.[1]

Clinical signs. The major clinical signs associated with all congenital heart defects include anorexia, reduced growth rate, exercise intolerance, lethargy, and weakness. Other signs such as dyspnea and cyanosis at rest or with exercise may suggest a specific defect. Signs of congestive heart failure may predominate. Tachycardia and a heart murmur may be present. The most common murmur associated with a VSD is a pansystolic murmur heard best on the right side over the tricuspid valve. Often it can be heard on both sides of the thorax. A PDA murmur also is often heard on both sides of the thorax, but it is loudest in the left third or fourth intercostal space at the level of the shoulder. The murmur is described as high-pitched and continuous throughout systole and diastole. Its intensity increases with increased heart rate, exercise, and excitement. A tetralogy of Fallot may cause both a VSD murmur or a murmur heard best over the pulmonic valve.

Diagnosis. Identification of a murmur in a young sheep or goat in conjunction with signs of failure to thrive is highly suggestive of congenital heart disease. Echocardiography is the diagnostic method of choice for noninvasive identification of cardiac anomalies and assessment of the hemodynamic significance of the shunt. Two-dimensional echocardiography can be used to image the VSD directly and measure the size of the defect. Color flow Doppler may be useful in observing the jet of regurgitant blood. A PDA and tetralogy of Fallot may be difficult to visualize with echocardiography. Clinical pathology findings are usually unremarkable with VSDs and PDAs, but tetralogy of Fallot may cause an increase in packed cell volume and hemoglobin concentration (polycythemia). Radiography may be used to diagnose congenital heart defects. Cardiomegaly, decreased pulmonary vascularity, and presence of an overriding aorta may be some of the radiographic findings. Cardiac catheterization can be used to provide supplemental information about congenital cardiac defects where applicable.

Treatment and prognosis. No treatment to correct congenital heart defects is economically viable in small ruminants. Prostaglandin inhibitors have been used successfully in humans to close PDAs, although their efficacy has not been evaluated in small ruminants. In the absence of clinical signs, animals can live productive lives with defects, but the prognosis is poor for animals with signs of congestive heart failure.

Prevention. Because the role of inheritance in congenital heart defects is unclear, affected animals should generally not be bred.[1]

ACQUIRED CARDIAC DISEASES

Heartwater Disease (Cowdriosis)

Heartwater disease is an acute, tick-borne septicemic disease caused by the rickettsial organism *Cowdria ruminantium*. All ruminants are susceptible, particularly Angora goats. The disease is not contagious and is transmitted by ticks of the genus *Amblyomma*, particularly *A. hebraeum* (the bont tick) and *A. variegatum*. The rickettsial organism is found in the intestinal epithelial cells of its vector. The host tick requires three blood meals to complete its life cycle; only the third host must be a large mammal. Infected ewes and does develop ovarian infections and pass *C. ruminantium* vertically to their offspring. The disease is largely confined to areas where ticks of the genus *Amblyomma* are prevalent, including sub-Saharan Africa, Madagascar, some islands in the Indian Ocean, the Caribbean, and Europe. Reports have described the recovery of infected ticks from imported tortoises in Florida.[2-4]

Pathogenesis. *C. ruminantium* multiplies in reticuloendothelial cells, particularly the capillary endothelial cells of the brain. Regional lymph nodes may serve as the primary replication sites after infection. Rupture of infected neutrophils and macrophages leads to release of the organism and circulation in the blood (parasitemia and vasculitis) with subsequent colonization of the vascular endothelium of body organs.[3,4]

Clinical signs. The incubation period in sheep and goats varies between 14 and 17 days. Depending on the susceptibility of the animal (Angora goats are exquisitely sensitive; lambs younger than 8 days and kids younger than 6 weeks are inherently resistant to *C. ruminantium*) and the virulence of the organism, three different clinical forms of heartwater disease have been identified. Peracute

cowdriosis is relatively rare and occurs most commonly in naive exotic breeds of ruminants in a heartwater-endemic area. Signs include sudden death with no premonitory signs or fever and convulsions. Occasionally severe diarrhea may be seen. The acute form is the most common. Symptoms include a sudden onset of pyrexia (as high as 107° F) followed by anorexia, depression, and respiratory distress, with resultant rapid breathing and cyanosis. Clinical signs may develop in a few days and include chewing movements, twitching of the eyelids, protrusion of the tongue, behavior changes, circling and high-stepping gait, wide-based stance, and muscle fasciculations. Hyperesthesia, nystagmus, frothing at the mouth, recumbency, seizures, and coma can occur terminally. Death usually occurs within 1 week of the onset of clinical signs. A mild or subacute form (heartwater fever) is seen in some indigenous breeds of sheep with high natural resistance to the disease. It is more common in older animals. This form is characterized by a transient fever. Animals with heartwater fever may serve as sources of infection for others because the rickettsial organisms do not clear for as long as 223 days in sheep and 8 days in goats.[2-4]

Diagnosis. Heartwater disease can be definitively diagnosed by identification of the tick vector and microscopic demonstration of *C. ruminantium* in histologic sections of brain cortex stained with Giemsa stain. Brain biopsies have been experimentally obtained from goats for antemortem diagnosis. The organism also can be found in the intima of large blood vessels and in sections of kidney glomeruli and lymph nodes. A common biologic test to confirm the diagnosis involves inoculation of fresh blood from a suspect animal into susceptible sheep. An indirect immunofluorescence test also is available.

Treatment. Early in the disease course, oxytetracycline (6 to 10 mg/kg intravenously [IV] every 12 hours for 3 to 4 days) may be helpful. Long-acting tetracyclines also are effective but must be used early in disease. Treatment is less effective in the later, neurologic stages of the disease.

Prevention. Tick control in pastures is the mainstay of cowdriosis prevention. This is difficult because *Amblyomma* ticks have developed ascaricide resistance and because ticks feed off many hosts and have a high rate of reproduction. Complete elimination of tick infestation is not desirable (or possible in some places) because exposure to low levels of the organism is effective in developing immunity. In some parts of South Africa, goat herds are given oxytetracycline every 14 days during the summer months. Controlled infection followed by antibiotic administration has been tried as a means of immunizing small ruminants. Such a method is effective in preventing disease caused by a homologous strain of *Cowdria* but has no effect against a heterologous strain. An attenuated live strain of *Cowdria* is available as a vaccine, but it has not been tested in field conditions. Immunity after disease is not life-long; susceptibility to reinfection varies between 6 and 58 months. Mortality rates in sheep range between 6% and 80% depending on the breed (Persian or Africander sheep versus Merino sheep). Mortality rates in Angora goats can exceed 90%.[2-4]

Nutritional Myodegeneration (White Muscle Disease)

Nutritional myodegeneration, or white muscle disease (WMD), produces two distinct syndromes: a cardiac form and a skeletal form (see Chapters 2 and 19). Both affect young, rapidly growing farm animals, but the cardiac form typically affects neonates in the first week of life. It is caused primarily by a dietary deficiency of selenium and/or vitamin E. Animals are most often affected if their dams consumed selenium-deficient diets during gestation.[5,6]

Pathogenesis. Deficiencies of selenium and vitamin E result in the destruction of cell membranes and proteins, impairing cellular integrity. Both nutrients are biologic antioxidants. In their absence, cell damage results from the presence of free radicals and peroxides liberated during normal cellular metabolism. Many animals deficient in selenium and/or vitamin E have no evidence of WMD, and sometimes both nutrients must be deficient to cause signs.[5,6]

Clinical signs. Clinical signs of both the cardiac and skeletal syndromes range from peracute to subacute. WMD often results in severe debilitation or sudden death. Small ruminants suffering from the cardiac form often exhibit referred respiratory signs because the cardiac, diaphragm, and intercostal muscles are affected. Respiratory signs include dyspnea, tachypnea, foamy or blood-tinged nasal discharge, profound weakness, recumbency, and sudden death. Auscultation often reveals cardiac murmurs and irregular rapid heartbeats. The clinical course is often short, with death often occurring within 24 hours. Small ruminants that survive the acute phase may fail to thrive because of residual cardiac damage and may exhibit signs of skeletal muscle involvement later in life.

Diagnosis. Definitive antemortem diagnosis of WMD is based on deficient whole blood levels of selenium and plasma levels of vitamin E. Plasma selenium concentrations are indicative of the current diet or recent injections, whereas whole blood concentrations (or glutathione peroxidase analysis) also include selenium incorporated into intracellular selenoenzymes several months previously. Therefore plasma is only useful if the diet has not changed.

Tissue samples of liver can be used to evaluate body stores of selenium. Ration analysis may help support a diagnosis. Postmortem lesions include white streaks in muscle fibers and pale areas that represent areas of acute coagulative necrosis or chronic fibrosis and calcification. Nonspecific clinical pathology findings that are suggestive of WMD include significant elevations in creatine kinase (CK), aspartate aminotransferase (AST), and lactate dehydrogenase (LDH). Evidence of dehydration and myoglobinuria may be present.

Treatment. The cardiac form of WMD carries a poor prognosis despite appropriate treatment. Injectable vitamin E and selenium preparations should be given parenterally and appropriate supportive care should be provided. The vitamin E content of combination supplements is insufficient to correct vitamin E deficiency. Both oral and injectable vitamin E products are available.[5,6]

Prevention. Prevention is aimed at proper supplementation of the dam either by salt mix or by total ration supplementation (0.1 to 0.3 ppm selenium in the diet). During late gestation, injectable vitamin E and selenium may be necessary[5,6] (see Chapters 2 and 9).

Vegetative Endocarditis

Acquired endocarditis is most common in adult small ruminants and is caused by infection, degenerative changes, inflammation, trauma, and valvular insufficiency caused by idiopathic dysfunction of one or more of the four heart valves. As a result of infectious, neoplastic, or inflammatory changes, vegetative lesions form on the cardiac valves and cause vegetative valvular endocarditis. Chronic active infections such as foot or liver abscesses, rumenitis, and omphalophlebitis can lead to sustained or recurrent bacteremia that predisposes the animal to develop bacterial endocarditis. Common bacterial isolates include *Arcanobacter (Actinomyces) pyogenes* and alpha-hemolytic *Streptococcus* species.[7]

Pathogenesis. Vegetative lesions on the valves interfere with normal blood flow and cause cardiac dysfunction. Dysfunction can result from leakage of blood caused by the inability of the valve to close properly or from interference with the ejection of blood by an obstructed orifice. The vegetative lesions also fragment easily, resulting in embolic showers that can create abscesses in distant sites such as the lungs, kidney, and joints.

Valvular incompetence results in volume overload of the recipient heart chamber. Eventually increased end diastolic volume of this chamber leads to dilatation and mild elevations in end diastolic pressure. Compensatory hypertrophy may result. Eventually the contractility of the chamber is impaired, leading to further elevations in end diastolic pressure and reduced compliance. Depending on the valve involved, other sequelae can include pulmonary venous hypertension and left-sided heart failure (with aortic and mitral regurgitation) or elevated central venous pressure and right-sided heart failure (with tricuspid regurgitation).

Clinical signs.   Affected animals initially show no clinical signs but have an audible heart murmur with the point of maximum intensity (PMI) over the affected heart valve in the direction of abnormal blood flow. The intensity of the murmur is not associated with the severity of the lesion. Chronic endocarditis can cause the clinical signs of cyclic or intermittent fever, weight loss, exercise intolerance, anorexia, and signs of congestive heart failure (tachycardia, respiratory distress, cough, jugular venous distention, subcutaneous edema, and ascites). Cattle may have diarrhea, decreased milk production, and lameness; these signs also may be encountered in small ruminants.

Diagnosis.   The best method of diagnosing vegetative endocarditis is a complete echocardiographic examination. Two-dimensional echocardiography is best for detecting valvular lesions and dysfunction and measuring ventricular function. Lesions must be at least 2 to 3 mm in diameter to be visible. M-mode ultrasonography may help detect chamber enlargement and a shortening fraction. Color flow, pulse wave, or continuous wave Doppler ultrasound may be useful to help quantitate the severity of valvular regurgitation.

In the absence of echocardiographic examination, a presumptive diagnosis can be based on thoracic auscultation. Systolic heart murmurs over the left or right heart apex or diastolic murmurs over the left base are suggestive of valvular incompetence.

Bacteriologic culturing of blood samples taken during febrile episodes and preferably before antibiotic administration may help determine the etiology of bacterial endocarditis. Other nonspecific clinical pathology findings include nonregenerative anemia, neutrophilia with or without a left shift, hyperglobulinemia, and hyperfibrinogenemia. Radiographic evidence includes generalized or focal cardiac enlargement and disseminated pneumonia. The ECG may indicate cardiac arrhythmias occurring as sequelae to chamber enlargement or underlying myocardial disease. Nonspecific tests such as cardiac catheterization for pressure measurements and nuclear angiocardiography may reveal myocardial dysfunction and cardiac enlargement, respectively, but may be cost prohibitive.

Treatment.   The treatment and prognosis depend on the cause, duration, and severity of the valvular lesion. When valvular incompetence is present, the prognosis is often guarded to poor. Degenerative lesions may be asymptomatic and often have a slow progression, contributing to the guarded prognosis. If no abnormalities are detected or minimal regurgitation is present on echocardiography, the prognosis is fair to good. Bacterial endocarditis should be treated with long-term broad-spectrum antibiotic administration. Treatment may last for weeks to months. Bactericidal antibiotics are chosen based on sensitivity patterns and the ability of the drug to penetrate tissue. Nevertheless, bacterial endocarditis has a guarded to grave prognosis even with long-term antibiotic administration.[7]

Plant Cardiotoxicity

Important plants that contain cardioactive glycosides (cardenolides) capable of poisoning livestock in North America include oleander *(Nerium oleander),* foxglove *(Digitalis purpurea),* Indian hemp or dogbane *(Apocynum cannabinum),* lily-of-the-valley *(Convallaria majalis),* laurels *(Kalmia* species), milkweed *(Asclepias* species), azalea *(Rhododendron* species), and ornamental succulent *(Cotyledon orbiculata).* Plant-derived drugs that affect the autonomic nervous system and cardiac function include atropine derived from *Atropa belladonna* and *Datura* species, muscarine derived from *Amanita muscaria,* ephedrine derived from *Ephedra* species, ergotamine derived from *Claviceps purpurea,* and nicotine derived from *Nicotiana* species. Alkaloids found in yews *(Taxus* species) and false hellebore *(Veratrum* species) have both direct and indirect cardiac effects.

Specific antidotes are rarely available for plant toxins. Therefore prevention is the most effective cure. In general, most toxic plants are unpalatable and grow in overgrazed pastures. The plants may be masked in hay, silage, and grain. Most plant toxicoses can be prevented by feeding adequate amounts of feed that is free of toxic plants and providing adequate grazing management, weed control, and proper harvest techniques for feeds. Goats are more inquisitive than sheep and therefore are more susceptible to plant toxicity through oral exploration of their environment.[8,9]

Pathogenesis.   The principal agents responsible for producing cardiotoxic effects in plants are cardioactive glycosides; many varieties exist. The concentration of glycosides within the plant varies with season, stage of maturity, part of the plant, and environmental conditions. Cardiac glycosides block cellular sodium-potassium ATPase, leading to sodium accumulation in excitable cells such as those found in nervous tissue and the myocardium. The result is increased myocardial contraction and altered heart rhythm. These glycosides also are potent gastrointestinal (GI) irritants.

As noted previously, agents found in plants that affect the autonomic nervous system also may affect cardiac function. The alkaloids in yews depress myocardial conduction by blocking sodium movement through membranes. The result is arrhythmias ranging from decreased chronotropic and inotropic effects to ventricular tachycardia or fibrillation. Nicotinic-acting alkaloids such as *Nicotiana* species cause toxicity by stimulating ganglions, then blocking them, leading to paralysis. Sheep are less susceptible to these effects than cattle. Tropane alkaloids such as belladonna contain atropine, which blocks acetylcholine at muscarinic nerve synapses. The cardiac effect is tachycardia.

Clinical signs. Many of the clinical signs of acute cardiac glycoside toxicosis in sheep and goats are the direct result of hypoxia caused by the inability of the heart to pump blood, as well as GI irritation. They may include nausea, abdominal pain, anorexia, increased salivation, catarrhal or hemorrhagic diarrhea, coma, convulsions, and sudden death. A variety of cardiac conduction abnormalities are seen, including bradycardia, tachycardia later in the disease course, dropped beats, heart block, and atrial or ventricular arrhythmias. Signs develop 4 to 12 hours after ingestion of the plant. If death does not occur, signs may persist for 2 or 3 days. Relapses may occur in ruminant species because of continued release of the glycoside from the rumen. Cardiac toxins often cause death before any clinical signs are noted.

Yew poisoning causes both cardiac and nervous system signs. Cardiac signs include bradycardia and cardiac arrest. Nervous system signs include depression, trembling, dyspnea, collapse, and sudden death. Subacute toxicity causes gastroenteritis and diarrhea.

Belladonna toxicosis causes GI atony, anorexia, rapid heart and respiratory rates, diarrhea, excess urination, vision impairment, and delirium. Death is uncommon. Nicotine-containing plants cause ataxia, weakness, central nervous system stimulation, tremors, bloating, and death from respiratory paralysis.[8,9]

Diagnosis. Definitive diagnosis of cardiotoxic plant ingestion requires a demonstration of the presence of cardiotoxic plants in the animal's pasture and rumen contents. Clinical signs are suggestive of ingestion of cardiotoxic plants but are not pathognomonic. Cardiac auscultation and electrocardiographic examination may suggest rhythm and rate disturbances. Necropsy lesions also are nonspecific and include hemorrhagic gastroenteritis and pale mottling of the heart with congestion and hemorrhage. Histologic evidence may include myocardial degeneration and necrosis. A human serum radioimmunoassay is available to assess exposure to digoxin or ouabain, but such tests are often host- and glycoside-specific and may not be practical for evaluating suspected animal poisoning. This test also may cross-react with oleander glycosides. Alkaloids can be identified by mass spectral chemistry in samples taken from poisoned animals.

Treatment. Elimination of continued exposure to the poisonous plant is an important part of treatment and prevention. A rumenotomy may be required to wash out the rumen and remove any remaining cardiotoxic plants before significant systemic absorption occurs. Transfaunation may help to reestablish rumen motility. Supportive care should include provision of fluids, minimization of stress, and administration of activated charcoal (2 g/kg) as well as beta-adrenergic blocking agents and antidysrhythmic drugs to treat cardiac dysrhythmias. Fab antibodies against cardiac glycosides have been used experimentally to treat digitalis and oleander toxicosis.[8,9]

Prevention. Prevention involves vigilant pasture care and examination of all feedstuffs. Generally animals do not consume these plants if other palatable, readily available food is present.

Ionophore Toxicity

Ionophores include monensin, lasalocid, salinomycin, and narasin. Some are approved for use as coccidiostats and some are used to improve feed efficiency in sheep, goats, chickens, and cattle. The toxicity of ionophores varies considerably among species, with horses being the most sensitive. Toxicoses commonly occur when sensitive species consume ionophore-containing feed formulated for another species and when errors are made in mixing. Ionophore toxicity is potentiated by concurrent administration of various antibiotics, including erythromycin, chloramphenicol, and sulfonamides. Even at therapeutic doses, monensin can potentiate selenium toxicity.[10]

Pathogenesis. Excessive ionophore ingestion causes preferential transport of specific ions, which results in altered ionic gradients and disturbed cellular physiology. Damage to the myocardium leads to fibrosis and resultant reduced performance or congestive heart failure. As dilated cardiomyopathy develops, changes in cellular metabolism occur, leading to ECG abnormalities and reduced cardiac output.[10] Compensation for reduced cardiac output includes activation of the renin-angiotensin-aldosterone system and increased arterial resistance. The result is increased ventricular preload (venous return) and afterload (arterial resistance), leading to pulmonary edema and further reduction in cardiac contractility. The ventricle dilates, further reducing cardiac output, and signs of heart failure occur.

Clinical signs. Signs in sheep acutely poisoned with monensin include lethargy, stiffness, muscular weakness, stilted gait, mild to moderate dyspnea, mild mucoid diarrhea, and recumbency. Sudden death may occur after stress or exercise. Cardiac auscultation may reveal an elevated heart rate with or without cardiac arrhythmias. Signs of congestive heart failure such as jugular venous distention, peripheral edema, and evidence of circulatory collapse may be present. Cardiac murmurs may be present and associated with ventricular dilation. Signs in goats may be similar. Dairy goats may exhibit decreased milk production.[10]

Diagnosis. Diagnosis is made by analyzing suspected feed for inappropriate ionophore concentrations. A presumptive diagnosis can be based on clinical signs and clinical pathology findings. These include evidence of skeletal and cardiac muscle injury, kidney damage, and increased erythrocyte fragility. Findings indicative of erythrocyte fragility include elevated concentrations of alkaline phosphatase, indirect bilirubin, blood urea nitrogen, CK, creatinine, LDH, and AST. Reductions in calcium and potassium concentrations and urine pH may occur. Abnormal values for the myocardial isoenzymes CK and LDH are highly suggestive of monensin toxicosis in conjunction with historical information. An ECG may demonstrate sinus tachycardia and other cardiac dysrhythmias. Echocardiography may be normal or show evidence of dilated cardiomyopathy with increased ventricular chamber size, decreased thickness of the interventricular septum and left ventricular free wall, and decreased myocardial function. Increased end-diastolic and end-diastolic dimensions of the left and right ventricles may be apparent, as well as increased left arterial size and an increased left atrial–to–aortic root dimension ratio. Cardiac catheterization may reveal elevated intracardiac pressures consistent with dilated cardiomyopathy. Postmortem findings include microscopic evidence of fibrosis, degeneration of the myocardium, and myocardial necrosis. Myopathy of skeletal muscles may be present. Evidence of congestive heart failure may be reflected in passive congestion of the liver and lungs.[10]

Treatment. No specific antidote or tested treatment is available for animals that have recently ingested ionophores. General management consists of administration of activated charcoal; provision of IV fluids to correct electrolyte imbalances, preserve renal function, and minimize shock (but not in amounts large enough to exacerbate congestive heart failure); specific treatment for dysrhythmias (digoxin, quinidine, vasodilators, diuretics); and stall rest. The prognosis for animals with dilated cardiomyopathy is poor.

Prevention. Prevention involves careful mixing of feeds containing ionophores and not giving animals feed formulated for other species. Proper concentrations of selenium in ionophore-treated feed are important to prevent selenium toxicosis.

PERICARDIAL DISEASE

Pericarditis

Pericarditis is pericardial inflammation that results in fluid or exudate accumulation between the visceral and parietal layers of the pericardium. Causes in large animals include trauma induced by penetration of an ingested foreign object (hardware disease), external wounds, hematogenous spread of infection (septicemia), extension of infection originating from the pulmonary cavity, and specific viral or neoplastic causes. This condition is rare in sheep and goats.

Pathogenesis. Pericarditis is classified as primarily effusive, constrictive, or a combination of both. Inflammation between the parietal and visceral layers of the pericardium results in fluid accumulation. Over time, pericarditis results in decreased cardiac distensibility, which causes increased ventricular end diastolic pressure. This in turn impairs the ability of the heart to fill during diastole. As a result, atrial pressures rise and venous return to the heart is reduced, impairing the perfusion of the myocardium. Reduced perfusion causes a depression in ventricular contractility, stroke volume, and ultimately cardiac output. Arterial pressures and renal blood flow decrease. The heart compensates initially through vasoconstriction, increased heart rate, and sodium retention, increasing vascular volume to maintain cardiac output.

Traumatic reticulopericarditis results from penetration of the reticular wall, diaphragm, and pericardial sac by a sharp metal object and ensuing septic inflammation. The foreign body is pushed through the cranial wall of the reticulum during reticular contractions or episodes of increased abdominal pressure such as parturition. (The pericardium and reticulum are in close proximity.) The foreign object allows bacteria from the reticulum to enter the pericardial sac. Cattle are often said to have "splashy" heart sounds referred to as a *washing machine murmur* because of gas and fluid accumulation in the pericardium. Acute, subacute, or chronic fibrinopurulent pericarditis results. After the pericardial sac becomes inflamed, the pathogenesis is similar to that of pericarditis from other causes. Because of their grazing habits, sheep are only rarely affected by traumatic reticulopericarditis. Goats may be slightly more prone to the condition because of their inquisitive nature and eating habits. Nontraumatic pericarditis usually results from sepsis.

Clinical signs. The most consistent clinical signs of pericarditis on auscultation include muffled heart sounds, tachycardia, and dampened or absent lung sounds in the ventral thorax. Loudness of heart sounds may alternate between loud and quiet beats (bigeminy). Dorsal lung sounds may be more pronounced. Nonspecific clinical signs include fever, anorexia, depression, and weight loss.

Signs of congestive heart failure may be apparent and include distended or pulsatile jugular veins, tachypnea or dyspnea, and exercise intolerance. Signs of chest pain such as abducted elbows and grunting or breath-holding on palpation and auscultation may be seen. Clinical signs depend on the speed of development of pericarditis and the volume of fluid accumulation.

Diagnosis. Definitive diagnosis of pericarditis is made by pericardiocentesis and echocardiography. The former technique enhances evaluation of effusion and allows the clinician to take samples for bacterial and fungal culture. It should be performed using echocardiography to guide aspiration. Echocardiography can be useful to evaluate cardiac function and visualize the site and extent of fluid and gas accumulation. Common findings include an echo-free space surrounding the right and left ventricular free walls and between the descending aorta and left ventricular posterior wall. If cardiac tamponade is present, right ventricular diastolic collapse and right atrial collapse will be apparent. Electrocardiographic findings associated with pericarditis include decreased amplitude of the QRS complexes, electrical alternans, and S-T segment elevation or slurring. A right-axis deviation may be noted in the standard limb leads. Clinical pathology findings are nonspecific and may include evidence of hemoconcentration, mild anemia, leukocytosis with an absolute neutrophilia and/or lymphopenia, and hyperfibrinogenemia. Hypoalbuminemia and hyperglobulinemia may be present. Frequently mild elevations in liver enzymes, creatinine, bilirubin, and serum urea nitrogen are seen. Elevations in the myocardial isoenzymes AST, CK, and LDH occur. Radiography of the thorax or reticulum and diaphragm may be helpful, particularly for diagnosing traumatic reticulopericarditis in ruminants. A metallic foreign body may be seen in the cranial reticulum and/or caudal thorax. Cardiomegaly may be seen with pericarditis and is caused by pericardial effusion obscuring the cardiac silhouette. An obscured vena cava and diaphragm, dorsal displacement of the trachea, and interstitial pneumonia may be noted.

Treatment. Treatment of traumatic reticulopericarditis is often unrewarding and not economically viable in most cases. When instituted it is frequently directed toward salvage and short-term survival. Removal of a foreign body by rumenotomy may prevent further complications but rarely is curative. Pericardial drainage can be performed repeatedly by means of pericardiocentesis, fifth rib resection, lavage, or pericardiectomy. However, often heart function does not return to normal after these procedures are performed. Thoracotomy and pericardiectomy by means of a split-rib technique may be effective in treating ruminants with traumatic, restrictive pericarditis. Treatment with long-term antibiotics is required. The prognosis for the treatment of nontraumatic pericarditis

is guarded. Indwelling chest tubes placed in the pericardial sac can enable drainage, lavage, and local infusion of antibiotics. These procedures can be performed once or twice a day. Treatment with systemic broad-spectrum antibiotics is indicated. Nonsteroidal antiinflammatory drugs (NSAIDs) are useful adjuncts, as are corticosteroids if no evidence of bacterial involvement is present. Diuretics may be helpful in the short term to relieve some of the signs of congestive heart disease. Fluids may help combat dehydration and signs of shock.

Prevention. In flocks in which this condition is a problem, small magnets can be administered before pregnancy to help prevent metallic foreign bodies from perforating the pericardial sac. However, because of the rare nature of this condition, their routine use is not warranted.

VASCULAR DISEASES

African Trypanosomiasis

People and animals can become infected with trypanosome protozoa. The trypanosomes can complete their developmental cycle only in tsetse flies (*Glossina* species). Trypanosomes multiply in blood, tissues, and body fluids of their vertebrate hosts and are transmitted between vertebrate hosts in the saliva of blood-sucking flies as they feed. The trypanosome species that are known to infect goats and sheep include *Trypanosoma congolense, T. vivax, T. brucei* subsp. *brucei, T. evansi,* and *T. simiae.* The first three are moderately pathogenic to these small ruminants, whereas the latter two are only mildly pathogenic.[11]

Pathogenesis. After entering through the skin, trypanosomes reach the bloodstream by way of the lymphatic system. The parasites multiply and the prepatent period lasts for 10 to 14 days after infection. The infection is characterized by periods of parasitemia followed by the absence of parasites. This pattern of infection occurs because of antigenic variation: trypanosomes vary the antigenic nature of their glycoprotein surface coat to evade the host's immune system. This ability of trypanosomes to alter their surface coat prolongs infection and is responsible for chronic disease. Some trypanosomes tend to invade extravascular spaces such as the ocular aqueous humor and cerebral spinal fluid. The pathogenicity of trypanosomes varies with the different host species. Trypanosomes may produce a hemolysin early in the course of the disease that causes anemia in the host. Later, increased phagocytic activity results in massive erythrocyte destruction. This may occur in the absence of parasitemia.[11]

Clinical signs. The clinical signs are variable and nonspecific and depend on the speed of onset of anemia and the degree of organ impairment. Entire herds may be affected. All aspects of production are affected—fertility, birth weights, lactation, weaning weights, growth, and survival. Trypanosomiasis may predispose the animal to other diseases that mask the underlying trypanosome infection.

Trypanosomiasis may be acute, subacute, or chronic, with the latter being the most common. Acute disease often causes abortion. Dairy goats may show a sudden drop in milk production. Depression, anorexia, and a stiff gait may be present. Physical examination reveals tachycardia, tachypnea, and a slight fever. Hyperemic mucous membranes and excessive lacrimation may be noted. Animals often become recumbent and anorexic and die within 1 to 3 weeks of the onset of clinical signs. If the animal survives, it may go on to the subacute phase, which includes listlessness, weight loss, enlargement of superficial lymph nodes, and a dull, dry hair coat. Affected animals have similar auscultation findings as those seen in other acute cardiac disease, as well as pale mucous membranes and a pronounced jugular pulse. The animal may linger for several weeks or months or go on to develop chronic disease. Affected animals show ill-thrift—dull, dry hair coats; inelastic skin; lethargy; emaciation; peripheral lymphadenopathy; pale mucous membranes; and exercise and stress intolerance. Death may occur many months or even years after infection and usually results from congestive heart failure. Subclinical trypanosomiasis causes acute episodes when animals are stressed by inadequate nutrition, increased production demands, or concurrent disease.[11]

Diagnosis. Diagnosis is difficult because the parasitemia is intermittent, clinical signs are nonspecific, and infection is not always synonymous with disease. Although a tentative diagnosis can be made on the basis of clinical signs, presence of vectors, and history of trypanocide use in the herd, a definitive diagnosis requires the appearance of trypanosomes on a fresh blood smear, a Giemsa-stained blood smear, or less commonly a lymph smear. Examination of the buffy coat of centrifuged blood with dark-field phase-contrast spore illumination is the most sensitive direct diagnostic method and is useful when parasite numbers are low. Pathogenic trypanosomes must be distinguished from more ubiquitous, nonpathogenic species particularly common in cattle such as *T. theileri*. Repeated sampling of individual animals is often necessary because parasitemia is intermittent. The diagnosis is supported by evidence of anemia on a complete blood count.

Indirect diagnostic methods include an indirect fluorescent antibody test (IFA) and the enzyme-linked immunospecific assay (ELISA). These tests are less useful for diagnosing a single clinical case but are useful in assessing herd infection. Both *T. congolense* and *T. brucei* readily infect rats and mice and can be used to diagnose the infection indirectly.[11]

Treatment. Treatment consists of the use of trypanocidal agents and supportive care. Animals with acute, subacute, and subclinical disease respond better to treatment than animals with chronic disease because of the irreversible damage to hematopoiesis caused by chronic infection. The therapeutic indices of trypanocides are low and vary with the host species. Trypanocide efficacy also varies with the species of trypanosome present; resistance to agents is common. Some trypanocides are irritating to the skin and may cause severe inflammation at the injection site. In sheep and goats with *T. brucei* infection, the trypanocide of choice is diminazene aceturate, and it should be used at a higher dosage rate (7 mg/kg intramuscularly or subcutaneously) than that recommended for cattle. Protection after trypanocide use usually lasts 2 to 4 months depending on the season. Animals must be rested before and after treatment. Supportive care consists of providing fluids, rest, good nutrition, and possibly blood transfusions.

Prevention. Vector control, stress and nutrition management, and selection of trypanosome-tolerant breeds of sheep and goats help control or prevent trypanosomiasis. No vaccine is available. Animals can be treated with insecticides (pyrethroids) to prevent bites by tsetse flies and other flies. Control consists of strategic use of trypanocides during the peak season. Constant parasitologic and clinical surveillance is essential to determine the efficacy of control measures.[11]

Shock

Pathogenesis. Shock is the result of many varied pathologic processes and, regrettably, is often the point at which veterinary attention is sought. Among the numerous important causes are sepsis, localized bacterial infections, myocarditis, dehydration, electrolyte and acid-base disturbances, and cardiovascular anomalies. Shock is caused by inadequate tissue perfusion and organ dysfunction and can result from inadequate vascular tone or integrity, poor cardiac output, and pooling of blood within capacitance vessels.

Shock begins with a hormone-mediated hyperdynamic phase that is characterized by bounding pulses, tachycardia with loud heartbeats, and decreased capillary filling times of mucous membranes. This phase is transient and often unnoticed, but it is quickly followed by the hypodynamic phase of circulatory failure.

Clinical signs. Most clinical abnormalities center around insufficient perfusion of organs or the inability of the cardiovascular system to maintain perfusion. Common signs include weakness, obtundation, cold extremities, tachycardia with a weak pulse, decreased urination and defecation, cyanotic or pale mucous membranes, and shallow breathing. Other signs are possible depending on the inciting cause.

Diagnosis. Most of the clinicopathologic changes reflect the inciting cause of shock, but others reflect the changes that occur with shock. The latter include organic acidosis, azotemia, and stress hyperglycemia. Diagnosis is by recognition of characteristic clinical signs and clinicopathologic abnormalities.

Treatment. Restoration of organ perfusion and function are the main goals of treatment. This is best accomplished through administration of IV fluids. A shock dose of approximately 8% of the animal's body weight should be given as an initial bolus. Any isotonic fluid is adequate in most emergency situations because of the positive effect such fluids have on vascular volume. Polyionic, pH-balanced fluids are the most useful. Continued therapy depends on the animal's response to the initial bolus. Oral and subcutaneous fluids are unlikely to restore adequate cardiovascular function in animals in shock. Vasoactive drugs may be helpful to increase blood pressure, but these should be used in conjunction with fluids if possible. Corticosteroids may be beneficial for nonseptic shock because of their antiinflammatory and membrane-stabilizing effects. Because most shock in small ruminants has an infectious origin, the usefulness of these drugs is limited. Other treatments for primary disease processes, including antimicrobial drugs, antitoxins, and antiinflammatory drugs, may be indicated in specific cases.

REFERENCES

1. Reef VB, McGuirk SM: Congenital cardiovascular disease. In Smith BP, editor: *Large animal internal medicine*, ed 2, St Louis, 1996, Mosby.
2. Hagan WA, Bruner DW, Timoney JH: Heartwater disease. In Hagan WA, Bruner DW, Timoney JF, editors: *Hagan and Bruner's microbiology and infectious diseases of domestic animals*, ed 8, Ithaca, NY, 1988, Comstock Publishing.
3. Commission on Foreign Animal Diseases: Heartwater. In Commission on Foreign Animal Diseases, editors: *Foreign animal diseases*, Richmond, VA, 1984, US Animal Health Association.
4. Oberem PT: Heartwater. In Howard JL, editor: *Current veterinary therapy*, ed 3, Philadelphia, 1993, WB Saunders.
5. Welker B: Nutritional myodegeneration. In Howard JL, editor: *Current veterinary therapy*, ed 3, Philadelphia, 1993, WB Saunders.
6. Maas J et al: Nutritional myodegeneration. In Smith BP, editor: *Large animal internal medicine*, ed 2, St Louis, 1996, Mosby.
7. Reef VB, McGuirk SM: Valvular heart disease. In Smith BP, editor: *Large animal internal medicine*, ed 2, St Louis, 1996, Mosby.
8. Fowler ME: Cardiotoxic plants. In Howard JL, editor: *Current veterinary therapy*, ed 3, Philadelphia, 1993, WB Saunders.
9. Galey FD: Glycosides. In Smith BP, editor: *Large animal internal medicine*, ed 2, St Louis, 1996, Mosby.
10. McCoy CP: Ionophores: monensin, lasalocid, salinomycin, and narasin. In Howard JL, editor: *Current veterinary therapy*, ed 3, Philadelphia, 1993, WB Saunders.
11. Commission on Foreign Animal Diseases: African trypanosomiasis. In Commission on Foreign Animal Diseases, editor: *Foreign animal diseases*, Richmond, VA, 1984, US Animal Health Association.

Chapter 16

Anesthetic Management

HUI-CHU LIN AND D.G. PUGH

Sheep and goats are similar in many ways to cattle species, both anatomically and physiologically. Although some of these animals may cost as much as purebred companion animals, often the small ruminant clinician is faced with the same economic issues and limited approved drugs for use in surgical procedures requiring anesthesia as the clinician in companion animal practice. Physical restraint and local anesthetic techniques are most commonly employed to provide immobility and analgesia for small ruminants. These animals perceive pain no differently than other species, and therefore analgesia for prevention and easing of pain is just as important as it is for other companion animals. Occasionally general anesthesia is required for surgical intervention. In these cases, balanced anesthetic technique should be employed to provide narcosis, analgesia, and muscle relaxation and thereby minimize the stress response induced by surgery and anesthesia.

At the time of this writing, only one anesthetic drug had been approved for use in goats (ophthalmic proparacaine) and one for use in sheep (thiopental sodium). Table 16-1 summarizes meat and milk withdrawal intervals recommended by the Food Animal Residual Avoidance Databank (FARAD) for some of the tranquilizers and injectable anesthetics used in an extra-label manner for sheep and goats.[1] Clinicians should consult with FARAD whenever using any unapproved drugs because withdrawal times are subject to change.

PREANESTHETIC PREPARATION

Domestic ruminants have a multicompartmental stomach with a large rumen that does not empty completely[2] and are therefore susceptible to complications associated with recumbency and anesthesia. Tympany, bloat, regurgitation, and aspiration pneumonia are common problems that should be anticipated and addressed with the proper precautions. When possible, adult animals should be fasted for 12 to 24 hours and water withheld for 8 to 12 hours before induction of anesthesia. The fasting of neonates is not recommended because of the potential for hypoglycemia.[2] In emergency situations, fasting may not be possible and precautions should be taken to avoid aspiration of gastric fluid and ingesta. This can be done effectively by endotracheal intubation and positioning of the head so that the throat latch area is elevated relative to the mouth and thoracic inlet, which prevents pooling of saliva and ruminal contents in the oral cavity.

Venipuncture and catheterization of the jugular vein are usually performed before anesthesia. A 16-gauge indwelling catheter is appropriate for adult sheep and goats and an 18-gauge catheter is suitable for younger animals. The technique for catheterization in sheep and goats is similar to that used in calves (Figures 16-1 and 16-2).

Intubation is more difficult to accomplish in sheep and goats than in many other animals because the mouth does not open widely, the intermandibular space is narrow, and the laryngeal opening is distant beyond the thick base of the tongue.[2] Intubation should be prompt and performed with the animal in sternal recumbency immediately after the induction of anesthesia. Intubation is best accomplished if an assistant pulls the mouth open by placing a loop of gauze around the upper jaw and a second loop around the lower jaw and tongue (Figure 16-3). At the same time the assistant should hyperextend the animal's neck. If the larynx cannot be visualized, the neck should be extended further.[3] The clinician uses a long laryngoscope blade (250- to 350-mm) to suppress the tongue base and epiglottis and enable visualization of the larynx. He or she then places the "guide tube" (preferably a 10 French, 22-inch-long polyethylene canine urethral catheter that is three times the length of the endotracheal tube), over which the endotracheal tube is slipped into

TABLE 16-1

THE FARAD RECOMMENDED WITHDRAWAL INTERVAL FOR SHEEP AND GOATS FOR SINGLE AND MULTIPLE TREATMENTS OF ANESTHETIC DRUGS*

DRUG	DOSE (mg/kg)	MEAT WITHDRAWAL INTERVAL (DAYS)	MILK WITHDRAWAL INTERVAL (HOURS)
Acepromazine	Up to 0.13, IV Up to 0.44, IM	7	48
Detomidine	Up to 0.08, IM, IV	3	72
Guaifenesin	Up to 100, IV	3	48
Ketamine	Up to 2, IV; 10, IM	3	48
Lidocaine with epinephrine	Infiltration, epidural	1	24
Ultra–short-acting barbiturates	Thiamylal, up to 5.5 Thiopental, up to 9.4	1	24
Xylazine	0.016 to 0.1, IV 0.05 to 0.3, IM 0.3 to 2.0, IM	10	120
Yohimbine	Up to 0.3, IV	7	72

From Craigmill AL, Rangel-Lugo M, Riviere JE: Extralabel use of tranquilizers and general anesthetics, *J Am Vet Med Assoc* 211:302, 1997.
*Whenever using unapproved pharmacologics in animals intended for meat or milk production, the clinician should check with federal authorities concerning proper withdrawal times.

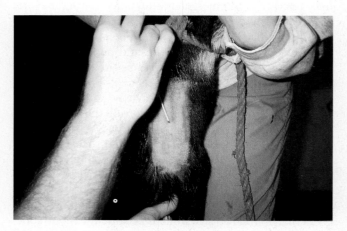

Figure 16-1 Distention of the right jugular vein for intravenous catheterization. In this case the goat is carefully restrained and the head is turned 30° to 45° to the left on the long axis and tilted up 15° to 20° from parallel to the ground.

place. This method makes endotracheal intubation much easier to achieve than with other methods (Figure 16-4). A cuffed endotracheal tube should be used to prevent regurgitation and aspiration of ruminal contents, and the animal should be maintained in sternal recumbency until the cuff is inflated.

PREANESTHETICS

Preanesthetic tranquilization or sedation is rarely needed in small ruminants. However, in larger or more vigorous animals the use of a tranquilizer or sedative may minimize the stress caused by forceful restraint, ease the induction process, and decrease the dose requirement of anesthetic, thereby preventing the possibility of disastrous hypotension (Table 16-2).

Phenothiazine Derivatives

Acepromazine maleate produces mild tranquilization without analgesia. This drug has minimal effects on heart rate and respiratory function. Its use may result in hypotension and increase the risk of regurgitation.[4,5] When administering acepromazine, the clinician should avoid using the coccygeal vein for intravenous (IV) injection because of the close proximity of the coccygeal artery.[2] Prolapse of the penis with the potential for trauma after the use of acepromazine sometimes occurs in horses and may occur in sheep and goats as well. Furthermore, the use of acepromazine is contraindicated in debilitated or hypovolemic animals.[4]

α₂ Agonists and Antagonists

α₂ agonists. Xylazine hydrochloride is probably the most popular α_2 agonist in large animal practice today. Ruminants are very sensitive to xylazine, with goats appearing to be more sensitive than sheep.[5] Xylazine is a potent sedative, analgesic, and muscle relaxant that is frequently used as an preanesthetic or anesthetic adjunct in ruminants. Xylazine alone produces dose-dependent effects from standing sedation to recumbency, immobi-

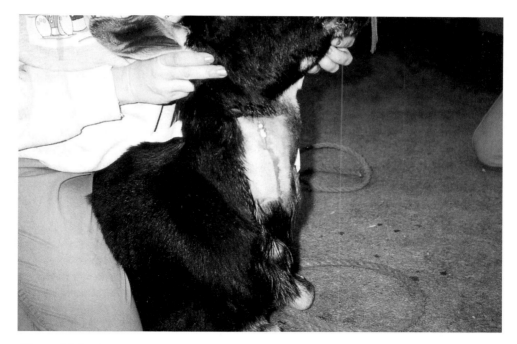

Figure 16-2 Intravenous catheterization of the right jugular vein. The esophagus is on the left side of the neck in most instances. Therefore many clinicians choose the right jugular furrow for catheter placement.

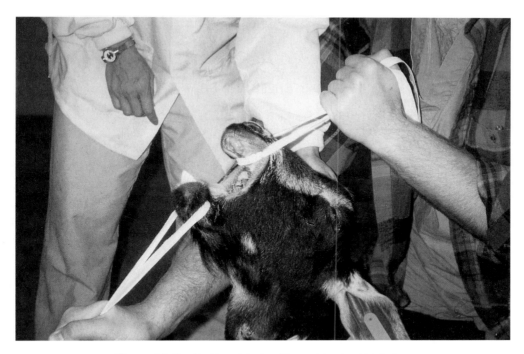

Figure 16-3 Position of the head for endotracheal intubation.

lization, and complete anesthesia. Xylazine may cause bradycardia, hypotension, hypoxemia, hypercapnia, pulmonary edema, hyperglycemia, hypoinsulinemia, increased urine production, and an oxytocin-like effect.[6] It should be used with extreme caution in animals with pre-existing cardiopulmonary disease or urinary tract obstruction. An up to six-fold increase in urine output is frequently observed after xylazine administration.[8] Administration of xylazine to ruminants in the final trimester of pregnancy may cause premature parturition

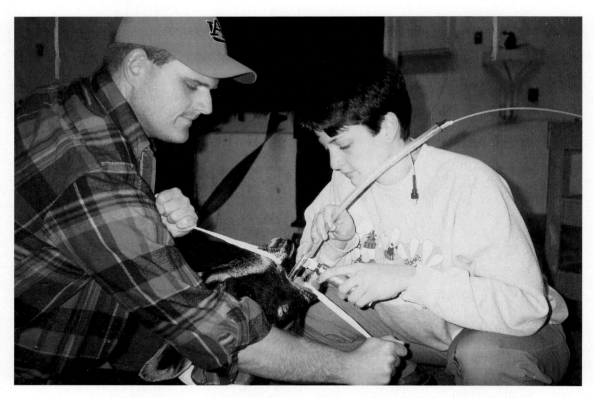

Figure 16-4   Endotracheal intubation with the aid of a guide tube and laryngoscope.

TABLE 16-2

DOSES OF PREANESTHETICS COMMONLY USED IN SHEEP AND GOATS

PREANESTHETICS	DOSAGE FOR SHEEP (mg/kg)	DOSAGE FOR GOATS (mg/kg)
Atropine	0.066, IV	0.066, IV
Glycopyrrolate	0.005 to 0.01, IM; 0.002 to 0.005, IV	0.005 to 0.01, IM; 0.002 to 0.005, IV
Acepromazine	Less than 50 kg: 0.1 to 0.2, IV	Less than 50 kg: 0.1 to 0.2, IV
	More than 50 kg: 0.05 to 0.1, IV or IM	More than 50 kg: 0.05 to 0.1, IV or IM
Xylazine	0.01 to 0.02, IV, standing sedation for 30 to 60 min; 0.1 to 0.2, IV, or 0.2 to 0.3, IM, recumbency for 60 min	0.01 to 0.02, IV, standing sedation for 30 to 60 min; 0.05 to 0.11, IV, or 0.11 to 0.22, IM, recumbency for 60 min
Detomidine	0.005 to 0.02, IV, or 0.01 to 0.04, IM, sedation for 45 to 60 min	0.005 to 0.02, IV, or 0.01 to 0.04, IM, sedation for 45 to 60 min
Medetomidine	0.001 to 0.007, IV, sedation; 0.04, IM, recumbency for 58 min	0.001 to 0.007, IV, sedation; 0.04, IM, recumbency for 58 min
Diazepam	0.25 to 0.5, IV, slowly	0.25 to 0.5, IV, slowly
Meperidine	N/A	10, IM
Butorphanol	0.05 to 0.5, IM, sedation 0.4, IV, sedation and ataxia	0.05 to 0.5, IM, sedation; 0.4, IV, sedation and ataxia
Xylazine and butorphanol	X: 0.1 to 0.2, IV B: 0.01 to 0.02, IV Deep sedation to recumbency for 60 min	X: 0.1 to 0.2, IV B: 0.01 to 0.02, IV Deep sedation to recumbency for 60 min

and retention of fetal membranes and should therefore be avoided.[7] Lateral recumbency has been reported to induce a significant decrease in partial pressure of arterial oxygen (PaO_2) in conscious sheep.[9] This hypoxemia can occur even when the animal remains standing during xylazine sedation.[10,11] Severe hypoxemia and pulmonary edema have been implicated as the causes of death in sheep that die under xylazine anesthesia.[12-14] Epidural administration of xylazine (0.07 to 0.1 mg/kg) with or without lidocaine into the sacrococcygeal space induces long-lasting good somatic analgesia for open castration in rams (8 hours without lidocaine) and correction of vaginal prolapse in ewes (24 hours with 0.5 mg/kg of lidocaine).[15,16] However, visceral analgesia induced by xylazine alone may not be sufficient for ligation of the spermatic cord.[15]

Detomidine hydrochloride, when administered at an IV dose of 0.02 mg/kg, produces sedation comparable to that provided by 0.04 mg/kg of xylazine.[17] Increasing the dose to 0.03 mg/kg induces recumbency in sheep, which is equivalent to xylazine at 0.15 mg/kg and medetomidine at 0.01 mg/kg.[18] The pharmacologic effects of detomidine are very similar to those of xylazine.[18] Ruminants appear to be less sensitive to detomidine than they are to xylazine. Unlike xylazine, detomidine at IV doses smaller than 0.04 mg/kg does not produce an oxytocin-like effect on the uterus in gravid cattle. Even though detomidine at doses higher than 0.04 mg/kg may increase the electrical activity of the uterine muscles, it does not induce the synchronization of the bursts of potentials that is characteristic of parturition. Detomidine is unlikely to induce abortion in pregnant ruminants at therapeutic doses[19,20] and therefore may be safer for pregnant sheep and goats.

Medetomidine hydrochloride in doses of 0.001 to 0.007 mg/kg IV induces dose-dependent sedation and analgesia; 0.005 mg/kg appears to produce analgesia in sheep comparable to that provided by 0.015 mg/kg of fentanyl.[21] At an intramuscular (IM) dose of 0.04 mg/kg, medetomidine induces recumbency for 58 minutes, as well as good analgesia and marked muscle relaxation for 30 to 45 minutes. Sheep usually recover within 1.5 to 2 hours after regaining the righting reflex.[22] In sheep anesthetized with medetomidine (0.02 mg/kg IV) and ketamine (2 mg/kg IV) and breathing room air, PaO_2, arterial pH, and arterial oxygen (O_2) saturation decrease and the partial pressure of arterial carbon dioxide ($PaCO_2$) increases significantly. Supplementation of 100% O_2 may improve PaO_2 and hemoglobin saturation.[23]

α_2 **antagonists.** The pharmacologic effects induced by xylazine, detomidine, or medetomidine can be effectively antagonized by an α_2 antagonist such as yohimbine, tolazoline, or atipamezole (Table 16-3). These antagonists can be used to shorten recovery time and prevent the significant adverse effects sometimes seen with agonists, especially accidental overdose. However, these drugs are not

without risks: the death of a sheep after administration of a large dose of yohimbine (0.8 mg/kg IV) has been reported.[24] When administering an antagonist, slow injection is recommended to avoid sudden awareness of pain and excitement on the part of the animal. Rapid injection of tolazoline has been reported to cause significant cardiac stimulation, tachycardia, increased cardiac output, vasodilation, coronary vasodilation, and gastrointestinal distress.[25] It has been hypothesized that ruminants are more sensitive to tolazoline than other species, and death has been reported in several animals after its use.[26] Nevertheless, the undesirable effects of α_2 antagonists are extremely rare in healthy animals when the drugs are administered by slow IV injection and at appropriate dosages.

Benzodiazepines

Diazepam is a minor tranquilizer. It produces mild sedation, hypnosis, decreased anxiety, and muscle relaxation. Diazepam is often used for its anxiolytic effect in high-risk animals because of its minimal cardiovascular and pulmonary effects at therapeutic doses. It also can be used in combination with ketamine to improve muscle relaxation during anesthesia.[27]

Opioid Analgesics

Meperidine hydrochloride is a synthetic opioid that has an analgesic potency of only 10% to 13% that of morphine. It produces mild sedation and analgesia. Its administration can be associated with histamine release.[28] In yearling goats, meperidine (10 mg/kg IM) can be used as a premedicant 10 minutes before induction of anesthesia with thiopental. After intubation this combination provides 20 minutes of surgical anesthesia with complete recovery in 90 minutes.[29]

Butorphanol tartrate is an opioid agonist/antagonist with an analgesic potency approximately five times higher than that of morphine. Butorphanol has a unique "ceiling

TABLE 16-3

DOSES OF α_2 ANTAGONISTS COMMONLY USED IN SHEEP AND GOATS

α_2 ANTAGONIST	DOSAGE FOR SHEEP (mg/kg)	DOSAGE FOR GOATS (mg/kg)
Atipamezole	0.125 to 0.2, slow IV	0.125 to 0.2, slow IV
Tolazoline	2, slow IV	2, slow IV
Yohimbine	0.125 to 0.22, slow IV	0.125 to 0.22, slow IV

effect"—that is, after effective action has been attained, further increases in dose do not increase or enhance the degree of desired pharmacologic effect.[30] Butorphanol may cause slight central nervous system (CNS) stimulation, especially when used in animals that are not in pain. Twitching of the facial muscles, lips, and head may occur.[31] Butorphanol can be given alone in sheep and goats to produce light sedation. No behavioral effects were seen with butorphanol given at 0.05 mg/kg IV in sheep, but ataxia was observed at 0.4 mg/kg IV, and excitement occurred at 0.1 to 0.2 mg/kg IV.[5,31,32] Butorphanol is frequently used in combination with a sedative or tranquilizer to produce good standing sedation for minor surgery and diagnostic procedures. It also can be administered postoperatively for pain relief. In sheep and goats, xylazine and butorphanol can be administered simultaneously to produce deep sedation and recumbency for as long as 60 minutes.[2]

ANESTHETICS (Table 16-4)

Injectable Anesthetics

Thiopental sodium can be used to induce anesthesia in sheep and goats; the depth of anesthesia and muscle relaxation is sufficient for endotracheal intubation. Additional incremental doses may be administered to prolong anesthesia.[2] A guaifenesin- (GG-) thiopental mixture can be administered to effect to induce and maintain short-term anesthesia. The final concentration of the mixture is 5% (50 mg/ml) GG and 0.2% (2 mg/ml) thiopental.[33] Thiopental causes minimal cardiovascular depression. A moderate tachycardia, slight decrease in mean arterial blood pressure, and short period of respiratory depression usually occur immediately after rapid induction of anesthesia with thiopental. Transient apnea is not uncommon during induction with thiopental, and spontaneous breathing returns within several minutes. In

---

TABLE 16-4

DOSES OF GENERAL ANESTHETICS COMMONLY USED IN SHEEP AND GOATS

ANESTHETIC	DOSAGE FOR SHEEP*	DOSAGE FOR GOATS*
Thiopental	10 to 16, IV	10 to 16, IV
Guaifenesin (5%) and thiopental (0.2%)	*Induction:* 2 ml/kg, IV, 50% to 75% calculated dose first *Maintenance:* 2.2 ml/kg/hr or to effect	*Induction:* 2 ml/kg, IV, 50% to 75% calculated dose first *Maintenance:* 2.2 ml/kg/hr or to effect
Guaifenesin (5%) and ketamine (0.1%)	*Induction:* 2 ml/kg, 50% to 75% calculated dose first *Maintenance:* 2.2 ml/kg/hr or to effect	*Induction:* 2 ml/kg, 50% to 75% calculated dose first *Maintenance:* 2.2 ml/kg/hr or to effect
Acepromazine and ketamine	A: 0.55, IV K: 2.2, IV	N/A
Xylazine and ketamine	X: 0.22, IM, wait 10 min K: 10 to 15, IM	X: 0.22, IM, wait 10 min K: 11, IM
Guaifenesin (5%), xylazine (0.01%), and ketamine (0.1% to 0.2%)	*Induction:* 0.67 to 1.1 ml/kg *Maintenance:* 2.2 ml/kg/hr or to effect	*Induction:* 0.67 to 1.1 ml/kg *Maintenance:* 2.2 ml/kg/hr or to effect
Medetomidine and ketamine	M: 0.02, IV K: 2, IV	M: 0.02, IV K: 2, IV
Diazepam and ketamine	D: 0.11, IV K: 4.4, IV; or D: 0.25 to 0.5, IV K: 4 to 7.5, IV	D: 0.11, IV K: 4.4, IV
Propofol	*Induction:* 3 to 4, IV; or *Induction:* 4 to 8, IV; *Maintenance:* 18 to 40 mg/kg/hr of IV infusion or to effect	*Preanesthetic:* detomidine, 0.01, IM and butorphanol 0.1, IM *Induction:* 3 to 5, IV *Maintenance:* 31 ml/kg/hr
Tiletamine and zolazepam (Telazol)	5.5, IV, anesthesia for 100 min 5.5, IV with butorphanol 0.1, IV, anesthesia for 100 min	5.5, IV, anesthesia for 100 min 5.5, IV with butorphanol 0.1, IV, anesthesia for 100 min

*Dose is in mg/kg unless stated otherwise.

case of prolonged apnea the animal should be intubated and ventilated until spontaneous breathing resumes.[34] Recovery from thiopental anesthesia relies mainly on redistribution of the drug from the brain to the peripheral tissues. Administration of a large dose or prolonged infusion may result in extremely prolonged recovery. Therefore maintenance of anesthesia with thiopental is not recommended if the surgery requires more than 1 hour.[34]

Ketamine hydrochloride, a dissociative derivative, is probably the most commonly used injectable anesthetic in sheep and goats. Acepromazine, diazepam, xylazine, and medetomidine can be used in combination with ketamine to enhance the degree of analgesia and muscle relaxation during anesthesia. Unlike other conventional anesthetics, ketamine does not depress cardiovascular function; instead, heart rate and arterial blood pressure increase during ketamine anesthesia as a result of central sympathetic stimulation. A mixture of ketamine (1 mg/ml) and GG can be used to maintain short-term anesthesia.[35] A combination of GG (50 mg/ml), ketamine (1 to 2 mg/ml), and xylazine (0.1 mg/ml), often referred to as *GKX* or *Triple Drip*, can be used both for induction and maintenance of anesthesia.[36]

Telazol (Fort Dodge Animal Health, Fort Dodge, Iowa) is a proprietary combination of tiletamine (dissociative) and zolazepam (benzodiazepine) in a 1:1 (weight:weight) ratio. Compared with ketamine, Telazol anesthesia produces better muscle relaxation, more profound analgesia, and longer lasting effects. In ruminants the induction of anesthesia after Telazol administration is rapid and smooth, and the recovery is usually gradual and prolonged.[14] Similar to ketamine, this drug causes cardiovascular stimulation rather than depression.[35] Hypoventilation and hypothermia may occur during Telazol-induced anesthesia. Assisted or controlled ventilation with O_2 supplementation may be required in cases of severe hypoventilation and hypoxemia. Animals should be placed in sternal recumbency with support throughout the recovery period.[14]

Propofol is a unique short-acting anesthetic. Structurally, this drug does not relate to any of the injectable anesthetics currently available in veterinary practice. Propofol is only slightly water-soluble and comes as an emulsion containing 10 mg of propofol, 100 mg of soybean oil, 22.5 mg of glycerol, and 12 mg of egg lecithin per ml in sterile glass ampules. Because this emulsion contains no preservative, after the ampule is opened, the contents should be used or discarded within 8 hours.[35] A single dose of propofol (2 mg/kg) induces approximately 10 minutes of anesthesia with complete recovery occurring in 20 to 30 minutes.[2,37] Propofol is best used for induction before inhalation anesthesia; it also can be used as a continuous infusion to maintain short-term anesthesia.[38-40] In goats a combination of detomidine, butorphanol, and propofol for induction and continuous IV infusion of propofol for maintenance provides adequate anesthesia for castration or ovariectomy.[41]

Inhalation Anesthetics

Inhalation anesthetics require expensive and specialized equipment for delivery to the patient. However, they allow veterinarians to perform complicated and prolonged surgery. Either halothane or isoflurane can be used effectively and safely in sheep and goats. Mask induction may not be a wise choice in healthy, adult animals but can be used in smaller or debilitated animals. A small animal anesthesia machine with a double carbon dioxide (CO_2) absorbent canister is usually adequate for most sheep and goats. The clinician should be aware of a rare condition called *halothane-induced hepatitis,* an acute, massive liver necrosis that sometimes occurs after halothane anesthesia in healthy goats, especially after prolonged exposure.[42,43] Clinical signs, including depression, inappetence, salivation, teeth grinding, head pressing, and icterus, usually occur within 24 hours. Serum concentrations of aspartate transaminase, bilirubin, alkaline phosphatase, creatinine, and blood urea nitrogen are significantly increased from normal ranges. Death usually occurs within 4 days and necropsy reveals centrilobular necrosis. Necrosis of the proximal renal tubules, abomasal ulceration, and hepatic encephalopathy have been observed in some cases.[42,43] Severe hypotension, hypoxemia, and hepatic hypoxia may encourage the reductive metabolism of halothane, leading to the production of toxic free radicals.[44] Therefore, maintaining adequate cardiovascular function and oxygenation through careful monitoring and supportive therapy are the keys to successful anesthesia.

Local Anesthetics

Local anesthetics produce their effects by blocking the propagation of action potentials along nerve axons in a reversible manner. These anesthetics can be injected into the tissue at the surgical site to produce local anesthesia or they can be administered in the perineural area of major nerves to produce regional anesthesia (see Chapter 6). In small ruminants, many surgical procedures are performed safely and painlessly under local or regional anesthesia. All local anesthetics have similar physical properties and molecular structures. Most of them are weakly basic tertiary amines with a hydrophilic end, a lipophilic end, and an intermediate hydrocarbon chain. They are generally available as acid solutions of the water-soluble salts. The acid salt is neutralized in the tissue, liberating the base, which then penetrates the cell membrane and interrupts the propagation of the action potential. This mechanism of action means that a local anesthetic is less effective in inflamed tissue with lower pH because less liberation of the basic form of the drug occurs.[45] Local anesthetics are classed as ester-link or amide-link drugs depending on the intermediate chain structure. Inactivation of ester-link local anesthetics (e.g., procaine, tetracaine) depends on hydrolysis by cholinesterase enzymes in the plasma and to a lesser extent in the liver. Metabolism of amide-link local anesthetics (e.g., lidocaine, bupivacaine, mepivacaine) relies on microsomal enzymes located primarily in the liver.[45] Lidocaine is probably the most popular local anesthetic used and may produce anesthesia for 0.75 to 2 hours. Because of its ability to induce vasoconstriction in the tissue around the injected area, epinephrine decreases systemic absorption of concurrently administered local anesthetics. Therefore epinephrine (1:200,000 to 1:50,000) at concentrations of 5 to 20 μg/ml can be incorporated with or added to lidocaine solution to prolong the duration of local anesthesia.[46] Mepivacaine (which lasts for 1.5 to 3 hours) and bupivacaine (which lasts for 4 to 8 hours) can be used for procedures that require a longer duration of local anesthesia.[45] Administration of a large single dose or repeated small doses of local anesthetics can result in toxicity in sheep and goats, especially in neonatal and young patients. Clinical signs of toxicity include nystagmus, muscle fasciculation, CNS stimulation progressing to opisthotonos and convulsions, hypotension, respiratory arrest, circulatory collapse, and death.[45] The maximum calculated safe dose of lidocaine was reported to be 13 mg/kg in one study.[47] In another study, accumulated IV doses of 5.8 mg/kg, 18 mg/kg, and 42 mg/kg induced signs of toxicity in adult, neonatal, and fetal sheep, respectively.[48] IV infusion of meperidine in sheep induced convulsions at doses of 7.5 to 7.9 mg/kg and cardiovascular collapse at doses as high as 52 to 69 mg/kg.[49] Bupivacaine is approximately four times more potent than lidocaine, and therefore a 0.5% solution produces the same degree of neuronal blockade as a 2% lidocaine solution.[50] Ewing[51] suggests using a maximum of 6 mg/kg of lidocaine or mepivacaine and 2 mg/kg of bupivacaine in small ruminants. With this maximum safe dose in mind, the clinician should dilute lidocaine and mepivacaine solutions to 1% and 0.5%, respectively, to prevent overdosage when using these drugs in lambs and kids.[51] Diazepam (0.1 mg/kg IV) or thiopental (5 mg/kg IV) should be administered if seizure activity or convulsions caused by accidental overdose persist longer than 1 to 2 minutes.[50,52]

PERIOPERATIVE MANAGEMENT AND RECOVERY

Monitoring During Anesthesia

Animals should be monitored continuously throughout anesthesia. Peripheral pulses should be palpable and an electrocardiogram, if available, should be used at all times. Recently, the use of capnograms to evaluate end-tidal CO_2 and pulse oximeters to assess arterial O_2 saturation have became part of the routine monitoring accessories used to ensure adequate ventilation and gas exchange.

TABLE 16-5

NORMAL VITAL SIGNS AND VALUES FOR ANESTHETIZED SHEEP AND GOATS

VITAL SIGN OP. VALUE	VALUES FOR SHEEP AND GOATS
Heart rate (beats/min)	80 to 150
Respiratory rate (breaths/min)	20 to 40
Systolic arterial pressure (mm Hg)	80 to 120
Mean arterial pressure (mm Hg)	75 to 100
Diastolic arterial pressure (mm Hg)	60 to 80
Partial pressure of arterial carbon dioxide ($PaCO_2$) (mm Hg)	28 to 36
Partial pressure of arterial oxygen (PaO_2) (mm Hg)	72 to 90
Arterial pH	7.48 to 7.58

From Riebold TW, Geiser DR, Goble DO: Clinical techniques for food animal anesthesia. In Riebold TW, Geiser DR, Goble DO, editors: *Large animal anesthesia: principles and techniques,* ed 2, Ames, IA, 1995, Iowa State University Press; Alon E et al: Effects of propofol and thiopental on maternal and fetal cardiovascular and acid-base variables in the pregnant ewe, *Anesthesiology* 78:562, 1993.

Samples for measurement of end-tidal CO_2 are collected directly at the connecting point between the breathing system (Y piece) of the anesthesia machine and the end of the endotracheal tube; the partial pressure of CO_2 is determined by infrared absorption. Normal end-tidal CO_2 should be closely related to alveolar CO_2, assuming the anesthetized patient is healthy and has no preexisting diffusion disturbance in the lung tissues. Arterial hemoglobin O_2 saturation is measured by pulse oximetry with the sensor clip placed on the lingual artery in the tongue or on the auricular artery in the ears. Normal arterial hemoglobin O_2 saturation should always be close to 98% to 100%. Indirect arterial blood pressures can be measured by a oscillometric blood pressure machine (Dinamap) with an inflatable pressure cuff placed on the coccygeal or dorsal metatarsal artery. Normal values for heart rate, respiratory rate, arterial blood pressures and various arterial blood gases are provided in Table 16-5. A balanced electrolyte solution (5 to 10 ml/kg/hr) should be administered IV for supportive hydration during anesthesia. Administration of 5% dextrose solution is required to prevent hypoglycemia in neonates and young animals. A circulating warm water blanket can be used to maintain body temperature during anesthesia and recovery.

Sheep and goats usually recover from anesthesia gradually and smoothly. Emergence delirium and premature attempts to stand seldom occur in these animals. They should be placed in sternal recumbency with support, if necessary, during the recovery period (Figure 16-5). If regurgitation occurred during anesthesia, the oral cavity

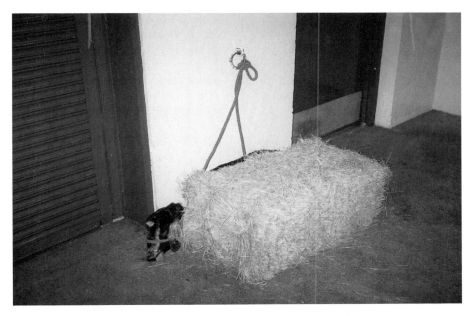

Figure 16-5   Sternal recumbency for postanesthetic recovery.

and pharynx should be lavaged to prevent aspiration of ruminal materials and subsequent aspiration pneumonia. The endotracheal tube should be left in place until the animal regains its chewing and coughing reflexes. It should be removed with the cuff inflated.

Influences of Pathophysiologic Alterations on Anesthesia

Obstructive urolithiasis is the inability to void urine normally because of obstruction of the urinary outflow tract by calculi (see Chapter 10). It occurs most frequently in young castrated goats. In cases of urethral obstruction without ruptured bladder, perineal urethrostomy can be performed under local infiltration or epidural analgesia. General anesthesia is induced for bladder repair, penile urethrostomy, and tube cystotomy.[53,54] Xylazine, detomidine, medetomidine, and other α_2 agonists are contraindicated in obstructive urolithiasis because their potent diuretic effects can result in bladder rupture before the obstruction can be relieved and the bladder emptied.[6] Most of the routine anesthetic regimen can be safely used in cases of obstructive urolithiasis and ruptured bladder. However, anesthetic dosage adjustments may be necessary depending on the animal's physical condition, particularly in animals with increased blood urea nitrogen and creatinine levels and/or hypoproteinemia.[53]

Caseous lymphadenitis in sheep and goats is a chronic contagious disease caused by *Corynebacterium pseudotuberculosis;* it is discussed in various chapters in this text. Airway obstruction may result from occlusion of the pharynx by the enlarged pharyngeal lymph nodes. In some cases, respiratory embarrassment is severe enough to cause

respiratory distress. Treatment of affected animals involves either draining or surgically removing the abscessed nodes. Depending on the size and invasiveness of the abscess, general anesthesia is sometimes required to ensure immobilization so that vital tissues (e.g., carotid artery, vagus nerve, esophagus) are not compromised during dissection.[55] Animals with respiratory embarrassment should be handled with great caution and with as little stress as possible. Stress and excitement may worsen the severity of respiratory embarrassment, resulting in severe hypoxemia and death. Induction of anesthesia and intubation to maintain the airway should be performed rapidly. Tracheal intubation may be difficult because the larynx may be obscured by the swollen pharyngeal tissues. Therefore the skin over the upper third of the trachea should be clipped and surgically prepared before the induction of anesthesia. Tracheostomy can be performed to ensure a patent airway should difficulty in endotracheal intubation occur. Tracheostomy and placement of a cuffed tracheostomy tube also can be performed under local anesthesia before the induction of general anesthesia. Anesthesia can be induced with either IV injectable anesthetics or inhalation anesthetics through the tracheostomy tube. The tracheostomy tube should be left in place for 48 to 72 hours after surgery if possible. If removal of the tracheostomy tube is necessary after completion of the surgery, the clinician should assess airway patency rostral to the tracheostomy tube by deflating the cuff and ensuring good air flow before removing the tube.[54]

Cesarean section is sometimes preformed as an elective surgery to save valuable fetuses and relieve dystocia in sheep and goats. The selection of suitable anesthetics and techniques is vital for the survival of the dam and fetus.

Pregnancy induces several physiologic changes that can affect the response to anesthesia. Because of hormonal changes, minute ventilation increases and the requirement for inhalation anesthetics decreases (by 25% for halothane, 32% for methoxyflurane, and 40% for isoflurane). Therefore induction of anesthesia is more rapid than it is in nonpregnant patients.[54] Heart rate and cardiac output increase because of the increased cardiac work required by pregnancy and at parturition. Consequently, cardiac reserves decrease and pulmonary congestion and heart failure may occur in animals that are exhausted or prone to shock because of prolonged and difficult delivery; animals with preexisting cardiovascular diseases also are at risk.[54] Furthermore, venous engorgement resulting from increased intraabdominal pressure from the enlarged uterus reduces the space available for local anesthetic administration by epidural injection, with resultant cranial migration of the anesthetics. This migration may result in sympathetic blockade, profound maternal hypotension, and reduction of uteroplacental perfusion. Therefore the dose of local anesthetic administered to produce adequate epidural anesthesia should be reduced to one third to one half that used in nonpregnant animals.[54] Drugs administered to induce or enhance uterine contraction during parturition (e.g., oxytocin) cause peripheral vasodilation and hypotension when administered in large or repeated doses and can result in decreased uterine perfusion to the fetus and decreased fetal viability. Fluid with balanced electrolytes should be administered to animals with severe hypotension before induction and during anesthesia.[54]

Either general anesthesia or local anesthesia is suitable for cesarean section. Selection of the anesthetic regimen should be based on maternal and/or fetal safety. Most anesthetics have physicochemical properties that allow them to cross the blood-brain barrier; these properties also permit them to cross the placenta, with resultant depression of the fetal CNS. The only exceptions are neuromuscular blocking agents such as succinylcholine, pancuronium, and atracurium. These drugs cannot cross the placenta as easily as other anesthetics because of their quaternary molecular structure. To ensure fetal viability, the intended incision site should be clipped and roughly prepared before induction, the period between induction of anesthesia and removal of the fetus should be as short as possible, and the anesthetic concentration should be kept to a minimum. For these reasons, in addition to economic concerns, local anesthesia is often chosen for this procedure. Local infiltration of anesthetic along the incision site and lumbosacral epidural or subarachnoid anesthesia are the two most commonly used techniques for cesarean section in most food animals. Procaine and tetracaine, which are esters of para-aminobenzoic acid, do not accumulate in the dam and fetus. Lidocaine, mepivacaine, bupivacaine, and etidocaine are amide-link local anesthetics that depend on hepatic microsomal enzymes for inactivation of drug effects.[45] Blood concentrations of these drugs decline slowly after absorption from the injection site. They can accumulate in the fetus and cause fetal depression when large doses are administered.[54]

Preanesthetic tranquilizers or sedatives are usually reserved for excited or unruly animals. General anesthetics with low lipid solubility, short duration of action, and minimal cardiovascular depression are preferred. Low doses of thiopental, a combination of xylazine and ketamine, or Triple Drip can be used for induction; anesthesia is maintained with Triple Drip IV infusion to effect or inhalation anesthesia (halothane or isoflurane). Tracheal intubation should be performed in these animals even when they are under injectable anesthesia for prevention of possible aspiration pneumonia and administration of supplemental O_2. Neonatal respiratory or CNS depression caused by anesthetic effects can be antagonized by the administration of doxapram or an α_2 antagonist immediately after delivery.

PERIOPERATIVE ANESTHETIC COMPLICATIONS

Regurgitation and Aspiration Pneumonia

Regurgitation can occur during both light (active regurgitation) and deep (passive regurgitation) anesthesia in ruminants in spite of preoperative fasting and withholding of water. Active regurgitation is a reflexive, protective mechanism of a body intent on rejecting unwanted materials from the pharynx, upper airway, and upper digestive tract. Passive regurgitation occurs when the esophageal muscles and transluminal pressure gradients relax as a result of the anesthetic effects. Aspiration of acidic stomach or gastric contents may result in aspiration pneumonia, which is characterized by reflex airway closure, bronchospasm, dyspnea, hypoxemia, and cyanosis. Pulmonary hemorrhage and/or edema may result from destruction of type II alveolar cells and pulmonary capillary lining cells after aspiration of large amounts of particulate material or extremely acidic material. In severe cases, animals die before an endotracheal tube can be placed to protect the airway. Therefore preoperative withholding of feed and endotracheal intubation with the cuff adequately inflated are recommended in all anesthetized ruminants for prevention of aspiration pneumonia.[56] Placing a sandbag or some other rolled padding beneath the animal's neck to elevate the occiput and avoiding vigorous manipulation of the rumen and other internal abdominal organs during surgery helps minimize the occurrence of aspiration pneumonia. If regurgitation occurs before intubation can be completed, the clinician should either quickly lower the animal's head or place the endotracheal tube in the esophagus and inflate the cuff to allow ruminal contents to flow out of the mouth while another tube is placed in the trachea.[2] IV aminophylline (2 to 4 mg/kg over a 5-minute period or 11 mg/kg over a 20-minute period) or other bronchodilators along with

100% O_2 can be administered to relieve bronchospasm at the time of aspiration. If the animal survives the initial insult, corticosteroids and broad-spectrum antibiotics are indicated for the treatment of pneumonia.[2,33]

Ruminal Tympany

Ruminal tympany is sometimes observed during anesthesia as a result of the accumulation of gas produced by fermentation of ingesta and the animal's inability to eructate (see Chapter 3). Pressure increases within the abdomen and on the diaphragm, resulting in reduced functional residual capacity of the lungs and impeded ventilation. Placing the animal in sternal recumbency immediately after anesthesia helps eliminate the accumulated gas in the rumen. However, decompression of the rumen may need to be performed while the animal is still anesthetized and the surgery is in progress. Passage of a stomach tube or insertion of a 12-gauge needle through the abdominal wall allows outflow of the accumulated gas, reducing the pressure in the abdomen and on the diaphragm and thereby improving ventilation. Most anesthetics, particularly α_2 agonists and opioid agonists, decrease gastrointestinal motility; an antagonist can be administered to treat the resultant ruminal tympany if necessary. Preoperative fasting reduces the amount of fermentable ingesta in the rumen and thereby decreases the chance for development of perioperative ruminal tympany.[56]

Hypoventilation

In conscious sheep, lateral recumbency alone can induce significant hypoxemia.[9] During anesthesia, severe hypoventilation and hypoxemia (characterized by a significant increase in $PaCO_2$ and decrease in PaO_2) may result from the abnormal surgical body position combined with the respiratory depressing effect of the anesthetic drugs. Ventilation should be assisted or controlled by squeezing the rebreathing bag with a positive pressure of 20 to 25 cm H_2O if an inhalation anesthetic is used. Supplemental O_2 also can be provided to sedated and recumbent animals through an orotracheal or endotracheal tube by using an O_2 demand valve, particularly if xylazine is part of the anesthetic regimen. Occasionally apnea may occur and persist throughout anesthesia. The anesthetist should ensure that the animal is under an adequate plane of anesthesia before instituting any drug treatment. A respiratory stimulant (doxapram 0.1 to 0.5 mg/kg IV) can be administered to initiate respiration. If the depression persists, doxapram can be administered as a continuous IV infusion (5 to 10 μg/kg/min).[57]

Cardiovascular Collapse

During anesthesia, prolonged decreases in pulse pressure, hypotension (mean arterial pressure less than 60 to 75 mm Hg), increases in capillary refill time, pale mucous membranes, and bradycardia (heart rate less than 70 to 80 beats/min) or tachycardia (heart rate greater than 150 beats/min) can lead to cardiovascular collapse. Causes of this perioperative collapse include significant endotoxin-induced peripheral vasodilation, severe hypovolemia resulting from dehydration and/or blood loss, and deep anesthesia resulting in profound myocardial depression. Treatment of impending cardiovascular failure should begin with correction of the causative disease status, rapid administration of supportive fluid (90 ml/kg), and reduction or even cessation of anesthesia.[57] Additional symptomatic treatment includes vasoactive drugs (e.g., dopamine, phenylephrine, ephedrine) for hypotension, inotropic drugs (e.g., dobutamine) for myocardial depression, chronotropic drugs (e.g., atropine, glycopyrrolate) for bradycardia, and antiarrhythmic drugs (e.g., lidocaine) for ventricular arrhythmias such as ventricular tachycardia or premature ventricular contractions. Dobutamine (1 to 5 μg/kg/min) is a β_1 agonist that increases cardiac output and arterial blood pressure by increasing myocardial contractility when administered at a low dosage. Dobutamine seldom increases heart rate, except in the presence of reduced total blood volume.[58] Dopamine is a dose-dependent, dopaminergic, β and α agonist. When administered at an IV infusion rate of 1 to 2 μg/kg/min, dopamine increases renal perfusion by stimulating dopaminergic receptors. Increasing the infusion rate to 2 to 10 μg/kg/min causes stimulation of β_1 receptors and a resultant increased heart rate. Vasoconstriction and the subsequent increase in arterial blood pressure mediated by stimulation of α_1 receptors are not evident until the infusion rate is greater than 10 μg/kg/min.[58] Phenylephrine (2 to 4 mg/kg IV bolus or 0.2 to 0.4 μg/kg/min via infusion) and ephedrine (22 to 66 μg/kg IV) have both been used to treat hypotension in anesthetized animals.[59] Ephedrine appears to have a longer duration of action (30 to 60 minutes) than dobutamine or dopamine, which may be undesirable if tachycardia occurs after ephedrine administration.[59]

Prolonged untreated cardiovascular collapse may result in cardiac arrest and death. Cardiopulmonary resuscitation (CPR) should follow the *ABC technique*. *A* entails opening of the *a*irway by endotracheal intubation, *B* is the initiation of controlled *b*reathing by squeezing an Ambu bag or using the rebreathing bag on the anesthesia machine (12 to 20 breaths/min), and *C* is the establishment of artificial *c*irculation by cardiac compression (80 to 100 compressions/min). After CPR has been instituted, an IV catheter should be placed if one is not already present. If the attempts at IV catheterization is unsuccessful, emergency drugs may be administered intratracheally through the endotracheal tube at 2 to 2.5 times the IV dose after dilution with sterile water or saline to a volume of 5 to 10 ml. Absorption of the drugs from the lung is sometimes significant enough to be more effective than IM, subcutaneous, or IV administration through a peripheral vein.[57] Emergency drugs and products frequently used during CPR include 100% O_2, balanced electrolyte solutions, atropine, lidocaine, and epinephrine. Depending on the animal's condition, the vasoactive drugs mentioned previously can be used in conjunction with emergency drugs. Electrical defibrillation is the most effective treatment for conversion of ventricular fibrillation, but it is not practical in field situations. Epinephrine (10 μg/kg IV) is usually the drug of choice for treatment of ventricular fibrillation. Epinephrine induces peripheral vasoconstriction and increases arterial diastolic blood pressure, intracranial and coronary blood flow, coarseness of ventricular fibrillation, and positive inotropic effect by stimulating α and β adrenoceptors. Potential side effects of epinephrine include increased myocardial and cerebral O_2 demand, post-resuscitation arrhythmia, and tachycardia. Lidocaine (0.5 to 2 mg/kg IV) may be used to treat the post-resuscitation ventricular arrhythmia.[57] Chemical defibrillation with IV potassium chloride (1 mg/kg) and acetylcholine (6 mg/kg) followed by administration of 10% calcium chloride (1 ml/10 kg) is recommended for treatment of ventricular fibrillation. Although it is ineffective in defibrillation, this technique usually converts fibrillation to asystole.[57] A normal sinus rhythm is actually more easily initiated from asystole.

The best treatment for perioperative complications is prevention, which requires a devoted and vigilant anesthetist. Careful preanesthetic evaluation and preparation and proper use of anesthetic regimens can prevent most anesthetic-related complications; close monitoring allows the anesthetist to recognize potentially dangerous situations quickly and institute corrective measures at an early stage. The clinician should keep in mind that "there is no safe anesthetic or anesthetic technique, only safe anesthetists."

SPECIFIC NERVE BLOCKS

Many of the local anesthetic techniques for specific surgeries are covered in the text as part of the surgical description. However, three commonly used local and regional anesthetic techniques are described in this chapter. The authors of this chapter perform caudal epidural anesthesia routinely and lumbosacral epidural anesthesia occasionally, but rarely use local anesthetic techniques for horn removal. When removing large horns from adult goats or rams, the authors prefer to use general anesthesia. However, on occasion local anesthesia for horn removal is warranted and therefore it is included here.

Caudal Epidural

If properly performed, caudal epidural anesthesia desensitizes the perineum, vulva, vagina, and rectum. To locate the injection site the clinician grasps the tail and locates the most cranial moveable intervertebral space. Location of this space is enhanced by "pumping" the tail. In sheep and goats the injection site is either in the inter-

space between the fifth sacral and first coccygeal vertebrae or between the first coccygeal and second coccygeal vertebrae. The area over the site is clipped and aseptically prepared. The needle (18- to 20-gauge, 4-cm) is placed into the correct interspace at a 90° angle to the skin. The needle (without an attached syringe) is pushed ventrally through the interarcuate ligament toward the floor of the neural canal.[60] A sight vacuum should be noted on entering the epidural space. If blood is visualized in the hub or flows from the needle, the needle should be withdrawn because it has been inappropriately placed into a venous sinus. As a general rule, 1 ml of 2% lidocaine per 45 kg of body weight is adequate and therefore a total dose of 1 to 2 ml is effective for most sheep and goats. The onset of analgesia occurs within 1 to 5 minutes, and the duration is about 1 hour.[1] This technique also is described in Chapters 3 and 6.

Lumbosacral Epidural Anesthesia

If properly performed, a lumbosacral epidural provides analgesia caudal to the diaphragm (abdominal wall caudal to the umbilicus, inguinal region, flank, and perineal area).[1] The site for injection can be palpated in some sheep and goats as a soft spot where the dorsal midline intersects an imaginary line drawn between the cranial borders of the two iliac wings[2] (Figure 16-6). In sheep and goats this lumbosacral space is located just caudal to the spinous process of the last lumbar vertebra. The skin over the space between the last lumbar vertebra and the first sacral vertebra is clipped and aseptically prepared. A needle (18- to 20-gauge, 4- to 9-cm) is advanced through the skin at a 90° angle. Occasionally a slight cranial movement of the needle is required. If cerebrospinal fluid or blood is encountered, the needle is in the subarachnoid space. In this case the needle should be withdrawn and the procedure should be attempted again. A slight vacuum should be noted on entering the epidural space. If local anesthetic is injected into the subarachnoid space, rear-limb paralysis occurs within 3 to 5 minutes.[60,61] After passing through the epidural space, the needle "pops" through the interarcuate ligament.[61] The syringe can then be injected slowly without resistance. A dosage of 0.3 to 0.5 ml of a 2% lidocaine hydrochloride solution per 10 kg of body weight is adequate for most surgeries.[61] The onset of analgesia and rear-limb paralysis occurs after 5 to 15 minutes and lasts 1 to 2 hours.[60,61]

Horn Anesthesia

As dehorning in adult goats and rams is a very bloody surgical procedure, general anesthesia should probably be used; however, some clinicians prefer local anesthesia. The administration of local anesthesia for dehorning sheep (rams) is similar technically to that provided for

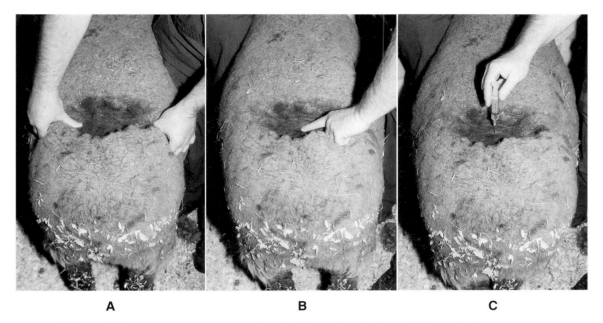

A   **B**   **C**

Figure 16-6   Lumbosacral anesthesia. The site is located on the dorsal midline, behind the most caudal lumbar vertebra and midway between the dorsal aspect of the iliac wings. **A,** The clinician's thumbs are pressing on the iliac wings. **B,** The index finger indicates the site to be injected. **C,** The clinician locates the site, places the needle about 90° to the skin, and injects the anesthetic agent without resistance.

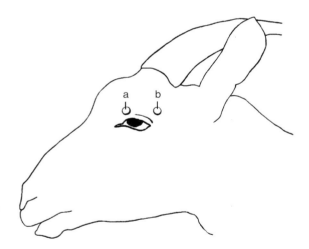

Figure 16-7   The location of the cornual branch of the intratrochlear nerve *(a)* and the cornual branch of the lacrimal nerve *(b)*. Local anesthetic can be infiltrated into these two areas to attain good analgesia of the horn and surrounding skin.

cattle.[62,63] In the ram local anesthetic (1 to 2 ml of 2% lidocaine) is injected at a depth of 1 to 2 cm just beneath the zygomatic ridge toward the horn. Another protocol entails the application of a 3- to 4-cm line block 1 or 2 cm from the base of the horn. The subcutaneous injection should be placed perpendicular to an imaginary line drawn along the shortest distance from the horn base to the eye. A third option is to place a ring block around one or both horns and adjacent tissue, infiltrating the tissue

with a local anesthetic. In one of the authors' experience (Dr. Pugh) the ring block has yielded the most reproducible results. Because of the potential for lidocaine toxicity, the 2% lidocaine should be mixed with an equal volume of sterile saline.[64]

In the goat the horn and immediately surrounding skin can be anesthetized by "blocking" the corneal branch of the lacrimal nerve. This nerve is anesthetized by injecting a local anesthetic (1 to 2 ml of 2% lidocaine 1.5 to 2 cm deep) adjacent to the caudal ridge of the base of the supraorbital process. The cornual branch of the intratrochlear nerve, which is located dorsomedial to the eye and adjacent to the margin of the orbit (Figure 16-7), can be palpated in some animals. Local anesthetic (1 to 2 ml of 2% lidocaine) can be administered there about 1 cm deep. By anesthetizing both of these anesthetic sites, good horn analgesia is attained.[63]

References

1. Craigmill AL, Rangel-Lugo M, Riviere JE: Extralabel use of tranquilizers and general anesthetics, *J Am Vet Med Assoc* 211:302, 1997.
2. Riebold TW: Ruminants. In Thurmon JC, Tranquilli WJ, Benson GJ, editors: *Lumb & Jones' veterinary anesthesia,* ed 3, Baltimore, 1996, Lea & Febiger.
3. Short CE: Preanesthetic medications in ruminants and swine, *Vet Clin North Am: Food Anim Pract* 2:553, 1986.
4. Gross ME, Booth NH: Tranquilizers, α_2-adrenergic agonists, and related agents. In Adams HR, editor: *Veterinary pharmacology and therapeutics,* ed 7, Ames, IA, 1995, Iowa State University Press.

5. Taylor PM: Anesthesia in sheep and goats, *In Pract* 13:31, 1991.
6. Greene SA, Thurmon JC: Xylazine—a review of its pharmacology and use in veterinary medicine, *J Vet Pharmacol Ther* 11:295, 1988.
7. Rosenberger G, Hempel E, Baumeister M: Contributions to the effect and applicability of Rompun in cattle, *Vet Med Rev* 2:137, 1996.
8. Thurmon JC et al: Effects of xylazine hydrochloride on urine in cattle, *Aust Vet J* 54:178, 1978.
9. Mitchell B, Williams JT: Respiratory function changes in sheep associated with lying in lateral recumbency and with sedation by xylazine, *Proc Assoc Vet Anaesth Great Br Ire* 6:30, 1976-1977.
10. Doherty TJ et al: Antagonism of xylazine-induced sedation by idazoxan in calves, *Can J Vet Res* 51:244, 1987.
11. Waterman AE, Nolan A, Livingston A: Influence of idazoxan on the respiratory blood gas changes in conscious sheep, *Vet Rec* 121:105, 1987.
12. Hsu WH, Schaffer DD, Hanson CE: Effects of tolazoline and yohimbine on xylazine-induced central nervous system depression, bradycardia, and tachypnea in sheep, *J Am Vet Med Assoc* 190:423, 1987.
13. Hsu WH et al: Effects of idazoxan, tolazoline, and yohimbine on xylazine-induced respiratory changes and central nervous system depression in ewes, *Am J Vet Res* 50:1570, 1989.
14. Lin HC et al: Telazol and xylazine anesthesia in sheep, *Cornell Vet* 83:117, 1993.
15. Scott PR et al: Assessment of xylazine hydrochloride epidural analgesia for open castration of rams, *Theriogenology* 42:1029, 1994.
16. Gessert ME, Scott PR: Combined xylazine and lidocaine caudal epidural analgesia injection in the treatment of ewes with preparturient vaginal or cervico-vaginal prolapse, *Agri-Pract* 16:15, 1995.
17. Ruckebusch Y, Allal C: Depression of reticulo ruminal motor functions through the stimulation of α_2-adrenoceptors, *Vet Pharmacol Therap* 10:1, 1987.
18. Celly CS et al:. Comparative cardiopulmonary effects of four α-2 adrenoceptor agonists in sheep, *Vet Surg* 22:545, 1993.
19. Pyörälä E et al: Detomidine to pregnant cows, *Nord Vet Med* 38:237, 1986.
20. Jedruch J, Gajewski Z: The effect of detomidine hydrochloride (Domosedan) on the electrical activity of the uterus in cows, *Acta Vet Scand* 82:189, 1986.
21. Muge DK et al: Analgesic effects of medetomidine in sheep, *Vet Rec* 135:43, 1994.
22. Mohammad FK, Zangana IK, Abdul-Latif AR: Medetomidine sedation in sheep, *J Vet Med* A40:328, 1993.
23. Tulamo R-M, Raekallio M, Ekblad A: Cardiovascular effects of medetomidine-ketamine anaesthesia in sheep, with and without 100% oxygen and its reversal with atipamezole, *J Vet Anaesth* 22:9, 1995.
24. Hsu WH, Schaffer DD, Hanson CE: Effects of tolazoline and yohimbine on xylazine-induced central nervous system depression, bradycardia, and tachycardia in sheep, *J Am Vet Med Assoc* 190:423, 1987.
25. Yellin TO, Sperow JW, Buck SH: Antagonism of tolazoline by histamine H_2-receptor blockers, *Nature* 253:561, 1975.
26. Read MR, Duke T, Toews AR: Suspected tolazoline toxicosis in a llama, *J Am Vet Med Assoc* 216:227, 2000.
27. Gray PR, McDonell WN: Anesthesia in goats and sheep, Part II: general anesthesia, *Cont Edu* 8:S127, 1986.
28. Flacke JW et al: Histamine release by four narcotics: a double blind study in humans, *Anesth Analg* 66:723, 1987.
29. Singh B, Kumar A: Meperidine as preanesthetic to thiopentone anesthesia in goats, *Ind J Anim Sci* 58:1279, 1988.
30. Murphy MR, Hugg CC, Jr: "Ceiling effect" of butorphanol (Stadol) as an anesthetic supplement [abstract], *Anesthesiology* 55:261, 1981.
31. Waterman AE, Livingston A, Amin A: Analgesic activity and respiratory effects of butorphanol in sheep, *Res Vet Sci* 51:19, 1991.
32. O'Hair KC et al: Cardiopulmonary effects of nalbuphine hydrochloride and butorphanol tartrate in sheep, *Lab Anim Sci* 38:58, 1988.
33. Thurmon JC, Benson GJ: Anesthesia in ruminants and swine. In Howard JL, editor: *Current veterinary therapy*, ed 3, Philadelphia, 1993, WB Saunders.
34. Thurmon JC, Tranquilli WJ, Benson GJ: Injectable anesthetics. In Thurmon JC, Tranquilli WJ, Benson GJ, editors: *Lumb & Jones' veterinary anesthesia*, ed 3, Baltimore, 1996, Lea & Febiger.
35. Lin HC: Dissociative anesthetics. In Thurmon JC, Tranquilli WJ, Benson GJ, editors: *Lumb & Jones' veterinary anesthesia*, ed 3, Baltimore, 1996, Lea & Febiger.
36. Lin HC et al: Effects of anesthesia induced and maintained by continuous intravenous administration of guaifenesin, ketamine, and xylazine in spontaneously breathing sheep, *Am J Vet Res* 54:1913, 1993.
37. Handel IG et al: Observations on the pharmacokinetics of propofol in sheep, *Proceedings of the Fourth International Congress of Veterinary Anaesthesia*, 1991, Utrecht University, Utrecht, Netherlands.
38. Waterman AE: Use of propofol in sheep, *Vet Rec* 122:26, 1988.
39. Reid J, Nolan AM, Welsh E: Propofol as an induction agent in the goats: a pharmacokinetic study, *J Vet Pharmacol Ther* 16:488, 1993.
40. Lin HC, Purohit RC, Powe TA: Anesthesia in sheep with propofol or with xylazine-ketamine followed by halothane, *Vet Surg* 26:247, 1997.
41. Carroll GL et al: Detomidine-butorphanol-propofol for carotid artery translocation and castration or ovariectomy in goats, *Vet Surg* 27:75, 1998.
42. Fetcher A: Liver diseases of sheep and goats, *Vet Clin North Am: Large Anim Pract* 5:525, 1983.
43. O'Brien TD et al: Hepatic necrosis following halothane anesthesia in goats, *J Am Vet Med Assoc* 189:1591, 1986.
44. Riebold TW, Geiser DR, Goble DO: Clinical techniques for food animal anesthesia. In Riebold TW, Geiser DR, Goble DO, editors: *Large animal anesthesia: principles and techniques*, ed 2, Ames, IA, 1995, Iowa State University Press.
45. Stoelting RK: Local anesthetics. In Stoelting RK, editor: *Pharmacology and physiology in anesthetic practice*, Philadelphia, 1987, JB Lippincott.
46. Skarda RT: Techniques in local analgesia in ruminants and swine, *Vet Clin North Am: Food Anim Pract* 2:621, 1986.
47. Scarratt WK, Trout HF: Iatrogenic lidocaine toxicosis in ewes, *J Am Vet Med Assoc* 188:184, 1986.
48. Morishima HO et al: Toxicity of lidocaine in adult, newborn, and fetal sheep, *Anesthesiology* 55:57, 1981.
49. Santos AC et al: Does pregnancy alter the systemic toxicity of local anesthetics?, *Anesthesiology* 70:991, 1989.
50. Hall LW, Clarke KW: General principles of local analgesia. In Hall LW, Clarke KW, editors: *Veterinary anaesthesia*, ed 9, London, 1991, Bailliere Tindall.
51. Ewing KK: Anesthesia techniques in sheep and goats, *Vet Clin North Am: Food Anim Pract* 6:759, 1990.

52. Alon E et al: Effects of propofol and thiopental on maternal and fetal cardiovascular and acid-base variables in the pregnant ewe, *Anesthesiology* 78:562, 1993.
53. Smith MC, Sherman DM: Urinary system. In Smith MC, Sherman DM, editors: *Goat medicine,* Philadelphia, 1994, Lea & Febiger.
54. Benson GJ: Anesthetic management of ruminants and swine with selected pathophysiologic alterations, *Vet Clin North Am: Food Anim Pract* 2:677, 1986.
55. Smith MC, Sherman DM: Subcutaneous swellings. In Smith MC, Sherman DM, editors: *Goat medicine,* Philadelphia, 1994, Lea & Febiger.
56. Steffey EP: Some characteristics of ruminants and swine that complicate management of general anesthesia, *Vet Clin North Am: Food Anim Pract* 2:507, 1986.
57. Kruse-Elliott KT: Management and emergency intervention during anesthesia, *Vet Clin North Am: Food Anim Pract* 12:563, 1996.
58. Riebold TW, Geiser DR, Goble DO: Anesthetic emergencies. In Riebold TW, Geiser DR, Goble DO, editors: *Large animal anesthesia: principles and techniques,* ed 2, Ames, IA, 1995, Iowa State University Press.
59. Klein L: Anesthetic complications of equine anesthesia, *Vet Clin North Am: Equine Pract* 6:665, 1990.
60. Purohit RC: Anesthesia. In Wolfe DF, Moll HD, editors: *Large animal urogenital surgery,* Baltimore, 1998, Williams & Wilkins.
61. Hooper RN: General surgical techniques for small ruminants: Part II, *Small Ruminants for the Mixed Animal Practitioner Western Veterinary Conference,* 1998, Las Vegas, NV.
62. George AN: A note on the anatomy of the horns of sheep, *Br Vet J* 111:391, 1955.
63. Greenough PR, Johnson L: The integumentary system: skin, hoof, claw, and appendages. In Oehme FW, Prier JE, editors: *Textbook of large animal surgery,* Baltimore, 1974, Williams & Wilkins.
64. Hooper RN: General surgical techniques for small ruminants: Part I, *Small Ruminants for the Mixed Animal Practitioner Western Veterinary Conference,* 1998, Las Vegas, NV.

Chapter 17

Flock Health

SEYEDMEHDI MOBINI, CINDY WOLF, AND D.G. PUGH

This chapter provides a brief overview of flock and herd health care programs for sheep and goats. Treatment and prevention of specific diseases are addressed in other chapters. In this chapter goat herd programs are covered first, followed by sheep flock programs.

GOATS

Herd Health Management

Herd health management and preventive medicine programs are designed to minimize potential adverse effects of predictable problems and to protect against unexpected ones.[1] The goal of a herd health program is to improve the goat herd's productivity through general husbandry, nutritional management, parasite control, vaccination, and environmental management.[2] An understanding of various management practices and common disease problems is helpful to accomplish this goal.

Because of their remarkable adaptability, goats are maintained over a more diverse range of production systems than any other domestic livestock species. Goat production can be divided into dairy, fiber, meat, pet, and show production. The largest body of information about goat herd health management and preventive medicine focuses on dairy and fiber-producing goats. Still, with the recent expansion of the meat goat industry in North America, development of herd health protocols in this area is desirable. Herd health management programs must be designed to fit an individual herd and vary according to the herd size, its purpose, and the owner's production goals.[2] In an attempt to organize information applicable to goat herd health into a simple, usable, and easily remembered format, herd health management practices are divided into groups of dry does and does in late pregnancy, kidding does, kids and weanlings, and bucks.

Dry Does and Does in Late Pregnancy

The major disease problems in this group are pregnancy toxemia, abortion, and pseudopregnancy. Goats that are over-conditioned during this period are at risk of pregnancy toxemia, vaginal prolapse, and dystocia.[1,3] The primary objective for these animals is proper nutritional management, avoidance of obesity in early gestation, and provision of adequate nutrients to support the rapid growth of the fetus in the final trimester.[1] Supplement feeding where needed should commence at the beginning of the final trimester of pregnancy and be increased steadily until parturition. Obesity, however, should be avoided. To protect pregnant does from infectious abortion, no new animals should be introduced into the group.

Management Practices
- Vaccinate for abortion diseases (if the herd has a history of abortion) 1 month before the start of breeding.
- Perform pregnancy diagnosis on all bred does 45 to 60 days after breeding.
- Prevent over-conditioning and provide plenty of exercise for parturient does.
- Do not mix any new animals with pregnant does.
- In areas or on farms with a history of infectious abortion, consider adding ionophores and/or tetracyclines to feeds or mineral mixtures.
- Give yearly vaccination boosters of toxoids for *Clostridium perfringens* type C and D and *C. tetani* 30 days before kidding. This helps protect the doe and ensures high levels of antibodies to protect the newborn kid.
- Deworm 30 days before kidding and continue deworming through the birthing season for meat and fiber goats. Pregnant does experience a preparturient nematode parasite egg rise and exhibit

increased shedding of parasite eggs around kidding. The authors of this chapter avoid levamisole and albendazole for the deworming of pregnant does. Monitor fecal egg count during this period.

- Infuse mammary glands of dairy goats with half a tube of dry cow antibiotic products at the time of dry off (40 to 60 days before parturition).
- Trim feet as needed. Avoid hoof disease late in gestation.
- In deficient areas, administer vitamin E and selenium to does 30 to 45 days before kidding. Ensure adequate selenium intake with a free-choice mineral mixture.
- Provide a clean, dry, draft-free area for maternity pens, or a well-drained, clean pasture with shelter.
- Assess body condition score of does. Scores of 2.5 to 3.5 (on a 5-point system) are desirable.[1,4]
- Periodically check pregnant does' urine for ketones with urine sticks in herds experiencing pregnancy toxemia. If an individual or a large percentage of the animals examined have higher than normal ketone values, take steps to correct the problem (e.g., feed niacin and/or ionophores, feed more grain, force more exercise).

Kidding Does

Kidding should be a well-anticipated event and not an unexpected surprise.[1] Where possible the pregnant doe must be given adequate exercise until the time for kidding. Kidding does should be moved to a clean pen or pasture as parturition nears. The udders of dairy goats should be clipped 2 weeks before the due date. Being prepared for routine processing of kids at birth, including navel dipping, colostrum feeding, and readiness to respond to emergencies, reduces neonatal losses.[5] A timed induction of parturition using prostaglandins (PGF$_{2\alpha}$ 2.5 to 20 mg IM) is one management option to ensure does are attended at birth.

Great emphasis should be placed on kid-rearing techniques that reduce neonatal mortality and diseases that inhibit the rapid, efficient growth of young kids. The major obstacles to newborn kids' survival are hypothermia, hypoglycemia, and infectious diseases resulting from delayed or inadequate colostral intake. Failure of passive transfer of maternal antibodies to newborn kids leads to an increased incidence of disease and death. Caprine arthritis-encephalitis virus (CAEV) infection is a major concern in dairy goats. Newborn dairy kids should be a focus of CAEV control programs because the virus is primarily spread from infected does to susceptible kids by colostrum and milk. To help prevent the spread of CAEV, colostrum can be heat-treated at 56° C (133° F) for 60 minutes before being fed. The mammary form of CAEV infection often occurs at the onset of lactation. The udder appears normal but is firm, and hypogalactia or agalactia are usually present.[1,6]

Management Practices
- Tape the teats of does that are CAEV-positive to prevent accidental nursing of kids.
- Clean dams' teats and strip milk from each teat to ensure the presence of colostrum.
- In dairy goats, dry off kids and separate them from their dams.
- Dip the navel cord with tincture of iodine immediately after birth.
- Ensure that kids receive colostrum within 4 hours of birth. In dairy goats feed 60 ml of pasteurized colostrum by bottle or stomach tube within 1 hour of birth. Continue colostrum feeding for 3 to 4 days.
- Examine kids for congenital defects.
- Ensure that does pass the placenta within 12 hours of parturition.
- In dairy breeds, disbud and castrate kids at 4 to 10 days. Meat goat owners may prefer to leave horns on their goats. In meat goats the age of marketing determines the need for castration. For pet or show goats, castration should be delayed until after puberty.
- In deficient areas, inject kids with vitamin E and selenium at 1 to 2 weeks.
- Properly identify kids (e.g., by ear tag or neck collar).
- Begin coccidiosis prevention at the second week of life and parasite control at 1 month.
- Vaccinate kids at 1 to 2 months for *C. perfringens* type C and D and administer *C. tetani* toxoids if the dams were vaccinated during the final month of pregnancy. If the dams were not vaccinated, begin kid vaccination at 1 week of age and repeat vaccination in 3 or 4 weeks.
- Expose kids to hay and grain early in life to promote rumen development.

Kids and Weanlings

Weaning may occur at 6 to 12 weeks in dairy goats or orphaned kids, depending on the feeding and management system. Meat goats are usually weaned at 4 to 6 months.[1,4] Common diseases encountered during the weaning period include pneumonia, coccidiosis, and gastrointestinal (GI) nematode parasites. In finishing programs in which young bucks are fed high-concentrate feed, conditions such as bloat, urinary calculi, and enterotoxemia are frequently encountered. The authors have diagnosed cases of urinary calculi in male Boer kids as young as 2 to 3 months. Providing a continuous supply of clean, fresh water and increasing the concentration of salt in the ration to a maximum of 4% are helpful management tools to prevent calculi. Prophylactic use of urinary acidifiers also has been advocated. The continuous administration of ammonium chloride at a level of 1% to

2% of the diet is recommended in castrated and intact bucks. Polioencephalomalacia can occur under intensive management conditions. Weaned meat goat kids consuming rations containing high levels of concentrates or grains are highly susceptible. Causes of polioencephalomalacia include thiamine deficiency, inhibition of thiamine activity, and sulfate contamination of water or feed. Increasing the roughage and decreasing the grain portion of the diet, decreasing sulfate ingestion, and possibly including thiamine in the diet are all good therapeutic tools.

Management Practices
- Separate doe kids from intact buck kids before 3 or 4 months to avoid unwanted breeding.
- Provide coccidiostats in feed or water and maintain good sanitary practices.
- Monitor fecal egg counts (McMaster's score higher than 100 eggs per gram) and deworm as needed.
- Provide free-choice hay when feeding concentrates.
- Examine the external genitalia for abnormalities such as intersex.
- Maintain a 2:1 dietary calcium–to–phosphorus ratio and provide high levels of salt (up to 4% salt) and 1% to 2% ammonium chloride in the diets of bucks and wethers to prevent urinary calculi. Allow for sufficient trace mineral intake (e.g., selenium, zinc), particularly in deficient areas. Ensure that drinking water is clean, fresh, and readily available.

Bucks

Bucks are too often neglected and omitted from herd health management practices. Urolithiasis is probably the most important disease condition in bucks. Although they are more common in castrated males, urinary calculi also have been observed in intact males (especially meat goats); they can result in the bucks' destruction as breeding animals. Providing fresh water, increasing salt concentration in the diet to 2% to 4%, and using urine acidifiers are as important in the herd health management of bucks as they are in the management of kids and weanlings.

Bucks become very aggressive during the breeding season and can injure workers and one another. They urinate on their faces and forelimb during breeding season, which can cause severe urine scald, secondary bacterial dermatitis, and stench.

Management Practices
- Allow exercise.
- Vaccinate the bucks at the same time as the does (*C. perfringens* type C and D and *C. tetani* toxin).
- Trim feet as needed.
- Perform breeding soundness examination 1 to 2 months before breeding. Determine body condition scores and maintain animals at a score of 3 to 3.5.
- Monitor fecal egg counts and deworm as needed. Deworm 1 month before breeding season.
- Apply petroleum jelly to any urine-scalded areas of the head and back of front legs.
- Maintain a 2:1 ratio of dietary calcium to phosphorus and provide a high level of salt (up to 4%) and 1% to 2% ammonium chloride in the diet to prevent urinary calculi. Ensure that drinking water is clean, fresh, and readily available.

Vaccination Protocol

Enterotoxemia and tetanus. A minimal vaccination program for goats includes vaccinations against *C. perfringens* type C and D (enterotoxemia) and *C. tetani*.[1,2,7-9] Some multivalent clostridial vaccines, including those against blackleg, malignant edema, and bacillary hemoglobinuria, are used in goats. These are unusual diseases in goats, and vaccination to prevent them is usually not economically justified, but many vaccines contain seven or eight bacterins in one shot. Vaccination site considerations include the potential for development of blemishes, lameness, and site reactions that require trimming at slaughter or cause poor performance in the show ring. Subcutaneous injection in the caudolateral neck region or behind the elbow is often preferred. Injection over the ribs is an alternative for adult animals.[9] All the animals should be vaccinated initially with clostridial and tetanus toxoid products and receive a second vaccination in 3 to 4 weeks. Pregnant does should receive their annual vaccination 1 month before parturition. Bucks, yearlings, and other adults should receive annual boosters at the same time to streamline animal handling. Animals that are fed large amounts of concentrate may need to receive a booster vaccination every 6 months. This can be accompanied by vaccination of does a month before breeding.

Kids from immunized dams should be vaccinated at 1 to 2 months and given a booster 3 to 4 weeks later. Kids from nonimmunized dams should be vaccinated at 1 to 3 weeks and given a booster 3 to 4 weeks later. A *C. perfringens* type C and D antitoxin is available for treatment in case of failure of passive transfer of colostral antibodies and for use in endemic areas. Similarly, *C. tetani* antitoxin is available and should be used before surgeries (e.g., castration, dehorning) and parturition, if the previous vaccination status of the animal is unclear. The dosage of the tetanus antitoxin for young kids is 150 to 250 units and 400 to 750 units for adult goats.[2,5] A basic vaccination protocol for goats is shown in Box 17-1.

Contagious ecthyma. Goats should be vaccinated to protect against contagious ecthyma only if the disease has been identified in the herd.[2,7] Because the vaccine is a live virus, herds not exposed to the disease should not be vaccinated because the virus may survive in the environment

BOX 17-1

BASIC VACCINATION PROGRAM FOR GOATS

PREGNANT DOES
- Vaccinate does during last month of pregnancy for *Clostridium perfringens* type C and D and *C. tetani*.

KIDS
- Immunize kids from immunized dams at 1 to 2 months of age for *Clostridium perfringens* type C and D and *C. tetani;* repeat immunization in 3 to 4 weeks.
- Immunize kids from non-immunized dams at 1 to 3 weeks of age for *Clostridium perfringens* type C and D and *C. tetani;* repeat immunization twice at 3- to 4-week intervals.

BUCKS AND YEARLINGS
- Immunize bucks and yearlings at the same time pregnant does are vaccinated, with emphasis on *Clostridium* species.
- In endemic areas, vaccines for rabies, and leptospirosis may be of value.

BREEDING DOES
- Vaccinate breeding does for *Chlamydia* and *Campylobacter* before breeding, and repeat in mid-gestation.

for long periods and act as a source of herd infection. After the environment becomes contaminated by the vaccine-virus or through natural infection, vaccination is warranted. During outbreaks, disinfection of goat handling and working areas after the animals' lesions have cleared is recommended if the owner elects not to vaccinate. In a herd in which the showing or buying of goats is a regular practice, vaccination of the original animals is recommended 6 months before they are to be commingled with animals from outside the herd. The initial vaccination for contagious ecthyma should include all animals in the herd. After the initial vaccination, only new kids and unvaccinated purchased animals should be vaccinated.[2,7] The preferred site for vaccination is inside the ear pinna or beneath the tail.[1] The skin is lightly scarified, and the virus suspension is applied. Scabs appear at the vaccination site within 1 to 3 days and indicate successful immunization. Persons exposed to the vaccine can become infected. Proper precautions such as wearing gloves during vaccine administration and properly disposing of vaccine containers reduce human health risks. Vaccines can cause severe lesions in humans if they are accidentally self-injected.

Caseous lymphadenitis. Caseous lymphadenitis is a common disease of goats that causes abscesses at the lymph nodes and results in poor production, weight loss, and death. A vaccine is usually available singly or in combination with *C. perfringens* type C and D and *C. tetani* vaccines for sheep. The value of this vaccine in controlling caseous lymphadenitis in goats has been questioned.[1] The vaccine itself can cause severe local or systemic reactions in infected goats and may interfere with some forms of serologic testing.[5,9] However, either autogenous or commercial vaccines may reduce the number and severity of lesions in individual animals (see Chapter 8).

Other vaccines. Vaccines for some diseases of goats are commercially available only for sheep and cattle but may be beneficial on an as-needed basis. Vaccines against abortion-causing diseases are not commonly administered to goats. In the United States, *Chlamydia* and *Toxoplasma* are the most commonly identified infectious causes of abortion in goats. *Campylobacter,* which is one of the most common causes of abortion in sheep, is relatively uncommon in North American goats.[10] *Listeria* also should be considered a potential cause of abortion in meat goats.[11]

Sheep vaccines against chlamydiosis can be used in goats if the disease is a problem in a particular herd. Initially, all breeding adults and replacement yearlings should be vaccinated 60 days and 30 days before the breeding season. In successive years, all adults should be vaccinated 2 to 4 weeks before the start of the breeding season. A combined vaccine against *Chlamydia* and *Campylobacter* for sheep can be used in the rare event that *Campylobacter* is a problem in a particular goat herd. The efficiency of these vaccines is questionable because several biotypes of these two diseases exist and vaccines against one biotype may not be cross-protective.

No vaccine against *Toxoplasma* is presently available for use in sheep or goats and commercial vaccines against listeriosis are not available in the United States. Autogenous biologics may be prepared by the practitioner or a licensed facility and may be valuable tools in some management systems. An autogenous bacterin developed from six different isolates of a listeriosis outbreak in Georgia reduced the incidence of abortion in a meat goat herd.[11] Cattle leptospirosis vaccines can be used in goats that are kept near cattle or hogs or housed in an area where confirmed *Leptospira* abortion is a problem in other species.[7] Pinkeye in goats is usually caused by *Mycoplasma* and *Chlamydia* and no vaccine is currently available to prevent this condition. *Moraxella bovis,* a causative organism of pinkeye in cattle, can rarely cause keratoconjunctivitis in goats. Therefore cattle pinkeye vaccine is of little benefit in goats. No rabies vaccine is approved for use in goats in the United States. Vaccination of valuable breeding stock or pets with a killed vaccine approved for sheep is advisable in endemic areas.[1]

Some cattle respiratory vaccines are occasionally used by goat producers and veterinarians. The efficacy of these vaccines and their value in reducing respiratory disease complex for goats are questionable. Bovine K99 *Escherichia coli* vaccine has been demonstrated to produce increased K99-specific antibodies in doe serum and colostrum. However, confirmation of K99 *E. coli* in outbreaks of kid diarrhea is currently limited.[1]

Nutritional Management

Based on body size, goats have larger nutritional requirements than other ruminants. They have an almost unique browsing and foraging ability and consume a wide variety of grass, legume, weed, and browse species as food.[12] Goats seem to prefer about 50% browse, 20% grasses and legumes, and 20% forage in their diets. Good-quality grass forage and minimal grain feeding with a trace mineral and salt supplement and fresh water is generally sufficient to meet most nutritional requirements of goats, particularly those kept as pets.[1] Dairy goats with high genetic potential for milk production benefit from relatively high levels of grain feeding during early lactation. Does in late gestation and early lactation and breeding bucks also may benefit from the feeding of concentrates, particularly if forage quality and quantity is poor. However, excessive grain feeding can result in health problems. The likely cost benefit of feeding grain to some meat goats, with respect to feed-induced health problems, is not sufficient to warrant this practice.

Flushing, or increasing the feed intake of does 3 to 4 weeks before and during the breeding season, increases the ovulation rate, particularly in animals of moderate body condition. Flushing can be accomplished by providing high-quality pasture free choice, supplement grain feeding, or creep grazing pasture. Pregnant does should receive supplemental feed 4 weeks before and after kidding. Over- or under-conditioning can predispose females to pregnancy toxemia. Free access to legumes should be limited during the final trimester of gestation (particularly in dairy goats) to prevent excessive calcium intake, which can predispose to milk fever.[1] Pregnant animals in selenium-deficient areas should receive dietary supplementation or vitamin E and selenium injections during the final months of pregnancy. A complete, loose, trace mineralized salt containing selenium should be offered free choice year-round to all goats. Salt and/or mineral blocks designed for cattle may not be suitable for goats, particularly in deficient areas or for growing or lactating goats.

Proper feeding of colostrum is crucial to the health and survival of the kid. Properly treated, slow-pasteurized colostrum should be used in dairy herds for CAEV control. If goat colostrum is not available, heat-activated cattle colostrum can be used. A creep feeding starter ration and good-quality hay should be provided to kids from the first week of life to promote rumen development. Adult bucks and wethers should be fed a ration similar to one that is appropriate for nonpregnant, nonlactating does. Bucks should be on urinary calculi prevention programs. Body condition scores can be used to monitor the long-term energy intake of goats. Because of their curiosity and browsing habits, goats are exposed to toxic plants but are not likely to eat fatal quantities of any given plant. However, when feed supply is scarce, they are at risk of toxicity. Also, confined goats may be at higher risk of consuming anything within their reach, including toxic plants.

Production Management

In dairy goat operations the monitoring of milk and udder health is an important aspect of production management. Complete animal records are important for both dairy and fiber-producing goat operations. Records can be kept on individual animals by a card file or computer system. Dairy Herd Improvement Association (DHIA) records should be kept for dairy goats, both for individual animals and the herd as a whole. Animal identification is imperative if individual animal records are to be kept. Dairy goats are usually identified by neck tags and/or ear tattoos. Plastic ear tags are more commonly used in meat goats.

Facilities

The most important aspect of facility management for most types of goats is fencing. The two goals of a fence are to keep goats in and predators out. Both of these goals are very difficult. A 6- by 12-inch woven wire, 48-inch tall fence is the most suitable perimeter fencing for horned goats. Electric fencing also can be used for the perimeter or for cross-fences. Ease of handling requires the use of working pens. Furthermore, goats require some shelter from inclement weather, especially at or around kidding or after shearing (especially for Angora goats). Shelters provide shade in summer and protect animals from wind, rain, and snow in winter. Goats tolerate cold weather rather well as long as they are dry and can move out of the wind.

Feeders are necessary for supplemental feeding of grain or concentrates and for allowing free access to minerals. They should be constructed in such a way that goats cannot lay or defecate in them. A feeder space of 1.5 to 2 feet per adult goat will usually suffice. Goats prefer fresh, clean water and should have access to a constant supply. Predator control should never be overlooked, particularly for pastured meat or pet goats. Guard dogs (Great Pyrenees) are commonly used, but donkeys and llamas also have predator control value. These other herbivores may become goat companions (i.e., llamas, donkeys).

Goats should be separated into groups based on production status. Males should be separated from females, and females of breeding age should be maintained separately from other animals. Meat goat kids should be kept in a "grow-out" group. Stocking rates for meat goats are around six to eight adults per adult cow/calf unit. As many as 10 adult goats can be maintained on the same land required to feed a cow and her calf, if the land is predominately browse. Although many space requirements have been suggested, one of the authors (Dr. Pugh) recommends for 55- to 110-lb (25- to 100-kg) goats that a minimum of 15 square feet (if kept alone) to 11.5 square feet (if kept in groups of five or more) should be made available. Goats weighing less than 60 lb should be allowed a minimum of 10 square feet (if kept alone) or 7.5 square feet (if kept in groups of five or more), whereas goats weighing more than 50 lb should have 20 square feet of space (if kept alone) or 15 square feet (if kept in groups of five or more). Overstocking predisposes the herd to losses from parasites, poor pasture forage production, and greater production costs. Pasture rotation is essential for the profitable farm.

Unproductive animals should be identified and culled. Does that fail to conceive, fail to carry their kids to birth, or fail to raise kids to weaning and those that produce kids with genetically undesirable traits should be culled. Any buck that fails to aggressively seek out and breed females should be culled. Herd improvement can be accomplished by focusing on increasing kidding percentage and rate of growth.

Finally, biosecurity is at the heart of a herd health program. Denying disease-causing organisms access to the herd is more economical than attempts at elimination. Biosecurity can be achieved by buying goats from herds free of contagious disease, performing pre-purchase examinations, testing for disease, instituting on-farm quarantine for a minimum of 30 days, retesting during quarantine, providing treatment with antibacterial agents and anthelmintics to address subclinical carrier states, and immunizing incoming goats against certain diseases.[2] Excellent immunity should be maintained in the nucleus herd by routine vaccination, deworming, and proper dietary intake in case of a breakdown in biosecurity.

Reproductive Management

Efficient reproductive management is essential to the profitability of a goat enterprise. Reproductive management of goats in the United States has focused primarily on milk and fiber production systems. However, the introduction of exotic meat goat breeds (South African Boer, New Zealand Kiko) is encouraging a greater emphasis on reproductive management to increase the number of offspring born and weaned.[13] The production of out-of-season kids and milk is desirable to take advantage of market premiums. Goats are seasonally polyestrous, but some degree of breed-specific variation does exist. The natural breeding season is August through March in North America. However, the peak breeding season of October through December results in kidding in January through March. The transition periods are approximately 2 months before and after the breeding season. The "deepest" anestrous period is April through May.[13]

Dairy goats are generally not expected to kid more than once per year because of selection for 10 months of lactation. They frequently have numerous offspring and low neonatal mortality because of the intense rearing practices under which they are kept.[7] Selective hand-mating or artificial insemination is the usual breeding practice in dairy goats.

Goals for reproductive efficiency in meat goats include high fertility (greater than 90%), optimal litter size (1.5 to 2 kids), high survival to weaning (more than 90%), and kidding intervals of less than 12 months. Establishing the time of mating marks the commencement of the annual production cycle. It can be calculated based on the desired date of parturition in a given region to take advantage of good spring pasture. The bucks should be left with does for 32 days (one and a half reproductive cycles), resulting in kids being born within a month. This short kidding period should produce a uniform kid crop and streamline weaning and other herd health management practices. After 32 days with the does, the bucks' job is finished for the year. Pregnancy diagnosis 45 to 60 days after buck removal is an important component of reproductive management.

Controlled accelerated kidding programs (three kid crops every 2 years) require out-of-season breeding. Proper nutrition, intense management, early weaning, and some hormonal manipulation are required for such programs to be successful. If enhanced production is the aim of the breeding program, at least 20% of the breeding females should be replaced annually. The kidding percentage can be increased by retaining female replacements that are twins and the daughters of twins. Selection of highly fertile males also contributes to the attainment of this goal.

Parasite Control

GI nematodes are the most serious problem affecting goat production worldwide.[14,15] Economic losses caused by GI nematodes are related to decreased production, costs for treatment and prophylaxis, and animal death. Effective control of internal parasites of goats is one of the most difficult challenges facing the veterinary practitioner. The major GI nematode of fiber and meat goats is *Haemonchus contortus* (barber's pole worm).[7,16,17] In dairy goats, several other GI nematodes such as *Ostertagia, Trichostrongylus,* and *Nematodirus* species may significant in certain geographic areas.[7,14] In addition to *Haemonchus* infestation, coccidiosis can be a major problem in recently weaned meat and dairy kids.[17] GI nematodes have similar life cycles. *Haemonchus* thrives in warm, moist conditions. The survival time of the infective stage is short during hot summers (30 to 60 days) and prolonged during the winter (4 to 8 months).[17] The degree of infestation varies with the management system employed. Goats kept in dry lots (e.g., dairy goats) may have minimal problems with GI nematodes. Kids grazing on range land pastures seem to be less affected by coccidiosis, but in confined quarters they are very susceptible to infestation. Meat goats grazing land with adequate brush and tall weeds suffer little exposure to infective parasitic larvae. These browsing goats develop little immunity and are highly susceptible to infection if they then graze infested pastures. Parasite infestation may be insignificant in dry years and in certain range land areas. Parasites are a continual problem in moist, temperate areas.[7] *Haemonchus* has the ability to undergo hypobiosis, or become metabolically inactive, within the host during adverse weather conditions.[17] This dormancy results in better parasite survival and increased transmission from spring to fall. Implementation of a control program for GI parasites of goats requires a working knowledge of the important parts of their life cycle.

Prevention, rather than cure, is the philosophy used in developing control programs against GI nematodes. It must be assumed that "worms" cannot be eradicated but may be limited to the point where they do not cause serious economic loss to the producer.[16,17] A combination of management and treatment is necessary to achieve control. Feeding practices that decrease stocking rates and lessen pasture contamination help minimize parasite infestation. Drought, inclement weather, and lack of adequate forage (or pasture) may increase animal concentration and encourage parasitism. Therefore, when animals are fed supplemental feeds, owners should take care to minimize the intake of nematode larvae. Feeders that minimize fecal contamination of feedstuffs should be used. Feed should never be placed on the ground.[14] Goats flock together and tend to bed down in the same place nightly. This allows a heavy parasite population to develop in concentrated areas. Several approaches for the use of anthelmintics in control regimens are summarized in Box 17-2.

Few dewormers are approved for goats in the United States, but extra-label use of anthelmintics designed for cattle is not uncommon.[18] Dewormers and coccidiostats used in goats are listed in Tables 17-1 and 17-2, respectively. Anthelmintics should only be administered orally to goats. Clinicians and owners should keep in mind that anthelmintics may be metabolized at different rates by goats than by cattle or sheep. Unless a dose has been established for goats, the animals should generally receive a dose 1.5 times larger than that given to sheep.[16] Effective anthelmintics should only be used for approximately 1 year before rotation to another class of dewormer. Because of the increasing resistance of parasites to anthelmintics, goats must be examined after deworming so clinicians and owners can determine whether the drugs

BOX 17-2

A SUMMARY RECOMMENDATION FOR PARASITE CONTROL*

1. Make certain that the anthelmintic or combination of anthelmintics used on the farm actually works (kills at least 90% of the variable worms). Check for resistance with fecal egg counts before and after deworming.
2. Use strategic deworming. Deworm the flock while the parasites are in hypobiosis and are being transmitted at low levels (i.e., the winter). This reduces the frequency of exposure to deworming products.
3. Employ pre- and post-birthing deworming starting 1 month before birthing at 2- to 4-week intervals and ending 2 to 4 weeks after the final lamb or kid is born.
4. Tactical dewormings (based on increased levels of parasite eggs or 10 to 14 days after rainfall) enhance the effectiveness of a parasite program.
5. Use clean or safe pastures when possible: the aftermath of crops, annual forage, and rotational grazing or co-grazing with cattle or horses. Permanent Pastures Promote Parasites.
6. Deworm new animals and place them in a non-pasture environment such as a dry lot or barn after treatment for as long as 72 hours before moving them to a safe pasture.
7. Rotate anthelmintics yearly if effective drugs are available.
8. Do not under-dose animals. Dose for the heaviest animal in a group.
9. Identify and select individuals resistant to internal parasites.

*The reader is encouraged to review more in-depth recommendations in Chapter 4.

used are effective. This can be accomplished by a fecal egg count reduction test. Fecal samples are collected on the day of deworming and 10 to 14 days later. McMaster's floatation (see Chapter 3) is performed on both samples, and the numbers of parasite eggs per gram (EPG) are compared. If the drop in EPG is less than 90%, anthelmintic resistance is present and the animals should be switched to another class of dewormer.[16] Assessment of fecal egg count is a valuable tool for parasite control programs in goats. A McMaster's EPG count of 500 to 1000 in the spring or early summer or more than 2000 in the fall suggests serious infection. Regular egg counts help the veterinarian determine when animals are to be dewormed. Perhaps the most overlooked component of a

BOX 17-3

Generic Management Calendar for Spring Kidding and Lambing

January
Evaluate range and forage conditions; monitor body condition of does and ewes and supplement if necessary; ensure adequate intake of minerals, salt, and water; vaccinate during the final month of gestation for clostridial disease and any other endemic diseases.

February
Begin supplemental feeding of pregnant females and consider pre-birthing shearing; begin birthing; check teats for milk and identify lambs and kids; ensure lambs and kids ingest adequate colostrum; institute pre- and post- birthing strategic deworming; maintain an ionophore in feed or mineral mixture before and after birthing to decrease *Coccidia* contamination of pasture.

March
Separate singles from twins; confine and feed females with their lambs and kids as needed; feed does and ewes to maintain milk production; continue strategic deworming program.

April
Continue to feed a supplement to lactating does and ewes; monitor for parasites.

May
Wean small, stunted lambs and kids; discontinue supplemental feeding of does and ewes; monitor internal parasites (with fecal samples and McMaster's).

June
Continue parasite control program.

July
Monitor internal parasites; watch for signs of heat stress; wean lambs and kids.

August
Continue parasite control program; continue weaning lambs and kids and supplement replacement does, ewes, bucks, and rams; select replacement males and females; evaluate and cull unsound and inferior animals; perform breeding soundness evaluation of males. Criteria for culling include the following:
- Poor or slow growth
- Barren females (missed one season)
- Unsound teats or udders (too big or too small)
- Poor dentition
- Structural defects (feet, leg, or back abnormalities)
- Testicles that are small or soft or have other abnormalities (animal fails a breeding soundness evaluation)
- Unthriftiness (caused by old age or chronic disease)

September
Begin supplemental feeding of females and males on fresh green pasture with ½ lb feed/head/day for 2 to 3 weeks before and after males are placed with females; continue parasite control program.

October
Begin breeding; maintain good male-to-female ratio, depending on pasture size and conditions; continue supplemental feeding of females for 2 to 3 weeks after start of breeding season.

November
Evaluate range and forage conditions; determine females' body condition and plan winter supplemental and feeding program; control internal and external parasites; remove some of males' feed to regain body condition; determine pregnancy status and number of fetuses.

December
Watch body condition of does and supplement feed if needed; monitor internal and external parasites.

TABLE 17-1

ANTHELMINTIC PRODUCTS AND DOSAGES*

ACTIVE AGENT	DOSAGE	ROUTE
Albendazole	10 mg/kg	PO
Doramectin	0.3 mg/kg	PO
Eprinomectin	0.5 mg/kg	PO
Fenbendazole	10 mg/kg	PO
Ivermectin	0.3 mg/kg	PO
Levamisole	8 mg/kg	PO
Morantel tartrate	10 mg/kg	PO
Moxidectin	0.5 mg/kg	PO
Oxfendazole	10 mg/kg	PO

*See also Appendix I.

TABLE 17-2

COCCIDIOSTATS FOR USE IN GOATS FOR HERD PROBLEMS

CHEMICAL NAME	TRADE NAME	DOSE
Amprolium*	Corid	42 g/100 gallon water
Monensin†	Rumensin	15 to 20 g/ton of feed
Lasalocid	Bovatec	25 g/ton of feed
Decoquinate†	Decox	27 g/ton of feed

*Do not use for more than 28 days.
†Approved for use in goats in the United States.

well-managed parasite control program is the identification and selection of parasite-resistant goats or at least animals that are apparently less susceptible. Individuals with the lowest EPG in a herd may have the most resistance.[16] A generic herd health program is provided in Box 17-3.

REFERENCES

1. Smith MC, Sherman DM: *Goat medicine,* Philadelphia, 1994, Lea & Febiger.
2. Olcott BM: Production medicine and health problems in goats. In Howard JL, Smith B, editors: *Current veterinary therapy in food animal practice,* ed 4, Philadelphia, 1999, WB Saunders.
3. Mobini S: Herd health management practices for goats, *Vet Tech J* 16:238, 1995.
4. Pugh D: Small ruminant medicine and nutrition, *Proceedings of the Southern Georgia Veterinary Medical Association,* 1999, Fort Valley, GA.
5. Mobini S: Herd health management practices for meat goat production, *Proceedings of the Southeast Region Meat and Goat Producers Symposium,* 1996, Tallahassee, FL.
6. Rings DM: Basic neonatology, *Proceedings of the American Veterinary Medicine Association,* 1999, New Orleans, LA.
7. Bretzlaf K: Production medicine and health programs for goats. In Howard JL, editor: *Current veterinary therapy in food animal practice,* ed 3, Philadelphia, 1993, WB Saunders.
8. East NE: Vaccination programs for sheep and goats. In Smith BP, editor: *Large animal internal medicine,* ed 2, St Louis, 1996, Mosby.
9. Council on Biologies and Therapeutic Agents: Vaccination guidelines for small ruminants, *J Am Vet Med Assoc* 205:539, 1994.
10. Mobini S: Infectious causes of abortion in the goat. In Youngquist B, editor: *Current therapy in large animal theriogenology,* Philadelphia, 1997, WB Saunders.
11. Wiedmann M et al: Molecular investigation of a listeriosis outbreak in goats caused by an unusual strain of *Listeria monocytogenes, J Am Vet Med Assoc* 215:369, 1999.
12. Terrill T: Grazing habits and diet selection of goats, *Proceedings of the Symposium on Meat Production from Goats in Georgia,* 1998, Fort Valley, GA.
13. Mobini S: Reproductive management in goats, *Proceedings of the North American Veterinary Conference,* 2000, Orlando, FL.
14. Pugh DG, Mobini S, Hilton CD: Control programs for gastrointestinal parasites in sheep and goats, *Comp Cont Ed Pract Vet,* 20(4):S112, 1998.
15. Miller JE: Parasites affecting goats in the Southeast, *Proceedings of the Conference on Goat Production Market Opportunity South,* 1995, Baton Rouge, LA.
16. Craig TM: Control of gastrointestinal nematodes of sheep and goats in North America, *Proceedings of the American Association of Small Ruminant Practitioners Symposium on the Health and Disease of Small Ruminants,* 1996, Nashville, TN.
17. Craig TM: Goats—condominiums for parasites: What should a producer do?, *Proceedings of the Fourteenth Annual Goat Field Day,* 1999, Langston, OK.
18. Mobini S: Practice tips related to medications in goats, *Proceedings of the North American Veterinary Conference,* 2000, Orlando, FL.

SHEEP

Many of the herd health protocols and basic ideas discussed in the section on goats are applicable for sheep flock health. Each chapter of this book also describes health care practices that are applicable for sheep. Therefore the following section is an abbreviated discussion of flock health. A generic herd and flock health program is provided in Box 17-3.

Definition of Flock Health

Flock health programs target the production groups and needs present in an operation throughout the year. Although flock health programs focus on populations of animals, the needs of individual sheep are not intentionally ignored. Instead, they are better addressed through proactive approaches. Because the demands of various stages of production are anticipated and addressed, the sheep are better off than those in a flock that does not have a well-timed and well-thought-out health program in place. The aim of a flock health program is to improve the overall health and welfare of the flock, including decreasing losses from disease. Successful programs increase both the productivity and the profitability of the flock. The use and analysis of production, health, and financial records are the best ways to gauge the success of the program. Flock health programs vary in their intensity because different breeds of sheep, production levels, and environments dictate different approaches. Regardless of the approach used, flock health programs should include a written component that addresses the whole year at a time.

Flock health programs are developed for multiple uses. They may be used by an individual operation or incorporated into operations for the control and eradication of specific diseases either by voluntary or mandatory cooperation with state and federal animal health officials. Programs used by individual operators are generally planned annual approaches that address the following:

- Prevention of common disease conditions through the use of appropriate vaccination schedules
- Management strategies that minimize risk factors for disease occurrence
- Provision of appropriate levels of nutrition for the stage of production
- Assessment of metabolic status and productivity

In order to provide correct advice the veterinarian must have a sound knowledge base regarding the sheep industry and the individual production system. The client and veterinarian should work out the details of a record-keeping system.

Veterinary visits are usually timed to occur with major production events (e.g., before breeding; in mid-pregnancy; before, during, and after lambing; in mid-summer). During the first visit the veterinarian assigns a body condition score to the ewe flock. He or she then makes nutritional and feeding management recommendations to optimize the ovulation rate at breeding. Evaluation of the rams should include a physical and fertility examination (see Chapter 6). A written record should indicate the ram's body condition score and weight, problems identified on the physical examination, an action plan to address any problems that are crucial to breeding, and whether the ram passed or failed the fertility examination. The mid-pregnancy visit primarily focuses on ultrasound pregnancy determination and fetal counting and aging. Based on these results the veterinarian can develop a plan to feed the ewes appropriately and economically based on fetal numbers and stage of pregnancy. This visit can be crucial in preventing metabolic disease in late pregnancy and assisting the farmer in making the operation profitable. The pre-lambing visit entails a review of the nutrition of the late-gestation ewe so that she can perform up to her genetic potential at lambing. Properly fed ewes produce maximal amounts of colostrum and milk, give birth to thrifty lambs without difficulty, and demonstrate excellent mothering abilities. The final 2 months of pregnancy are crucial to successful lamb rearing. During this visit the veterinarian can review strategies to prevent disease such as vaccinating against clostridial diseases 4 weeks before lambing and providing a clean environment. The management plan at lambing time, including the layout and use of facilities, also should be reviewed. This plan should include a component to educate personnel to recognize when intervention is needed for lambing problems.

Minimum standards and target production parameters for morbidity, mortality, culling, and growth rates should be set. Box 17-4 provides a list of target production parameters. At this time a quality assurance program should be designed for the flock. To date, the sheep-packing industry has not required producers to participate in flock quality assurance programs, but such programs exist and will become more common in the future as a result of consumer demand. Quality assurance programs educate producers in good production practices. They encourage cooperation between practitioners and area producers for the betterment of the operation and the sheep.

Biosecurity Aspects of Flock Health Programs

Biosecurity programs are geared to control infectious disease. They include management steps to reduce the likelihood of introduction of a new disease from an external source. Another benefit of a biosecurity program is that it reduces the spread of infectious disease already present in the flock. Scientifically sound approaches regarding the introduction of new sheep into a flock are required to prevent the introduction of new diseases into the resident sheep population. Practical biosecurity programs include purchasing animals directly from the farm of origin, transporting them in clean and disinfected transport vehicles, housing them in true isolation facilities while following practical isolation practices for 1 month, and regularly observing for conditions such as pruritus, lameness, external lumps, and unexplained weight loss. In addition, isolated sheep should be started

---

BOX 17-4

Production Targets

Pregnancy	
Ewes	More than 95%
Ewe lambs	More than 75%
Visible abortion	Less than 5%
Lambing	
Ewes	More than 90%
Ewe lambs	More than 70%
Stillbirths	Less than 2%
Weaning	More than 95%

on the flock's regular vaccination program, dewormed with an effective anthelmintic, and have their feet trimmed and visually inspected for footrot. Even before performing a visual examination and obtaining the history of the flock of origin, the producer or clinician may wish to give them a foot bath for 15 minutes in a 10% solution of zinc sulfate. During isolation the sheep may be serologically tested for diseases of concern to the buyer. If the sheep were tested for various diseases before purchase, the buyer should request the official test forms and results to check the results and test dates. Wherever practical, sheep should be thoroughly examined for obvious clinical manifestations of contagious or infectious diseases such as sore mouth, pinkeye, external parasites, caseous lymphadenitis, scrapie, footrot, strawberry footrot, and dermatophilosis.

Vaccination Programs

Through regular and correct usage, vaccines are designed to reduce the incidence and/or severity of a specific disease. Few vaccines can completely prevent disease. However, when used properly, their beneficial effects far outweigh their drawbacks. Local veterinarians can provide advice on prevalent diseases that are preventable by vaccination. Farms in different areas have different needs. The local veterinarian should work with the producer to design a farm-specific vaccination program for ewes, young lambs, market or feedlot lambs, replacement breeding stock, and rams. His or her knowledge of prevalent diseases in the area and diagnostic laboratory data are the best bases for developing a vaccination program. Vaccination should proceed according to label directions because the timing of doses is crucial to optimal protection.

Clostridial diseases are the only universal group of diseases that all sheep should be vaccinated against. Decisions regarding the inclusion of other vaccines in an individual flock health program should be based on knowledge of prevalent diseases in the area and the needs of the particular flock. In areas where a disease is known to occur but no vaccine is available, risk factors for that disease should be controlled with proper management. Sheep that are frequently exhibited are at greater risk of contracting contagious and infectious diseases. For this reason they should be vaccinated against more diseases than sheep in a closed flock.

Other diseases that have a labeled sheep vaccine available in the United States include some infectious causes of abortion such as *Campylobacter* species and *Chlamydia psittaci;* multisystemic diseases such as caseous lymphadenitis, musculoskeletal diseases such as footrot, neurologic diseases such as rabies, and integumentary diseases such as sore mouth. If past history indicates that the flock is at risk of a disease, such vaccines can be included in an immunization program. A generic vaccination program for sheep is provided in Box 17-5. It can be modified for the individual farm.

Internal Parasite Control Programs

Programs that control internal parasites must be tailored to the region of the country where the flock resides. The program also must take into account whether the flock is confined or pastured. The epidemiology of pathogenic sheep nematodes and protozoan species depends on the climate of the region. Successful programs implement regular monitoring of the efficacy of anthelmintics, sheep-friendly handling equipment for anthelmintic delivery such as well-designed pens and chutes, and use of automatic syringes and/or drench guns. Other components of a parasite control program include the use of

---

BOX 17-5

BASIC VACCINATION PROGRAM FOR SHEEP

PREGNANT EWES
- In endemic areas, vaccinate ewe lambs or previously vaccinated animals against *Campylobacter* and *Chlamydia* abortion in midgestation.
- Vaccinate for *Clostridium* species (*C. perfringens* type C and D, *C. novyi, C. sordelli, C. chauvoei, C. septicum, C. tetani*) in the last month of pregnancy.
- Repeat *Chlamydia* and *Campylobacter* vaccinations for previously unvaccinated animals and give yearly booster to other ewes 2 to 4 weeks after birth.

LAMBS
- Immunize lambs from immunized dams at 1 to 2 months for *Clostridium* species (*C. perfringens* type C and D, *C. novyi, C. sordelli, C. chauvoei, C. septicum, C. tetani*); repeat immunizations in 3 to 4 weeks.
- Immunize lambs from nonimmunized dams at 1 to 3 weeks for *Clostridium* species (*C. perfringens* type C and D, *C. novyi, C. sordelli, C. chauvoei, C. septicum, C. tetani*); repeat immunizations twice at 3- to 4-week intervals.

Rams and yearlings can be vaccinated at the same time as ewes, with an emphasis on *Clostridium* species. Vaccines against rabies and leptospirosis may be given in endemic areas.

multiple measures to minimize the buildup of nematode eggs on pasture; this can be achieved by deworming ewes with larvicidal doses during winter housing, 4 weeks after spring turn-out, and 3 weeks into lambing. Control also is enhanced by the use of management practices that reduce reliance on chemical anthelmintics such as grazing *clean* ground with weaned lambs, "vacuuming" nematode eggs by grazing the previous year's sheep pastures with cows or horses, and selecting for and breeding nematode-resistant sheep (see Chapter 4).

When circumstances dictate that the flock graze close to the ground and nutritional input is marginal, nematode infestation may accelerate and clinical parasitism in stressed sheep is likely. The veterinarian and producer should develop an annual calendar that details the entire flock health program. The producer should record details about any procedures performed on the production groups. Box 17-2 summarizes recommendations to improve parasite control. Tables 17-1 and 17-2 show some commonly used anthelmintics and coccidiostats, respectively.

External Parasite Control Programs

Keds and biting lice are the prevalent external parasites of sheep. Many sheep flocks have not introduced these parasites. In these flocks, all newly purchased sheep should be treated prophylactically while they are in isolation to prevent parasite introduction. In flocks where either parasite is endemic, all sheep on the property should be treated at the same time so that one group does not serve as a reservoir for reintroduction. Treated sheep should be kept out of any contaminated buildings for 2 weeks because buildings also can serve as reservoirs during this time. Further treatments should not be necessary after the whole flock is properly treated. The flock should be monitored for ectoparasite infestation after reintroduction from carrier sheep or improperly applied whole flock treatment. An external parasite control program is described in Chapter 8.

Flock Health Monitoring

Program records should include a flock inventory divided into production groups:

- Ram-to-ewe ratios at breeding
- Pregnancy rates
- Lambing percentages
- Ewe and ram mortality numbers and reasons
- Pre- and post-weaning lamb mortality rates and reasons
- Ram morbidity and treatment outcomes (especially those that pertain to breeding use)

The average body condition score of the ewe flock should be recorded at breeding, lambing, and weaning (see Chapter 2). If target scores are not achieved, the producer and veterinarian need to determine why and make appropriate management changes. If the correct changes are implemented, future scores should reflect improved production.

If mortality rates exceed targets, representative sheep should be necropsied. Gross findings can be clarified by ancillary laboratory-based tests, if necessary. Fortunately, common sheep diseases that affect production are often straightforward to diagnose based on gross necropsy findings.

Culling Practices

Culling practices should be based on genetics, productivity, poor fertility, substandard growth, parasite and disease susceptibility, and disease (e.g., footrot, caseous lymphadenitis, scrapie, ovine progressive pneumonia). Not all sick or thin animals survive to the point of culling. Each operation must have a plan for carcass disposal. Carcass disposal procedures should be legal in the area and state, environmentally friendly for the size of the animal and number of carcasses, and practical for the producer. Many states legally permit sheep composting (Box 17-6). A sheep of any size will turn into compost if the procedure is done correctly. Sheep composting fulfills the previously described criteria. Some diseased carcasses may by law require incineration (e.g., scrapie, foot-and-mouth disease).

Neonatal Care

The phrase "sip, dip, strip, and clip" regarding management of the newborn lamb is sound advice for beginning and advanced clinicians and owners alike. A practitioner should **strip** the wax plug from the teat so the lamb can **sip** colostrum, as well as **clip** and **dip** the umbilicus in 7% iodine or another antiseptic or astringent (e.g., solutions of chlorhexidine, povidone iodine). Owners and practitioners should be able to recognize normal maternal and neonatal behavior as well as normal appearing and functioning mammary glands. The recognition of normal traits and conditions allows abnormal ones to be detected and dealt with appropriately. Equipment and facilities should be prepared and organized before the start of lambing. Records to guide improvements in management should be kept and used. Regardless of whether animals are raised in confinement or on pasture, periparturient ewes should be grouped together based on expected lambing dates and fetal numbers, if available. These groupings enable tailored levels of feeding, which are economically justifiable, minimize the occurrence of metabolic disease, and prevent fetal under- or over-nutrition. The result is the birth of more viable lambs. When lamb losses occur, representative cases should be necropsied by the local veterinarian and management changes should be based on the necropsy findings.

Sheep or Goat Composting

- A 5- to 10-square foot enclosure or container makes a good composter. The sides (e.g., corrugated wire, fine wire mesh) should have enough holes to allow for maximal airflow during the composting process.
- The composter should be placed separate from the flock but in an area where water is easily attainable to keep the composted material moist. All runoff should be kept out of the flock's water supply.
- The carcass, aborted material, or offal should be placed in the composter so 1 foot of sawdust separates it from the ground and the sides. The carcass should then be covered with 1 to 1.5 feet of sawdust. Approximately 1 cubic foot of sawdust is required for every 10 lb of carcass weight. Green or freshly cut sawdust is superior for composting.
- Water should be added to attain a water-to-dry matter ratio between 50:50 and 60:40. During very rainy seasons, the composter should be covered to prevent excessive water accumulation.
- A 2- to 4-foot-long thermometer should be placed into the stack and the temperature monitored. The temperature should be maintained at 130° F for 1 week to destroy most pathogenic bacteria. If the composter's temperature drops below 100° F, water should be added and the material aerated (i.e., stirred, forked).
- The material can be safely placed on the pasture after 21 to 30 weeks. However, in the case of animals dying of scrapie, the owner should notify local, state, or federal authorities and follow their guidelines (e.g., incineration).

Adapted from Estienne MJ: Disposing of dead goats, *Practical Goat Farming Seminar*, 1998, Salisbury, MD (http://www.sheepandgoat.com/compost.html).

Shearing Management

Shearing is the most stressful experience for a sheep. The handling set-up should be designed so that handling stress is minimized. Many preventive health procedures are often performed at shearing. These include pre-lambing vaccination against clostridial diseases, especially *C. perfringens* type C and D and *C. tetani*. Ewes should be vaccinated against colibacillosis (where used) approximately 30 days before lambing on farms where previous neonatal lamb diarrhea cases are known or suspected to be caused by pathogenic *E. coli*. Other procedures frequently performed at shearing include sorting out noncompetitive sheep or those with abscesses or mastitis, foot trimming, and deworming. All procedures need to be considerate of the sheep and the shearers. Freshly trimmed feet can lacerate a shearer if the sheep kicks. The owner should be encouraged to be present at shearing, listen to the shearers' observations, and consider this information in conjunction with other professional opinions. Pre-lambing shearing of ewes may decrease the incidence of pregnancy toxemia, improve the desire of the ewe to seek shelter on cold days (with the resultant moving of lambs to warm, dry environments), decrease the maintenance requirements of the ewe (because of less fleece weight), and enhance the likelihood that newborns will nurse the udder instead of the ewes' wool.

Most small flock facilities lack a permanent shearing set-up. Therefore many shearers shear on sheets of plywood or pieces of indoor/outdoor carpet that they carry in their trucks and use every day on numerous farms. Owners should provide their own shearing surfaces instead of using surfaces that have been on many farms and can transmit bacteria, fungi, and even viruses.

Foot Care

Part of the annual care of sheep should include assessment of the condition and length of their hooves. Depending on the terrain and rainfall in the area, some flocks do not require annual foot trimming, but most flocks in the Midwestern and eastern regions of the United States do. The timing of this procedure is not important as long as the feet are not allowed to grow long and predispose the animals to other foot problems such as toe abscesses and footrot. Many farm flocks trim the ewes' feet around lambing time while they are in confinement and being handled regularly. Many range flocks only require foot trimming of a few individual animals. Many sheep wear their feet down adequately on dry, rough terrain, and some breeds are predisposed to slower foot growth. Rams should have their feet trimmed 4 to 8 weeks before breeding. Their feet should definitely not be trimmed in the week before the start of breeding in case overzealous trimming causes temporary lameness. A generic footrot prevention program is provided in Box 9-1.

Facility Design and Function

Sheep housing should be designed and constructed for proper ventilation and efficient manure handling.

Water Availability and Design

Water is an essential nutrient of all ages of sheep. It should be palatable and readily available. Cleanliness, taste, impurities, and temperature all affect palatability. Key times during which the quality of the water supply has a direct influence on the productivity or health of the sheep include the lambing and finishing phase, late pregnancy, and lactation (see Chapter 2).

Role of Management in Maintaining Health

The level of management determines the success and sustainability of a farming operation. Excellent managers make most decisions correctly relative to the care of their flock. Accordingly, the flock responds by meeting target production goals. In today's economic environment, sound management decisions are based on a combination of records and observational subjective findings.

Specific Diseases Introduced by Carrier Sheep

Sheep can carry and introduce into a flock a number of diseases that are not visible to the naked eye. These disease conditions include footrot, chlamydia, campylobacteriosis, and anthelmintic-resistant nematode infestation. In general, tests for these diseases do not exist or are not financially feasible for whole flocks. Therefore all animals introduced into the flock should undergo a complete physical examination and be quarantined from the rest of the flock for 21 to 30 days to minimize the introduction of new diseases.

Commonly Used Drugs in Sheep and Goats: Suggested Dosages*

VIRGINIA R. FAJT AND D.G. PUGH

DRUG	SHEEP	GOATS
Acepromazine maleate (see Chapter 16, Tables 16-1 and 16-2	0.03 to 0.05 mg/kg IV[1] 0.05 to 0.10 mg/kg IM[1]	0.03 to 0.1 mg/kg IV[1,2] 0.05 to 0.1 mg/kg IM[1] 0.2 mg/kg IM for tetany[2]
Acetic acid (5% solution)	0.5 to 1.0 L/head PO for ammonia toxicosis[3]	
Albendazole	5 mg/kg PO for nematodes and tapeworms[4] 7.5 mg/kg PO for flukes[4] 10 mg/kg PO for cestodes[5]	7.5 mg/kg PO[6]
Ammonium chloride	0.5% of diet for prevention of urinary calculi[7] 100 to 200 mg/kg PO BID to prevent urolithiasis[8]	
Ammonium molybdate	100 mg/head/day PO to prevent copper toxicity[9] 20 mg/L in sole source of drinking water to prevent copper toxicity[9] 100 mg/head/day PO for copper toxicity[10]	
Ammonium tetrathiomolybdate	3.4 mg/kg SC for 5 days to treat copper toxicity[9] 50 to 100 mg/head PO twice weekly[10]	

*Some of the drugs and uses listed in this appendix may be illegal, unavailable, or extra-label in the United States or other countries. It is the responsibility of attending veterinarians to be familiar with the laws governing drugs in their practice areas. The clinician should be cognizant of and take steps to reduce drug residues in food animals.

SC, subcutaneously; *IM,* intramuscularly; *IV,* intravenously; *IP,* intraperitoneally; *PO,* per os (orally); *IU,* international units; *BID,* twice a day; *TID,* three times a day.

When no dosage was available for sheep or goats, a general "ruminant dose" was provided if available. If a dose is provided only for sheep and not for goats, unless the drug appears to be contraindicated or toxic to goats, one of the authors (Dr. Pugh) usually extrapolates the sheep dose for use in goats, or vice versa. Some of the anesthetic dosages listed here are the same as seen in Chapter 16 and are referenced as such. For anesthetics that have different dosages, the clinician may choose to review the dosages listed in Chapter 16 and compare the two.

Continued

DRUG	SHEEP	GOATS
Amoxicillin–clavulanic acid	20 mg/kg IM or IV TID[4]	20 mg/kg IM or IV TID[4]
Amoxicillin trihydrate	10 mg/kg IM TID[11]	10 mg/kg IM TID[11]
Ampicillin sodium	10 to 20 mg/kg IV or IM BID[11]	10 to 20 mg/kg IV or IM BID[11]
Ampicillin-sulbactam	10 mg/kg IM every 12 to 24 hrs[11]	10 mg/kg IM every 12 to 24 hrs[11]
Amprolium	10 to 60 mg/kg orally in water or feed once a day for 14 to 21 days to treat coccidiosis in lambs[12]	25 to 40 mg/kg PO daily for 5 days for treatment; 5 mg/kg daily PO for 21 days for prevention[14]
	100 to 200 ppm or 10 mg/kg/day in water for 5 days for coccidiosis[13]	
	25 to 40 mg/kg PO daily for 5 days for treatment; 5 mg/kg daily PO for 21 days for prevention[14]	
Antivenin polyvalent	10 to 200 ml IV[15]	
Aspirin		100 mg/kg PO BID[2]
Atipamezole (see Chapter 16, Table 16-3)	0.125 to 0.2 mg/kg IV slowly	0.125 to 0.2 mg/kg IV slowly
Atropine (see Chapter 16, Table 16-2)	0.06 to 0.10 mg/kg IV to prevent bradycardia during anesthesia[16]	0.02 to 0.1 mg/kg IV to prevent bradycardia during anesthesia[2,16]
	0.25 to 0.50 mg/kg (one fourth IV, then rest IM or SC) for organophosphate poisoning[17]	0.25 to 0.50 mg/kg (one fourth IV, then rest IM or SC) for organophosphate poisoning[17]
Boldenone undecylenate	50 to 100 mg IM once (or repeat treatment in 3 weeks) for adjunctive therapy of anemia[18]	50 to 100 mg IM once (or repeat treatment in 3 weeks) for adjunctive therapy of anemia[18]
Buprenorphine	6 μg/kg IV for 4 to 8 hours of pain relief[1]	
Butorphanol	0.05 to 0.50 mg/kg IM for sedation and analgesia[16]	0.05 to 0.50 mg/kg IM for sedation and analgesia[16]
Calcium borogluconate	50 ml of 20 mg calcium/ml solution IV, 50 ml SC to treat hypocalcemia[19]	60 to 100 ml of 20% to 25% solution for hypocalcemia[2]
	100 ml of 20% solution IV to treat acute oxalate poisoning[9]	
Calcium gluconate		1 g calcium ions/45 kg (50 to 100 ml of 10% to 23% calcium ion solution) IV for hypocalcemia[20]
Carprofen	4 mg/kg SC for postoperative analgesia[1]	
Ceftiofur sodium	1.0 to 2.2 mg/kg IM every 24 hours[11]	1.0 to 2.2 mg/kg IM every 24 hours[11]
Charcoal (activated)	0.5 kg PO for plant poisoning[21]	
	2 to 9 g/kg PO[15]	
Chloral hydrate	No specific dosage for sheep or goats is reported but 50 to 70 mg/kg IV is reported for ruminants[22]	
Chlorpromazine	0.55 to 4.4 mg/kg IV[24]	2.0 to 3.5 mg/kg IV[24]
	2.2 to 6.6 mg/kg IM[24]	
Chlortetracycline	80 mg/head/day to reduce the incidence of abortion caused by *Campylobacter fetus*[23]	
Cloprostenol	125 to 150 μg at 9- to 11-day interval for estrus synchronization[25]	125 μg for luteolysis and estrus synchronization[26]
		150 μg IM for pregnancy termination[27]
Clorsulon	7 mg/kg PO for flukes[2]	7 mg/kg PO for flukes[2]

DRUG	SHEEP	GOATS
Closantel	10 mg/kg PO for flukes and *Oestrus ovis*[4]	
Decoquinate	2 mg/kg orally throughout gestation to prevent abortion caused by *Toxoplasma gondii*[28]	0.5 mg/kg in feed for at least 28 days for coccidiosis[13]
	100 ppm in complete feed for coccidiosis control in lambs[12]	
	2 mg/kg PO during pregnancy to reduce lamb mortality from toxoplasmosis[29]	
	0.5 mg/kg in feed for at least 28 days for coccidiosis[13]	
Detomidine (see Chapter 16, Tables 16-1 and 16-2)	0.005 to 0.02 mg/kg IV for standing sedation[16]	0.005 to 0.02 mg/kg IV
	0.03 mg/kg IV for recumbency[16]	0.01 to 0.04 mg/kg IM
Dexamethasone	15 to 20 mg IV or IM to induce parturition[19,12] or to terminate pregnancy[27]	20 to 25 mg IM after 141 days for pregnancy termination[27]
	0.1 to 1 mg/kg IV or IM for inflammation[22]	0.44 mg/kg IM once as an antiinflammatory[2]
Dexamethasone sodium phosphate	1 to 2 mg/kg IV as a mediator inhibitor in circulatory shock therapy[30]	1 to 2 mg/kg IV as a mediator inhibitor in circulatory shock therapy[30]
Dextrose (glucose)	60 to 100 ml of 50% solution IV for treatment of pregnancy toxemia[19]	1 g every 4 hours IV until recovery (ketosis)[20]
	5 to 7 g IV for pregnancy toxemia[31]	
	10 ml/kg of 20% solution intraperitoneally for weak lambs[2]	
Diazepam (see Chapter 16, Tables 16-2 and 16-4)	0.5 to 2.0 mg/kg[1]	0.5 to 1.0 mg/kg IV or 2 mg/kg IM for premedication before ketamine anesthesia[2]
	0.25 to 0.50 mg/kg IV for sedation without analgesia[16]	0.04 mg/kg IV to stimulate appetite[2]
	0.25 to 0.50 mg/kg IV in combination with ketamine for induction[16]	0.25 to 0.50 mg/kg IV for sedation without analgesia[16]
		0.5 to 1.5 mg/kg IV for tetany[2]
Digoxin	In ewes, 0.025 mg/kg IV every 8 hours three times for loading dose, 0.005 to 0.015 mg/kg every 12 hours for maintenance[18]	
	In lambs, 0.04 mg/kg IV every 8 hours three times for loading dose, 0.008 to 0.025 mg/kg every 12 hours for maintenance[18]	
Dinoprost (prostaglandin $F_{2\alpha}$)	15 mg IM twice at 9- to 11-day interval for estrus synchronization[25]	2.5 to 20 mg IM for induction of parturition[32]
	5 to 10 mg IM to terminate pregnancy between days 5 and 50[27]	5 mg IM or SC for retained placenta[33]
		5 to 10 mg IM for luteolysis and estrus synchronization[6]
Dopamine	2 to 10 μg/kg/min IV drip as inotrope, 5 to 10 μg/kg/min IV drip as vasopressor[30]	2 to 10 μg/kg/min IV drip as inotrope, 5 to 10 μg/kg/min IV drip as vasopressor[30]

Continued

DRUG	SHEEP	GOATS
Doramectin	200 µg/kg SC for lungworms, *Cooperia*, and gastrointestinal parasites, 300 µg/kg SC for *Nematodirus* and psoroptic mites[4]	200 µg/kg[6] (Anecdotal reports suggest this dosage may not be clinically effective against some nematode parasites in sheep and goats and the clinician may need to increase this dosage by 1.5 to 2 times)
EDTA (calcium EDTA)	75 mg/kg IV slowly every 24 hours (may be given for the first 48 hours as divided doses every few hours) for lead poisoning[9] 55 to 90 mg/kg slowly IV or IM BID for 3 to 5 days for lead poisoning[34]	
Enrofloxacin	5 mg/kg IV or IM every 24 hours[11]	
Epinephrine (1:1000 sol)	A dosage of 0.02 to 0.03 mg/kg SC, IM, or IV for use in ruminants has been reported[22]	
Eprinomectin	0.5 mg/kg PO	0.5 mg/kg PO
Erythromycin	3 to 5 mg/kg IM every 8 to 12 hrs[11] 4 mg/kg IM for treatment of virulent footrot caused by *Dichelobacter nodosus*[35]	3 to 5 mg/kg IM every 8 to 12 hrs[11]
Estradiol cypionate	1 to 2 mg IM weekly for pseudoestrus in females; used to tease male for semen collection	1 to 2 mg IM weekly
Febantel	5 mg/kg PO[4]	5 mg/kg PO[2]
Fenbendazole	5 mg/kg PO[4] (Anecdotal reports suggest that this dosage may not be clinically effective and 10 to 20 mg/kg PO may be required to control nematode parasites in sheep and goats)	5 mg/kg PO[6]
Fenprostalene		500 µg IM for pregnancy termination[27]
Florfenicol	20 mg/kg IM every 48 hours[11]	20 mg/kg IM every 48 hours[11]
Flunixin meglumine	1.1 to 2.0 mg/kg IV or IM[1] 0.3 to 1.0 mg/kg IV as a mediator inhibitor in circulatory shock[30]	1 mg/kg IV or IM every 24 hours for pain relief[2] 0.3 to 1.0 mg/kg IV as a mediator inhibitor in circulatory shock[30]
Follicle-stimulating hormone (see Chapter 6)	Six doses at 12-hour intervals beginning 2 days before progestin removal, with the last dose given 12 hours after progestin removal, for a total dose of 18 to 22 mg for superovulation[36]	Decreasing doses BID for 2 to 4 days before progestin removal for a total dose of 18 to 20 mg (e.g., 5, 4, 4, 3, 2, and 2 mg)[37] or 3 mg BID for 3 days before progestin removal for superovulation[37]
Furosemide	2 to 5 mg/kg PO or 1 to 2 mg/kg IV or IM every 12 to 24 hours for heart failure[18] 5 to 10 mg/kg IV for anuria[8]	2 to 5 mg/kg PO or 1 to 2 mg/kg IV or IM every 12 to 24 hours for heart failure[18] 5 to 10 mg/kg IV for anuria[8]
Glycerol monoacetate (Monoacetin)	0.55 ml/kg IM every half hour for several hours as an antidote to fluoracetate poisoning	

DRUG	SHEEP	GOATS
Griseofulvin	7.5 to 60 mg/kg PO for 7 to 20 days for dermatophytosis[38]	
Guaifenesin-ketamine-xylazine (see Chapter 16, Tables 16-1 and 16-4)	0.5 to 1.0 mg/kg IV for induction, 2 ml/kg/hr for maintenance (concentrations in the solution are 50 mg/ml guaifenesin, 1 to 2 mg/ml ketamine, and 0.1 mg/ml xylazine)[16]	
Hypertonic saline (7%)	4 ml/kg IV over 5 to 10 minutes[30]	4 ml/kg IV over 5 to 10 minutes[30]
Insulin	20 to 40 units IM of repository insulin for pregnancy toxemia[31]	
Iron (ferrous sulfate)	0.5 to 2.0 g/day PO for up to 2 weeks[18]	0.5 to 2.0 g/day PO for up to 2 weeks[18]
Ivermectin	200 μg/kg PO or SC[4] 200 μg/kg SC, two doses at a 7-day interval for psoroptic mites[4]	200 μg/kg[6] (Anecdotal reports suggest that this dosage may be clinically ineffective in sheep and goats, and more than 300 μg/kg may be needed for nematode parasite control)
Ketamine (see Chapter 16, Tables 16-1 and 16-3)	5 to 15 mg/kg IM for induction in combination with xylazine[16] 4.0 to 7.5 mg/kg IV in combination with diazepam[16] 2 to 10 mg/kg IV or IM[1]	11 mg/kg IV or IM[2] 5 to 15 mg/kg IM for induction in combination with xylazine[16]
Ketoprofen	3 mg/kg IV or IM every 24 hours[39]	3 mg/kg IV or IM every 24 hours[39]
Lasalocid	30 ppm in complete feed for coccidiosis control in lambs[12] 1 mg/kg/day, 20 to 30 g/ton PO for coccidiosis[13]	0.5 to 1.0 mg/kg/day[11]
Levamisole	8 mg/kg PO[40] (Anecdotal reports suggest that this dosage may be clinically ineffective for nematode parasite control in sheep and goats, and 12 mg/kg PO may be needed)	8 mg/kg PO[40]
Lidocaine (2%) (see Chapter 16, Table 16-1)	1 to 2 mg/kg IV over 60 seconds for ventricular arrhythmias[18] 0.3 to 0.4 mg/kg/minute IV infusion for 15 minutes, followed by 0.1 to 0.2 mg/kg/minute for 45 minutes for arrhythmias[18]	2 to 4 ml for caudal epidural anesthesia[2] (see Chapter 16 for possible toxicity of this drug)
Lincomycin hydrochloride	10 to 20 mg/kg IM every 12 to 24 hrs[11]	10 to 20 mg/kg IM every 12 to 24 hrs[11]
Lincomycin/spectinomycin	5 mg/kg lincomycin and 10 mg/kg spectinomycin for treatment of virulent footrot caused by *Dichelobacter nodosus*[35]	
Magnesium	50 to 100 ml IV of solutions containing 1.5 to 4 g of magnesium boroglyconate, chloride, or gluconate for treatment of hypomagnesemic tetany[41]	

Continued

DRUG	SHEEP	GOATS
Mannitol	0.25 to 1.5 g/kg IV over 5 minutes for diuresis[8]	0.25 to 1.5 g/kg IV over 5 minutes for diuresis[8]
Mebendazole	15 mg/kg PO[4]	
Medetomidine (see Chapter 16, Tables 16-2 and 16-4)	0.001 to 0.007 mg/kg IV 0.04 mg/kg IM for recumbency	0.001 to 0.007 mg/kg IV 0.015 to 0.04 mg/kg IM for recumbency
Melengesterol acetate	0.125 mg BID for 8 to 14 days for estrus synchronization[25]	
Methocarbamol		22 mg/kg IV for tetany[2]
Methohexitone (methohexital)	4 mg/kg IV for anesthesia[1]	
Methylene blue	10 mg/kg IV for treatment of nitrate toxicity[9]	
Metoclopramide	0.1 mg/kg IM or IV BID[42]	
Midazolam	4 mg/kg IM or IV[1]	
Mineral oil	0.5 to 1.0 L PO for treatment of bloat[43]	
Monensin sodium	15 mg/head/day orally throughout gestation to prevent abortion caused by *Toxoplasma gondii*[12] 11 to 22 ppm in complete feed for coccidiosis control in lambs[12]	1 mg/kg/day PO, 10 to 30 g/ton for coccidiosis[13]
Morantel tartrate	10 mg/kg PO[44]	10 mg/kg PO[6]
Moxidectin	200 to 500 µg/kg PO or SC for nematodes[4,22] 200 µg/kg SC for psoroptic mites[4]	500 µg/kg PO[22]
Nandrolone phenproprionate	50 to 100 mg IM every 7 to 10 days for adjunctive therapy of anemia[18]	50 to 100 mg IM every 7 to 10 days for adjunctive therapy of anemia[18]
Neomycin soluble powder	12 mg/kg BID PO in water for treatment and control of colibacillosis caused by *Escherichia coli* susceptible to neomycin[45]	12 mg/kg BID PO in water for treatment and control of colibacillosis caused by *E. coli* susceptible to neomycin[45]
Neostigmine methylsulfate	0.01 to 0.02 mg/kg SC[24]	0.01 to 0.02 mg/kg SC[24]
Netobimin	7.5 mg/kg PO for adult nematodes and developing larvae, 20 mg/kg PO for arrested larvae and flukes[4]	
Niacin		1 to 2 g/head/day PO for 1 to 2 weeks prepartum and 10 to 12 weeks postpartum for prevention of ketosis[20]
Nitroxynil	10 mg/kg SC for flukes and nonhematogenous nematodes[4]	
Norgestomet 6 mg implant	One half implant (3 mg) for estrus synchronization[25]	One half (3 mg) or full implant (6 mg) for estrus synchronization[26]
Oxfendazole	5 mg/kg PO[4] 4.5 mg/kg PO for cestodes[5]	5 mg/kg PO[6] (Anecdotal reports suggest that this dose may be clinically ineffective and 10 mg/kg PO may be more effective in gastrointestinal nematode control of sheep and goats)
Oxyclozanide	15 mg/kg PO for flukes and tapeworms[4]	

DRUG	SHEEP	GOATS
Oxytetracycline hydrochloride	10 mg/kg IV or IM BID for at least 7 days for listeriosis[46] 10 mg/kg IV or IM every 12 to 24 hrs[11]	10 mg/kg IV or IM every 12 to 24 hrs[11]
Oxytetracycline (in feed)	250 to 300 mg/head/day orally to prevent abortion caused by *Campylobacter* species and *Chlamydia psittaci*[28] 200 to 400 mg/head/day orally to prevent abortions caused by *Leptospira interrogans*[28] 10 mg/lb/day PO for treatment of bacterial enteritis caused by *Escherichia coli* and bacterial pneumonia caused by *Pasteurella multocida* susceptible to oxytetracycline[47]	400 to 500 mg/head/day PO for 2 weeks orally for control of abortion caused by *Chlamydia* and *Campylobacter*[48]
Oxytetracycline (long-acting)	20 mg/kg IM every 48 to 72 hours[11]	20 mg/kg IM every 48 to 72 hours[11] 20 mg/kg IM twice a week in the last 4 to 6 weeks of gestation to prevent abortion caused by *Chlamydia* and *Campylobacter*[49]
Oxytocin	30 to 50 IU IV, IM, or SC for obstetric use[49]	10 to 20 IU IM every 2 hours for retained placenta[33] 10 to 20 IU IM for uterine inertia or to stimulate uterine contractions after dystocia[50]
Penicillamine	50 mg/kg/day PO to increase fecal elimination of copper[9] 52 mg/kg/day PO for 6 days[10]	
Penicillin G, potassium or sodium	20,000 to 40,000 IU/kg IV every 6 hours[11]	20,000 to 40,000 IU/kg IV every 6 hours[4]
Penicillin G procaine	20,000 to 45,000 IU/kg IM every 24 hrs[11] 70,000 IU/kg for virulent footrot caused by *Dichelobacter nodosus*[35] 44,000 IU/kg IM or SC BID for 7 to 14 days, followed by 7 to 14 days of 22,000 IU/kg BID for listeriosis[46] 50,000 IU/kg IM for clostridial infections[15]	20,000 to 45,000 IU/kg IM very 24 hrs[11]
Pentobarbital (pentobarbitone)	10 to 30 mg/kg IV or IP to control seizures[9] 24 to 33 mg/kg IV (to effect) for anesthesia[1]	
Phenylbutazone		10 mg/kg PO every 24 hours for pain relief[2]
Poloxaline	2 g/head/day in feed or molasses blocks or 10 g/45 kg to prevent or treat bloat[43]	
Praziquantel	10 to 15 mg/kg PO for tapeworms[24]	10 to 15 mg/kg PO for tapeworms[24]

Continued

DRUG	SHEEP	GOATS
Pregnant mare serum gonadotropin (equine chorionic gonadotropin, eCG, or PMSG)	250 to 400 IV and up to 500 IU for out-of-season breeding 1000 to 1500 IU 48 to 72 hours before progestin removal for superovulation[36] 300 to 500 IU at the time of progestin removal before artificial insemination[51] 150 to 250 IU simultaneously with first dose of follicle-stimulating hormone to improve consistency of superovulation[36]	200 to 600 IU for estrus synchronization[26] 500 to 1500 IU 24 to 48 hours before progestin removal[37]
Propofol (see Chapter 16, Table 16-4)	4.0 to 6.0 mg/kg IV for induction[16] 3 to 4 mg/kg IV[1]	4.0 to 6.0 mg/kg IV for induction[16]
Propylene glycol	60 ml of 600 mg/ml solution orally for mild signs of pregnancy toxemia (noncomatose)[19] 100 to 200 ml PO 2 to 4 times/day for pregnancy toxemia[31]	1 to 2 oz PO for treatment of ketosis[20]
Pyrantel pamoate	25 mg/kg PO[16]	25 mg/kg PO[6]
Salinomycin	200 ppm in complete feed for coccidiosis control in lambs[12] 11 to 16 g/ton in feed for period of risk[11]	11 to 16 g/ton in feed for period of risk[11]
Selenium	0.75 mg/head SC at birth in selenium-deficient areas if ewes have not been supplemented[12] 0.1 to 0.3 mg/kg of total ration dry matter to supplement ewes in selenium-deficient areas[12] 3 mg/45 kg every 14 days for a maximum of four doses in the last trimester of pregnancy in selenium-deficient areas[12]	
Sodium bicarbonate	2 L of isotonic (1.3%) solution IV for treatment of pregnancy toxemia (70-kg ewe)[19]	25 g/doe/day PO after parturition for acidosis prevention[20]
Sodium iodide	1 g/14 kg IV, repeated at 3- to 7-day intervals for dermatophytosis[38] 70 mg/kg IV every 7 to 10 days[52]	
Sodium nitrate	10 to 20 mg/kg IV for hydrocyanic (prussic) acid poisoning[9]	
Sodium sulfate (anhydrous)	1 g/head/day PO for copper toxicity in combination with ammonium molybdate[10]	
Sodium thiosulfate	0.5 mg/kg IV for hydrocyanic (prussic) acid poisoning[9]	
Stanozolol	25 to 50 mg IM weekly up to four doses for adjunctive therapy of anemia[18]	25 to 50 mg IM weekly up to four doses for adjunctive therapy of anemia[18]
Sulfamethazine	110 mg/kg PO daily for 5 days for treatment of coccidiosis[14]	110 mg/kg PO daily for 5 days for treatment of coccidiosis[14]
Sulfaquinoxaline	8 to 70 mg/kg PO for 5 days for treatment of coccidiosis[14]	8 to 70 mg/kg PO for 5 days for treatment of coccidiosis[14]

DRUG	SHEEP	GOATS
Sulfonamides	50 mg/kg (100 mg/kg loading dose) PO or in water every 24 hours[11]	50 mg/kg (100 mg/kg loading dose) PO or in water every 24 hours[11]
Testosterone proportionate	25 mg IM three times a week for adjunctive therapy of anemia[18]	25 mg IM three times a week for adjunctive therapy of anemia[18]
Thiabendazole	44 mg/kg PO[53] (Anecdotal reports suggest that this drug may only rarely be clinically effective for sheep and goats)	44 mg/kg PO[6]
Thiamine	2 mg/kg IM BID for up to 13 days to reduce clinical signs of lead poisoning[34] 10 to 20 mg/kg IM or SC (or IV in dextrose or other isotonic fluid) TID for at least 3 days[54]	10 to 20 mg/kg IM or SC (or IV in dextrose or other isotonic fluid) TID for at least 3 days[54] 50 to 60 mg/head/day in feed[53]
Thiopental sodium (see Chapter 16, Tables 16-1 and 16-4)	10 to 16 mg/kg IV for anesthesia[1]	10 to 20 mg/kg IV for induction of anesthesia[2]
Thiophanate	100 mg/kg PO for lungworms and *Nematodirus*, 50 mg/kg PO for gastrointestinal nematodes[4]	
Tiletamine-zolazepam (Telazol) (see Chapter 16, Table 16-4)	2.0 to 4.0 mg/kg IV for induction; administer additional as needed to prolong anesthesia[16]	5.5 mg/kg IV for general anesthesia[2]
Tilmicosin	10 mg/kg SC[11]	(Anecdotal reports suggest that the use of this drug may result in death in some goats)
Tolazoline (see Chapter 16, Table 16-3)	2 to 4 mg/kg slow IV, titrate to effect[24]	1.5 to 2 mg/kg IV to reverse xylazine[2] 2.1 mg/kg IV to reverse xylazine-ketamine anesthesia[2]
Triclabendazole	10 mg/kg PO for flukes[4]	5 to 15 mg/kg PO for flukes[2]
Trimethoprim-sulfonamide	24 to 30 mg/kg IM every 12 to 24 hours[11]	24 to 30 mg/kg IM every 12 to 24 hours[11]
Tylosin	20 mg/kg IM every 12 hours[11]	20 mg/kg IM every 12 hours[11]
Vitamin B$_{12}$ (cyanocobalamin)	1000 μg/head IM for deficiency[18]	1000 μg/head IM for deficiency[18]
Vitamin K$_1$ (phylloquinone)	0.5 to 2.5 mg/kg IM for poisoning by warfarin and related compounds[24]	0.5 to 2.5 mg/kg IM for poisoning by warfarin and related compounds[24]
Xylazine (see Chapter 16, Tables 16-1, 16-2, and 16-4)	0.05 to 0.2 mg/kg IV or IM[1] 0.1 to 0.2 mg/kg IV or 0.2 to 0.3 mg/kg IM for light planes of general anesthesia and for induction[16]	0.03 to 0.04 mg/kg IV for brief procedures[2] 0.05 mg/kg IV or 0.10 mg/kg IM for painful procedures[2] 0.22 mg/kg IM followed 10 minutes later by 11 mg/kg ketamine IM for general anesthesia[2] 0.05 mg/kg IV or 0.1 mg/kg IM for light planes of general anesthesia and for induction[16]
Yohimbine (see Chapter 16, Table 16-3)	0.125 to 0.22 mg/kg slow IV	0.125 mg/kg IV to reverse xylazine[2]

References

1. Scott EW: Anaesthesia and common surgical procedures. In Martin WB, Aitken ID, editors: *Diseases of sheep,* ed 3, Oxford, UK, 2000, Blackwell Science.
2. Smith MC, Sherman DM: *Goat medicine,* Malvern, PA, 1994, Lea & Febiger.
3. Haliburton JC: Nonprotein nitrogen-induced ammonia toxicosis in ruminants. In Howard JL, Smith RA, editors: *Current veterinary therapy 4: food animal practice,* Philadelphia, 1999, WB Saunders.
4. McKellar QA: Pharmacology and therapeutics. In Martin WB, Aitken ID, editors: *Diseases of sheep,* ed 3, Oxford, UK, 2000, Blackwell Science.
5. Herd RP: Cestode infections in cattle, sheep, goats, and swine. In Howard JL, Smith RA, editors: *Current veterinary therapy 4: food animal practice,* Philadelphia, 1999, WB Saunders.
6. Olcott BM: Production medicine and health problems in goats. In Howard JL, Smith RA, editors: *Current veterinary therapy 4: food animal practice,* Philadelphia, 1999, WB Saunders.
7. Hinds FC: Dietary management in sheep. In Howard JL, Smith RA, editors: *Current veterinary therapy 4: food animal practice,* Philadelphia, 1999, WB Saunders.
8. Langston VC: Therapeutic management of urinary diseases. In Howard JL, Smith RA, editors: *Current veterinary therapy 4: food animal practice,* Philadelphia, 1999, WB Saunders.
9. Angus KW: Plant poisoning in Britain and Ireland. In Martin WB, Aitken ID, editors: *Diseases of sheep,* ed 3, Oxford, UK, 2000, Blackwell Science.
10. George LW, Carlson GP: Copper toxicosis. In Smith BP, editor: *Large animal internal medicine,* St Louis, 1996, Mosby.
11. Menzies PI: Antimicrobial drug use in sheep and goats. In Prescott JF, Baggot JD, Walker RD, editors: *Antimicrobial therapy in veterinary medicine,* ed 3, Ames, IA, 2000, Iowa State University press.
12. Menzies PI, Bailey D: Lambing management and neonatal care. In Youngquist RS, editor: *Current therapy in large animal theriogenology,* Philadelphia, 1997, WB Saunders.
13. Speer CA: Coccidiosis. In Howard JL, Smith RA, editors: *Current veterinary therapy 4: food animal practice,* Philadelphia, 1999, WB Saunders.
14. Uhlinger CA: Coccidiosis in food animals. In Smith BP, editor: *Large animal internal medicine,* ed 2, St Louis, 1996, Mosby.
15. White SD: Bacterial skin diseases. In Howard JL, Smith RA, editors: *Current veterinary therapy 4: food animal practice,* Philadelphia, 1999, WB Saunders.
16. Riebold TW: Tuminants. In Thurmon JC, Tranquilli WJ, Benson GJ, editors: *Lumb and Jones' veterinary anesthesia,* Baltimore, 1996, Williams & Wilkins.
17. Plumlee KH: Toxicology of organic compounds. In Smith BP, editor: *Large animal internal medicine,* ed 2, St Louis, 1996, Mosby.
18. Constable PD: Therapeutic management of cardiovascular diseases. In Howard JL, Smith RA, editors: *Current veterinary therapy 4: food animal practice,* Philadelphia, 1999, WB Saunders.
19. Menzies PI, Bailey D: Diseases of the periparturient ewe. In Youngquist RS, editor: *Current therapy in large animal theriogenology,* Philadelphia, 1997, WB Saunders.
20. East NE. Metabolic diseases of the puerperal period. In Youngquist RS, editor: *Current therapy in large animal theriogenology,* Philadelphia, 1997, WB Saunders.
21. Casteel SW: Hepatotoxic plants. In Howard JL, Smith RA, editors: *Current veterinary therapy 4: food animal practice,* Philadelphia, 1999, WB Saunders.
22. Howard JL: *Current veterinary therapy: food animal practice 2,* Philadelphia, 1986, WB Saunders.
23. Arrioja-Dechert A, editor: *Compendium of veterinary products,* Port Muron, MI, 1999, North American Compendiums.
24. Plumb DC: *Veterinary drug handbook,* ed 3, White Bear Lake, MN, 1999, Pharma Vet Publishing.
25. Keisler DH, Buckrell BC: Breeding strategies. In Youngquist RS, editor: *Current therapy in large animal theriogenology,* Philadelphia, 1997, WB Saunders.
26. Bretzlaff KN: Control of the estrous cycle. In Youngquist RS, editor: *Current therapy in large animal theriogenology,* Philadelphia, 1997, WB Saunders.
27. Momcilovic D: Elective termination of pregnancy. In Howard JL, Smith RA, editors: *Current veterinary therapy 4: food animal practice,* Philadelphia, 1999, WB Saunders.
28. Menzies PI, Miller R: Abortion in sheep: diagnosis and control. In Youngquist RS, editor: *Current therapy in large animal theriogenology,* Philadelphia, 1997, WB Saunders.
29. Buxton D: Toxoplasmosis and neosporosis. In Martin WB, Aitken ID, editors: *Diseases of sheep,* ed 3, Oxford, UK, 2000, Blackwell Science.
30. Streeter RN, McCauley C: Circulatory shock. In Howard JL, Smith RA, editors: *Current veterinary therapy 4: food animal practice,* Philadelphia, 1999, WB Saunders.
31. Rook JS. Pregnancy toxemia of ewes. In Howard JL, Smith RA, editors: *Current veterinary therapy 4: food animal practice,* Philadelphia, 1999, WB Saunders.
32. Braun W, Jr: Induced abortion and parturition in the goat. In Youngquist RS, editor: *Current therapy in large animal theriogenology,* Philadelphia, 1997, WB Saunders.
33. Braun W, Jr: Periparturient infection and structural abnormalities. In Youngquist RS, editor: *Current therapy in large animal theriogenology,* Philadelphia, 1997, WB Saunders.
34. Casteel SW: Lead poisoning. In Howard JL, Smith RA, editors: *Current veterinary therapy 4: food animal practice,* Philadelphia, 1999, WB Saunders.
35. Egerton JR: Foot-rot and other foot conditions. In Martin WB, Aitken ID, editors: *Diseases of sheep,* ed 3, Oxford, UK, 2000, Blackwell Science.
36. Buckrell BC, Pollard J: Embryo transfer in sheep. In Youngquist RS, editor: *Current therapy in large animal theriogenology,* Philadelphia, 1997, WB Saunders.
37. Flores-Foxworth G: Reproductive biotechnologies in the goat. In Youngquist RS, editor: *Current therapy in large animal theriogenology,* Philadelphia, 1997, WB Saunders.
38. Semrad SD, Moriello K: Dermatophytosis (ringworm). In Howard JL, Smith RA, editors: *Current veterinary therapy 4: food animal practice,* Philadelphia, 1999, WB Saunders.
39. Damian P, Craigmill AL, Riviere JE: Extralabel use of nonsteroidal anti-inflammatory drugs, *J Am Vet Med Assoc* 211:860, 1997.
40. Corwin RM: Anthelmintic therapy. In Howard JL, Smith RA, editors: *Current veterinary therapy 4: food animal practice,* Philadelphia, 1999, WB Saunders.
41. Goff JP: Ruminant hypomagnesemic tetanies. In Howard JL, Smith RA, editors: *Current veterinary therapy 4: food animal practice,* Philadelphia, 1999, WB Saunders.

42. Rings DM: Abomasal emptying defect in sheep. In Howard JL, Smith RA, editors: *Current veterinary therapy 4: food animal practice*, Philadelphia, 1999, WB Saunders.

43. Gumbrell RC: Other enteric conditions. In Martin WB, Aitken ID, editors: *Diseases of sheep*, ed 3, Oxford, UK, 2000, Blackwell Science.

44. Kimberling CV: *Jensen and Swift's diseases of sheep*, ed 3, Philadelphia, 1988, Lea & Febiger.

45. Arrioja-Dechert A: Pharmacia & Upjohn, Neomix 325 soluble powder. In Arrioja-Dechert A, editor: *Compendium of veterinary products*, Port Huron, MI, 1999, North American Compendiums.

46. Finley MR, Dennis SM: Listeriosis (circling disease, silage sickness). In Howard JL, Smith RA, editors: *Current veterinary therapy 4: food animal practice*, Philadelphia, 1999, WB Saunders.

47. Arrioja-Dechert A: Pfizer Animal Health, Terramycin type A medicated article. In Arrioja-Dechert A, editor: *Compendium of veterinary products*, Port Huron, MI, 1999, North American Compendiums.

48. Mobini S: Infectious causes of abortion. In Youngquist RS, editor: *Current therapy in large animal theriogenology*, Philadelphia, 1997, WB Saunders.

49. Arrioja-Dechert A: Anthony Products Co. Oxytocin injection. In Arrioja-Dechert A, editor: *Compendium of veterinary products*, Port Huron, MI, 1999, North American Compendiums.

50. Braun W, Jr: Parturition and dystocia in the goat. In Youngquist RS, editor: *Current therapy in large animal theriogenology*, Philadelphia, 1997, WB Saunders.

51. Mylne MJA, Hunton JR, Buckrell BC: Artificial insemination in sheep. In Youngquist RS, editor: *Current therapy in large animal theriogenology*, Philadelphia, 1997, WB Saunders.

52. Smith BP: Actinomycosis (lumpy jaw). In Smith BP, editor: *Large animal internal medicine*, ed 2, St Louis, 1996, Mosby.

53. Herd RP, Zajac AM: Nematode infections in cattle, sheep, goats, and swine. In Howard JL, Smith RA, editors: *Current veterinary therapy 4: food animal practice*, Philadelphia, 1999, WB Saunders.

54. George LW: Polioencephalomalacia (polio, cerebrocortical necrosis). In Smith BP, editor: *Large animal internal medicine*, ed 2, St Louis, 1996, Mosby.

Practical Fluid Therapy

CHRISTINE B. NAVARRE

1. ESTIMATING PERCENT (%) DEHYDRATION

PERCENT (%) DEHYDRATION*	CLINICAL SIGNS
5%	Minimal depression, skin tent only a few seconds, minimal enophthalmos, mucous membranes still moist, capillary refill slightly greater than 2 seconds
8%	Obvious depression, skin tent 2 to 4 seconds, obvious enophthalmos, mucous membranes have a purple tint and are tacky, capillary refill 3 to 4 seconds
10%	Severe depression, weakness, possible recumbency, skin tent remains for several seconds, severe enophthalmos, mucous membranes dark and dry, capillary refill more than 4 seconds, cold extremities

*These are estimates only. Other factors may change the physical examination parameters and mimic dehydration. For example, severe weight loss can cause enophthalmos, and chronic debilitation makes the skin less elastic and causes prolonged tenting. Also, certain diseases cause excess salivation, which keeps the mucous membranes moist, even during dehydration.

2. USE OF PACKED CELL VOLUME AND TOTAL PROTEIN (PCV/TP)

The PCV and TP can be used as tools to assess dehydration but **should not** replace an estimation from physical examination. An elevated PCV is rarely caused by anything but dehydration. However, elevated protein can occur with severe, chronic inflammation. Also, an animal with anemia and hypoproteinemia in conjunction with dehydration can have a normal PCV/TP. Therefore PCV/TP is most useful in monitoring the progress of fluid therapy.

3. CALCULATING A FLUID DEFICIT FROM DEHYDRATION

% dehydration × body weight in kg = fluid deficit in liters

For example, a 50-kg animal with 8% dehydration needs 4 liters of fluid.

For neonates the calculated fluid deficit in liters (usually less than 1) should be converted to milliliters. For example, a 5-kg lamb with 10% dehydration needs 0.5 liters, or 500 milliliters.

4. CALCULATION OF MAINTENANCE NEEDS

After treating deficits and dehydration, maintenance needs should be met if the animal is not taking in fluids on its own.

Maintenance for adults and neonates = approximately 1 ml/lb/hr
A 10-lb kid needs 10 ml/hour

If the animal has diarrhea, the clinician should give two times maintenance and assess rate daily with physical examination and PCV/TP, adjusting rate as needed. For diuresis with renal disease, the clinician can give two times maintenance and assess daily with physical examination, PCV/TP, and creatinine concentrations, adjusting rate as needed.

CAUTION: Small ruminants on continuous fluid therapy are inclined to become hypoproteinemic quickly.

Diligent assessment of total protein is needed to prevent this.

5. CALCULATION OF BICARBONATE NEEDS

To correct metabolic acidosis, a total carbon dioxide (CO_2) measurement from a chemistry panel or blood gas or an evaluation of base deficits from blood gas assessments are needed.

Rule of thumb. The clinician should correct half of the calculated deficit if the acidosis results from dehydration only. The entire deficit may be corrected if the dehydration is from neonatal diarrhea (not adults) or rumen acidosis.

Adults: Body weight in kg × 0.3 ×
base deficit = bicarbonate deficit in mEq
Neonates: Body weight in kg × 0.5 ×
base deficit = bicarbonate deficit in mEq

Base deficit can be substituted with (normal total CO_2 − measured total CO_2). The normal range for total CO_2 is usually 20 to 30, so the clinician can use 20 to 25 mmol/L to be conservative. Commercial bottles of sodium bicarbonate define the mEq of bicarbonate/ml of fluid, making the calculation of the total ml of this solution easy. Solutions of 5% sodium bicarbonate can be given without dilution if dehydration needs are corrected at the same time. Alternatively, 1.3% isotonic bicarbonate can be given.

A 100-kg ewe with a base deficit of 8:
100 kg × 0.3 × 8 = 240 mEq bicarbonate needed
1.3% sodium bicarbonate has 0.156 mEq/L,
so 240/0.156 = approximately 1.5 liters
5% sodium bicarbonate has 0.6 mEq/ml, so 240/0.6 = 400 milliliters
8% sodium bicarbonate has 1 mEq/ml, so 240/1 = 240 milliliters

If no total CO_2 or base deficit is available. If the animal is only 5% to 8% dehydrated, correcting the fluid deficit and the primary problem are usually sufficient. If the animal is 10% dehydrated, some supplementation is needed:

If no neonatal diarrhea or rumen acidosis is present, the clinician can give 2.5 mEq/kg body weight of bicarbonate. If neonatal diarrhea or rumen acidosis is present, 5 mEq/kg body weight of bicarbonate can be given.

6. HELPFUL CONVERSIONS AND TIPS*

1 level teaspoon of most salts (e.g., NaCl, $NaHCO_3$) is approximately 5 g.
Isotonic $NaHCO_3$: 13 g/L, or 1.3%, or 156 mEq/L of HCO_3 (312 mEq/L total for both Na and HCO_3). Approximately 3 teaspoons of baking soda/L water is isotonic sodium bicarbonate.
Isotonic saline: 9 g/L noniodized table salt. Approximately 2 teaspoons of NaCl/L water is isotonic saline.
Supplemental potassium: 10 to 20 mEq/L, or 1 g/L (14 mEq/L). Supplemental potassium can be provided by 1/2 teaspoon lite salt/L of water (lite salt is half sodium chloride and half potassium chloride).
Supplemental glucose can be provided with a 1% to 2% dextrose solution (20 ml of 50% dextrose/L for each 1% of dextrose needed).
Calcium borogluconate can be supplemented at 25 ml/L.

EASY IV FORMULA FOR NONDIARRHEIC DEHYDRATED ANIMALS

Balanced isotonic electrolyte solution for base fluid (e.g., lactated Ringer's, Ringer's, plasmalyte)
Add 1 g/L KCl (14 mEq/L)
Add 15 g dextrose/L (30 ml of 50%/L) = 1.5% dextrose
Add 25 ml/L calcium borogluconate for *adults only*

EASY IV FORMULA FOR NEONATAL DIARRHEA

Calculate fluid deficit and give three quarters of the previous fluid and one quarter as isotonic sodium bicarbonate.

EASY PO FORMULA FOR NEONATAL DIARRHEA

2 teaspoons noniodized table salt
1 teaspoon lite salt
50 ml 50% dextrose
Add to 1 qt or L of water

CAUTION: The use of commercially prepared products for IV and oral use is strongly recommended. These tips for using table salts and baking soda are approximations of commercial products and should be given only in emergency situations and only one time. If fluid therapy continues, commercial products should be used. The IV use of nonsterilized salts and water is strongly discouraged because bacteremia and endotoxemia from pyrogens may lead to infection or adverse reactions.

EASY PO FORMULA FOR ADULTS

8 teaspoons noniodized table salt
2 teaspoons lite salt
100 ml calcium solution
Add to 1 gal or 4 L of water

HYPERTONIC SALINE SOLUTION (HSS)

HSS can be used in severe hypovolemic shock situations—either from severe hemorrhage or dehydration. It temporarily improves cardiac output. The clinician can give 4 ml/kg body weight rapid IV push of a 7% solution. If hemorrhage has occurred, it may be exacerbated when blood pressure increases after administration of HSS. The clinician should consider blood transfusion after administering HSS for hemorrhage. If dehydration is present, HSS should be followed with IV isotonic or oral fluids in both neonates and adults. HSS often increases the animal's drive for water intake, so many adult animals will consume oral fluids or water and not need to have fluids administered to them.

Normal Values and Conversions

D.G. PUGH

ERYTHROCYTE PARAMETERS

PARAMETER	Sheep		Goats	
	RANGE	MEAN	RANGE	MEAN
Hematocrit (packed cell volume [PCV]) %	27 to 45	35	22 to 38	28
Hemoglobin (Hb) g/dl	9 to 15[1,2]	11.5[1]	8 to 12[1,2]	10[1]
Erythrocytes (red blood cells [RBCs]) $10^6/\mu l$	9 to 15[1,2]	12[1]	8 to 18[1,2]	13[1]
Mean corpuscular volume (MCV) fl	28 to 40[1,2]	34[1]	16 to 25[1,2]	19.5[1]
Mean corpuscular hemoglobin (MCH) pg	8 to 12[1,2]	10[1]	5.2 to 8[1,2]	6.5[1]
Mean corpuscular hemoglobin concentration (MCHC) g/dl	31 to 34[1,2]	32.5[1]	30 to 36[1,2]	33[1]
Platelet count, $N \times 10^3/\mu l$	205 to 705[2] 800 to 1100[1]	500[1]	300 to 600[1,2]	450[1]
RBC diameter (μm)	3.2 to 6.0[1]	4.5	2.5 to 3.9	3.2
RBC life (days)	125		140 to 150	
Myeloid:erythroid ratio (M/E)	0.7[1] 0.8 to 1.7[2]		0.77 to 1.7[1] 0.7 to 1[2]	

LEUKOCYTE PARAMETERS, PLASMA PROTEIN, AND FIBRINOGEN

PARAMETER	Sheep			Goats		
	PERCENTAGE	RANGE	MEAN	PERCENTAGE	RANGE	MEAN
White blood cell count (WBC) n/μl		4000 to 12,000[2]			4000 to 13,000[2]	
Segmented neutrophils (seg) (%) n/μl	10 to 50[2]	700 to 6000[1,2]	2400[1]	30 to 48[1]	1200 to 7200[1,2]	3250[1]
Banded neutrophils (band) (%) n/μl		0			0	
Lymphocytes (lymph) (%) n/μl	40 to 75[2]	2000 to 9000[1,2]	5000[1]	50 to 70[1]	2000 to 9000[1,2]	5000[1]
Monocytes (mono) (%) n/μl	6 to 6[2]	0 to 750[1,2]	200[1]	0 to 4[1]	0 to 550[1,2]	250[1]
Eosinophils (eos) (%) n/μl	0 to 10[2]	0 to 1000[2]	400[1]	1 to 8[1]	50 to 650[1,2]	450[1]
Basophils (baso) (%) n/μl	0 to 3[2]	0 to 300[1,2]	50[1]	0 to 1[1]	0 to 120[1,2]	50[1]
Plasma protein (PP) g/dl		6 to 7.5[1,2]			6.0 to 7.5[1,2]	
Fibrinogen (mg/dl)		100 to 500[1,2]			100 to 400[1,2]	

TABLE C

SERUM BIOCHEMICAL VALUES

VALUE	SHEEP	GOATS
Acetone mmol/l	0 to 1.72[3]	
Acetylcholinesterase U/l	640[3]	270[3]
Albumin, g/dl	2.4 to 3.0[2,3]	2.7 to 3.9[2,3]
Alkaline phosphatase (ALP) U/l	68 to 387[2,3]	93 to 387[2,3]
Arginase (ARG) U/l	0 to 14[3]	
Aspartate aminotransferase (AST, SGOT) U/l	60 to 280[2,3]	167 to 513[2,3]
β-hydroxybutyrate (β-OHB) mmol/l	normal: <0 to 7 moderate: 0.8 to 1.6 severe underfeeding: 1.7 to 3.0 pregnancy toxemia: >6.5	
Bicarbonate (HCO_3^-) mmol/l	20 to 25[3]	
Bilirubin, total mg/dl	0.1 to 0.5[2,3]	0.10 to 1.71[3]
Bilirubin, unconjugated (UCB) mg/dl	0 to 0.12[3]	
Bilirubin, conjugated (direct) mg/dl	0 to 0.27[2,3]	
Cholesterol mg/dl	52 to 76[1]	80 to 130[1]
Carbon dioxide, total (TCO_2) mmol/l	21 to 28[3]	25.6 to 29.6[3]
Creatinine phosphokinase (CPK) U/l	8 to 13[3]	0.8 to 9[2,3]
Creatinine mg/dl	1.2 to 1.9[3]	1 to 1.82[2,3]
Gamma-glutamyl transferase (GGT) U/l	44 ± 11[2] 20 to 52[3]	20 to 56[3]
Globulin g/l, g/dl	3.5 to 5.7[3]	2.7 to 4.1[3]
Glucose mg/dl	50 to 80[2,3]	50 to 75[2,3]
Glutamate dehydrogenase (GD) U/l	20[3]	
Hemoglobin mg/dl	90 to 140[3]	80 to 120[3]
Icterus index	2 to 5[3]	2 to 5[3]
Isocitrate dehydrogenase (ICD) U/l	0.4 to 8.0[3]	
Lactate dehydrogenase (LDH) U/l	238 to 440[2] 88 to 487	123 to 392[2,3]
Lactate mmol/l	1 to 1.33[3]	
Protein, total serum g/dl	6 to 7.9[3]	6.4 to 7[2,3]
Sorbitol dehydrogenase U/l	5.8 to 27.9[3]	14 to 23.6[3]
Blood urea nitrogen (BUN) mg/dl	8 to 20[2,3]	10 to 20[2,3]

TABLE D

SERUM ELECTROLYTE AND MINERAL CONCENTRATIONS

PARAMETER	SHEEP	GOATS
Calcium mg/dl	11.5 to 12.8[1]	8.9 to 11.7[1]
Phosphate mg/dl	5.0 to 7.3[1]	4.2 to 9.1[1]
Magnesium mg/dl	2.2 to 2.8[1]	2.8 to 3.6[1]
Sodium mEq/l	139 to 152[1]	142 to 155[1]
Chloride mEq/l	95 to 103[1]	99 to 110.3[1]
Potassium mEq/l	3.9 to 5.4[1]	3.5 to 6.7[1]
Bicarbonate (HCO_3^-) mEq/l	20 to 25[1]	
Iron μmol/l	29.7 to 39.7[3]	
μg/dl	162 to 222[3]	
Copper μmol/l	9.13 to 25.2[3]	
Lead μmol/l	0.24 to 1.21[3]	0.24 to 1.21[3]
μg/dl	5 to 25[3]	5 to 25[3]

TABLE E

VITAMINS AND MINERALS IN SERUM AND LIVER (SHEEP)

MEASURED ELEMENT	DEFICIENT	ADEQUATE	TOXIC
Vitamin A (serum) ng/ml[7]	Newborn <20	30 to 100	
	Yearling <150	225 to 500	
	Adult <150	225 to 500	
Vitamin A (liver) μg/g dry weight[7]	Newborn <20	50 to 100	
	Yearling <40	100 to 500	
	Adult <40	300 to 1100	
Vitamin E (liver) μg/dl dry weight[7]	Newborn <3	7 to 35	
	Yearling <10	20 to 40	
	Adult <10	20 to 40	
Selenium (serum) ng/ml[7]	Newborn <20	50 to 90	
	Yearling <50	80 to 120	
	Adult <50	110 to 160	
Zinc (serum) ppm	0.22 to 0.45[8]	0.8 to 2[7,8]	30 to 50
Zinc (liver) mg/kg (dry weight)		105 to 250	>400
Copper (serum) mg/kg	<0.6	0.7 to 2.0[7,8]	3.3 to 20
Copper (liver) mg/kg (dry weight)	0.5 to 4.0	88 to 350[7]	250 to 400
Iron (serum) mg/kg (as soluble element)		1.6 to 2.2[7]	
Iron (liver) mg/kg (dry weight)		105 to 1050	
Manganese		7 to 15	
Molybdenum		1.5 to 6	

TABLE F

CEREBROSPINAL FLUID[3]

PARAMETER	SHEEP	GOATS
White blood cells number/μl	0 to 5	0 to 4
Erythrocytes number/μl		
Calcium mg/dl	5.1 to 5.5	4.6
Magnesium mg/dl	2.2 to 2.8	2.3
Chloride mg/dl	128 to 148	116 to 130
Phosphorus mg/dl	1.2 to 2	
Potassium mg/dl	3.0 to 3.3	3.0
Sodium mg/dl	145 to 157	131
Hydrogen ion (pH)	7.3 to 7.4	
Glucose mg/dl	52 to 85	70
Total protein mg/dl	29 to 42	12

TABLE G

URINALYSIS

TEST	NORMAL RESULTS
Color	Pale yellow
Glucose	Negative
Ketones	Negative
Protein	Negative to trace
Specific gravity	1.015 to 1.045
Bilirubin	Negative
Turbidity	Clear
Crystals	Rare
Casts	Occasional hyaline
Epithelial cells	Occasional
Gamma-glutamyl transferase (GGT)	<40 U/l
Red blood cells (RBC)	<5
White blood cells (WBC)	<5

TABLE H

PARACENTESIS[4,5]

CHARACTERISTIC	NORMAL VALUE
Odor	None
Color	Colorless to yellow
Turbidity	Clear to slightly turbid
Total protein g/dl	≤ 3
Neutrophils	<10,000
Specific gravity	<1.018

TABLE I

SYNOVIAL FLUID[6]

CHARACTERISTIC	NORMAL	INFLAMMATION OR LOW-GRADE INFECTION	SEPTIC	DEGENERATIVE JOINT DISEASE
Color	Clear	Yellow to red	Yellow to red	Yellow
Clarity	Transparent	Translucent	Cloudy	Transparent
Leukocytes/μl	<200	2000 to 10,000	30,000 to 100,000	200 to 2000
Neutrophils %	<25	>75	>75	25
Viscosity	Very viscous	Poor	Poor	Variable

TABLE J

CONVERSIONS[9]

PREFIX	VALUE
Milli-	1/1000
Centi-	1/100
Deci-	1/10
Deca-	10
Necto-	100
Kilo-	1000

TABLE K

MISCELLANEOUS CONVERSIONS[9]

CONVERSION	MULTIPLY BY
grain to milligrams	64.799
ounces to grams	28.35
pounds to grams	453.6
pounds to kilograms	0.4536
tons to metric tons	0.9
grams to ounces	0.035
kilograms to pounds	2.205
metric tons to tons	1.102
mg/lb to g/ton	2
g/lb to g/ton	2000
lb/ton to g/ton	453.6
mg/g to mg/lb	453.6
mg/kg to mg/lb	0.4536
mcg/kg to g/lb	0.4536
ppm to mg/lb	0.4536
mg/lb to ppm	2.2046
ppm to g/ton	0.907
g/ton to g/lb	0.0005
g/ton to lb/ton	0.0022
g/ton to %	0.00011
% to g/ton	9072.2
g/ton to ppm	1.1
% to ppm	Divide by 10,000
ppm to %	10,000

TABLE L

ENGLISH TO METRIC AND METRIC TO ENGLISH CONVERSION

VALUE	CONVERTED EQUIVALENT
1 oz	28.5 g
1 lb	16 oz
1 kg	1000 g
1 ton	2000 lb
	1.07 kg
1 metric ton	1000 kg
	2205 lb
	1.102 ton
1 mg/kg	1 ppm

TABLE M

EQUIVALENT VALUES FOR CAPACITY OR VOLUME[9]

VALUE	EQUIVALENT
a cubic cm	1 milliliter
1 US pint	28.875 cubic inches
	0.5 quarts
	0.47316 liter
1 US quart	57.75 cubic inches
	2 US pints
	0.9463 liter
1 US gallon	231 cubic inches
	8 US pints
	4 US quarts
	3.7853 liters
1 liter	2.1134 US pints
	1.057 US quarts
	0.2642 US gallon
1 bushel	2150.42 cubic inches
	1.244 cubic feet
	9.309 US gallons

BOX A

CENTIGRADE TO FAHRENHEIT AND FAHRENHEIT TO CENTIGRADE

To change centigrade to Fahrenheit, multiply the degrees in centigrade by 1.8, then add 32 to the number.

Example: 40° C

(1.8) (40) + 32 = 104° F

To change Fahrenheit to centigrade, subtract 32 from the degrees in Fahrenheit, then multiply that number by 0.556.

Example: 104° F

(104 − 32) (0.556) = 40° C

REFERENCES

1. Kramer JW: Normal hematology of cattle, sheep, and goats. In Feldman BF, Zinkl JG, Jain NC, editors: *Schlam's veterinary hematology,* ed 5, Philadelphia, 2000, Williams & Wilkins.
2. Duncan JR, Prasse KW: *Veterinary laboratory medicine—clinical pathology,* ed 2, Ames, IA, 1986, Iowa State University Press.
3. Kaneko JJ, Harvey JW, Bruss ML: *Clinical biochemistry of domestic animals,* ed 5, San Diego, CA, 1997, Academic Press.
4. Belknap EB, Navarre CB: Differentiation of gastrointestinal diseases in adult cattle, *Vet Clin North Am: Food Anim Pract* 16(1):63, 2000.
5. Kopcha M, Schultze AE: Peritoneal fluid. Part II. Abdominocentesis in cattle and interpretation of non neoplastic samples, *Comp Cont Ed Pract Vet* 13(4):703, 1999.
6. Orsini JA: Septic arthritis (infectious arthritis). In Smith BP, editor: *Large animal internal medicine,* ed 2, St Louis, 1996, Mosby.
7. Braselton WE: Animal Health Diagnostic Laboratory, personal communication, Michigan State University.
8. D'Andrea G, Robert S: Veterinary Diagnostic Laboratory, personal communication, Auburn University.
9. Ensminger ME, Oldfield JE, Heinemann WW: *Feeds and nutrition,* ed 2, Clovis, CA, 1990, Ensminger Publishing.

*The letter *t* following the page number indicates a table; *f* indicates a figure; *b* indicates a box.